Head and Neck Surgery

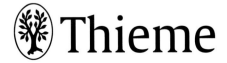

Head and Neck Surgery

Series Editors

Professor Emeritus Milind V. Kirtane, M.S. (ENT)
Seth G. S. Medical College & KEM Hospital
P. D. Hinduja National Hospital & Research Centre
Breach Candy Hospital
Prince Ali Khan Hospital
Saifee Hospital
Mumbai, India

Chris E. de Souza, M.S., D.O.R.L., D.N.B., F.A.C.S.
ENT Consultant
Lilavati Hospital
Holy Family Hospital
Holy Spirit Hospital
Tata Memorial Hospital
Mumbai, India

Visiting Assistant Professor
Department of Otoloaryngology,
SUNY Brooklyn, New York, USA
Department of Otolaryngology
LSUHSC, Shreveport
Louisiana, USA

Volume Editors

Gady Har-El, M.D., F.A.C.S.
Chairman
Department of Otolaryngology – Head and Neck Surgery
Lenox Hill Hospital
New York, New York, USA

Professor
Departments of Otolaryngology and Neurosurgery
SUNY Downstate Medical Center
Long Island College Hospital
Brooklyn, New York, USA

Cherie-Ann O. Nathan, M.D., F.A.C.S.
Professor and Chairman
Department of Otolaryngology – Head and Neck Surgery
Louisiana State University-Health
Shreveport, Louisiana, USA

Director
Head and Neck Surgical Oncology
Feist-Weiller Cancer Center
Shreveport, Louisiana, USA

Terry A. Day, M.D., F.A.C.S.
Professor and Director
Department of Head and Neck Tumor Center
Wendy and Keith Wellin Endowed Chair in Head
and Neck Surgery
Charleston, South Carolina, USA

Vice Chairman
Department of Otolaryngology – Head and Neck Surgery
Hollings Cancer Center
Medical University of South Carolina
Charleston, South Carolina, USA

Shaun A. Nguyen, M.D., M.A., C.P.I.
Associate Professor
Director of Clinical Research
Department of Otolaryngology
Medical University of South Carolina
Charleston, South Carolina, USA

Thieme Medical and Scientific Publishers Private Limited
A-12, Second Floor, Sector - 2
Noida, Uttar Pradesh - 201 301, India
Email: customerservice@thieme.in
www.thieme.com

Thieme
Delhi • Stuttgart • New York

Thieme Medical and Scientific Publishers Private Limited
A-12, Second Floor, Sector - 2
Noida, Uttar Pradesh - 201 301, India

Managing Editor: Sangeeta P.C.
Assistant Manager - Publishing: Kumar Kunal
National Sales and Marketing Manager: Harish Singh Bora
Chief Executive Officer: Ajit Kohli

Head and Neck Surgery / [edited by] Gady Har-El, Cherie-Ann O. Nathan, Terry A. Day, Shaun A. Nguyen.

Includes bibliographical references and index.

ISBN 978-93-82076-03-2

Har-El, Gady. II. Nathan, Cherie-Ann O. III. Day, Terry A. IV. Nguyen, Shaun A.

Important note: Medical knowledge is ever changing. As new research and clinical experience broaden our knowledge, changes in treatment and drug therapy may be required. The authors and editors of the material herein have consulted sources believed to be reliable in their efforts to provide information that is complete and in accord with the standards accepted at the time of publication. However, in view of the possibility human error by the authors, editors, or publishers of the work herein or changes in medical knowledge, neither the authors, editors, nor publishers, nor any other party who has been involved in the preparation of this work, warrants that the information contained herein is in every respect accurate or complete, and they are not responsible for any errors or omissions or for the results obtained from use of such information. Readers are encouraged to confirm the information contained herein with other sources. For example, readers are advice to check the product information sheet included in the package of each drug they plan to administer to be certain that the information contained in this publication is accurate and that changes have not been made in the recommended dose or in the contraindications for administration. This recommendation is of particular importance in connection with new or infrequently used drugs. Some of the product names, patents, and registered designs referred to in this book are in fact registered trademarks or proprietary names even though specific reference to this fact is not always made in the text. Therefore, the appearance of a name without designation as proprietary is not to be construed as a representation by the publishers that it is in the public domain.

5 4 3 2 1

ISBN: 978-93-82076-03-2
eISBN: 978-93-82076-09-4

Head and Neck Surgery
Published by Thieme Medical and Scientific Publishers Private Limited
A-12, Second Floor, Sector - 2, Noida, Uttar Pradesh - 201 301, India
Email: customerservice@thieme.in
www.thieme.com
Printer: Gopsons Papers Limited, Noida

Head and Neck Surgery

Table of Contents

Foreword

It is my privilege to have been invited to provide the Foreword to this head and neck surgery book, edited by colleagues with a list of contributors from a variety of backgrounds, many of whom I have known for years. Their collective experience cannot be questioned and all the chapters written by them are the products of the learning curve that we have witnessed over the past 25 to 30 years.

Although the principles of head and neck surgery have changed dramatically, many of the problems still remain. When considering these basic principles, they have skillfully set the scene for all the complex sites within the head and neck region. Each section provides current "state-of-the-art" management followed by a most important resume of the increasing improvements in rehabilitation and reconstruction, vital if patients are to be returned to a meaningful quality of life in society.

The most challenging task in writing any book is to anticipate the future. The chapters are filled with educational pearls, visionary facts, and detailed treatment recommendations, all presented in a clear and concise manner that includes both critical and contrasting points of view. This excellent work chronicles the breadth and depth of understanding that now exists with etiologic approaches, diagnostic techniques, and rehabilitation, all of which have helped enhance the quality of life of this unfortunate patient population. This volume spans the broad categories and treatment options of all other tumors of the head and neck region.

This book is, to my knowledge, a most important and timely account of our present knowledge of both the principles and present-day practice of the management of the varied neoplasms that affect the head and neck region.

This book covers the broad range of management of head and neck neoplasms from thyroid to paraganglioma and from skull base to trachea. This book has an exciting feature that includes the rehabilitation of patients with head and neck tumors including dental, prosthetic, and swallowing rehabilitation. Finally, the book reaches the cutting edge of our specialty with a section entitled, "Emerging Technologies and Therapeutics in Head and Neck Surgery."

My congratulations therefore, to the editors and the authors for their contributions that will benefit the treatment of patients with head and neck malignancies and in addition help enhance the knowledge required for residents, fellows, and all practicing specialists involved in head and neck surgery.

Patrick J. Gullane, C.M., M.D., F.R.C.S.C., F.A.C.S., F.R.A.C.S. (Hon.), F.R.C.S. (Hon.)
Otolaryngologist-in-Chief, University Health Network/Toronto General Hospital
Wharton Chair Head and Neck Surgery, Princess Margaret Hospital
Professor and Chair, Department of Otolaryngology-Head and Neck Surgery
University of Toronto
Canada

A Note from Series Editors

This volume deals with conditions of the head and neck. Head and neck surgery has changed remarkably since the days of Chevalier Jackson. This has been possible primarily because of the incredible leaps in technology, optics, and biomedical engineering. This in no way diminishes the achievements and accomplishments of the giants such as Chevalier Jackson. Biomedical engineering and technology has expanded the ability of head and neck surgeons to treat many conditions that were once considered untreatable. This has also come at a price. As technology improves and newer generation of instruments evolves, so does the cost factor. Insurers insist on cutting costs and impose their will on the manner in which a head and neck surgeon will practice and interfere with choice of technology for the diagnosis, evaluation, and management of a patient. Head and neck surgeons are placed in a unique and uncomfortable condition. What should they do for the patient keeping all these limitations in mind? As yet there is no clear answer and only as time goes by will an equilibrium evolve and solutions be found.

The editors and authors have kept all these unique situations in mind while writing this book. This book serves to help the head and neck surgeon of today to be effective, competent, and capable of facing and solving any challenge the future might pose as they search for ways and means for the treatment of their patients.

Milind V. Kirtane, M.S.
Chris E. de Souza, M.S., D.O.R.L., D.N.B., F.A.C.S.

Contributors

Nishant Agrawal, M.D.
Department of Otolaryngology – Head and Neck Surgery
Johns Hopkins Hospital
Baltimore, Maryland, USA

Moran Amit, M.D.
The Laboratory for Applied Cancer Research
Tel Aviv Sourasky Medical Center
Tel Aviv, Israel

Vijay Anand, M.D., F.A.C.S.
Departments of Otolaryngology – Head and Neck Surgery
Weill Cornell Medical College
New York Presbyterian Hospital
New York, New York, USA

Hassan Arshad, M.D.
Departments of Head and Neck Surgery, and Plastic and Reconstructive Surgery
Roswell Park Cancer Institute
Buffalo, New York, USA

R. Bryan Bell, M.D., D.D.S., F.A.C.S.
Department of Surgery
Providence Cancer Center
Robert W. Franz Cancer Research Center
Providence Portland Medical Center
Portland, Oregon, USA
Department of Surgery
Legacy Emanuel Medical Center
Portland, Oregon, USA
Department of Oral and Maxillofacial Surgery
Oregon Health and Science University
Portland, Oregon, USA

Benjamin S. Bleier, M.D.
Department of Otology and Laryngology
Massachusetts Eye and Ear Infirmary
Harvard Medical School
Boston, Massachusetts, USA

J. Kenneth Byrd, M.D.
Department of Otolaryngology
University of Pittsburgh Medical Center
Pittsburgh, Pennsylvania, USA

Trinitia Y. Cannon, M.D.
Division of Head and Neck Surgery
Department of Otorhinolaryngology
University of Oklahoma Health Sciences Center
Oklahoma City, Oklahoma, USA

Eric R. Carlson, D.M.D., M.D.
Department of Oral and Maxillofacial Surgery
The University of Tennessee Cancer Institute
University of Tennessee Medical Center
Knoxville, Tennessee, USA

William R. Carroll, M.D.
Division of Otolaryngology
Section of Head and Neck Oncology
Department of Surgery
The University of Alabama at Birmingham
Birmingham, Alabama, USA

Kundan S. Chufal, M.D.
Department of Oncology
Batra Hospital and Medical Research Centre
New Delhi, Delhi, India

S. Lewis Cooper, M.D.
Department of Radiation Oncology
Medical University of South Carolina
Charleston, South Carolina, USA

Betsy K. Davis, D.M.D., M.S.
Departments of Otolaryngology – Head and Neck Surgery, and Oral and Maxillofacial Surgery
Medical University of South Carolina
Charleston, South Carolina, USA

Terry A. Day, M.D., F.A.C.S.
Department of Otolaryngology – Head and Neck Surgery
Hollings Cancer Center
Medical University of South Carolina
Charleston, South Carolina, USA

A. K. D'Cruz, M.S., D.N.B., F.R.C.S.
Department of Head and Neck Surgery
Tata Memorial Hospital
Mumbai, Maharashtra, India

Ilana Doweck, M.D.
Department of Otolaryngology – Head and Neck Surgery
Carmel Medical Center
Haifa, Israel

Brent R. Driskill, M.D.
Department of Otolaryngology – Head and Neck Surgery
Naval Medical Center Portsmouth
Portsmouth, Virginia, USA

Raghav C. Dwivedi, M.R.C.S., D.O.H.N.S., M.S., F.I.C.S., Ph.D.
Head and Neck Unit
Royal Marsden Hospital
London, United Kingdom

Department of Otolaryngology and Head and Neck Surgery
Addenbrooke's Hospital
Cambridge University Hospitals NHS Foundation Trust
Cambridge, United Kingdom

Joel B. Epstein, D.M.D., M.S.D., F.R.C.D.(C), F.D.S.R.C.S.(Ed.), Dip. A.B.O.M.
Division of Oral Medicine
Department of Surgery
City of Hope National Medical Center
Duarte, California, USA
Division of Dentistry
Department of Surgery
Cedars Sinai Health System
Los Angeles, California, USA

Boban M. Erovic, M.D., P.D.
Department of Otolaryngology – Head and Neck Surgery
Medical University of Vienna
Waehringer Gürtel
Vienna, Austria

Tanya Fancy, M.D.
Department of Otolaryngology
West Virginia University Hospitals
Morgantown, West Virginia, USA

Dan M. Fliss, M.D.
Departments of Otolaryngology – Head and Neck Surgery and Maxillofacial Surgery
Tel Aviv Sourasky Medical Center
Tel Aviv University
Tel Aviv, Israel

Paul Friedlander, M.D.
Department of Otolaryngology – Head and Neck Surgery
Tulane University
New Orleans, Louisiana, USA

Valerie A. Fritsch, M.D.
Department of Otolaryngology – Head and Neck Surgery
Medical University of South Carolina
Charleston, South Carolina, USA

Mustafa Gerek, M.D.
Department of Otolaryngology – Head and Neck Surgery
Gülhane Military Medical Academy
Ankara, Turkey

G. E. Ghali, D.D.S., M.D., F.A.C.S.
Departments of Oral and Maxillofacial Surgery – Head and Neck Surgery
Louisiana State University Health Sciences Center
Shreveport, Louisiana, USA

Ziv Gil, M.D., Ph.D.
Department of Otolaryngology – Head and Neck Surgery
Rambam Medical Center
The Technion – Israel Institute of Technology
Haifa, Israel

M. Boyd Gillespie, M.D.
Department of Otolaryngology – Head and Neck Surgery
Medical University of South Carolina
Charleston, South Carolina, USA

Joshua D. Hornig, M.D., F.R.C.S.(C)
Division of Head and Neck Surgical Oncology
Department of Otolaryngology – Head and Neck Surgery
Medical University of South Carolina
Charleston, South Carolina, USA

Gilad Horowitz, M.D.
Tel Aviv Sourasky Medical Center
Tel Aviv University
Tel Aviv, Israel

Jennifer L. Hunt, M.D., Med.
Department of Pathology and Laboratory Medicine
University of Arkansas for Medical Sciences
Little Rock, Arkansas, USA

Jonathan Irish, M.D., M.Sc., F.R.C.S.C., F.A.C.S.
Departments of Otolaryngology – Head and Neck Surgery and Surgical Oncology
Princess Margaret Hospital
University of Toronto
Toronto, Ontario, Canada

Rehan A. Kazi, M.S., D.N.B., F.A.C.S., F.R.C.S., Ph.D.
Institute of Head and Neck Studies and Education [InHanse]
University Hospital Coventry
Coventry, United Kingdom

Andrzej L. Komorowski, M.D., Ph.D.
Department of General Surgery
Hospital Virgen del Camino
Sanlúcar de Barrameda, Cádiz, Spain

David I. Kutler, M.D.
Department of Otolaryngology – Head and Neck Surgery
Weill Cornell Medical College
New York, New York, USA

Eric J. Lentsch, M.D.
Department of Otolaryngology – Head and Neck Surgery
Medical University of South Carolina
Charleston, South Carolina, USA

Ryan J. Li, M.D.
Department of Otolaryngology – Head and Neck Surgery
Johns Hopkins Hospital
Baltimore, Maryland, USA

Derrick T. Lin, M.D., F.A.C.S.
Division of Cranial Base Center
Department of Otology and Laryngology
Massachusetts Eye and Ear Infirmary
Harvard Medical School
Boston, Massachusetts, USA

J. Scott Magnuson, M.D.
Department of Head and Neck Surgery
Head and Neck Surgery Center
Celebration Health Florida Hospital
Celebration, Florida, USA

Barry T. Malin, M.D., M.P.P.
Department of Otolaryngology
Medical University of South Carolina
Charleston, South Carolina, USA

Ariel E. Marciscano, B.S., M.S.I.V.
New York University School of Medicine
New York, New York, USA

Michael R. Markiewicz, D.D.S., M.P.H., M.D.
Departments of Oral and Maxillofacial Surgery
Oregon Health and Science University
Portland, Oregon, USA

Rosemary Martino, Ph.D.
Departments of Speech Language Pathology and Otolaryngology – Head and Neck Surgery
University of Toronto
Toronto, Ontario, Canada
Health Care Outcomes Research
Toronto Western Research Institute
University Health Network
Toronto, Ontario, Canada

Edward D. McCoul, M.D., M.P.H.
Department of Otolaryngology – Head and Neck Surgery
Weill Cornell Medical College
New York, New York, USA

Oleg Militsakh, M.D.
Division of Head and Neck Surgery
Department of Otolaryngology
Nebraska Medical Center
Nebraska Methodist Hospital
Omaha, Nebraska, USA

Jason Jay Miller, M.D., D.M.D., F.A.C.S.
Department of Plastic and Reconstructive Surgery
University of Nebraska Medical Center
Omaha, Nebraska, USA

Anupam Mishra, M.B.B.S., M.S., D.N.B., Dip. Can. Prev. (NIH)
Department of Otolaryngology and Head and Neck Surgery
Chhatrapati Shahuji Maharaj Medical University
King George Medical University
Lucknow, Uttar Pradesh, India

Allen O. Mitchell, M.D., F.A.C.S.
Naval Medical Center Portsmouth
Portsmouth, Virginia, USA

Nadia G. Mohyuddin, M.D.
Bobby R. Alford Department of Otolaryngology – Head and Neck Surgery
Baylor College of Medicine
Houston, Texas, USA

David Myssiorek, M.D., F.A.C.S.
Department of Otolaryngology – Head and Neck Surgery
New York University Clinical Cancer Center
New York, New York, USA

Brendan P. O'Connell, M.D.
Department of Otolaryngology – Head and Neck Surgery
Medical University of South Carolina
Charleston, South Carolina, USA

Matthew O. Old, M.D.
Department of Otolaryngology – Head and Neck Surgery
The James Cancer Hospital and Solove Research Institute
Wexner Medical Center
Ohio State University
Columbus, Ohio, USA

Gregory W. Randolph, M.D., F.A.C.S.
Departments of Otolaryngology and Laryngology
Harvard Medical School
Massachusetts Eye and Ear Infirmary
Massachusetts General Hospital
Boston, Massachusetts, USA

Madhup Rastogi, M.D.
Department of Radiation Oncology
Dr. Ram Manohar Lohia Institute of Medical Sciences
Lucknow, Uttar Pradesh, India

David J. Reisberg, D.D.S., F.A.C.P.
Division of Prosthodontics and Maxillofacial Prosthetics
Department of Surgery
The Craniofacial Center
College of Medicine
The University of Illinois Hospital and Health Sciences Systems
Chicago, Illinois, USA

Ohad Ronen, M.D.
Department of Otolaryngology – Head and Neck Surgery
Lady Davis' Carmel Medical Center
Ruth and Bruce Rappaport Faculty of Medicine
The Technion – Israel Institute of Technology
Haifa, Israel

Nicholas J. Sanfilippo, M.D.
New York University School of Medicine
New York, New York, USA

Suhail I. Sayed, M.S., D.O.R.L.
Division of Head Neck Services
Department of Surgical Oncology
Tata Memorial Hospital
Mumbai, Maharashtra, India

Rodney J. Schlosser, M.D.
Division of Rhinology and Sinus Surgery
Department of Otolaryngology – Head and Neck Surgery
Ralph H. Johnson VA Medical Center
Medical University of South Carolina
Charleston, South Carolina, USA

Theodore H. Schwartz, M.D., F.A.C.S.
Departments of Neurosurgery, Otolaryngology, Neurology and Neuroscience
Weill Cornell Medical College
New York Presbyterian Hospital
New York, New York, USA

**Crispian Scully, C.B.E., M.D., Ph.D., M.D.S., M.R.C.S., F.D.S.R.C.P.S., F.F.D.R.C.S.I., F.D.S.R.C.S., F.R.C.P.A.T.H.,
F.Med.Sci., F.H.E.A., F.U.C.L., F.S.B., D.Sc., D.Ch.D., D.Med. (HC), Dhc.**
Department of Maxillofacial Diagnostic
Medical and Surgical Sciences
Eastman Dental Institute
University College London
London, United Kingdom

Anand Sharma, M.D.
Department of Radiation Oncology
Medical University of South Carolina
Charleston, South Carolina, USA

Michael C. Singer, M.D.
Department of Otolaryngology – Head and Neck Surgery
Henry Ford Hospital
Detroit, Michigan, USA

Chaz L. Stucken, M.D.
Department of Otolaryngology – Head and Neck Surgery
Mount Sinai School of Medicine
New York, New York, USA

Emily Z. Stucken, M.D.
Department of Otolaryngology – Head and Neck Surgery
New York Presbyterian Hospital
Weill Cornell Medical Center
Columbia University Medical Center
New York, New York, USA

Theodoros N. Teknos, M.D.
Department of Otolaryngology – Head and Neck Surgery
Ohio State University
Columbus, Ohio, USA

David J. Terris, M.D., F.A.C.S.
Department of Otolaryngology
Georgia Health Thyroid Center
Georgia Health Sciences University
Augusta, Georgia, USA

Ralph P. Tufano, M.D., M.B.A., F.A.C.S.
Division of Head and Neck Endocrine Surgery
Department of Otolaryngology – Head and Neck Surgery
Multidisciplinary Thyroid Tumor Center
Johns Hopkins University School of Medicine
Johns Hopkins Hospital
Baltimore, Maryland, USA

R. Michael Tuttle, M.D.
Division of Endocrinology Service
Department of Medicine
Memorial Sloan – Kettering Cancer Center
New York, New York, USA

Jonathan Brett Wallach, M.D.
Mount Sinai School of Medicine
Elmhurst Hospital Center
Elmhurst, New York, USA

David R. White, M.D.
Department of Otolaryngology – Head and Neck Surgery
Medical University of South Carolina
Charleston, South Carolina, USA

Ryan Winters, M.D.
Department of Otolaryngology – Head and Neck Surgery
Tulane University
New Orleans, Louisiana, USA

Wojciech M. Wysocki, M.D., Ph.D.
Department of Surgical Oncology
Institute of Oncology
Maria Skłodowska – Curie Memorial Cancer Center
Kraków, Poland

Robert J. Yawn, M.D.
Department of Otolaryngology and Communication Sciences
The Vanderbilt Bill Wilkerson Center
Vanderbilt University Medical Center
Nashville, Tennessee, USA

Jose P. Zevallos, M.D.
Bobby R. Alford Department of Otolaryngology – Head and Neck Surgery
Baylor College of Medicine
Houston, Texas, USA

SECTION I: Site-Specific Approach to Head and Neck Cancer

A. Endocrine Neoplasms of the Head and Neck

1 Benign Thyroid Disorders

Michael C. Singer and David J. Terris

Core Messages

- Accurate diagnosis is essential for appropriate management of benign thyroid disorders.

- Wide range of possible therapies range from observation to medications to surgery.

- Surgical approach is dictated by safety, efficacy, and technical feasibility.

- Customize surgical treatment for each patient and their disease characteristics rather than using a "one-size-fits-all" approach.

While thyroid cancer commands extensive clinical and research attention, benign thyroid disorders are significantly more common. In contrast to thyroid cancer, in which surgical intervention is the principal component of therapy, benign thyroid disorders can often be observed or managed medically. Patients may present with a wide range of symptoms, including endocrine, compressive, and even cosmetic concerns. Accurate diagnosis and assessment is important to select the most appropriate therapeutic regimen.

Benign thyroid disorders can be categorized in several ways. However, they are most often classified most broadly as either inflammatory/autoimmune disorders and nodular diseases.

Inflammatory and Autoimmune Disorders

The hallmark of inflammatory thyroid disorders is the lymphocytic infiltration that occurs in the gland. While these diseases share some common pathophysiologic mechanisms, they vary greatly in presentation. They may be acute, subacute, or chronic in nature.

An autoimmune etiology is the cause of several inflammatory thyroid conditions. In these autoimmune diseases, failure of the immune system to properly recognize self-leads to antibodies is generated against several different thyroid antigens. These autoantibodies can cause cell injury, as in Hashimoto thyroiditis (HT), or promote inappropriate thyroid cell hyperfunction, as in Graves disease (GD). Inflammatory and autoimmune thyroid disorders can therefore cause patients to be hyperthyroid, hypothyroid, or euthyroid. This status often dictates the treatment a patient receives.

Hashimoto Thyroiditis

HT, alternatively referred to as autoimmune or chronic lymphocytic thyroiditis, is the most common inflammatory disease of the thyroid and is the most frequent etiology of hypothyroidism in developed countries (in some regions, iodine deficiency is endemic and is the leading cause of hypothyroidism). Markedly more common in women (particularly during their third and fourth decade of life) than in men, HT affects approximately 2% of the general population.[1]

HT is an autoimmune disease that leads to several cell- and antibody-mediated processes that cause thyroid cell destruction. While several antibodies can be present in the disease, antibodies to thyroid peroxidase (previously referred to as antimicrosomal) and thyroglobulin are the most common. While a genetic predisposition to the development of the disease appears likely, supported by the frequent association with human leukocyte antigens DR5, DR3, and DRB8, the exact triggering mechanism and pathophysiology of HT remains unclear.[2] Irrespective of the mechanism, these processes lead to follicular cell injury and death, causing the associated findings.

In HT, the thyroid gland exhibits an extensive lymphocyte and plasma cell infiltrate that can form germinal centers. The follicular cells can become enlarged with abundant cytoplasmic mitochondria. These eosinophilic cells are referred to as Hürthle or oxyphil cells.

The overwhelming majority of these patients will present in a hypothyroid state, reflecting the reduced production of hormone caused by follicular cell destruction. However, patients can be euthyroid or even hyperthyroid particularly early in their disease course as a result of the release of thyroid hormone from damaged follicles. Symptoms are typically dictated by the functional status of the gland. While nodularity can develop, most commonly HT leads to the development of a diffusely enlarged, nontender, rubbery goiter. In fact, HT is a leading cause of goiter development. In certain cases, the goiter may have a fine nodular pattern. Later in the course of the disease, the gland can contract owing to fibrosis.

The diagnosis of HT is most often driven by clinical history and biochemical tests. In addition to standard thyroid function tests, evaluation for antiperoxidase and thyroglobulin antibodies may be performed. These are elevated in most patients, and antiperoxidase antibodies are the most specific findings for the diagnosis of HT.[3] However, in up to 10 to 15% of the HT cases, these antibodies will be absent. Ultrasound (US) should be considered in all patients with HT to determine whether thyroid nodules are present. In any patient who is hypothyroid or euthyroid, American Thyroid Association (ATA) guidelines recommends biopsy of nodules greater than 1 cm.[4]

Treatment for HT entails administration of thyroxine to achieve a euthyroid state. Surgery is reserved only for cases of compressive goiters or nodules concerning for possible malignancy. Importantly, patients with HT are at an increased risk of developing B-cell lymphoma of the thyroid, and any rapid increase in the size of their gland should be carefully assessed.[5]

Acute Suppurative Thyroiditis

Acute suppurative thyroiditis (AST) is a rare entity that is most often caused by infection with gram-positive bacteria. *Staphylococcus* and *Streptococcus* species are most commonly involved, but infections with gram-negative bacteria can occur (fungal, mycobacterial, and parasitic organisms are the causative agents in rare cases).

Cases of AST are often seen in patients with a recent upper respiratory infection. Spread of infection to the gland can occur by lymphatic or hematogenous spread or by direct extension of an adjacent infection in the head and neck. In children or adults with recurrent episodes, consideration should be given to the possibility of a pyriform sinus fistula communicating with the thyroid gland.[6]

Patients with AST present with the standard signs of infection: thyroid pain and tenderness, fever, swelling, and possibly dysphagia and odynophagia. In addition to history and physical examination, a fine-needle aspiration (FNA) can be used to obtain specimens for culture and cytology. Patients are most commonly euthyroid. Appropriate antimicrobial therapy is curative in most instances.

Subacute Thyroiditis

Different forms of subacute thyroiditis (ST) can be classified by the presence or absence of pain. These disorders share a similar clinical hormonal pattern, more commonly affecting women and typically require medical management only. In most cases of ST, patients pass through several phases, initially enduring a period of thyrotoxicosis lasting variable

amounts of time (from several months to a year). This thyrotoxic state is due to the release of thyroid hormone from damaged follicles. This is usually followed by a brief euthyroid phase, followed by a period of hypothyroidism while the gland is in a reparative state. Eventually, most patients return to a euthyroid state.

Acute onset of pain is the hallmark of subacute granulomatous thyroiditis, also known as de Quervain thyroiditis or painful thyroiditis. The pain is centered over the thyroid gland, which is exquisitely tender to palpation. In many instances, the disease is preceded by an upper respiratory tract infection, leading some to propose an infectious etiology. In the acute phase, a markedly elevated erythrocyte sedimentation rate is often seen. Pathologically, a lymphocytic destruction of thyroid follicles occurs and multinuclear giant cells with granuloma formation can also be present. Spontaneous resolution occurs in most patients. However, the acute pain can be treated with a combination of steroids and salicylates.

Painless ST occurs in both sporadic and postpartum forms. While the etiology remains unclear, an autoimmune process is likely. A lymphocytic infiltration of the gland with destruction of follicles is seen. These patients may require medical treatment as they progress through their hyperthyroid or hypothyroid phases.

Riedel Thyroiditis

Riedel thyroiditis (RT), also known as Riedel struma or invasive fibrous thyroiditis, is a rare disorder that typically affects middle-aged women. An inflammatory process of unknown etiology first affects the thyroid gland, which becomes extremely firm owing to extensive fibrosis.[7] The fibrosis often extends beyond the capsule of the gland to involve the strap muscles, trachea, and esophagus. This disorder may be a part of a systemic disease that can involve the mediastinum, retroperitoneum, or orbit.

Beyond a firm neck mass, approximately one-third of the patients develop hypothyroidism from the loss of functional follicles. Given the typical examination findings and the aggressive, invasive nature of RT, differentiating it from malignancy is critical and frequently difficult. Open biopsy is often necessary to confirm the diagnosis.

While treatment with different medical therapies, including high-dose steroids and tamoxifen, has shown some benefit, optimal treatment has not yet been delineated.[8] Surgery has a limited role in RT. If patients develop constriction of the trachea or esophagus, leading to dyspnea or dysphagia, isthmusectomy or localized resection can be performed to relieve symptoms.

Graves Disease

In contrast to the inflammatory disorders Graves disease (GD) does not cause damage to the thyroid follicular cells. Rather, an autoimmune process leads to stimulation and growth of the thyroid gland. This causes true hyperthyroidism, in which elevated thyroid hormone levels are due to an excessive production of thyroid hormone by the gland. In the inflammatory disorders, thyrotoxicosis, a pathologic excess of thyroid hormone, can occur but is due to the release of stored hormone from damaged thyroid follicles.

In non-iodine–deficient areas, GD is the most common cause of hyperthyroidism, occurring more commonly in women than in men. A family history of GD or other inflammatory thyroid disorders increases the risk of developing GD.

The production of autoantibodies that target and activate thyroid-stimulating hormone (TSH) receptors is the hallmark of GD. While several types of antibodies are present in GD, these G1 subclass immunoglobulins, called thyroid-stimulating immunoglobulins (TSIs), appear to be the main cause of the manifestations of the disease. By acting as agonists at TSH receptors, follicular cells receive the errant message to enlarge and produce additional hormone.

The TSI stimulation leads to two of the main features of GD: hyperthyroidism and a diffusely enlarged goiter.[9] Many of the associated symptoms reflect the hyperthyroidism and are the same as in any patient with elevated thyroid hormone levels, including nervousness, tachycardia, hypertension, diarrhea, insomnia, weight loss, and heat intolerance. Graves ophthalmopathy, another of the characteristic manifestations of GD, is present in approximately 25 to 30% of the patients. An inflammatory infiltration of the orbit, which causes edema of the orbital muscles and periorbita, leads to proptosis (**Fig. 1.1**). If severe and untreated, this process can ultimately lead to optic nerve compression and blindness. Typical ocular signs include staring and lid lag. This infiltrative ophthalmopathy along with a dermopathy, known as pretibial myxedema, is unique to GD.

The diagnosis of GD is often ascertained with a history and physical examination, with symptoms and findings presenting in different combinations.[10] Laboratory evaluation will show an increased serum-free T4 and a decreased TSH level. If tested, approximately 95% of the patients with GD will have circulating TSIs in their serum. The presence of TSIs confirms the diagnosis of GD. In difficult diagnostic cases, a radionuclide thyroid scan can sometimes provide crucial data. In GD, a diffuse, increased uptake should be visualized on a thyroid scan. This contrasts with toxic nodular goiter, in which only the hyperfunctioning nodules (or nodule) will exhibit increased uptake. If thyrotoxicosis is resulting from some form of thyroiditis, the radioactive iodine uptake is typically low.

The goal of the treatment in GD is the restoration of a euthyroid state (proper management of Graves ophthalmopathy is crucial and is beyond the scope of this chapter). While different mechanisms are used, both medical and surgical treatment options are directed at limiting the output of thyroid hormone by the gland. Careful attention must be given to avoid or protect against precipitation of thyroid storm during therapy. Treatment regimens are determined on a patient-by-patient basis, depending on the severity of the disease, size of the goiter, risks of complications, comorbidities, patient age, and patient preference.

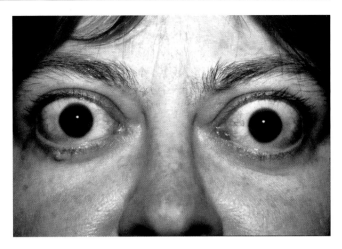

Figure 1.1 Proptotic ophthalmopathy characteristic of Graves disease.

Thionamide antithyroid drugs (ATDs), such as methimazole and propylthiouracil (PTU), decrease the synthesis of thyroid hormone. These medications interfere with the process of iodine organification and prevent the coupling of iodotyrosines necessary for the production of T4 and T3. In some patients, these medications can be used as a temporary measure before definitive treatment with surgery or radioactive iodine ablation. In many patients, ATDs can be used as their primary therapy. In approximately one-third of patients managed in this manner, remission of the disease occurs, typically after treatment for 6 months to 2 years. Spontaneous remission is more likely in patients with mild disease, small goiters, and low TSI levels. While in the past PTU was widely used, methimazole has become the preferred medication owing to its convenient once-daily dosing and the rare but dangerous risk of hepatotoxicity with PTU.[11] In patients who are pregnant, which is another appropriate situation for the use of these medications, PTU is used preferentially as it has less placental transmission to the fetus.

Treatment with beta-blockers, such as propranolol is often used as an adjunct to therapy with ATDs. Beta-blockers provide a dual benefit in patients with HT. First, they inhibit the peripheral conversion of T4 to T3. Second, and perhaps more importantly, they minimize or eliminate symptoms caused by the peripheral effects of hyperthyroidism.[12] These medications are often used preoperatively in these patients to mitigate the risk of thyroid storm during surgery.

To limit or eliminate the hyperfunctional activity of the thyroid gland in GD, ablative approaches can be used as an alternative to ATDs. Ablation of thyroid tissue can be achieved either with the use of radioactive iodine or through surgery. Radioactive iodine ablation in GD, using ^{131}I, is a widely used technique. Patients, particularly those with more severe disease, are often pretreated with ATDs to become euthyroid before ablation. In patients who have recurrent disease, or who are poor operative candidates, iodine ablation is often the preferred therapeutic regimen.[13] Radioactive iodine does not impact fertility, but its use is contraindicated during pregnancy. Pregnancy should be avoided for several months after it has been used.

An effective and safe alternative to radioactive iodine ablation is surgery. Thyroidectomy is a definitive technique for the management of disease in patients with large goiters that cause compressive symptoms, those whose goiters are so large that they will likely not be adequately treated by iodine therapy, in those with recurrent disease, in the setting of a concerning nodule(s), and for those patients preferring a surgical approach.[14] Historically, some surgeons performed less than a total thyroidectomy, leaving behind a remnant of the gland to prevent postoperative hypothyroidism. This approach has been abandoned, because in many patients the remaining tissue caused a recurrence of the GD. The currently accepted surgical approach is a total thyroidectomy. These patients should be treated preoperatively with ATDs to be rendered euthyroid at the time of surgery. In addition, for 7 to 10 days before surgery, potassium iodide solution (SSKI) or Lugol solution may be used to reduce gland vascularity and bleeding at the time of surgery (**Fig. 1.2**).[15] Both medical and surgical ablative approaches lead to permanent hypothyroidism, requiring lifelong thyroxine supplementation.

Nodular Thyroid Diseases

Nodular thyroid disease is much more common than inflammatory thyroid disorders. It is estimated that 5 to 10% of the populations of developed countries is affected by nodular disease.[16]

Patients can develop single or multiple nodules, which may cause an array of symptoms and complications. Two fundamental questions must be considered when treating these patients. The first issue to be considered is whether one is dealing with a nodule(s) that is hyperfunctional (toxic) or not. The second key factor, which should determine the approach to treatment, is whether benign or malignant disease is more likely present. While other factors are considered, such as the presence of compressive symptoms, appropriate management is best dictated by determining whether benign or malignant disease is present and whether the nodules are hyperfunctional or not.

Nodules

Autopsy studies have shown that up to 50% of the cadavers have at least a single nodule in their thyroid gland.[17] A patient can have a solitary nodule or multinodular disease. In either case, similar diagnostic and therapeutic algorithms are used.

Nodules can present in several ways. In some patients, nodular disease causes the development of a goiter, an enlarged thyroid gland. Other patients will seek medical evaluation owing to symptoms of hyperthyroidism. Many nodules are identified on routine physical examinations in completely asymptomatic patients. More recently, the widespread use of radiographic imaging has led to

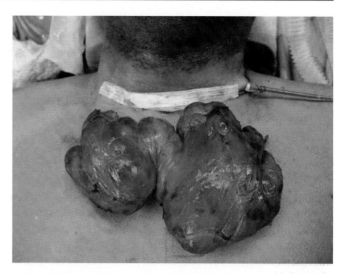

Figure 1.2 Graves disease patients develop highly vascular goiters as shown in this figure.

the incidental identification of a large number of thyroid nodules.

While the development of diffuse goiter is associated with iodine deficiency, the etiology of solitary nodules or multinodular goiters (MNGs) is less clear. A multifactorial process is likely involved, including environmental (such as certain foods) and genetic factors.[18]

Evaluation of patients with nodular thyroid disease requires a detailed history and physical examination. A history of radiation exposure, change in voice, rapid nodular growth, presence of compressive symptoms (such as dysphagia or dyspnea), and a family history of thyroid disease or cancer should be elicited. Physical examination should focus on both the thyroid gland and the cervical lymph nodes. While the protocols for evaluation of nodules differ greatly among physicians, most evaluate thyroid function with laboratory studies and perform some form of radiographic imaging. This approach should be used for both single and multiple nodules. The 2009 ATA guidelines on thyroid nodules strongly recommended that the initial evaluation of a newly identified thyroid nodule(s) should include a TSH level and diagnostic US.[4] The TSH level will provide evidence for a toxic or nontoxic nodule. A low TSH level suggests hyperthyroidism. In this setting, a radionuclide thyroid scan may be appropriate. As malignancy is rare in toxic or "hot" nodules, biopsy can potentially be avoided. A normal or high TSH level indicates a euthyroid or hypothyroid state. A nodule present in patient with a euthyroid or hypothyroid requires US and, in most instances, biopsy.[19]

Toxic Nodules

Toxic nodules, the incidence of which is much higher in iodine-deficient areas, represent approximately 10% of the nodules that are identified. In these nodules, TSH regulation of the thyroid gland is lost and thyroid hormone production continues unchecked. In the setting of hyperthyroidism, a thyroid nodule or MNG can be evaluated with a radionuclide scan. A solitary adenomatous nodule will appear as a single "hot" focus of uptake with decreased surrounding uptake owing to suppression of the remainder of the gland. A toxic MNG will have a heterogeneous appearance on radionuclide imaging, with alternating areas of hyperfunction and hypofunction.

The incidence of malignancy in a hot nodule is rare. The reported rate is less than 5%.[20] Biopsy, such as with FNA, can therefore be avoided in these patients.

Hyperthyroidism caused by toxic nodules—whether single or multiple—is a distinct disorder from GD. This condition is sometimes referred to as Plummer disease. While different in pathophysiology, treatment for these patients is similar to those with GD and may include ATDs, radioactive iodine ablation, surgery, or some combination thereof. However, aside from rare cases in which ablative alternatives are not possible, there is no role for long-term care with ATDs in patients with toxic nodules. This is due to the fact that, in contrast to GD, there is no possibility of spontaneous remission of the disease. Radioactive iodine ablation for toxic MNG typically requires high-dose treatment as compared with treatment for solitary toxic nodules or GD. In older patients, radioactive iodine is typically used for both single and multiple toxic nodules. Thyroidectomy is appropriate in children, in patients with large nodules, when the gland causes compressive symptoms, or in patients in whom there is a suspicion of malignancy.

Nontoxic Nodules

Nontoxic nodular disease is an extremely common entity, encompassing both solitary nodules and MNGs. For each condition, the most important factor to be assessed is whether the nodule(s) represent malignant or benign disease.[21] Benign nodules are most often colloid nodules, degenerative cysts, or follicular neoplasms. After their functional status has been determined by the TSH level, these patients should undergo a diagnostic US.

Solitary Nodules

Diagnostic US can provide extensive information in patients with nodular disease. It can help determine the size, structure, and vascularity of a nodule. While radiographic characteristics cannot determine whether a nodule is benign or malignant, the presence or absence of certain qualities, such as a cystic or spongiform appearance, can alter the level of suspicion for malignancy.

In these patients, biopsy, in the form of FNA, is often performed following the initial work-up.[22] The use of US to guide needle placement can increase the diagnostic accuracy of FNA. Although a benign result on FNA is generally reliable, false-negative benign results do occur and patients should continue to be monitored. Nodules smaller than 1 cm in size should not routinely be biopsied, unless concerning radiographic features (e.g., irregular margins or microcalcifications) are present or the patient

has a history of radiation exposure or a family history of thyroid cancer.

If a nodule has been determined to be benign, surgical intervention is not necessary unless other indications are present. While less common than with MNGs, large solitary nodules can cause compressive symptoms. Patients should be queried about symptoms of dysphagia, odynophagia, and dyspnea, particularly when supine. In certain patients, cosmetic concerns can arise owing to a solitary nodule and need to be considered.

Multinodular Goiters

Adequate iodine intake is closely related to the development of MNG. In iodine-deficient areas, goiter development can be considered endemic in a region when more than 5% of the children between 6 and 12 years of age are affected. Sporadic goiters occur in iodine-sufficient areas. While in certain clinical respects solitary nodules and MNGs are similar, several essential questions regarding the management of MNGs must be addressed.

There is some degree of debate regarding the incidence of malignancy in the setting of MNG and consequently experts disagree how best to assess these patients for the presence of malignancy. Research appears to show that the risk of cancer is the same in patients with solitary nodules and those with MNG. Most experts agree that FNA should be used in patients with MNG; however, there is no clear consensus on which nodules should be selected for biopsy. Some argue that the "dominant" nodule in each half of the gland should be biopsied. Others suggest that any nodule over 1 cm with suspicious radiographic appearance warrants biopsy evaluation.[4]

As with solitary nodules, other indications for surgery must be considered in patients with MNG. Compressive symptoms can be significant and even life-threatening. In addition to questioning patient regarding possible symptoms, certain findings on examination can suggest significant compression due to the goiter. Possible deviation of the airway should be assessed during laryngoscopy. In an effort to elicit the Pemberton sign (facial flushing, extended neck and facial veins, and respiratory distress), patients should be asked to raise both hands simultaneously over their heads as high as possible. This sign is indicative of thoracic outlet obstruction and may be caused by a substernal goiter, in which the goiter has descended into the mediastinum. Substernal goiters can often enlarge over many years without causing significant symptoms (**Fig. 1.3**). However, symptoms, including airway obstruction, can develop precipitously. Most authors agree that even relatively small substernal goiters should be removed, given the potential risk of severe complications and the increasing technical difficulty of thyroidectomy (including the need for possible sternotomy) as these goiters enlarge (**Fig. 1.4**). A marked cosmetic deformity caused by an MNG is another relative indication for thyroidectomy.

The extent of surgery required for patients with MNG (with no malignancy shown on biopsy) is debated.[23–25] Some authors argue that for unilateral disease, a hemi-thyroidectomy and isthmusectomy is an adequate treatment.

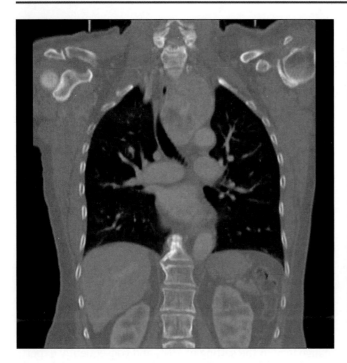

Figure 1.3 A coronal view of a computed tomography scan showing significant substernal extension of a multinodular goiter.

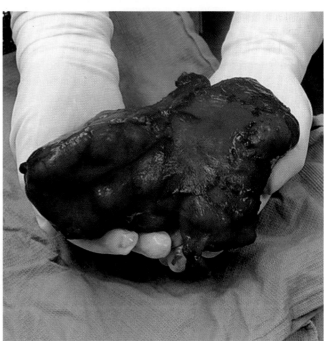

Figure 1.4 A multinodular goiter that had a large substernal component causing compressive symptoms.

However, others believe that a total thyroidectomy is the appropriate surgery for these patients, as their risk of developing goitrous enlargement of the contralateral lobe in the future is significant.

Surgical Treatment

While certain benign thyroid disorders are observed or treated medically as discussed above, thyroidectomy is a key component of management for many of these diseases. The past decade has seen significant changes in the approach to thyroidectomy. Minimally invasive and minimal incision techniques have been described and popularized. Therefore, not all patients require the incision and extensive dissection used in conventional thyroidectomy. The type of thyroidectomy performed should be determined on a case-by-case basis and should consider the safety, efficacy, and technical feasibility of that procedure for each individual patient.

Conventional thyroidectomy techniques should be used for larger MNGs and substernal goiters. To safely remove these goiters while minimizing the risk of complications, wide exposure is needed. Conventional thyroidectomy approaches provide the greatest exposure to facilitate visualization needed to ease dissection and perform safe surgery. In most patients with GD requiring thyroidectomy, conventional techniques should be used for similar reasons. Patients with GD are particularly apt to have hypervascular glands, and bleeding can be problematic. These cases are sometimes made more challenging by the loss of easily dissectible fascial plains owing to the inflammation caused by the disease.

Minimally invasive, nonendoscopic thyroidectomy, which involves smaller incisions (between 3 and 6 cm),

can be used in cases of small MNG or toxic goiters. While these diseases do not meet the criteria for safe and feasible minimally invasive video-assisted thyroidectomy (MIVAT) or transaxillary robot-assisted thyroidectomy, they can often be addressed while avoiding the larger incision and more extensive dissection of conventional thyroidectomy.

MIVAT or transaxillary robot-assisted thyroidectomy are newer techniques that can be used in patients with solitary nodules. MIVAT, performed through a 1.5- to 2-cm incision, and transaxillary robot-assisted thyroidectomy, achieved using an incision placed in the axilla, provide significant benefits over conventional thyroidectomy techniques. MIVAT is indicated in patients with a thyroid volume less than 20 mL, nodule size less than 2.5 to 3 cm, and no history of thyroiditis. These techniques are ideal for patients requiring a total thyroidectomy for cancer or in those needing a lobectomy for diagnostic purposes.

Conclusions

To summarize, benign thyroid conditions are common. Accurate diagnosis is important and may require several laboratory and/or radiographic assessments. The treatment required varies considerably, ranging from expectant observation to medical therapy (radioactive iodine and medicines) and sometimes including surgery.

References

1. Singer PA. Thyroiditis. Acute, subacute, and chronic. Med Clin North Am 1991;75(1):61–77
2. Weetman AP. Autoimmune thyroiditis: predisposition and pathogenesis. Clin Endocrinol (Oxf) 1992;36(4):307–323

3. Baker BA, Gharib H, Markowitz H. Correlation of thyroid antibodies and cytologic features in suspected autoimmune thyroid disease. Am J Med 1983;74(6):941–944

4. Cooper DS, Doherty GM, Haugen BR, et al; American Thyroid Association (ATA) Guidelines Taskforce on Thyroid Nodules and Differentiated Thyroid Cancer. Revised American Thyroid Association management guidelines for patients with thyroid nodules and differentiated thyroid cancer. Thyroid 2009;19(11): 1167–1214

5. Holm LE, Blomgren H, Löwhagen T. Cancer risks in patients with chronic lymphocytic thyroiditis. N Engl J Med 1985;312(10): 601–604

6. Miyauchi A, Matsuzuka F, Kuma K, Takai S. Pyriform sinus fistula: an underlying abnormality common in patients with acute suppurative thyroiditis. World J Surg 1990;14(3):400–405

7. Schwaegerle SM, Bauer TW, Esselstyn CB Jr. Riedel's thyroiditis. Am J Clin Pathol 1988;90(6):715–722

8. Few J, Thompson NW, Angelos P, Simeone D, Giordano T, Reeve T. Riedel's thyroiditis: treatment with tamoxifen. Surgery 1996;120(6):993–998, discussion 998–999

9. Weetman AP. Graves' disease. N Engl J Med 2000;343(17): 1236–1248

10. Alsanea O, Clark OH. Treatment of Graves' disease: the advantages of surgery. Endocrinol Metab Clin North Am 2000;29(2): 321–337

11. Emiliano AB, Governale L, Parks M, Cooper DS. Shifts in propylthiouracil and methimazole prescribing practices: antithyroid drug use in the United States from 1991 to 2008. J Clin Endocrinol Metab 2010;95(5):2227–2233

12. Geffner DL, Hershman JM. Beta-adrenergic blockade for the treatment of hyperthyroidism. Am J Med 1992;93(1):61–68

13. Takáts KI, Szabolcs I, Földes J, et al. The efficacy of long term thyrostatic treatment in elderly patients with toxic nodular goitre compared to radioiodine therapy with different doses. Exp Clin Endocrinol Diabetes 1999;107(1):70–74

14. Palit TK, Miller CC III, Miltenburg DM. The efficacy of thyroidectomy for Graves' disease: a meta-analysis. J Surg Res 2000;90(2):161–165

15. Lennquist S, Jörtsö E, Anderberg B, Smeds S. Betablockers compared with antithyroid drugs as preoperative treatment in hyperthyroidism: drug tolerance, complications, and postoperative thyroid function. Surgery 1985;98(6):1141–1147

16. Rojeski MT, Gharib H. Nodular thyroid disease. Evaluation and management. N Engl J Med 1985;313(7):428–436

17. Mortensen JD, Woolner LB, Bennett WA. Gross and microscopic findings in clinically normal thyroid glands. J Clin Endocrinol Metab 1955;15(10):1270–1280

18. Hegedüs L, Bonnema SJ, Bennedbaek FN. Management of simple nodular goiter: current status and future perspectives. Endocr Rev 2003;24(1):102–132

19. Marqusee E, Benson CB, Frates MC, et al. Usefulness of ultrasonography in the management of nodular thyroid disease. Ann Intern Med 2000;133(9):696–700

20. Senyurek Giles Y, Tunca F, Boztepe H, Kapran Y, Terzioglu T, Tezelman S. The risk factors for malignancy in surgically treated patients for Graves' disease, toxic multinodular goiter, and toxic adenoma. Surgery 2008;144(6):1028–1036, discussion 1036–1037

21. Mazzaferri EL. Management of a solitary thyroid nodule. N Engl J Med 1993;328(8):553–559

22. Ravetto C, Colombo L, Dottorini ME. Usefulness of fine-needle aspiration in the diagnosis of thyroid carcinoma: a retrospective study in 37,895 patients. Cancer 2000;90(6):357–363

23. Cohen-Kerem R, Schachter P, Sheinfeld M, Baron E, Cohen O. Multinodular goiter: the surgical procedure of choice. Otolaryngol Head Neck Surg 2000;122(6):848–850

24. Delbridge L, Guinea AI, Reeve TS. Total thyroidectomy for bilateral benign multinodular goiter: effect of changing practice. Arch Surg 1999;134(12):1389–1393

25. Marchesi M, Biffoni M, Tartaglia F, Biancari F, Campana FP. Total versus subtotal thyroidectomy in the management of multinodular goiter. Int Surg 1998;83(3):202–204

2 Benign Parathyroid Disorders

David J. Terris and Michael C. Singer

Core Messages

- Accurate preoperative diagnosis is essential for appropriate management of benign parathyroid disorders.

- Technological advances have improved diagnostic and management capabilities.

- Directed surgery, with minimally invasive techniques, can be used in most cases of primary hyperparathyroidism.

Advances in clinical laboratory science, radiographic techniques, and medical technology have changed management of parathyroid diseases dramatically over the past two decades. Patients with parathyroid dysfunction are being diagnosed earlier and with greater precision. At the same time, technical innovations have allowed for the development of directed, minimally invasive parathyroidectomy (MIP) techniques. These advances allow most patients with primary hyperparathyroidism (HPT), the most common benign parathyroid disorder, to be identified when still asymptomatic and managed with minimally invasive procedures.

The parathyroid glands are an essential component of the calcium homeostasis system. The production and release of parathyroid hormone (PTH), by the parathyroid chief cells, is directly regulated by serum calcium levels. In response to relative hypocalcemia, PTH is excreted. PTH influences the kidneys to increase calcium reabsorption, promotes resorption and calcium release by the bones, and enhances the absorption of calcium in the intestines by increasing renal activation of vitamin D.

Embryology and Anatomy

Knowledge of the embryologic development and resulting anatomic positioning of the parathyroid glands is essential in managing patients with parathyroid disease. The inferior parathyroid glands and the thymus gland originate from the third branchial pouches and arches, respectively. By descending in concert with the thymus gland, these parathyroid glands move caudally in the neck to a position inferior to the pair of glands derived from the fourth pharyngeal pouches. Thus, the superior parathyroid glands are fourth pouch derivatives, while the inferior glands are from the third pouches.

Several embryologic factors can make localization of the parathyroid glands challenging. The superior pair of glands typically remains intimately associated with the posterolateral aspect of the mid-to-superior segment of the thyroid gland.[1] The inferior parathyroid glands most often are located near the inferior poles of the thyroid. However, the lengthy migration of the parathyroid glands during embryologic development causes a high risk of aberrantly located glands. Ectopic glands, present in 15 to 20% of the patients, can be located at any position along their developmental course of descent. Glands have been identified from the angle of the mandible to the level of the aortic arch. Ectopic positioning of the superior glands is less common as they have only a limited migratory course. In contrast, the inferior glands, which travel a prolonged distance and are embryologically colocated with the thymus, are more likely to be ectopic. Because of their embryologic codevelopment, intrathyroidal and intrathymic positioning should always be considered when confronted with ectopic parathyroid glands.

A second embryologic confounder of parathyroid localization is the significant incidence of subnumerary or supernumerary glands. Approximately 2 to 5% of the patients have five or more glands. A similar percentage of patients have been reported to have fewer than four glands.

Typically, the inferior thyroid artery supplies both the superior and inferior parathyroid glands. Alternatively, an anastomotic branch between the inferior and superior thyroid arteries may supply the superior glands. In a coronal plane, the superior glands generally are more posterior than the inferior glands. Consequently, the superior glands tend to be deep to the recurrent laryngeal nerve (RLN), while the inferior glands are usually superficial to the nerve.

Advances in Diagnosis and Management

Before the early 1970s, physicians did not routinely screen patients for elevated calcium levels. Calcium levels are now routinely assessed, leading to early identification of patients with hypercalcemia.

PTH assays were first introduced in the 1960s, but it was not until the 1990s when they achieved a high degree of accuracy and reproducibility. For the first time, these assays allowed a definitive diagnosis of primary HPT to be made. More importantly, patients with primary HPT could be diagnosed rapidly and early in their disease course. Modifications of these immunoradiometric PTH assays produced the first "rapid" PTH tests, which could be used intraoperatively to assess the physiologic success of parathyroidectomy. The immunochemiluminometric, rapid assays that are now widely used by surgeons provide results within 8 to 10 minutes. While different protocols for the use of intraoperative PTH levels have been described, they all rely on the short half-life of PTH to quickly assess the impact of gland excision.[2,3]

Before the development of advanced radiologic localizing techniques, patients with primary HPT required bilateral neck exploration. Effective modalities that can distinguish enlarged, hyperfunctioning glands are now available. By singling out hyperfunctional glands, more focused procedures can be used in place of four-gland exploration.

Radionuclide imaging of the parathyroids was introduced in the late 1970s. Until the early 1990s, radionuclide imaging used two imaging agents that had different uptake characteristics by the thyroid and parathyroid glands. Subtracting the uptake of one agent from the other provided imaging of the hyperfunctional parathyroid tissue. In 1992, Taillefer et al described the use of technetium-99m sestamibi (^{99m}Tc-sestamibi) as a single agent in a dual-phase technique.[4] Both thyroid and parathyroid tissue take up ^{99m}Tc-sestamibi. However, hyperfunctional parathyroid tissue retains ^{99m}Tc-sestamibi for longer than normal thyroid or parathyroid glands. Two images are taken: the first 10 to 15 minutes after injection of the ^{99m}Tc-sestamibi and the second 1.5 to 3 hours after the first. Taking advantage of the differential washout rates, the first image is subtracted from the second. This highlights the prolonged uptake by the hyperfunctional parathyroid tissue (**Fig. 2.1**). Dual-phase ^{99m}Tc-sestamibi is highly specific and sensitive for the identification of single-gland adenomas

(90% or better). Cases of double adenomas and ectopically located glands are also effectively assessed by ^{99m}Tc-sestamibi imaging. Four-gland hyperplasia is less accurately identified by using this imaging technique. By combining ^{99m}Tc-sestamibi imaging with single-photon emission computed tomography, greater three-dimensional localization can be achieved.[5,6]

High-resolution ultrasonography (US) aids in localizing parathyroid adenomas in primary HPT. When used by an experienced operator, US has a high sensitivity and specificity for diagnosis of adenomas (**Fig. 2.2**). It can be particularly useful in patients with concurrent thyroid nodules or possible intrathyroidal parathyroid adenomas. The anatomic details provided by US complement the physiologic findings seen on radionuclide imaging.

These radiologic techniques have fostered the development of directed parathyroidectomy approaches. Performing safe and effective, minimally invasive, directed parathyroidectomies has also been promoted by several new surgical tools.

Performing minimally invasive video-assisted parathyroidectomy (MIVAP) relies on the use of high-resolution endoscopes, which provide detailed and magnified images of the operative bed (**Fig. 2.3**). With this clarity, anatomic structures are readily identifiable.

Skin adhesives, which alleviate the need for suture placement, are well suited for MIP incisions. Their use can shorten operative time, eliminate the need for suture removal, and provide excellent cosmetic outcomes.

Benign Parathyroid Disorders

The overwhelming majority of parathyroid disorders manifest themselves as HPT. While cases of hypoparathyroidism do occur, they are rare and, in most instances, are due to iatrogenic causes, such as thyroidectomy. HPT is classified as primary, secondary, or tertiary based on the underlying etiology. Primary HPT, in

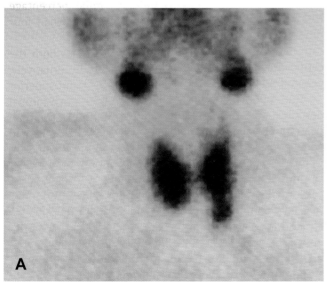
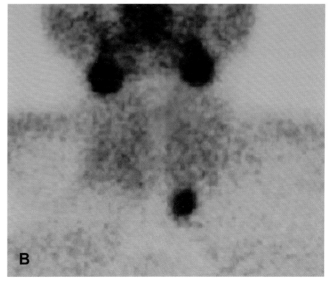

Figure 2.1   Images showing a "light-bulb" sestamibi scan, with an intense focus on tracer uptake, in a patient with a parathyroid adenoma. (A) Early-stage image and (B) late or washout scan.

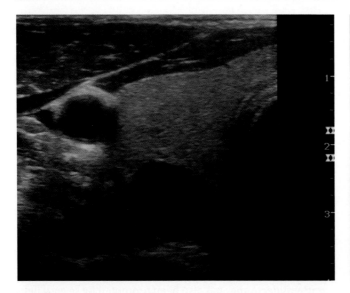

Figure 2.2 A transverse image of an ultrasonography of a parathyroid adenoma extending deep into the thyroid gland.

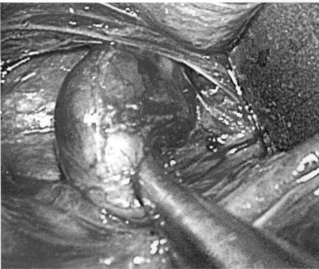

Figure 2.3 An endoscopic view of a parathyroid adenoma in situ. Note the magnification and anatomic detail.

which production of PTH by the parathyroid glands continues despite normal or elevated calcium levels, is the most common cause of hypercalcemia in the general population. This disease is managed surgically in most patients. In cases of secondary HPT, PTH production is driven by systemic hypocalcemia. In the majority of cases, secondary HPT results from hypocalcemia caused by chronic renal failure (**Fig. 2.4**). Correction of the underlying hypocalcemia will resolve the reactive HPT. Tertiary HPT develops when the parathyroid glands remain autonomously hyperactive even after correction of long-standing hypocalcemia. Patients with long-standing vitamin D deficiency will sometimes develop tertiary HPT after their deficiency is corrected. Surgical management, most often in the form of total or subtotal parathyroidectomy, is frequently used.

This chapter focuses on the diagnosis and management of primary HPT, given its predominant frequency and surgical nature.

Primary Hyperparathyroidism

The prevalence of primary HPT in the general population is estimated to be approximately 0.1 to 1%. Women, particularly older than 60 years, are between two and three times more likely to be affected than men.

Between 80 and 85% of the cases of primary HPT result from the development of a single adenoma. However, double adenomas, which can cause significant diagnostic and management challenges, are present in 2 to 3% of the patients. Multigland hyperplasia, from chief cell hyperplasia, is the cause of 12 to 15% of the cases of primary HPT.

Solid sheets of relatively uniform, polygonal chief cells are present in most adenomas. In hyperplasia, all four glands are affected. Differentiating adenomas from hyperplastic glands can be aided by the presence of any normal parathyroid tissue. While adenomas often have a thin rim

of normal parathyroid tissue at their periphery, hyperplastic glands contain no normal tissue.

Both adenomatous and hyperplastic pathology chief cells have decreased sensitivity to systemic calcium levels. The overactivity of proto-oncogenes and the loss of function of tumor suppressor genes are believed to contribute to the pathogenesis of primary HPT. Overexpression of the *PRAD 1* proto-oncogene (cyclin D1) is believed to occur in at least some adenomas. The biallelic loss of the tumor suppressor gene *MEN1* leads to the development of multiple endocrine neoplasia (MEN) syndrome type 1, but also likely occurs in some sporadic cases of primary HPT.

Historically, patients with HPT were not identified until they were symptomatic, often with significant sequelae. Currently, however, because of the advances in laboratory studies previously described, most patients with primary HPT are identified when still asymptomatic. If the disease has progressed, multiple organ systems can be affected. Patients can have genitourinary, rheumatologic, gastrointestinal, cardiovascular, and psychiatric symptoms in addition to generalized weakness and fatigue (**Table 2.1**).

The laboratory and radiologic advances previously described have promoted more accurate diagnosis. Paramount to the diagnosis of primary HPT are hypercalcemia and nonsuppressed PTH levels.[7] Importantly, when evaluating patients for HPT, the physiologically active ionized calcium should be considered. Only approximately 45% of calcium is ionized, with the remainder mostly bound to proteins (usually albumin) and some complexed with phosphate or citrate. In the setting of hypercalcemia, a PTH level at the high end of the normal range should be considered inappropriate and warrants additional evaluation. To differentiate primary HPT from familial hypocalciuric hypercalcemia, a generally benign, nonoperative condition, a 24-hour total urine calcium level and calcium clearance are sometimes required.

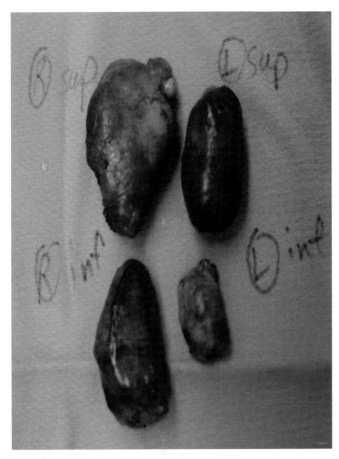

Figure 2.4 Parathyroid glands removed from a patient with secondary hyperparathyroidism. Asymmetric hyperplasia of all four glands is typical.

The potential association with MEN syndromes should be considered in any patient with parathyroid disease.

As previously described, the use of radionuclide scanning and high-resolution US to localize the diseased gland in patients with primary HPT has become an important preoperative step. US is often used in tandem with sestamibi imaging. Surgeon-performed US can be especially beneficial,

Table 2.1 Signs and Symptoms of Primary Hyperparathyroidism

System	Signs/Symptoms
Systemic	Weakness, fatigue, weight loss
Gastrointestinal	Abdominal pain, constipation, nausea, vomiting, peptic ulcer disease, pancreatitis
Rheumatologic	Bone pain, osteoporosis, brown tumors of bone, arthralgia, myalgia, gout
Renal	Nephrolithiasis, polyuria, polydipsia, renal failure
Cardiovascular	Hypertension, cardiac arrhythmias
Psychiatric	Depression, dementia, confusion

as it provides to them directly detailed anatomic information. The diagnostic accuracy of both sestamibi and US in cases of multigland hyperplasia is limited. Magnetic resonance imaging and computed tomography have limited application for patients with primary HPT. Their use can be beneficial in cases of ectopic glands or reoperative cases. Recently, the use of four-dimensional computed tomography, which provides both functional and anatomic information in one modality, for the localization of parathyroid adenomas has been described. The most appropriate and effective uses of this technique are unclear at this time, and additional studies are required to delineate its benefits.

Treatment/Surgery

Primary HPT is managed surgically in the vast majority of patients. Surgical intervention is curative and mitigates the risk of future sequelae. Supportive medical therapy is available for patients who are not operative candidates.[8] Recently, selective embolization via angiography of parathyroid adenomas has been performed successfully in some centers.[9]

Bilateral neck exploration with four-gland exploration has been the gold standard for the management of primary HPT. It is effective for the treatment of both adenomatous and hyperplastic pathology. In the setting of a single or possible double adenoma, one or two glands could be excised. In the case of hyperplastic disease, either a subtotal or a total parathyroidectomy with reimplantation of a portion of one gland can be performed. Four-gland exploration remains the appropriate procedure for patients with suspected hyperplasia.[10]

Surgical management of parathyroid adenomas no longer requires bilateral neck exploration in most cases. As described previously, with the current radiologic techniques, most adenomas can be localized before surgery and targeted for removal. Several different MIP techniques for directed parathyroidectomy have emerged. These approaches provide the benefits of less pain, faster recovery times, ambulatory care, and smaller incisions, while being as effective (over 90% cure rate) and even safer than a conventional parathyroidectomy.[11,12] Less dissection may reduce the risk of recurrent nerve injury and minimizes trauma to the nonpathologic parathyroid glands, thereby limiting the potential for postoperative hypoparathyroidism.

The MIP techniques use an incision of 2 cm or less. To assess efficacy of the surgery, intraoperative PTH levels are measured in most MIP approaches. The incision can be made in the midline or in the area directly over the suspected pathologic gland. Only limited or no subplatysmal flaps need to be elevated. Blunt dissection is used to identify, skeletonize, and excise the gland. A focused lateral approach that uses a similar technique but starts with an incision made more laterally has been described. Coming from this lateral orientation, posteriorly located adenomas may be more easily accessed. In radio-guided MIPs, similar techniques are used but dissection is directed by increased levels of radioactive tracer.[13,14] Preoperatively, [99mTc]-sestamibi is administered to the patient. This is taken up most avidly by the pathologic gland. After the incision is made, a gamma probe is used to guide the dissection. Subsequent to removal, the gamma probe is used to confirm increased uptake in the excised gland and the absence of additional hyperactivity in the neck.

An endoscopic approach to the parathyroids was first described in 1996.[15] Some surgeons continue to use only endoscopic approaches, which require gas insufflation. We prefer the MIVAP approach because it affords several benefits.[16,17] In contrast to the previously described MIP techniques, MIVAP is performed with excellent visualization of the anatomy. In addition, the field of view during MIVAP is in the same orientation as classical parathyroidectomy, providing a familiar working environment for the surgeon. Finally, MIVAP avoids multiple incisions and risks associated with the use of gas insufflation inherent only in endoscopic approaches, **Table 2.2** lists the indications and contraindications for MIVAP.

Surgical Considerations

To achieve the most cosmetically pleasing incision, the incision site is marked in the preoperative holding area. The actual position of the proposed incision and its relationship to natural skin creases is best assessed with the patient sitting upright. A blood specimen can be drawn at this time to check a preincision, rapid PTH level.

In most cases, general anesthesia is used. However, on the basis of patient preference and medical condition, MIVAP can be performed under local anesthesia. The patient is placed on the operating table in the supine position without significant neck extension. When working on the thyroid or parathyroid glands in video-assisted procedures, hyperextension creates a poor angle for work with the endoscope. It can also lead to unnecessary postoperative neck and back pain.

Appropriate positioning in the operating room is critical in MIVAP to facilitate the procedure. The operating table is rotated 180 degrees to allow room for the surgeon, assistants, and equipment. The surgeon stands at the patient's right side, with the camera assistant across the table and a second assistant positioned at the head of the patient. Monitors for the endoscopic portion of the case are placed to provide easy viewing for the surgeon, assistants, and nurses.

Table 2.2 Indications and Contraindications for Minimally Invasive Video-Assisted Parathyroidectomy

Indications
• Parathyroid adenoma < 3 cm in diameter
• Clear preoperative localization
• Thin to normal size neck
Contraindications
• Thyroid > 25 mL
• Previous neck surgery
• Possible parathyroid carcinoma

A 1.5-cm horizontal incision is made at the previously marked site through the skin and subcutaneous tissues. The platysma is often avoided in this area as the incision is made between the insertions of the muscle. No subplatysmal flaps are elevated in MIVAP. With electrocautery, the strap muscles are separated in the midline from the sternal notch to the thyroid notch.

Blunt dissection, a crucial technique in endoscopic procedures, is used to develop a plane between the strap muscles and the thyroid gland ipsilateral to the pathologic parathyroid gland. Retractors, held by the second assistant, are then placed to retract the muscles laterally and the thyroid gland medially.

A 5-mm, 30-degree endoscope, held by the first assistant, is then inserted into the wound. With endoscopic visualization, blunt dissection is used to identify the adenoma and mobilize it. The vascular pedicle, usually limited in caliber, is then ligated with either vascular clips or monopolar cautery. The gland can then be extracted through the incision. An intraoperative PTH level should be checked 5, 10, and 15 minutes after the excision of the gland.

Loose reapproximation of the strap muscles is achieved with the use of a single 3–0 Vicryl, figure-of-eight suture. No drains are used. A single subdermal, 4–0 Vicryl suture is placed to appose the wound edges, and the skin is sealed with a skin adhesive. A single, horizontal Steri-Strip is placed over the wound.

If surgery is uneventful and the postanesthesia recovery is smooth, most patients are discharged 1.5 to 2 hours after surgery. All patients are placed on a 3-week taper of Os-Cal D, mitigating the risk of postoperative hypocalcemia. One month after surgery, calcium levels are assessed.

Postoperative Complications

The rate of complications with all parathyroidectomy techniques is low. Standard postoperative complications, such as hematoma or infection, are rare. Injury to the RLN occurs in approximately 1% of the cases. These injuries are temporary in most instances. Revision surgery does have higher rates of nerve injury.

Postoperatively, a period of temporary hypocalcemia from transient hypoparathyroidism occurs in a significant number of cases. This is most often due to suppression of the normal parathyroid glands by the pathologic gland. After removal, the remaining glands will return to normal function after a variable period of time. If postoperative hypocalcemia does occur, levels typically reach a nadir 48 to 72 hours after surgery. Some surgeons use PTH levels to try to determine which patients are at risk for postoperative hypoparathyroidism. To facilitate ambulatory care, in our practice patients are discharged on calcium supplementation to alleviate any risk of this complication. If a total parathyroidectomy with autotransplantation was performed, patients should be expected to remain hypoparathyroid until the transplanted tissue begins to function, often within 3 to 6 months.

Hungry bone syndrome, a severe form of postoperative hypocalcemia, can occur rarely. Patients above 50 years of age and those with long-standing disease, severe osteopenia, elevated preoperative alkaline phosphatase levels, and large adenomas are most at risk of experiencing this complication. After surgery, badly depleted bones act as a calcium sponge causing potentially critical hypocalcemia. Aggressive calcium and electrolyte supplementation is required to prevent paresthesias, tetanies, seizures, and cardiac arrhythmias.

Controversy over the Management of Asymptomatic Patients

Primary HPT is a disease that requires surgical intervention for cure. There is consensus among experts that any patient who is symptomatic or presents with end-organ injury requires surgery.

However, as mentioned, currently the vast majority of patients diagnosed are asymptomatic. There has been some debate regarding which of these patients should undergo surgery and who can be observed (or in some instances treated medically).[18] Some argue that the disease of most asymptomatic patients does not progress and therefore many patients should be observed. A convening of the Consensus Development Conference on the Management of Asymptomatic Primary Hyperparathyroidism held in 2001, under the auspices of the National Institutes of Health, addressed this issue and established guidelines for surgical intervention. Since then, additional studies have provided evidence of the risks for untreated, asymptomatic patients and of the benefits provided by surgery. Several studies have shown that untreated, asymptomatic patients are at significant risk in the long term of developing decreased bone density and fractures. Parathyroidectomy has been shown to reduce this risk and lead to increased bone density. When followed-up for a long period, a large number of these asymptomatic patients also progress and develop impaired renal function and nephrolithiasis. Again, these risks are removed with surgery. The third meeting of the Consensus Development Conference supported by several American and international endocrine and surgical societies, held in 2008, established revised guidelines for surgery in these patients.[19,20] According to those guidelines, surgery should be considered in patients who meet one or more of the following criteria: age less than 50 years, serum calcium 1.0 mg/dL above the upper limit of normal, glomerular filtration rate less than 60 mL/min, bone densitometry T score less than –2.5, and/or previous fracture fragility.

References

1. Akerström G, Malmaeus J, Bergström R. Surgical anatomy of human parathyroid glands. Surgery 1984;95(1):14–21
2. Ito F, Sippel R, Lederman J, Chen H. The utility of intraoperative bilateral internal jugular venous sampling with rapid parathyroid hormone testing. Ann Surg 2007;245(6):959–963
3. Seybt MW, Loftus KA, Mulloy AL, Terris DJ. Optimal use of intraoperative PTH levels in parathyroidectomy. Laryngoscope 2009;119(7):1331–1333
4. Taillefer R, Boucher Y, Potvin C, Lambert R. Detection and localization of parathyroid adenomas in patients with hyperparathyroidism using a single radionuclide imaging procedure with technetium-99m-sestamibi (double-phase study). J Nucl Med 1992;33(10):1801–1807
5. Akram K, Parker JA, Donohoe K, Kolodny G. Role of single photon emission computed tomography/computed tomography in localization of ectopic parathyroid adenoma: a pictorial case series and review of the current literature. Clin Nucl Med 2009;34(8):500–502
6. Eslamy HK, Ziessman HA. Parathyroid scintigraphy in patients with primary hyperparathyroidism: ^{99m}Tc sestamibi SPECT and SPECT/CT. Radiographics 2008;28(5):1461–1476
7. Khan AA, Bilezikian JP, Potts JT Jr; Guest Editors for the Third International Workshop on Asymptomatic Primary Hyperparathyroidism. The diagnosis and management of asymptomatic primary hyperparathyroidism revisited. J Clin Endocrinol Metab 2009;94(2):333–334
8. Wüthrich RP, Martin D, Bilezikian JP. The role of calcimimetics in the treatment of hyperparathyroidism. Eur J Clin Invest 2007;37(12):915–922
9. Miller DL, Doppman JL, Chang R, et al. Angiographic ablation of parathyroid adenomas: lessons from a 10-year experience. Radiology 1987;165(3):601–607
10. Moalem J, Guerrero M, Kebebew E. Bilateral neck exploration in primary hyperparathyroidism—when is it selected and how is it performed? World J Surg 2009;33(11):2282–2291
11. Norman J, Chheda H, Farrell C. Minimally invasive parathyroidectomy for primary hyperparathyroidism: decreasing operative time and potential complications while improving cosmetic results. Am Surg 1998;64(5):391–395, discussion 395–396
12. Pellitteri PK. Directed parathyroid exploration: evolution and evaluation of this approach in a single-institution review of 346 patients. Laryngoscope 2003;113(11):1857–1869
13. Mariani G, Gulec SA, Rubello D, et al. Preoperative localization and radioguided parathyroid surgery. J Nucl Med 2003;44(9):1443–1458
14. Shaha AR, Patel SG, Singh B. Minimally invasive parathyroidectomy: the role of radio-guided surgery. Laryngoscope 2002;112(12):2166–2169
15. Gagner M. Endoscopic subtotal parathyroidectomy in patients with primary hyperparathyroidism. Br J Surg 1996;83(6):875
16. Casserly P, Kirby R, Timon C. Outcome measures and scar aesthetics in minimally invasive video-assisted parathyroidectomy. Arch Otolaryngol Head Neck Surg 2010;136(3):260–264
17. Miccoli P, Berti P, Conte M, Raffaelli M, Materazzi G. Minimally invasive video-assisted parathyroidectomy: lesson learned from 137 cases. J Am Coll Surg 2000;191(6):613–618
18. Eigelberger MS, Cheah WK, Ituarte PH, Streja L, Duh QY, Clark OH. The NIH criteria for parathyroidectomy in asymptomatic primary hyperparathyroidism: are they too limited? Ann Surg 2004;239(4):528–535
19. Bilezikian JP, Khan AA, Potts JT Jr; Third International Workshop on the Management of Asymptomatic Primary Hyperthyroidism. Guidelines for the management of asymptomatic primary hyperparathyroidism: summary statement from the third international workshop. J Clin Endocrinol Metab 2009;94(2):335–339
20. Udelsman R, Pasieka JL, Sturgeon C, Young JE, Clark OH. Surgery for asymptomatic primary hyperparathyroidism: proceedings of the third international workshop. J Clin Endocrinol Metab 2009;94(2):366–372

3 Differentiated Thyroid Carcinomas

Andrzej L. Komorowski, Wojciech M. Wysocki, Raghav C. Dwivedi, and Rehan A. Kazi

Core Messages

- Differentiated thyroid carcinomas (DTCs) are the most common endocrine malignancy in humans.

- DTCs generally have good prognosis.

- The cornerstone of treatment is surgery.

- Minimally invasive techniques are emerging as newer options in the treatment of these tumors.

Thyroid malignancies account for approximately 1 to 1.5% of all malignancies in humans. It is also the most common among all endocrine malignancies and accounts for 90% of cases. Of these, differentiated thyroid carcinomas (DTCs) alone constitute approximately 95% of the disease bulk. There are three major types of DTCs: papillary thyroid carcinoma (PTC; **Fig. 3.1**), follicular thyroid carcinoma (FTC; **Fig. 3.2**), and Hürthle cell tumors. These three variants collectively account for approximately 90% of all DTC cases. The most commonly encountered DTC is papillary thyroid cancer (constitutes 80 to 85% of all cases), followed by follicular thyroid cancer (10 to 20% of all cases) and Hürthle cell cancer (2 to 5% of all DTC cases). The disease is more commonly encountered in women than in men, with a woman to man ratio of 3:1 in most of the studies. Production and secretion of thyroglobulin is the characteristic feature of all types of DTCs. The serum level of this hormone supports correct diagnosis, helps in surgical radicality assessment, and serves as an early biochemical recurrence marker. More than 80% of the patients diagnosed with DTC have good or even excellent prognosis, with approximately 99% 20-year survival rates. However, the remaining 20% of the patients have a less favorable course of disease, with 10-year rates ranging between 20 and 50%.[1]

Epidemiology and Risk Factors

In the United States, approximately 20,000 new cases of thyroid carcinoma are diagnosed each year. Some 200,000 patients with thyroid carcinoma are followed-up each year in the United States, and nearly 1500 die from this disease annually.

The age at diagnosis ranges between 45 and 50 years. Less than 10% of all DTCs are found in patients younger than 21 years. The clinical course of DTC in children younger than 10 years is less favorable than in older individuals, as is in patients older than 65 years. This fact is not reflected in the current AJCC/TNM (American Joint Committee on Cancer/Tumor-Node-Metastasis) classification, and it also results in poorer outcomes for the whole stage I and II groups (all patients younger than 45 years and independent of extension of the disease are classified as stage I or II; see below for details).[2]

Various environmental, hormonal, and genetic factors play a role in the development of DTC. The risk of developing DTC is associated with radiation exposure: therapeutic irradiation (e.g., treatment for Hodgkin lymphoma in childhood/adolescence), accidental irradiation (e.g., after explosion in Chernobyl in 1986, 100-fold higher DTC incidence has been noted in several contaminated regions of Belarus and Ukraine), and occupational and geological irradiation. The peak risk of developing DTC is seen 20 to 30 years after irradiation. It is estimated that about 10% of the DTCs may be radiation induced.[3] The risk of developing thyroid carcinoma rises linearly with increasing radiation doses. At doses higher than 20 Gy, complete ablation of the thyroid tissue supervenes.

One of the factors that cause the development of a DTC is iodine intake. Interestingly, PTC is more common in regions with high iodine intake, while FTC is common in iodine-deficient regions.[4] Other environmental factors that possibly play a role in thyroid carcinoma development are retinol, vitamin C, and vitamin E.

Approximately 3 to 5% of PTC are inherited as an autosomal dominant trait and are supposed to be more clinically aggressive than the sporadic ones. Familial FTC is extremely rare. In general, familial DTC may be associated with familial adenomatous polyposis, Gardner syndrome, Cowden syndrome, Carney syndrome, or multiple endocrine neoplasia type I.

Among genetic mutations that are linked to the pathogenesis of DTC are *RAS, RET/PTC*, BRAF, PAX8/PPARγ, *TRK, MET. RAS* oncogens are most commonly identified in DTC (up to 80% of FTC, 50% of PTC, and 12% of Hürthle cell carcinoma).[4] BRAF proteins are found exclusively in PTC (up

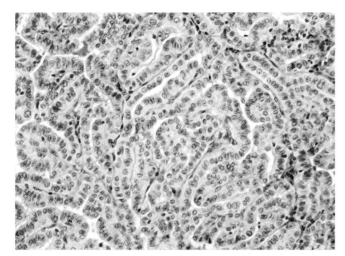

Figure 3.1 Microphotograph of the classical-type papillary carcinoma. Note the papillary structures and distinctive nuclear features of the tumor. Hematoxylin and eosin stain, magnification ×400.

Image courtesy: Prof. Janusz Ryś, Cancer Center Kraków, Poland.

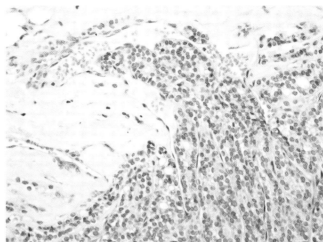

Figure 3.2 Microphotograph of follicular carcinoma. Note the vascular invasion in the peripheral portion of the tumor. Hematoxylin and eosin stain, magnification ×200.

Image courtesy: Prof. Janusz Ryś, Cancer Center Kraków, Poland.

to 70% of the cases). Tyrosine kinase oncogenes (*RET, TRK, MET*) are also typical for PTC (*RET* in 50%, *TRK* in 20%, *MET* in up to 80% of the cases). The only tyrosine kinase oncogene found in FTC (10% of the cases) is *MET*. FTC is also associated with PAX8/PPARγ.[5]

Pathology

Cytology

According to the Bethesda System for Reporting Thyroid Cytopathology, each thyroid fine-needle aspiration biopsy (FNAB) report should begin with a general diagnostic category. The diagnostic categories are given in **Table 3.1**.

PTC has characteristic cytological features, which can be easily recognized in aspirates from FNAB. Typically, there is a large number of cells that may be grouped into clusters and monolayers or formed papillary arrangements (**Fig. 3.1**). Other important features that help distinguish PTC from follicular cells are crowding, overlapping, and molding. The defining and diagnostic features of PTC are seen in the nuclei of cancer cells—enlarged nuclei containing dusty (powderlike) chromatin (ground glass nuclei).

Contrary to PTC, cytological diagnosis of FTC is often impossible because of microscopic similarity to adenoma. Smears contain numerous clusters of glandular cells, usually arranged in ringlike (follicular) or rossette-like acinar structures (**Fig. 3.2**). The presence of nuclear atypia does not necessarily imply malignant behavior of tumor. Therefore, the diagnosis of malignancy has to be based on histological and not cytological evaluation. The cytological diagnosis of follicular neoplasm implies obligatory surgical excision and microscopic examination of specimen.

Histopathology

The role of frozen section in the evaluation of thyroid nodules is limited. Artificial changes in microscopic appearance of cells make the assessment of the nuclear features virtually impossible.

Papillary Thyroid Carcinoma

PTC accounts for 80 to 85% of all cases of malignant epithelial tumors of thyroid. Multifocality is found in 20 to 30% of the cases; however, in some series it can reach 80% depending on the extent of the gland that has been evaluated and the thickness of sections used. Multifocality may be associated with intraglandular metastases, but data from the studies of the clonal rearrangements or X chromosome inactivation patterns support rather the simultaneous growth of multiple primary tumors in most patients. Patients with PTC generally have an excellent prognosis with 95% 10-year survival.

PTC presents a variety of macroscopic patterns. Most commonly, it presents as a gray-white mass with irregular margins. Calcifications may also be noticed on gross examination. PTC can present as solid and/or cystic tumor; however, entirely cystic papillary carcinoma is a rare finding. PTC can involve the whole lobe of thyroid gland and infiltrate into periglandular fat, invade skeletal muscles, and adjacent organs (esophagus, larynx, and trachea). When carcinoma's dimension is less than 1 cm in diameter, it is called "papillary microcarcinoma."

The World Health Organization (WHO) classification of thyroid tumors specifies 16 histological types of PTCs (including conventional variant). The histological division is based on the growth patterns, cytological features of tumor cells, and the type of tumor stroma. All papillary carcinomas present the typical nuclear features that are required for the diagnosis of PTC (*see* section on Cytology). Histological

Table 3.1 Bethesda System for Reporting Thyroid Cytopathology with Risk of Malignancy

Diagnostic Categories of FNAB	Risk of Malignancy (%)
Nondiagnostic or unsatisfactory specimen	1–4
Benign Consistent with a benign follicular nodule Consistent with Hashimoto thyroiditis Consistent with granulomatous thyroiditis	0–3
Atypia of undetermined significance or follicular lesion of undetermined significance	5–15
Follicular neoplasm or suspicious for a follicular neoplasm	15–30
Suspicious for malignancy Suspicious for papillary carcinoma Suspicious for medullary carcinoma Suspicious for metastatic carcinoma Suspicious for lymphoma	60–75
Malignant Papillary thyroid carcinoma Poorly differentiated carcinoma Medullary thyroid carcinoma Undifferentiated (anaplastic) carcinoma Squamous cell carcinoma Carcinoma with mixed features Metastatic carcinoma Non-Hodgkin lymphoma	97–99

FNAB, fine-needle aspiration biopsy.

variants of PTC and their respective clinical behavior are listed in **Table 3.2**.

A special variant of PTC that requires separate description because of its clinical importance is a papillary microcarcinoma. This term is reserved for incidentally found neoplasm measuring 10 mm in diameter or less. Typically, this type of PTC is characterized by relatively benign clinical course; however, in children it can behave more aggressively. Irrespective of the size of the tumor, up to 11% of the papillary microcarcinomas can be lymph-node positive. The features of papillary microcarcinoma suggestive of more aggressive behavior and implying prompt surgery are as follows:

- Tumors located near the trachea or on the dorsal surface of thyroid (these carcinomas will show dorsal extension and invade the adjacent organs).
- Features of high-grade tumor in cytological material (FNAB).
- Presence of regional lymph-node or distant metastasis, and
- Increase in the size of the tumor and/or appearance of node metastasis during observation.

Follicular Thyroid Carcinoma

By definition, it is a malignant epithelial tumor that shows a follicular differentiation (follicle formation) and a lack of characteristic nuclear features of papillary carcinoma (*see* section on Cytology). FTC accounts for 10 to 15% of the thyroid malignancies. FTC is more common in women and usually occurs later in life compared with PTC. It has much lower frequency of lymph-node metastasis compared with PTC (less than 5%), but distant metastasis (mainly to lung and bone) are more frequent at presentation (20 to 33%).[6]

Follicular carcinomas usually present as encapsulated solid tumors of larger than 1 cm diameter. The color varies from gray-tan to brown. The capsule can be noticed in some cases. Minimally invasive carcinomas are practically identical on gross examination with follicular adenomas.

Morphology of FTC is variable and includes tumors with follicles filled with colloid and neoplasms, which have solid and trabecular growth patterns. Diagnosis of malignant growth is based on the presence of vascular and/or capsular invasion. Architecture and cytological atypia are not essential for the diagnosis. Generally, FTC is divided into two main groups according to the extent of tumor invasiveness: minimally invasive (with limited infiltration of the tumor capsule or extension through the tumor capsule and/or vascular invasion) and widely invasive follicular carcinoma. The latter category includes carcinomas with distinct and wide infiltration of the thyroid tissue and/or blood vessels. "Capsular invasion" should be recognized with the penetration of tumor cells only through the capsule (not in the site of previous FNAB). "Vascular invasion" means the presence of intravascular tumor cells covered by endothelium or associated with thrombus; it refers to the vessels only within or beyond the capsule. Some authors also use the term "grossly encapsulated angioinvasive follicular carcinoma" to describe tumor in which both capsular invasion and vascular invasion are present (as opposed to minimally invasive carcinoma with only capsular invasion). Histological variants of FTC and their respective clinical behavior are presented in **Table 3.2**.

Survival rates for FTC vary from 70 to 95% and are little lower than for PTC. Prognostic factors that are related to unfavorable prognosis include age greater than 45 years, oncocytic variant of FTC, malignant infiltration beyond the thyroid, tumor size greater than 4 cm, and the presence of distant metastases.

Hürthle Cell Carcinoma

The WHO classification lists Hürthle cell carcinoma as a variant of FTC ("oncocytic variant of FTC"; *see* **Table 3.2**); however, it is frequently considered a separate pathologic entity characterized by distinct microscopic appearance and clinical behavior. Hürthle cell carcinoma or oncocytic variant of FTC comprises approximately 5% of the malignant thyroid tumors, and in contrast to FTC, the frequency of nodal metastases in this neoplasm is approximately 30%.

There is no evidence that pathogenesis of Hürthle cell carcinoma is different from that of conventional FTC, although *H-Ras* mutations are more often found in this type of tumor than in FTC.

Table 3.2   Histological Variants of PTC and FTC and Their Respective Prognosis

Type	Prognosis
PTC subtypes	
• Classical PTC (the most frequent; presents typical papillary architecture)	Good
• Follicular PTC	Similar as in the classical type
• Macrofollicular PTC	Similar to other follicular variants, with lymph-node metastases present in ~20% and distant metastases in 7% of the cases
• Oncocytic cell	Not known
• Clear cell	Not known
• Diffuse sclerosing	Similar as in the classical type (despite high incidence of regional lymph-node and distant metastases)
• Tall cell	Poor
• Columnar cell	Poor
• Solid	Poor
• Cribriform	Not known (usually associated with FAP or Gardner syndrome)
• With fascitis-like stroma	Similar as in the classical type
• With focal insular component	Not known
• With squamous cell or mucoepidermoid carcinoma	Poor
• With spindle and giant cell carcinomas	Not known
• Combined papillary and medullary carcinomas	Not known
• Papillary microcarcinoma	Good (but in up to 11% cases, lymph-node metastasis can be present)
FTC subtypes	
• Encapsulated FTC with microscopic capsular invasion (no vascular invasion is present) = minimally invasive follicular carcinoma	Very low probability (less than 5% of the cases) of metastases, recurrences, or tumor-associated mortality
• Encapsulated FTC with angioinvasion (capsular invasion is present or absent)	Metastases, recurrences, or tumor-associated mortality in 5–30% of the cases
• Widely invasive follicular carcinoma	Metastases, recurrences, or tumor-associated mortality in 50–55% of the cases
• Oncocytic cell (Hürthle cell)	Nodal metastases in ~30% of the cases
• Clear cell	Not known
• Mucinous variant	Not known
• FTC with signet-ring cells	Not known

PTC, papillary thyroid carcinoma; FAP, familial adenomatous polyposis; FTC, follicular thyroid carcinoma.

Macroscopically, Hürthle cell tumors have characteristic brown mahogany color (different from the color of other thyroid tumors) and are encapsulated. The morphological changes within the tumor, such as hemorrhage, cystic areas, infarction, fibrosis, and cellular atypia, can be associated, but not exclusively, with previous FNAB.

The tumor is built almost exclusively of oncocytic cells (at least 75% of all tumor cells). The growth pattern can be follicular or solid/trabecular. The Hürthle cells have deeply eosinophilic and granular cytoplasm; their nuclei are round and hyperchromatic with prominent nucleoli. Similar to FTC, the differentiation between Hürthle cell adenoma and carcinoma is based on the same criteria of capsular and/or vascular invasion. The malignant tumors are divided into minimally invasive and widely invasive variants.

Patients with Hürthle cell carcinoma are considered to have a poorer prognosis compared with patients with FTC and PTC. The frequency of lymph-node metastases as well as of distant metastases is higher than in non-Hürthle DTC. A lower uptake of radioactive iodine also makes the treatment of these tumors more challenging.

Patient Evaluation

Eliciting a detailed patient history is of immense importance. Besides the general history, the clinician should always ask the patient about important specific symptoms pertaining to thyroid disease. These include dysphagia, dyspnea, voice change (hoarseness), cough, sensation of a mass in the neck, change in weight, tremor, unusual sweating, mood changes, and palpitations. These help in establishing the diagnosis and in evaluating the extent of the disease process.

It is also important to ask about a family history of thyroid disorders and previous radiation exposure. As stated before, it is estimated that as many as 3 to 5% of all DTCs can occur in the familial settings. Patients with familial colon poliposis, those with Cowden disease, and those with Gardner syndrome also have a higher risk of developing a DTC.

Clinically apparent thyroid nodules can be found in approximately 4 to 7% of the adult population. It is important to bear in mind that of these nodules, malignancy will eventually be found in 5 to 12% of the patients with single nodules and in 3% of the patients with multiple nodules.

The clinical examination of a patient starts with visual inspection of the neck while it is slightly extended and the patient seated comfortably on an examination chair. During palpation it is customary to stand behind the patient. The examiner should place his or her hands on the patient's neck so that the index fingers are just below the cricoid cartilage. Then, the examiner asks the patient to swallow so that the isthmus can be palpated. Examination is continued, with the examiner moving his or her fingers downward and laterally. The examiner should look for single nodules fixed to surrounding tissues with hard consistency. Palpable cervical lymph nodes can also be noted in some cases.

Finding the lower borders of the thyroid may at times be difficult because it can be partially or totally retrosternal; further extension of the neck may help.

Cervical spine flexibility should also be assessed to ensure hyperextension of the neck during surgery (only minimally invasive techniques do not require neck hyperextension to ensure adequate visualization; see below). Examination of larynx and vocal cords mobility should also be performed and documented, especially with more advanced tumors.

Algorithm for the Evaluation of a Thyroid Nodule

Because the autopsy series suggests that up to 50% of the general population can have thyroid nodules, it is of utmost importance to identify those lesions that are potentially harmful. Furthermore, a vast majority of thyroid nodules that are being seen and investigated by clinicians are incidental, asymptomatic findings. It is therefore crucial

to not overdiagnose and overtreat otherwise healthy individuals who happen to have a completely benign thyroid nodule. The algorithm presented in **Fig. 3.3** should help in correctly addressing these issues.

Laboratory Tests and Imaging Studies

The screening test for the evaluation of thyroid function is a must when evaluating any thyroid nodule. It is sufficient to start with the estimation of serum thyroid-stimulating hormone (TSH) level. In the case of subnormal TSH serum levels (i.e., < 0.5 mIU/L), one should proceed to T3 and T4 serum levels evaluation and a radionuclide scan should be obtained. The serum TSH level serves as a screening test for thyroid function. The evaluation of T3 and T4 can confirm the diagnosis of hyperthyroidism, and radionuclide scan will identify hyperfunctioning nodules. The evaluation of thyroid nodules with radionuclide scan (it has been estimated that 16% of the nonfunctioning nodules and 9% of the normal-functioning nodules on radionuclide scan are malignant, while hyperfunctioning nodules only occasionally harbor a malignancy) is no longer used as a first-line diagnostic tool in thyroid cancer.

Obtaining a thyroid ultrasound is an essential step for the exact characterization of the mass, and best results are achieved when it is performed by a dedicated neck ultrasonologist. The decision whether ultrasound-guided FNAB should follow is based on several factors, as shown in **Fig. 3.3**. If the decision on FNAB is taken, the laboratory tests for hemostatic function become mandatory.

Until recently, it was presumed that the size of thyroid nodule as seen on ultrasound should be a threshold for biopsy. This approach has changed, and currently the decision concerning the biopsy is based on features other than the tumor size. The ultrasonic features of a thyroid nodule that warrant an FNAB are calcification, irregularity (irregular halo), solid lesion, and hypervascularity.

The possible general categories of FNAB of a thyroid mass are as follows:

- Benign.
- Malignant (PTC, medullary thyroid carcinoma, anaplastic thyroid carcinoma).
- Indeterminant (follicular neoplasm; this can mean FTC and follicular adenoma). and
- Insufficient/nondiagnostic specimen (15 to 25% of all FNABs).

The FNAB result should be reported by using Bethesda System for Reporting Thyroid cytopathology (*see* **Table 3.1**). The diagnostic accuracy of FNAB is estimated at greater than 95%, and its false-negative rates are around –5%. FNAB is more accurate for lesions measuring 1 to 4 cm in diameter. Smaller lesions are difficult to sample accurately, while larger lesions have greater sampling error. As mentioned before, the FNAB is able to provide definitive diagnosis of PTC due to characteristic nuclear changes. It is unfortunately unable to distinguish between FTC and follicular adenoma,

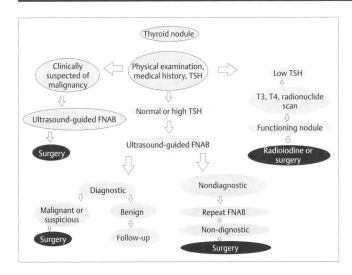

Figure 3.3 Algorithm for the evaluation and diagnosis of a thyroid nodule. FNAB, fine-needle aspiration biopsy; TSH, thyroid-stimulating hormone.

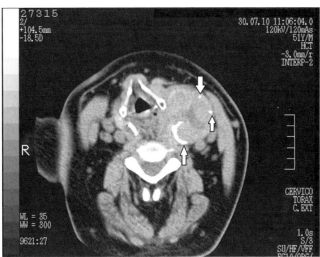

Figure 3.4 Computed tomographic scan of a large left thyroid lobe tumor. Note the calcifications within the left thyroid lobe tumor.

Image courtesy: Dr. Abdenour Ghouila, Hospital Virgen del Camino, Sanlúcar de Barrameda, Spain.

and therefore the diagnosis of FTC requires a histological proof of capsular invasion and/or vascular invasion. If the FNAB result suggests follicular neoplasm, thyroid lobectomy should be performed to permit full histological evaluation of the tumor. In approximately 20% of the lobectomy specimens in patients operated on because of FNAB suggesting follicular neoplasm, the final diagnosis confirms FTC. Undetermined or insufficient FNAB requires repetition of FNAB (*see* algorithm in **Fig. 3.3**).

Computed tomography (**Fig. 3.4**) is used in the evaluation of patients with advanced tumors to define the degree of invasion into adjacent structures such as trachea, esophagus, and great vessels as well as to define the intrathoracic extension of the tumor/gland.

Special attention should be paid to patients with tumors found incidentally (incidentalomas) during positron emission tomography (PET), as these lesions have higher percentage of being malignant (30 to 50%) and tend to present more aggressive histological characteristics.[1]

Staging of Thyroid Cancer

Once DTC is diagnosed, it is obligatory to correctly stage the patient according to the current version of the AJCC/TNM classification. The 2010 version is presented in **Tables 3.3** and **3.4**. It is important to note that DTC is the only cancer in which age at diagnosis is one of the factors defining the stage of the disease.

Other systems used for DTC staging include the following classifications: AGES (age, grade, extent, size), AMES (age, metastasis, extent, size), MACIS (metastasis, age, completeness of resection, invasion, size), and National Thyroid Cancer Treatment Cooperative Study, which includes size, multifocality, invasion, differentiation, cervical metastases, and extracervical metastases.

Pearl

- Age is an important factor in the staging of differentiated thyroid carcinomas.

Surgical Technique

The primary treatment of DTC is surgery. The possible approaches include total thyroidectomy (removal of both the lobes: isthmus lobe and pyramidal lobe) or a near-total thyroidectomy (a complete removal of thyroid lobes, leaving less than 1 g of the glandular tissue). Most surgeons recommend ipsilateral thyroid lobectomy in patients with occult papillary thyroid cancers (< 1 cm; i.e., papillary microcarcinoma) and in patients with minimally invasive follicular thyroid cancers. It is suggested that this should also be a treatment of choice for noncompliant patients and for patients who do not have access to thyroid hormone.

The authors prefer total thyroidectomy in the majority of patients with DTCs. It is also to be underlined that total or near-total thyroidectomy with radioiodine ablation (see below) will increase the sensitivity of serum thyroglobulin evaluation as a marker in the long-term follow-up for recurrent disease. Total thyroidectomy removes all subclinical foci of the carcinoma in the contralateral lobe (present in up to 85% of the cases). Less extensive resections are characterized by recurrent disease occurring in the thyroid remnant in up to 7% of the patients and 50% of the patients dying from the recurrent disease.[7] Finally, several large, retrospective studies have shown improved survival in patient treated with extensive surgery and radioiodine treatment over patients treated with less extensive procedures. However, the total thyroidectomy in

Table 3.3   Definitions of TNM

Primary tumor (T)	
• Tx	Primary tumor cannot be assessed
• T0	No evidence of primary tumor
• T1	Tumor ≤ 2 cm in greatest dimension, limited to the thyroid
• T1a	Tumor ≤ 1 cm, limited to the thyroid
• T1b	Tumor > 1 cm but not > 2 cm in greatest dimension, limited to the thyroid
• T2	Tumor > 2 cm but not > 4 cm in greatest dimension, limited to the thyroid
• T3	Tumor > 4 cm in greatest dimension, limited to the thyroid or any tumor with minimal extrathyroid extension (e.g., extension to sternothyroid muscle or perithyroid soft tissues)
• T4a	Moderately advanced disease; tumor of any size extending beyond the thyroid capsule to invade subcutaneous soft tissues, larynx, trachea, esophagus, or recurrent laryngeal nerve
• T4b	Very advanced disease; tumor invades prevertebral fascia or encases carotid artery or mediastinal vessels
Regional lymph nodes (N)[a]	
• Nx	Regional lymph nodes cannot be assessed
• N0	No regional lymph-node metastasis
• N1	Regional lymph-node metastasis(-es)
• N1a	Metastasis(-es) to level VI (pretracheal, paratracheal, and prelaryngeal/Delphian lymph nodes)
• N1b	Metastasis(-es) to unilateral, bilateral, or contralateral cervical (levels I, II, III, IV, or V) or retropharyngeal or superior mediastinal lymph nodes (level VII)
Distant metastasis(-es) (M)	
• M0	No distant metastasis
• M1	Distant metastasis(-es)

[a]Regional lymph nodes are central compartment, lateral cervical, and upper mediastinal lymph nodes.
TNM, tumor-node-metastasis.

inexperienced hands brings higher risk of complications.[8] This is probably why surgeons from low-volume hospitals are less likely to choose a total thyroidectomy compared with surgeons from high-volume centers.[9] Given the risks of complications of total thyroidectomy and the fact that the large proportion of patients has indeed a low risk of recurrent disease, the key for deciding on the extension of surgery should be identification of patients who would benefit from more radical approach. Currently, it is agreed that there is no survival benefit of total or near-total thyroidectomy in low-risk patients with occult PTC less than 1 cm (micro-PTC) or with microinvasive FTC.

The aims of surgical treatment of DTC are as follows:

• Eradicate primary tumor
• Eradicate nodal disease
• Minimize surgery-related mortality
• Permit accurate staging
• Facilitate radioiodine therapy
• Permit long-term surveillance with radioactive iodine, whole-body scan, and thyroglobulin assay
• Minimize the risk of disease recurrence and dissemination

In general, the indolent nature of DTC would require long-term follow-up to show differences in outcome between different treatment options. Thus, decisions on the type of surgery, the extent of lymph-node dissection, and the method of adjuvant treatment are based on the results of retrospective series.

Central Compartment Nodes

Certain controversies exist regarding the extent and necessity of central compartment lymph-node dissection. However, it is clear that central compartment (neck level VI) neck dissection for patients with clinically involved central or lateral neck lymph nodes should accompany total thyroidectomy. Prophylactic (without clinically involved nodes) central compartment neck dissection may be performed in patients with papillary thyroid cancer, especially for advanced primary tumors (T3, T4).[10]

Meta-analysis on prophylactic central compartment neck dissection showed that in experienced hands it is not associated with higher morbidity than thyroidectomy alone (with the exception of transient hypoparathyroidism).[11]

In the case of small papillary cancers (T1/T2) and most follicular cancers, the near-total or total thyroidectomy without prophylactic central compartment neck dissection can be considered appropriate.

Principles of Surgical Techniques

General principles that apply to all thyroid operations as follows:

• Good exposure of the thyroid gland.
• Meticulous dissection of the ipsilateral thyroid compartment.
• Proper identification of anatomic structures (parathyroid glands, laryngeal nerves).
• Surgery in a dry operative field without bleeding (suction should be avoided).
• Ligation of all thyroid vessels close to the gland.
• Wise use of energy-based tools for hemostasis and tissue dissection (e.g., diathermy, ultracision).

Table 3.4   AJCC/TNM Stage Grouping

Stage	Tumor (T)	Node (N)	Metastasis (M)
Papillary and follicular thyroid cancer (younger than 45 years)			
• I	Any T	Any N	M0
• II	Any T	Any N	M1
Papillary and follicular thyroid cancer (45 years and older)			
• I	T1	N0	M0
• II	T2	N0	M0
• III	T3	N0	M0
	T1	N1a	M0
	T2	N1a	M0
	T3	N1a	M0
• IVA	T4a	N0	M0
	T4a	N1a	M0
	T1	N1b	M0
	T2	N1b	M0
	T3	N1b	M0
	T4a	N1b	M0
• IVB	T4b	Any N	M0
• IVC	Any T	Any N	M1

AJCC/TNM, American Joint Committee on Cancer/Tumor-Node-Metastasis.

The meta-analysis of randomized clinical trials showed that thyroid surgery performed with harmonic scalpel results in shorter operative time and lower rates of transient hypocalcemia.[12] Similar results have been seen with LigaSure.[13]

In patients who undergo thyroid lobectomy (e.g., patient with follicular neoplasm on FNAB) and scheduled for second surgery, it is important to perform the second intervention either within 1 week after primary operation or after 3 months. The second thyroid surgery performed between 1 week and 3 months after primary surgery is linked to an important rise in postoperative complications. This is caused by the inflammation that makes correct identification of important anatomic structures more difficult.

Pearl

- Total thyroidectomy remains the treatment of choice in a vast majority of patients with differentiated thyroid carcinoma.

Minimally Invasive Procedures

In recent years, a variety of minimally invasive techniques have been adopted for the treatment of different diseases in numerous locations. This trend is also present in thyroid surgery. Among the minimally invasive procedures used for the treatment of DTC, minimally invasive video-assisted thyroidectomy (MIVAT; **Fig. 3.5**), transaxillary endoscopic approach, and transoral endoscopic approach are worth mentioning.

The MIVAT is becoming popular in dedicated thyroid centers. This is probably because it has several advantages and only a few disadvantages. The advantages and disadvantages of this technique are presented in **Table 3.5**.[14]

Other minimally invasive approaches to thyroid include sophisticated and technically demanding procedures such as transaxillary approach[15] also using the da Vinci robotic system[16] or transoral approach (the only approach that can be considered the true natural orifice surgery but remains in an experimental phase)[17] are of interest for academic surgeons and may bring benefit to patients and doctors in the future.

Pearl

- Minimally invasive techniques in thyroid cancer surgery are emerging but can be offered only to a selected group of patients with nonadvanced differentiated thyroid carcinoma.

Surgical Complications

Recurrent Laryngeal Nerve Injury

Permanent recurrent laryngeal nerve injury occurs in up to 2 to 3% of thyroid operations. If only one nerve is affected, this results in a breathy voice. If both nerves are injured (0.15% of thyroid surgery), this leads to critical airway obstruction. To avoid tracheostomy, widening of the posterior glottis with laser surgery or Lichtenberg operation can be performed.

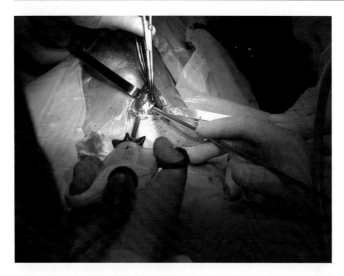

Figure 3.5 Thyroidectomy using the minimally invasive video-assisted thyroidectomy technique.

Image courtesy: Prof. Istvan Gal, Telki International Private Hospital, Telki, Hungary.

Superior Laryngeal Nerve Injury

The superior laryngeal nerve should be identified and preserved when dissecting superior pole vessels. It is important to exercise caution during this maneuver as the position of the nerve in relation to vessels may vary. The exact incidence of permanent injury to superior laryngeal nerve is unknown. This is because the dysfunction caused by this injury is noted only in professional voice users that in the case of nerve injury lose their ability to reach higher pitches. Some studies of advanced diagnostic techniques indicate that the rate of this injury can be as high as 5 to 28%.

Parathyroid Glands Injury

The damage of parathyroid glands by complete excision or by compromising their blood supply results in hypocalcemia. The risk of temporary hypocalcemia is 5% and that of permanent is 0.5%. If the injury to a parathyroid is suspected during surgery, this should mandate reimplantation of a minced gland into sternocleidomastoid or brachioradialis muscle. In the case of injury of suspected parathyroid tissue, a portion of the tissue should be sent for frozen section while the remaining portion is kept in a cold, sterile saline solution. If the presence of the parathyroid tissue is confirmed, the rest of the gland is minced and implanted as described above. This technique is of vital importance because the distinction of the parathyroid gland from a lymph node can sometimes be quite difficult.

The most common cause of postoperative hypocalcemia is injury to the vascular pedicle of the parathyroid glands. It is therefore important to bear in mind that around 80% of the superior parathyroid glands are situated within 1 cm of the intersection of the recurrent laryngeal nerve and the inferior thyroid artery. It is of importance that the dissection of inferior thyroid artery is performed in a careful manner to preserve lateral vascular pedicle and parathyroid vascular supply. It is sometimes necessary to spare a small portion of the thyroid tissue to avoid destroying the parathyroid pedicle.

Hematoma

The massive hematoma filling the closed space within the operation field can be diagnosed by sudden breathing difficulties and asphyxia in a recently operated patient. If this, occurs the surgeon has to remove the stitches immediately to decompress the hematoma (sometimes even bedside) and proceed with the revision of hemostasis. In a meta-analysis of randomized clinical trials comparing drains with no drains after thyroid surgery, it has been shown that drains do not influence the frequency of hematoma formation and may be associated with longer hospital stay. However, these results were based on studies performed on patients with goiters without lymph-node dissection.[18] This, together with a fear of large, asphyxiating hematoma makes a large number of surgeons reluctant to leave any drains after thyroid procedures.

Table 3.5 Advantages and Disadvantages of MIVAT

Advantages	Disadvantages
Magnification due to employment of the endoscope: this allows an optimal visualization of superior and recurrent laryngeal nerves as well as parathyroid glands	Long learning curve (at least 30 procedures)
The possibility to explore both sides with a small (1.5–3 cm) incision in the anterior neck	The procedure has to be performed by three surgeons working simultaneously
No neck hyperextension	
The surgical steps are the same as for an open procedure	
Operation can be easily converted to a conventional open procedure	

MIVAT, minimally invasive video-assisted thyroidectomy.

Other Surgical Complications

Injuries to other structures such as the vagus nerve, spinal accessory nerve, trachea, esophagus, carotid artery, and thoracic duct occur occasionally. The risk of these injuries is higher with more advanced tumors.

Adjuvant Treatment

After the surgical treatment of DTC, radioiodine treatment is generally used. The goal of radioiodine treatment is to ablate any residual thyroid tissue. This allows serum thyroglobulin measurements or radioactive iodine scanning to be used in the follow-up. The second goal of this treatment is to destroy any residual carcinoma cells that may be harbored in a thyroid remnant. As stated before, the size of the thyroid remnant should be as small as possible. A meta-analysis showed that the size of the thyroid remnant is determinantal in predicting total thyroid ablation with radioiodine.[19]

The mechanism of the action of radioiodine is based on the fact that thyrocytes as well as well-differentiated carcinoma cells trap and organify iodine. The ability to trap iodine is much higher in normal thyrocytes and therefore it is so important to minimize the size of the thyroid remnant. Excising all thyroid tissue by means of total thyroidectomy and destroying the remaining thyrocytes with radioiodine treatment can improve the diagnostic and therapeutic utility of radioiodine because it will only be taken-up by metastatic or recurrent foci. Furthermore, the elimination of all thyrocytes allows the use of serum thyroglobulin level as a marker of a recurrent disease. Because thyroglobulin is produced by normal thyroid tissue in a sane individual, any rise in thyroglobulin in a patient without any remaining thyroid cells becomes highly sensitive and specific of DTC recurrence in the form of local failure or metastatic disease.[20]

The initial radioiodine scan is performed 4 to 12 weeks after surgery. Most commonly used protocol consists of 2 mCi of the initial scanning dose followed by the ablative dose of 30 to 100 mCi. The dose can be higher for patients at high risk for disease recurrence and can reach 300 mCi. Uptake seen after total thyroidectomy should be less than 1%. After radioiodine treatment, the whole-body radioiodine scan should be negative; that is, no foci of thyroid cells uptaking radioiodine should be present. This allows the radioiodine scan to become a surveillance method for the early detection of recurrent disease.

Whether all patients operated for DTC are supposed to receive adjuvant treatment with radioiodine is still a matter of debate. It is generally agreed that patients with small (< 1 cm) papillary carcinomas do not need to receive radioiodine therapy. Patients with tumors larger than 4 cm (T3/T4) and/or with lymph-node metastasis (N1) are, on the other hand, clear candidates for adjuvant therapy. In the intermediate group (tumors between 1 and 4 cm, without lymph-node involvement), the decision if the radioiodine therapy should be applied is left at the discretion of the clinician in charge. Radioiodine treatment is also used in the treatment of patients with disseminated disease and locally inoperable tumors.[21]

> **Pearl**
>
> - After surgery for differentiated thyroid carcinoma, adjuvant treatment with radioiodine is recommended for more advanced cases.

Thyroid Hormone Suppression

TSH stimulates the growth and activity of both normal and malignant thyrocytes. This forms the theoretical basis for TSH suppression therapy in patients with DTC after the initial surgical treatment. The effect of TSH suppression therapy on the likelihood of disease progression, recurrence, and death has been evaluated in a large meta-analysis (> 4000 patients with DTC). The results showed that the patients receiving TSH suppression had a decreased risk of the above-mentioned events.[22]

TSH suppression treatment also has negative consequences. The treatment consists of causing subclinical thyrotoxicosis and therefore may cause bone mineral loss, osteoporosis, and cardiovascular abnormalities. The degree of TSH suppression is linked to the risk of recurrence. It is advisable to maintain the TSH level just below 0.1 mU/L in patients with high risk of recurrence and between 0.1 and 0.5 mU/L in patients with low risk of recurrence.

External Beam Radiation

There are limited indications for the application of external beam radiotherapy in the treatment of patients with DTC. However, it should be considered in the case of radioiodine-resistant DTCs and present with residual disease or nonresectable tumors. It is also used in palliative setting. There is no uniform dose and fractionation scheme.

Surveillance

After the termination of DTC treatment, each patient should begin a strict follow-up scheme. It should be clearly stated that the follow-up of patients with DTC has to be lifelong because recurrent disease can appear as late as 50 years after the initial treatment (although most recurrences occur within first 5 years). It is advisable that the follow-up visits take place in a center specialized in the treatment and follow-up of patients with thyroid cancer. There are differences between several institutions as regards the detailed program of follow-up; however, we practice the following:

- During the first 2 years after treatment, clinical evaluation is repeated every 3 to 6 months.
- Afterward, annual visits are planned if patients remain symptom-free.

The follow-up of low-risk patients should be based mainly on TSH-stimulated serum thyroglobulin level measurements and neck ultrasound. An annual chest X-ray should also be performed. As mentioned before, in patients who undergo total or near-total thyroidectomy and subsequent radioiodine treatment, the evaluation of the serum thyroglobulin level is highly specific for disease recurrence and thus the single most important tool in the surveillance. The test becomes even more sensitive when performed after TSH stimulation. TSH-stimulated serum thyroglobulin levels are obtained by withdrawing hormone supplementation or by administering recombinant human TSH. The National Comprehensive Cancer Network suggests using levels of greater than 10 ng/mL in TSH-stimulated serum and greater than 5 ng/mL in non–TSH-stimulated serum as thresholds for the suspicion of recurrent disease.

The main problem in measuring serum thyroglobulin levels in the follow-up of patients with DTC lies in the fact that approximately 25% of the patients with DTC will have thyroglobulin antibodies. This means that to determine whether the thyroglobulin levels can be reliably interpreted, one should perform evaluation of serum thyroglobulin antibodies.

Dilemmas

Which Thyroid Nodules to Operate?

This question is addressed extensively in **Fig. 3.1**. It should also be remembered that tumors found on PET scan have higher propensity to malignancy and as such have got to be operated.

Total Thyroidectomy or Hemithyroidectomy?

The authors advocate total thyroidectomy in all patients with papillary carcinoma larger than 1 cm and all patients with follicular carcinoma (**Table 3.6**). The central compartment node clearance needs to be done if clinically suspected. The prophylactic central compartment

Table 3.6 Clinical Situations when Total Thyroidectomy Is Indicated

Primary thyroid carcinoma is > 4 cm in size
Contralateral thyroid nodules are present
Regional or distant metastases are present
The patient has a personal history of radiation therapy to the head and neck
The patient has a first-degree family history of DTC
Age < 15 years or > 45 years
There is evidence of extrathyroid extension
Pathology reports an aggressive variant of DTC

DTC, differentiated thyroid carcinoma.

dissection is safe only if the surgeon is confident with the technique.

Method of Recurrent Laryngeal Nerve Localization

The following methods of recurrent laryngeal nerve preservation can be considered:

- Visual nerve identification (**Fig. 3.6**).
- Use of magnifying glasses to facilitate nerve visualization.
- Nerve palpation (against the tracheal wall).
- Visual nerve identification with the aid of an intraoperative nerve monitoring system.

In a large randomized clinical trial involving 1000 recurrent laryngeal nerves at risk, it has been shown that visual identification of the nerve results in a similar risk of permanent injury as intraoperative neuromonitoring. Thus, it can be stated that visual identification of a nerve by an experienced surgeon is a reliable method of avoiding permanent nerve injury.[23]

> **Pearl**
>
> - Laryngeal nerve localization is strongly advised.

Conclusions

DTCs are malignant tumors with a relatively good prognosis. Treatment of this disease is surgical, with total thyroidectomy with or without central compartment neck dissection being suitable for the majority of patients. Adjuvant treatment with radioiodine is suitable for patients with larger tumors and with lymph-node involvement.

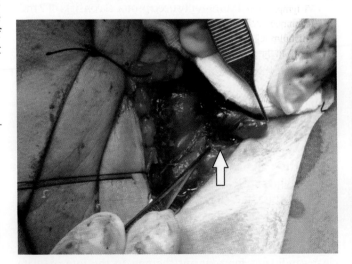

Figure 3.6 Visualization of the left laryngeal recurrent nerve.

Image property: Servicio de Cirugia General, Hospital Virgen del Camino, Sanlúcar de Barrameda, Spain. Printed with permission.

Clinical Pearls

- Not all thyroid nodules should be treated.
- Differentiated thyroid carcinoma has good prognosis.
- Surgery is the cornerstone of treatment.
- Adjuvant treatment with radioiodine is recommended only for more advanced tumors.

References

1. Iyer NG, Shaha AR. Management of thyroid nodules and surgery for differentiated thyroid cancer. Clin Oncol (R Coll Radiol) 2010;22(6):405–412
2. Amdur RJ, Mazzaferi EL. Incidence and prognosis of differentiated thyroid cancer. In: Amdur RJ, Mazzaferi EL, eds. Essentials of Thyroid Cancer Management. New York: Springer; 2005: 121–140
3. Caron NR, Clark OH. Well differentiated thyroid cancer. Scand J Surg 2004;93(4):261–271
4. Busnardo B, De Vido D. The epidemiology and etiology of differentiated thyroid carcinoma. Biomed Pharmacother 2000;54(6):322–326
5. Segev DL, Umbricht C, Zeiger MA. Molecular pathogenesis of thyroid cancer. Surg Oncol 2003;12(2):69–90
6. D'Avanzo A, Treseler P, Ituarte PH, et al. Follicular thyroid carcinoma: histology and prognosis. Cancer 2004;100(6):1123–1129
7. Kebebew E, Clark OH. Differentiated thyroid cancer: "complete" rational approach. World J Surg 2000;24(8):942–951
8. Sosa JA, Bowman HM, Tielsch JM, Powe NR, Gordon TA, Udelsman R. The importance of surgeon experience for clinical and economic outcomes from thyroidectomy. Ann Surg 1998;228(3): 320–330
9. Bilimoria KY, Bentrem DJ, Linn JG, et al. Utilization of total thyroidectomy for papillary thyroid cancer in the United States. Surgery 2007;142(6):906–913, discussion 913, e1–e2
10. Grodski S, Cornford L, Sywak M, Sidhu S, Delbridge L. Routine level VI lymph node dissection for papillary thyroid cancer: surgical technique. ANZ J Surg 2007;77(4):203–208
11. Chisholm EJ, Kulinskaya E, Tolley NS. Systematic review and meta-analysis of the adverse effects of thyroidectomy combined with central neck dissection as compared with thyroidectomy alone. Laryngoscope 2009;119(6):1135–1139
12. Melck AL, Wiseman SM. Harmonic scalpel compared to conventional hemostasis in thyroid surgery: a meta-analysis of randomized clinical trials. Int J Surg Oncol 2010; Article ID 396079: doi:10.1155/2010/396079
13. Cakabay B, Sevinç MM, Gömceli I, Yenidogan E, Ulkü A, Koç S. LigaSure versus clamp-and-tie in thyroidectomy: a single-center experience. Adv Ther 2009;26(11):1035–1041
14. Miccoli P, Materazzi G, Berti P. Minimally invasive thyroidectomy in the treatment of well differentiated thyroid cancers: indications and limits. Curr Opin Otolaryngol Head Neck Surg 2010;18(2): 114–118
15. Jeong JJ, Kang SW, Yun JS, et al. Comparative study of endoscopic thyroidectomy versus conventional open thyroidectomy in papillary thyroid microcarcinoma (PTMC) patients. J Surg Oncol 2009;100(6):477–480
16. Kang SW, Lee SC, Lee SH, et al. Robotic thyroid surgery using a gasless, transaxillary approach and the da Vinci S system: the operative outcomes of 338 consecutive patients. Surgery 2009;146(6):1048–1055
17. Benhidjeb T, Wilhelm T, Harlaar J, Kleinrensink GJ, Schneider TA, Stark M. Natural orifice surgery on thyroid gland: totally transoral video-assisted thyroidectomy (TOVAT): report of first experimental results of a new surgical method. Surg Endosc 2009;23(5):1119–1120
18. Samraj K, Gurusamy KS. Wound drains following thyroid surgery. Cochrane Database Syst Rev 2007;(4):CD006099
19. Doi SA, Woodhouse NJ. Ablation of the thyroid remnant and ^{131}I dose in differentiated thyroid cancer. Clin Endocrinol (Oxf) 2000;52(6):765–773
20. Karam M, Gianoukakis A, Feustel PJ, Cheema A, Postal ES, Cooper JA. Influence of diagnostic and therapeutic doses on thyroid remnant ablation rates. Nucl Med Commun 2003;24(5):489–495
21. Pacini F, Schlumberger M, Harmer C, et al. Post-surgical use of radioiodine (^{131}I) in patients with papillary and follicular thyroid cancer and the issue of remnant ablation: a consensus report. Eur J Endocrinol 2005;153(5):651–659
22. McGriff NJ, Csako G, Gourgiotis L, Lori C G, Pucino F, Sarlis NJ. Effects of thyroid hormone suppression therapy on adverse clinical outcomes in thyroid cancer. Ann Med 2002;34(7-8):554–564
23. Barczyński M, Konturek A, Cichoń S. Randomized clinical trial of visualization versus neuromonitoring of recurrent laryngeal nerves during thyroidectomy. Br J Surg 2009;96(3):240–246

4 Management of High-Risk Thyroid Cancer

Ryan J. Li, Nishant Agrawal, R. Michael Tuttle, and Ralph P. Tufano

Core Messages

- Patients with differentiated thyroid carcinomas comprise a heterogeneous group in terms of both patient demographics and natural history of the disease.

- An educated assessment of recurrence and mortality risk directs patient care to the safest, most specific, and most effective treatments and follow-up schedule.

- Risk stratification is an ongoing process that begins at the time of initial diagnosis and continues throughout long-term follow-up.

The management of differentiated thyroid carcinoma (DTC) is complicated by the broad spectrum of disease presentations. The physicians involved in the care of these patients must jointly develop a logical treatment plan based on an individual patient's presentation and define therapeutic goals clearly. As with other types of cancers, patient morbidity is related not only to the disease process but also to the treatment modalities used, each with known complication rates, toxicities, and likelihood of success. Complications related to treatment are profoundly important in DTC, given the frequently asymptomatic nature of this disease, as well as the excellent prognosis in the majority of cases. For example, the cohort of patients younger than 20 years has an overall disease-specific mortality rate of 1%, rising to only 5% in young and middle-aged adults.[1] Notably, disease-specific mortality rises to 20 to 30% in older adults, a fact that already shows the importance of risk stratification in determining appropriate treatment and follow-up for patients with DTC.[1] Physicians involved in the care of patients with thyroid cancer have worked extensively to develop treatment plans for patients with DTC based on important risk factors related to both individual patient characteristics and predicted behavior of individual tumors.[2] Although all patients with DTC may have been previously recommended for total thyroidectomy, radioiodine ablation, and a standard follow-up schedule, there has been an outpour of clinical studies demonstrating the importance of treatment planning that adjusts for patients' risk profiles.[2,3]

Ultimately, any risk stratification model should be able to predict the probability of different patients with DTC to achieve specific end points. There are logical questions to ask: (1) What is the risk that clinically evident persistence or recurrence will occur? (2) What is the risk of dying from this disease?[2] Tuttle et al suggest that the initial surgery and the consequent risk of initial therapy failure are most consequential in answering these two questions. The American Thyroid Association (ATA) emphasizes that the assessment of risk in individual patients must be an ongoing process as more information is gleaned from outcomes of treatment and diagnostic tests during follow-up.[3]

Assigning Risk for Recurrent and Persistent Disease Following Initial Treatment

The 2009 revised ATA guidelines for the management of DTC recommend a three-level stratification for the risk of recurrent disease.[3] This is based on the results of previous large studies examining the correlation between tumor characteristics and treatment outcomes. It seems reasonable that this stratification can identify patients at low or high risk of persistent disease as well. Patients at low risk of disease recurrence include those with (1) no locoregional or distant metastatic disease, (2) complete resection of all macroscopic tumors at the time of surgery, (3) no locoregional direct tumor invasion (i.e., no extrathyroidal extension), (4) no aggressive tumor histology, and (5) tumor less than 1 cm in size. Tumor histologies in DTC that are considered more aggressive include tall cell, insular, and columnar cell variants. If [131]I (radioactive iodine, RAI) is given, the first posttreatment RAI whole-body scan (RxWBS) should show no uptake outside the thyroid surgical bed to validate that this patient population is at low risk for recurrence.[4–6] As mentioned, low-risk patients should have a primary tumor less than 1 cm in size. These so-called microcarcinomas carry a very low recurrence risk, approximating 3.8% in one large study. This study included 445 patients with microcarcinomas treated with thyroid lobectomy (9.2%) or total thyroidectomy (90.8%), neck dissection (49.7%), and radioiodine ablation (87.4%).[7] Patients who fit this descriptive cohort may be of any age. Recurrence is unlikely in these patients because the risk of failing initial therapy is low.[2] Studies have also demonstrated the low risk of recurrence predicted by findings on posttreatment studies. At 6- and 12-month follow-up, a normal neck ultrasound and undetectable serum thyroglobulin (Tg) level after recombinant human thyroid-stimulating hormone (TSH) stimulation predict a less than 0.5% probability of future disease.[8,9] These diagnostic modalities are examined further below in several sections..

Patients with DTC at an intermediate risk of disease recurrence include those with microscopic direct extrathyroidal extension of the primary tumor (found at initial surgery), metastases to cervical lymph nodes, ^{131}I uptake apart from the thyroid bed on RxWBS, vascular invasion of tumor, and/or aggressive tumor histology. Primary tumor size ranges from 1 to 4 cm. There is an intermediate risk of failing initial therapy in this group.[2,3,10,11] The age range may again be broad for the intermediate risk group, although the American Joint Commission on Cancer (AJCC) differentiates patients younger than 45 years from patients older than 45 years, the latter being at higher risk of recurrent disease and decreased survival.[12]

Patients with DTC at high risk of disease recurrence include those having macroscopic extrathyroidal tumor extension, incomplete resection of primary tumor, and/ or distant metastases.[3] It is also proposed that there is a higher risk of recurrence if serum Tg levels are elevated out of proportion to findings on an RxWBS after RAI.[13] Other factors implicated in high risk of disease recurrence are primary tumor size greater than 4 cm and age at diagnosis of greater than 45 years. Consistent with the above trend, the risk of failing initial therapy is high in this cohort and thus the high risk of disease recurrence[2] or persistence.

Risk Stratification for Survival in Patients with Differentiated Thyroid Carcinoma

The AJCC and the International Union Against Cancer (UICC) developed a tumor staging system in an effort to predict patient survival in DTC.[14] As in many other types of cancers,

DTC can be staged by using tumor characteristics, nodal status, and the presence or absence of distant metastasis (tumor-node-metastasis), with some of this information attained during initial surgery. In addition, age at diagnosis has proven significant in predicting disease-specific survival, as it also does in predicting recurrence. A multitude of other staging systems have modified the AJCC/UICC guidelines to account for additional risk factors for increased mortality. Ultimately, the risk of disease-specific mortality is well assessed by these stratification models. A total of 70 to 85% of patients with DTC have a low risk for disease-specific mortality; these are patients with T1–T3 and M0 tumors in the AJCC/UICC staging system. Few patients are found to have T4 and/or M1 disease and are associated with higher mortality.[15]

Tuttle et al have classified risk of death into very low, low-, intermediate-, and high-risk categories. Again, the emphasis rests on the failure of initial therapy as a correlate to disease-specific mortality (**Table 4.1**).[2] As with the AJCC/UICC staging system—age at diagnosis, primary tumor size, lymph node metastasis, and distant metastasis factor into the risk of death. In addition, completeness of tumor resection at initial surgery and histopathological findings (e.g., aggressive histology and vascular invasion) of the surgical specimen are considered predictors of mortality.

Using Risk Stratification to Individualize Treatment Regimens

With an understanding of the individual patient and tumor characteristics that contribute to the success of treatment—and therefore a reduction in the likelihood of death or disease recurrence—decisions regarding specific modalities of therapy can be made. Surgical resection of disease, RAI therapy, and TSH suppression continue to be the mainstays of therapy for DTC, with external beam radiation therapy (EBRT) and systemic chemotherapy having limited efficacy.[3] Except for the low-risk categories (i.e., subcentimeter primary tumors), total thyroidectomy remains the initially

Table 4.1   Risk-Adjusted Approach to Longitudinal Follow-Up

Risk of Recurrence	Suppressed Tg (mo)	Stimulated Tg (mo)	Neck US (mo)	Other Imaging
Low	6, 12, 24	Not required	12–24	Not required
Intermediate	Every 6	12–18	6–12	Consider DxWBS if suppressed Tg > 1 ng/mL and/or stimulated Tg > 10 ng/mL
High	Every 6	12–18	6–12	Consider DxWBS if suppressed Tg > 1 ng/mL and/or stimulated Tg > 10 ng/mL; consider FDG-PET if DxWBS negative with elevated Tg

Tg, thyroglobulin; mo, month; US, ultrasound; DxWBS, diagnostic whole-body scan; FDG-PET, fluorodeoxy-D-glucose-positron emission tomography.

recommended treatment. **Table 4.2** summarizes a risk-adjusted approach to treatment.

Postoperatively, RAI may be given for reasons other than for ablation of any remaining (remnant) disease. After total or near-total thyroidectomy, RAI serves the additional purpose of ablating any remaining normal thyroid tissue with iodine-uptake capabilities. In all risk categories, this may improve the accuracy of initial staging, tumor surveillance with future diagnostic whole-body scans (DxWBSs) that utilize RAI, and serum Tg measurements that depend on the presence of normal or cancerous thyroid tissue for production.[3] Many large studies demonstrate a significant reduction in recurrence rate and disease-specific mortality with postoperative RAI treatment, particularly in the intermediate- and high-risk categories.[16-18] The ATA recommends using the minimum RAI activity (i.e., dose) that achieves complete remnant ablation, as defined by post-RAI undetectable stimulated serum Tg levels (see further for details), and/or lack of RAI uptake on a subsequent DxWBS. This is often in the range of 30 to 100 mCi. However, as the risk of recurrence and/or disease-specific mortality increases, higher RAI activity is considered, for example, in the range of 100 to 200 mCi. For example, patients with aggressive histologies (vascular invasion, tall cell, insular, or columnar cell variants) may receive higher RAI doses.[19-27]

The third modality, used after surgery for the treatment of DTC, is TSH suppression. In normal thyroid physiology, TSH promotes cell growth and synthesis of thyroid-specific functional proteins such as the sodium–iodide symporter.[3,28] Suppression of TSH and its physiologic or pathophysiologic effects are crucial for the postoperative management of DTC. Meta-analyses of outcomes in TSH-suppressed patients with DTC showed a significant reduction in adverse clinical outcomes.[3,29] The aggressiveness with which TSH levels should be suppressed also varies with risk strata as do surgery and RAI. For all but the low-risk categories of disease-specific mortality and recurrence, serum TSH levels should remain below 0.4 mU/L, a level just below the lowest normal value (0.5 mU/L). In intermediate- and high-risk patients, the preferred goal is less than 0.1 mU/L. Taking this a step further, in a large prospective study using the National Thyroid Cancer Treatment Cooperative Study staging system, higher risk patients (stages III and IV) with TSH suppression to undetectable levels demonstrated improved overall survival compared with low levels of suppression.[30]

EBRT is rarely used in patients with DTC. It is variably given for locally advanced tumors with residual disease, significant local invasion, and aggressive variants.[31-33] Similarly, EBRT is considered in older patients (> 60 years of age) with extrathyroidal extension in which all gross disease has been resected or in patients with aggressive histologic variants.[34,35] It does not replace the role of either primary surgery or RAI treatment. However, there are rare instances in which postoperative residual disease is not amenable to further surgery, and RAI has also failed, at which time EBRT may be beneficial.

Chemotherapy is used even less frequently than EBRT in DTC, and there is a paucity of data supporting its use. The anthracycline derivative doxorubicin has been used previously for radiosensitization, in preparation for EBRT, as it is used in cancers of other organs.[13]

Surgery in Higher Risk Differentiated Thyroid Carcinoma

Management of the Primary Tumor

Surgical management of thyroid lesions provides the opportunity for definitive diagnosis, cancer staging, and often curative treatment. Alternatively, it may be the first stage of a multimodality treatment regimen. It may prepare a patient for RAI therapy and eliminate any remaining gross thyroid tissue to facilitate serum Tg monitoring.[3] Near-total thyroidectomy is defined as a resection of thyroid tissue leaving less than 1 g of thyroid remnant in situ, usually in the region of the recurrent laryngeal nerve (RLN) at Berry ligament. Subtotal thyroidectomy is rarely recommended and leaves more than 1-g cuff of thyroid tissue in situ. Near-total or total thyroidectomy is recommended for patients of all risk profiles with DTC. However, the few patients who present with a tumor less than 1 cm in size which is unifocal, have no extrathyroidal extension, and no lymph node metastases may have adequate surgical management with a hemithyroidectomy. Patient age and history are important as well: a history of neck irradiation or age above 45 years would exclude a patient from less than near-total thyroidectomy.[3] In all patients, preoperative awake fiberoptic laryngoscopy should be performed to assess vocal cord function, which is a surrogate measure of RLN function. Tumor involvement of one RLN makes meticulous preservation of the contralateral RLN critical to preserve glottic function and avoid potentially permanent tracheostomy.

Patients with aggressive local disease invading the upper aerodigestive tract should be recommended for surgical

Table 4.2 Risk-Adjusted Approach to Treatment

Risk of Recurrence	Initial Surgical Procedure	RAI Remnant Ablation	TSH Suppression (mU/L)
Low	Lobectomy or total thyroidectomy	Not required	< 0.4
Intermediate	Total thyroidectomy	For selected patients	< 0.1
High	Total thyroidectomy	Yes	< 0.1

RAI, radioactive iodine; TSH, thyroid-stimulating hormone.

resection of all gross disease, if possible. Extrathyroidal extension to the strap muscles will require sacrifice of these structures with relative impunity. In contrast, intraoperative discovery of extrathyroidal disease invading the RLN, trachea, larynx, or esophagus may significantly increase the extent of resection. These findings may require strategies such as tracheal resection with primary reanastomosis, total laryngectomy, or laryngopharyngoesophagectomy. Alternatively, for more superficial invasion, an experienced surgeon may elect to shave the tumor off trachea or esophagus.[36–39]

Management of Cervical Lymph Nodes

Fine-needle aspiration (FNA) biopsy is routinely performed for suspicious thyroid nodules. When a diagnosis of DTC is made, a neck ultrasound should be performed to evaluate cervical lymph node status, again with FNA of any suspicious lesions. Neck ultrasound has proven to be an invaluable diagnostic instrument in the management of DTC and is often the imaging study of choice when a palpable thyroid lesion is discovered on physical examination. As many as 20 to 50% of the patients with DTC present with cervical lymph node involvement.[40–42] In expert hands, ultrasound has a high sensitivity for detecting locoregional nodal disease, which may lead to changes in the treatment regimen, although some metastatic lymph nodes posterior to the thyroid gland may not be discovered until the time of surgery.[43–46] Ultrasound has also improved the accuracy of FNA biopsy. Locoregional metastases may be detected by ultrasound even in cases in which the primary tumor is small and intrathyroidal,[3,47] leading to the classification of a patient in either the intermediate-risk or the high-risk category for disease-specific mortality and/or recurrence. When cervical metastatic disease is known preoperatively, the surgical plan extends beyond thyroidectomy to central and/or lateral compartment lymph node dissections.[3]

Findings suspicious for nodal metastasis on diagnostic neck ultrasound include node short axis 5 mm or greater, hypoechogenicity, cystic change, calcifications, peripheral vascularity, loss of nodal fatty hilus, and rounded, rather than oval shape. In one study of 19 patients with DTC, many of these findings were highly specific, but only peripheral vascularity demonstrated reasonable sensitivity (86%).[46]

As discussed in "Assigning Risk for Recurrent and Persistent Disease Following Initial Treatment," the presence of cervical lymph node metastases (regional metastases) places a patient in the intermediate to high risk of initial treatment failure and disease recurrence,[2,47] although not necessarily at higher risk of dying from the disease. Some studies have shown a small, but statistically significant increase in mortality in patients with papillary thyroid cancer with lymph node metastases,[48] whereas another study supported this finding only in patients older than 45 years. Lymph node metastases may portend a poorer prognosis in follicular cancer as well.[49] Thus, intermediate- to high-risk patients with evidence of metastatic central or lateral neck nodes are recommended to undergo dissection at the time of initial thyroid surgery. Some patients with larger and demonstrably more invasive primary tumors on preoperative imaging may also undergo central or lateral neck dissection "prophylactically."[3,50-54]

If locoregional (cervical) metastases are detected on follow-up (i.e., recurrent disease), the ATA recommendation is for comprehensive central and/or lateral neck dissection, depending on disease location. This does not differ from the recommendation for the management of locoregional disease identified at the time of initial diagnosis. A caveat to this treatment is for patients presenting with both locoregional and distant recurrence—does neck dissection improve outcome in these patients? More studies are required to answer this question, and currently neck dissection in patients with distant recurrences seems reasonable at least to help prevent or palliate airway compromise from locoregional invasion.[3]

Although patient selection is not always clear-cut when recommending cervical lymph node dissection (patient with distant metastatic disease), evidence supports comprehensive compartmental dissections rather than "berry picking" procedures when the decision is made to resect locoregional disease.[55]

Surgical Management of Locoregional Persistent or Recurrent Disease

Patients with persistent or recurrent thyroid cancer may pose a surgical challenge. Soft tissue scarring and fibrosis may obscure the surgical planes of the neck, placing vital structures at the risk of injury, including the RLNs, parathyroid glands, the aerodigestive tract, and great vessels. The methodical approach taken with initial thyroid and lateral neck surgery becomes more challenging with alteration of anatomic landmarks. Locoregional recurrent disease may manifest in the thyroid bed, paratracheal lymph nodes, and/or lateral neck nodes, with invasion of adjacent structures such as the esophagus or trachea. Although complication rates in primary thyroid surgery range from 1 to 2%,[56-58] these rates can be significantly higher in revision surgery. The surgeon needs to carefully consider the risks and benefits of revision thyroid surgery in light of the potentially devastating complications as well as questionable impact on the prognosis for individual patients.[59]

Shaha emphasized the need for an optimally planned primary thyroid surgery to minimize the potential need for revision surgery.[59] In planning initial surgery for known thyroid cancer, the surgeon should make an informed decision regarding the extent of the thyroid resection, considering extrathyroidal extension of tumor, RLN involvement, central and lateral neck node involvement, and, importantly whether radioiodine therapy will be implemented postoperatively. Leaving a large thyroid remnant or performing hemithyroidectomy may render RAI ineffective for treating metastatic disease.[60-62]

When a patient presents with persistent or recurrent locoregional disease, the same considerations need to be acknowledged as in primary surgery. Neck ultrasound and computed tomography (CT) imaging are used to clinically stage the neck, and FNA biopsy should confirm that lesions found on examination or radiographic imaging are indeed cancer persistent/recurrent. Lymph node recurrences less than 1 cm in size are frequently observed with serial ultrasound every 6 months, and those without progression in size may not require surgical resection.[59] When CT imaging is used, a possible use of postoperative RAI therapy should be considered, in which case iodinated contrast should be avoided. Positron emission tomography (PET) imaging is selectively used in patients with poorly differentiated thyroid carcinoma, who are unlikely to have a satisfactory treatment response to postoperative RAI. With knowledge of avid PET uptake, even greater emphasis should be placed on complete tumor resection and/or consideration of postoperative EBRT rather than RAI.

When available, operative and pathology reports from the initial surgery should be reviewed in detail. The operative report may document difficult tumor resection due to the involvement of vital structures such as the trachea, esophagus, or RLN. It may also report nerve sacrifice or parathyroid gland devitalization and the need for reimplantation. The pathology report will describe the level of differentiation and aggressiveness of the histology, which is helpful for prognostic purposes. Preoperative fiberoptic laryngoscopy is essential to evaluate true vocal cord motion. If the mobility of one vocal cord is impaired, surgical manipulation in the vicinity of the contralateral RLN risks bilateral vocal cord paresis and even the potential need for permanent tracheostomy. If laryngeal, tracheal, or esophageal involvement is of concern, intraoperative endoscopy of the aerodigestive tract will provide further information on frank invasion or compression of these structures and help determine the extent of surgical resection.[59]

Intraoperatively, identification of the parathyroid glands may be difficult, but is certainly worth the meticulous dissection to prevent significant postoperative hypocalcemia.[63] As they are most commonly perfused by the inferior thyroid artery, reoperative thyroid bed and central compartment dissection requires careful preservation of this vessel and its branches to prevent devascularization. Occasionally, the superior thyroid artery also supplies the parathyroid glands, and thus judicious dissection throughout the thyroid bed, minimizing the ligation of blood vessels, is ideal.[59]

Role of Postoperative Radioactive Iodine in Patients with High-Risk Differentiated Thyroid Carcinoma

As stated in "Using Risk Stratification to Individualize Treatment Regimens," postoperative RAI has several crucial therapeutic purposes. In many patients with DTC, it can be used to ablate residual normal thyroid tissue, improving the interpretability of serum Tg measurements during follow-up. RAI can also serve as an adjuvant therapy to treat suspected microscopic residual cancer. If persistent disease is known to be present, postoperative RAI may be given for definitive ablation.

As discussed earlier in this chapter, postoperative RAI ablation may facilitate initial staging and follow-up of patients with DTC in any risk category. This is because RAI has the ability to ablate remnant normal thyroid tissue that will interfere with both Tg measures and RxWBSs. Multiple studies have shown that RAI improves overall survival when given to intermediate- and high-risk cohorts.[64] It is also postulated that patients with aggressive histologies, regardless of other risk factors, may also have improved outcomes with postoperative RAI[65] and may benefit from higher doses than do low-risk patients.

Preparing for RAI ablation therapy requires meticulous planning. Most patients will be status post near-total or total thyroidectomy. They likely will be taking thyroid hormone replacement with levothyroxine (LT_4) or triiodothyronine (LT_3), which are used both as hormone supplements and in TSH suppression for oncologic purposes. In most DTCs, RAI uptake by normal and cancer cells is improved by increasing TSH levels before the administration of RAI. This is because both normal and cancer cells express the TSH receptor on their plasma membranes.

Stimulation of the TSH receptor leads to the upregulation of the sodium iodide symporter and greater RAI uptake. ATA recommendations are for withdrawal of LT_4 therapy for 2 to 4 weeks, or LT_3 for 2 weeks, with a goal TSH of greater than 30 mU/L right before RAI is given.[66] LT_4 therapy may be restarted 2 to 3 days after RAI is given.[3] A low-iodine diet (< 50 μg/d of iodine) and avoidance of iodine exposure (e.g., amiodarone [Cordarone] and CT with intravenous contrast) are also encouraged.[67–69] Withdrawal of thyroid hormone may or may not lead to symptomatic hypothyroidism. Furthermore, some patients are unable to increase TSH production appropriately when thyroid hormone is withdrawn. An alternative to thyroid hormone withdrawal is the administration of recombinant human TSH (thyrotropin [Thyrogen]), with both strategies showing equal efficacy in facilitating RAI uptake. Recurrence rates were comparable at least in one short-term follow-up study.[2] Several methods for dosing RAI are currently utilized, including empiric fixed amounts[70,71] and quantitative tumor dosimetry. The method chosen for a particular patient often depends on patient staging. A patient with distant metastases may be treated with the quantitative method rather than an empiric dosing, although further study of this practice is needed.

Thyroid-Stimulating Hormone Suppression in Patients with High-Risk Differentiated Thyroid Carcinoma

Tuttle describes the need for more aggressive suppression of TSH levels in patients with high-risk DTC, as summarized in "Using Risk Stratification to Individualize Treatment Regimens."

Recall that TSH receptors are present on both normal thyroid and DTC cells and that binding TSH promotes cell growth as well as expression of Tg and the sodium iodide symporter. Whether Tuttle's risk stratification system or another model such as the National Thyroid Cancer Treatment Cooperative Study Group (NTCTCSG) staging system is used, evidence supports the benefit of maintaining TSH levels below 0.1 mU/L in intermediate- and high-risk patients (NTCTCSG stages II and III/IV, respectively).[2,64] Large studies have shown a survival advantage with this practice. To achieve these levels of TSH suppression requires titration of thyroid hormone replacement therapy. In doing so, there must always be cognizance of individual patients' tolerances of hyperthyroidism, which usually is subclinical. Published examples of adverse effects include precipitation of atrial fibrillation in older patients, osteoporosis in postmenopausal women, and angina in patients with known coronary artery disease.[3,72]

Rational Approach to Follow-Up after Initial Treatment

As with treatment decisions, posttreatment follow-up is designed to address each patient's risk profile, again for disease-specific mortality, recurrence, and probability of failed initial therapy.[2] Tuttle suggests that the first 2 years following initial treatment will frequently elucidate which patients have been cured of disease, which have persistently low burden of disease, and which have persistent or progressive disease that requires the closest of follow-up. **Table 4.1** summarizes a risk-adjusted approach to longitudinal follow-up.

Regardless of risk profile, all patients treated for DTC should undergo neck ultrasound to evaluate the thyroid bed and cervical lymph node chains at the 1- and 2-year marks after the completion of initial therapy. Serum Tg levels should be checked in all patients every 6 months for the first year. This biannual schedule should continue for all but the low-risk cohorts. This latter cohort also does not require a stimulated Tg level, a sensitive test that is recommended for all higher risk patients to detect recurrent or persistent disease. Based on the results of the suppressed and/or stimulated Tg levels, imaging studies may be ordered to localize disease. A suppressed Tg level of greater than 1 ng/mL, or a stimulated Tg level of greater than 10 ng/mL, may be compelling enough to order a DxWBS. Confounders of these quantitative values need to be acknowledged, especially anti-Tg antibodies (in 25% of the patients with thyroid cancer and 10% of the general population),[73,74] which may falsely reduce the measured Tg level, and heterophile antibodies, which may falsely elevate the Tg level.[75]

Finally, a subset of intermediate- and high-risk patients may benefit from additional imaging beyond neck ultrasound. More aggressive tumors with poorer differentiation in older patients may have decreased ability to uptake RAI and produce Tg. Another known scenario is when Tg levels are abnormally elevated, and a DxWBS using RAI is negative for disease localization.[76] In both these cases, dedifferentiation of tumor is suggested by the lack of RAI uptake. Fluorodeoxy-D-glucose-positron emission tomography (FDG-PET), and often combination positron emission tomography-computed tomography (PET-CT), imaging of the head, neck, and chest is used, leading to further treatment decisions (surgery, EBRT, chemotherapy) that have a higher likelihood of success than, say, additional RAI therapy.[77]

Thyroglobulin Monitoring after Initial Treatment of Patients with High-Risk Differentiated Thyroid Carcinoma

Serum Tg measurements remain integral to the assessment of residual disease after initial therapy as well as to long-term tumor surveillance for patients with DTC. The frequency with which Tg levels are obtained increases with higher risk patients. It is important to follow the trend in Tg levels over serial measurements, because individual levels are often difficult to interpret (e.g., minimally elevated Tg).[3,8,78] Both nonstimulated Tg levels and TSH-stimulated Tg levels are obtained, the latter at longer intervals. To detect Tg levels, tumor cells must be able to produce and secrete this protein and this ability can be diminished in aggressive or poorly differentiated tumors.[3] It is difficult to predict which of these higher risk tumors will behave in this manner. Therefore, it is also important to utilize data from other studies (ultrasound, CT, DxWBS, FDG-PET) during follow-up.

Another confounding variable is the presence of serum anti-Tg antibodies. Recall that these antibodies may falsely lower the measured Tg level, making this measure a poor surrogate marker of persistent or recurrent disease. Alternatively, heterophile antibodies may falsely elevate the measured Tg level. Although not accepted widely at present, the measurement of Tg mRNA may circumvent this problem altogether, and there is interest in developing a reliable and standardized assay for this strategy.[79-83] At present, anti-Tg antibody levels should be measured with each serial Tg level to interpret the latter value accurately.

Neck Ultrasound after Initial Treatment of Patients with High-Risk Differentiated Thyroid Carcinoma

Postoperative ultrasound should be performed in all patients with DTC, generally first at 6 to 12 months after the initial treatment and then annually or at more frequent intervals for the first 2 years, depending on the risk profile of the patient for recurrent disease. The ATA recommends that patients with clinically significant lymph nodes greater than 5 mm in smallest diameter should undergo FNA biopsy, as well as Tg measurement of needle aspirate fluid, under ultrasound guidance.[2,3]

Role of DxWBS and Posttreatment RxWBS Using Radioactive Iodine in Patients with High-Risk Differentiated Thyroid Carcinoma

DxWBSs using RAI have value in some patients at risk for recurrent or persistent disease, locally and/or metastatically. However, the ATA recognizes that a pre-DxWBS using RAI has low value in most instances, with potential to confound the interpretation of subsequent scans, and interferes with treatment.[84–93] For example, the dose (activity) of ^{131}I for a DxWBS is much lower than that for the RAI treatment (1 to 10 mCi vs. 100 to 200 mCi). However, it may be of sufficient activity to cause "stunning" of remnant thyroid tissue and residual cancer cells.[92] RAI ablation may be suboptimal if remnant tissue and residual cancer cells are unable to maximally uptake ^{131}I at the time of treatment. Studies have shown that this "stunning" effect does not occur if the RAI therapy is administered within 72 hours of the DxWBS. However, evaluating remnant normal thyroid tissue and residual cancer is critical to risk-stratify patients, and the ability of a low-dose, pre-DxWBS using RAI to perform this function has been questioned.[88]

Alternatively, a posttreatment RxWBS may be performed. Essentially, a higher "loading dose" of ^{131}I is received by the patient because of the activity required for a therapeutic effect. Therefore, observable uptake on an RxWBS is theoretically improved compared with that on a pretreatment DxWBS. The improved sensitivity of RxWBS over lower dose pretreatment scans makes RxWBS the preferred scan for most patients.[94–96]

Role of FDG-PET and PET-CT Studies in Follow-Up of Patients with High-Risk Differentiated Thyroid Carcinoma

The 2009 revised ATA guidelines for posttreatment follow-up of patients with DTC reexamine the role of FDG-PET imaging studies in the detection of recurrent or persistent disease.[3] The classic scenario in which FDG-PET and other radiologic studies have been used is in the patient with a posttreatment elevated Tg level that persists and/or progressively increases over time. In this scenario, a WBS may be performed and it may not show a significant RAI uptake. The concern in these cases is for metastatic disease that does not concentrate RAI. Neck ultrasound and chest CT with contrast are recommended to visualize the most common anatomic sites of metastatic DTC. If metastatic cervical lymph nodes in the central compartment had previously been treated, a CT or magnetic resonance imaging (MRI) of the neck should be considered to evaluate retropharyngeal disease that is undetectable by ultrasound. To further complicate this scenario, radiologic evidence of metastatic disease may be detected by these imaging modalities—ultrasound,

CT, and/or MRI; however, the degree of Tg elevation may be inconsistent with the size of the identified metastatic lesion(s). In other words, the detected lesion may not be large enough to explain a significant elevation in Tg. FDG-PET imaging may then be used for further localization of disease. The sensitivity of FDG-PET scanning may be more significant when Tg levels are greater than 10 ng/mL.[97,98] The accuracy of the scan may be improved significantly when integrated with CT imaging (PET-CT), with one comparative study showing an accuracy of 93% in PET-CT versus 78% for PET alone.[3,99]

As stated above, the role of FDG-PET imaging may extend beyond that of patients with the combination of elevated Tg levels, negative RxWBS, and other equivocal radiologic studies.[46,101] Utility of FDG-PET and PET-CT may be seen in poorly differentiated thyroid carcinomas with decreased ability to uptake RAI. For the same reason, Hurthle cell carcinoma may be staged and monitored more accurately with FDG-PET. In patients with known distant metastases, FDG-PET may aid in prognostication. In a patient being considered for RAI therapy, an avid uptake on FDG-PET may suggest that this patient is unlikely to concentrate RAI effectively. Finally, as it is used in cancers of other organs, FDG-PET may be used to assess treatment response after surgery, radiation therapy, and systemic chemotherapy or immunotherapy. ATA guidelines caution that patients with low-risk DTC are unlikely to benefit from such scans, where the risk of metastatic, recurrent, or persistent disease is low, and other nonmalignant pathology may confound results (e.g., reactive lymph nodes, suture line granulomas, and active muscle activity).[3] For these reasons, FDG-PET-positive lesions require biopsy, whenever possible, to confirm malignant disease.

Pearls and Pitfalls

- The prognosis for most patients with differentiated thyroid carcinoma (DTC) is excellent, with a disease-specific mortality of 1 to 5% in young to middle-aged adults. It increases significantly to 20 to 30% in older adults.

- Patients with DTC at the highest risk of persistent or recurrent disease include those older than 45 years, with primary tumors greater than 4 cm in size, evidence of macroscopic extrathyroidal tumor extension, incomplete resection of primary tumor, and/or distant metastases.

- The risk of failing initial therapy is greatest in this high-risk group. Long-term disease control is predicated on the success of initial therapy.

- Histopathological characteristics also separate patients into high- and low-risk cohorts.

- After DTC is diagnosed, neck ultrasound with fine-needle aspiration (FNA) biopsy of suspicious lymph

- nodes is essential to plan appropriate surgery to remove all gross neck disease. Up to 20 to 50% of patients with DTC have cervical lymph node metastases at the time of diagnosis.

- Sonographic lymph node characteristics suggestive of metastasis include long axis 1 cm or greater, short axis 5 mm or greater, hypoechogenicity, cystic appearance, punctuate calcifications, peripheral vascularity, loss of nodal fatty hilus, and round rather than oval shape. None of these characteristics has a high sensitivity for metastatic disease.

- Treatment intensity should be individualized according to a patient's risk of mortality and disease recurrence.

- Ultimately, total thyroidectomy, radioactive iodine (RAI) therapy, and thyroid-stimulating hormone (TSH) suppression therapy have all been found to independently increase survival in patients with DTC as a whole.

- Total thyroidectomy with removal of all gross normal and cancerous thyroid tissue (with a < 1 g remnant) is recommended for all but a minority of patients with DTC (microcarcinoma: < 1 cm primary tumor without aggressive features is surgically managed with hemithyroidectomy in some practices).

- Although more studies are needed to demonstrate improved survival, central and lateral neck dissections are recommended whenever gross pathologic disease involves these regions. Posttreatment tumor surveillance is aided by the elimination of all gross disease.

- Revision thyroid surgery has technical challenges related to distortion of normal anatomy, with considerable risk of injury to the recurrent laryngeal nerves and parathyroid glands. Only an experienced surgeon should attempt revision surgery of the thyroid bed.

- Removal of all gross thyroidal, central, and lateral neck pathologic tissue optimizes the therapeutic response to RAI.

- Suppression of TSH levels after thyroidectomy is an integral component of treatment. In high-risk patients, the preferred goal is less than 0.1 mU/L, compared with less than 0.4 mU/L in low-risk patients. Subclinical or even clinical hyperthyroidism may occur with thyroxine replacement, requiring diligent monitoring.

- Both thyroid hormone withdrawal and recombinant human TSH are reasonable options in preparing a patient for RAI therapy. Both strategies promote increased uptake of RAI into normal and cancerous thyrocytes.

- External beam radiation therapy and conventional chemotherapy have limited roles in contemporary management of DTC.

- Biannual neck ultrasound for the first posttreatment year followed by annual ultrasound is a reasonable plan for initial tumor surveillance, in conjunction with serial serum thyroglobulin (Tg) measures. Any clinically significant suspicious lymph nodes should undergo FNA, which can be sent for both cytopathology and Tg measurement.

- Tg antibodies, found in 10% of the general population and 25% of the patients with thyroid cancer, can produce spuriously low serum Tg levels. Measurements of Tg antibodies are essential when testing Tg levels.

- RAI whole-body scans can be used in the setting of persistently elevated Tg levels. Other imaging modalities to consider include ultrasound, computed tomography, magnetic resonance imaging, and fluorodeoxy-D-glucose-positron emission tomography (FDG-PET) scan.

- FDG-PET imaging modalities may become increasingly important in staging poorly differentiated thyroid carcinomas, as well as in aiding tumor surveillance after initial treatment. Poorly differentiated thyroid cancer often does not produce measurable Tg or demonstrate robust RAI uptake, rendering these more common tests inadequate to detect recurrent or metastatic disease.

- Clinically significant FDG-avid lesions warrant a biopsy whenever possible.

References

1. Hundahl SA, Cady B, Cunningham MP, et al. Initial results from a prospective cohort study of 5583 cases of thyroid carcinoma treated in the United States during 1996. U.S. and German Thyroid Cancer Study Group. An American College of Surgeons Commission on Cancer Patient Care Evaluation study. Cancer 2000;89(1): 202–217

2. Tuttle RM, Brokhin M, Omry G, et al. Recombinant human TSH-assisted radioactive iodine remnant ablation achieves short-term clinical recurrence rates similar to those of traditional thyroid hormone withdrawal. J Nucl Med 2008;49(5):764–770

3. Cooper DS, Doherty GM, Haugen BR, et al; American Thyroid Association (ATA) Guidelines Taskforce on Thyroid Nodules and Differentiated Thyroid Cancer. Revised American Thyroid Association management guidelines for patients with thyroid nodules and differentiated thyroid cancer. Thyroid 2009;19(11):1167–1214

4. Rouxel A, Hejblum G, Bernier MO, et al. Prognostic factors associated with the survival of patients developing loco-regional recurrences of differentiated thyroid carcinomas. J Clin Endocrinol Metab 2004;89(11):5362–5368

5. Schlumberger M, Berg G, Cohen O, et al. Follow-up of low-risk patients with differentiated thyroid carcinoma: a European perspective. Eur J Endocrinol 2004;150(2):105–112

6. Toubeau M, Touzery C, Arveux P, et al. Predictive value for disease progression of serum thyroglobulin levels measured in the postoperative period and after (131)I ablation therapy in patients with differentiated thyroid cancer. J Nucl Med 2004;45(6): 988–994

7. Mercante G, Frasoldati A, Pedroni C, et al. Prognostic factors affecting neck lymph node recurrence and distant metastasis in papillary microcarcinoma of the thyroid: results of a study in 445 patients. Thyroid 2009;19(7):707–716

8. Baudin E, Do Cao C, Cailleux AF, Leboulleux S, Travagli JP, Schlumberger M. Positive predictive value of serum thyroglobulin levels, measured during the first year of follow-up after thyroid hormone withdrawal, in thyroid cancer patients. J Clin Endocrinol Metab 2003;88(3):1107–1111

9. Cailleux AF, Baudin E, Travagli JP, Ricard M, Schlumberger M. Is diagnostic iodine-131 scanning useful after total thyroid ablation for differentiated thyroid cancer? J Clin Endocrinol Metab 2000;85(1):175–178

10. Akslen LA, LiVolsi VA. Prognostic significance of histologic grading compared with subclassification of papillary thyroid carcinoma. Cancer 2000;88(8):1902–1908

11. Prendiville S, Burman KD, Ringel MD, et al. Tall cell variant: an aggressive form of papillary thyroid carcinoma. Otolaryngol Head Neck Surg 2000;122(3):352–357

12. AJCC Cancer Staging Atlas. New York: Springer; 2006

13. Kim TY, Kim WB, Kim ES, et al. Serum thyroglobulin levels at the time of 131I remnant ablation just after thyroidectomy are useful for early prediction of clinical recurrence in low-risk patients with differentiated thyroid carcinoma. J Clin Endocrinol Metab 2005;90(3):1440–1445

14. Brierley JD, Panzarella T, Tsang RW, Gospodarowicz MK, O'Sullivan BA. A comparison of different staging systems predictability of patient outcome. Thyroid carcinoma as an example. Cancer 1997;79(12):2414–2423

15. Sherman SI, Brierley JD, Sperling M, et al. Prospective multicenter study of thyroiscarcinoma treatment: initial analysis of staging and outcome. National Thyroid Cancer Treatment Cooperative Study Registry Group. Cancer 1998;83(5):1012–1021

16. DeGroot LJ, Kaplan EL, McCormick M, Straus FH. Natural history, treatment, and course of papillary thyroid carcinoma. J Clin Endocrinol Metab 1990;71(2):414–424

17. Mazzaferri EL, Jhiang SM. Long-term impact of initial surgical and medical therapy on papillary and follicular thyroid cancer. Am J Med 1994;97(5):418–428

18. Samaan NA, Schultz PN, Hickey RC, et al. The results of various modalities of treatment of well differentiated thyroid carcinomas: a retrospective review of 1599 patients. J Clin Endocrinol Metab 1992;75(3):714–720

19. Bal C, Padhy AK, Jana S, Pant GS, Basu AK. Prospective randomized clinical trial to evaluate the optimal dose of 131 I for remnant ablation in patients with differentiated thyroid carcinoma. Cancer 1996;77(12):2574–2580

20. Barbaro D, Boni G, Meucci G, et al. Radioiodine treatment with 30 mCi after recombinant human thyrotropin stimulation in thyroid cancer: effectiveness for postsurgical remnants ablation and possible role of iodine content in L-thyroxine in the outcome of ablation. J Clin Endocrinol Metab 2003;88(9):4110–4115

21. Creutzig H. High or low dose radioiodine ablation of thyroid remnants? Eur J Nucl Med 1987;12(10):500–502

22. Doi SA, Woodhouse NJ. Ablation of the thyroid remnant and 131I dose in differentiated thyroid cancer. Clin Endocrinol (Oxf) 2000;52(6):765–773

23. Franzius C, Dietlein M, Biermann M, et al. [Procedure guideline for radioiodine therapy and 131iodine whole-body scintigraphy in paediatric patients with differentiated thyroid cancer]. Nucl Med (Stuttg) 2007;46(5):224–231

24. Hackshaw A, Harmer C, Mallick U, Haq M, Franklyn JA. 131I activity for remnant ablation in patients with differentiated thyroid cancer: a systematic review. J Clin Endocrinol Metab 2007;92(1):28–38

25. Jarzab B, Handkiewicz-Junak D, Wloch J. Juvenile differentiated thyroid carcinoma and the role of radioiodine in its treatment: a qualitative review. Endocr Relat Cancer 2005;12(4):773–803

26. Mäenpää HO, Heikkonen J, Vaalavirta L, Tenhunen M, Joensuu H. Low vs. high radioiodine activity to ablate the thyroid after thyroidectomy for cancer: a randomized study. PLoS One 2008;3(4):e1885

27. Rosário PW, Reis JS, Barroso AL, Rezende LL, Padrão EL, Fagundes TA. Efficacy of low and high 131I doses for thyroid remnant ablation in patients with differentiated thyroid carcinoma based on post-operative cervical uptake. Nucl Med Commun 2004;25(11):1077–1081

28. Brabant G. Thyrotropin suppressive therapy in thyroid carcinoma: what are the targets? J Clin Endocrinol Metab 2008;93(4): 1167–1169

29. McGriff NJ, Csako G, Gourgiotis L, Lori CG, Pucino F, Sarlis NJ. Effects of thyroid hormone suppression therapy on adverse clinical outcomes in thyroid cancer. Ann Med 2002;34(7–8):554–564

30. Hovens GC, Stokkel MP, Kievit J, et al. Associations of serum thyrotropin concentrations with recurrence and death in differentiated thyroid cancer. J Clin Endocrinol Metab 2007;92(7):2610–2615

31. Ford D, Giridharan S, McConkey C, et al. External beam radiotherapy in the management of differentiated thyroid cancer. Clin Oncol (R Coll Radiol) 2003;15(6):337–341

32. Wilson PC, Millar BM, Brierley JD. The management of advanced thyroid cancer. Clin Oncol (R Coll Radiol) 2004;16(8):561–568

33. Terezakis SA, Lee KS, Ghossein RA, et al. Role of external beam radiotherapy in patients with advanced or recurrent nonanaplastic thyroid cancer: Memorial Sloan-kettering Cancer Center experience. Int J Radiat Oncol Biol Phys 2009;73(3):795–801

34. Brierley J, Tsang R, Panzarella T, Bana N. Prognostic factors and the effect of treatment with radioactive iodine and external beam radiation on patients with differentiated thyroid cancer seen at a single institution over 40 years. Clin Endocrinol (Oxf) 2005;63(4):418–427

35. Sanders EM Jr, LiVolsi VA, Brierley J, Shin J, Randolph GW. An evidence-based review of poorly differentiated thyroid cancer. World J Surg 2007;31(5):934–945

36. Czaja JM, McCaffrey TV. The surgical management of laryngotracheal invasion by well-differentiated papillary thyroid carcinoma. Arch Otolaryngol Head Neck Surg 1997;123(5):484–490

37. Avenia N, Ragusa M, Monacelli M, et al. Locally advanced thyroid cancer: therapeutic options. Chir Ital 2004;56(4):501–508

38. Ge JH, Zhao RL, Hu JL, Zhou WA. [Surgical treatment of advanced thyroid carcinoma with aero-digestive invasion]. Zhonghua Er Bi Yan Hou Ke Za Zhi 2004;39(4):237–240

39. McCaffrey JC. Evaluation and treatment of aerodigestive tract invasion by well-differentiated thyroid carcinoma. Cancer Contr 2000;7(3):246–252

40. Chow SM, Law SC, Chan JK, Au SK, Yau S, Lau WH. Papillary microcarcinoma of the thyroid—prognostic significance of lymph node metastasis and multifocality. Cancer 2003;98(1):31–40

41. Ito Y, Uruno T, Nakano K, et al. An observation trial without surgical treatment in patients with papillary microcarcinoma of the thyroid. Thyroid 2003;13(4):381–387

42. Nam-Goong IS, Kim HY, Gong G, et al. Ultrasonography-guided fine-needle aspiration of thyroid incidentaloma: correlation with pathological findings. Clin Endocrinol (Oxf) 2004;60(1):21–28

43. Kouvaraki MA, Shapiro SE, Fornage BD, et al. Role of preoperative ultrasonography in the surgical management of patients with thyroid cancer. Surgery 2003;134(6):946–954, discussion 954–955

44. Pacini F, Molinaro E, Castagna MG, et al. Recombinant human thyrotropin-stimulated serum thyroglobulin combined with neck ultrasonography has the highest sensitivity in monitoring differentiated thyroid carcinoma. J Clin Endocrinol Metab 2003;88(8):3668–3673

45. Torlontano M, Crocetti U, Augello G, et al. Comparative evaluation of recombinant human thyrotropin-stimulated thyroglobulin levels, 131I whole-body scintigraphy, and neck ultrasonography in the follow-up of patients with papillary thyroid microcarcinoma who have not undergone radioiodine therapy. J Clin Endocrinol Metab 2006;91(1):60–63

46. Leboulleux S, Girard E, Rose M, et al. Ultrasound criteria of malignancy for cervical lymph nodes in patients followed up for differentiated thyroid cancer. J Clin Endocrinol Metab 2007;92(9):3590–3594

47. Leboulleux S, Rubino C, Baudin E, et al. Prognostic factors for persistent or recurrent disease of papillary thyroid carcinoma with neck lymph node metastases and/or tumor extension beyond the thyroid capsule at initial diagnosis. J Clin Endocrinol Metab 2005;90(10):5723–5729

48. Podnos YD, Smith D, Wagman LD, Ellenhorn JD. The implication of lymph node metastasis on survival in patients with well-differentiated thyroid cancer. Am Surg 2005;71(9):731–734

49. Zaydfudim V, Feurer ID, Griffin MR, Phay JE. The impact of lymph node involvement on survival in patients with papillary and follicular thyroid carcinoma. Surgery 2008;144(6):1070–1077, discussion 1077–1078

50. Cavicchi O, Piccin O, Caliceti U, De Cataldis A, Pasquali R, Ceroni AR. Transient hypoparathyroidism following thyroidectomy: a prospective study and multivariate analysis of 604 consecutive patients. Otolaryngol Head Neck Surg 2007;137(4):654–658

51. Caliskan M, Park JH, Jeong JS, et al. Role of prophylactic ipsilateral central compartment lymph node dissection in papillary thyroid microcarcinoma. Endocr J 2012;59(4):305–311

52. Roh JL, Park JY, Park CI. Total thyroidectomy plus neck dissection in differentiated papillary thyroid carcinoma patients: pattern of nodal metastasis, morbidity, recurrence, and postoperative levels of serum parathyroid hormone. Ann Surg 2007;245(4):604–610

53. Sywak M, Cornford L, Roach P, Stalberg P, Sidhu S, Delbridge L. Routine ipsilateral level VI lymphadenectomy reduces postoperative thyroglobulin levels in papillary thyroid cancer. Surgery 2006;140(6):1000–1005, discussion 1005–1007

54. Tisell LE, Nilsson B, Mölne J, et al. Improved survival of patients with papillary thyroid cancer after surgical microdissection. World J Surg 1996;20(7):854–859

55. Uchino S, Noguchi S, Yamashita H, Watanabe S. Modified radical neck dissection for differentiated thyroid cancer: operative technique. World J Surg 2004;28(12):1199–1203

56. Chao TC, Jeng LB, Lin JD, Chen MF. Reoperative thyroid surgery. World J Surg 1997;21(6):644–647

57. Levin KE, Clark AH, Duh QY, Demeure M, Siperstein AE, Clark OH. Reoperative thyroid surgery. Surgery 1992;111(6):604–609

58. Wilson DB, Staren ED, Prinz RA. Thyroid reoperations: indications and risks. Am Surg 1998;64(7):674–678, discussion 678–679

59. Shaha AR. Revision thyroid surgery—technical considerations. Otolaryngol Clin North Am 2008;41(6):1169–1183, x

60. Shaha AR. Controversies in the management of thyroid nodule. Laryngoscope 2000;110(2 Pt 1):183–193

61. Shaha AR. Thyroid cancer: extent of thyroidectomy. Cancer Control 2000;7(3):240–245

62. Shaha AR. Thyroid cancer: extent of thyroidectomy. Cancer Control 2000;7(3):240–245

63. Harness JK, Fung L, Thompson NW, Burney RE, McLeod MK. Total thyroidectomy: complications and technique. World J Surg 1986;10(5):781–786

64. Jonklaas J, Sarlis NJ, Litofsky D, et al. Outcomes of patients with differentiated thyroid carcinoma following initial therapy. Thyroid 2006;16(12):1229–1242

65. Jung TS, Kim TY, Kim KW, et al. Clinical features and prognostic factors for survival in patients with poorly differentiated thyroid carcinoma and comparison to the patients with the aggressive variants of papillary thyroid carcinoma. Endocr J 2007;54(2):265–274

66. Edmonds CJ, Hayes S, Kermode JC, Thompson BD. Measurement of serum TSH and thyroid hormones in the management of treatment of thyroid carcinoma with radioiodine. Br J Radiol 1977;50(599):799–807

67. Goslings BM. Proceedings: effect of a low iodine diet on 131-I therapy in follicular thyroid carcinomata. J Endocrinol 1975;64(3):30P

68. Maxon HR, Thomas SR, Boehringer A, et al. Low iodine diet in I-131 ablation of thyroid remnants. Clin Nucl Med 1983;8(3):123–126

69. Pluijmen MJ, Eustatia-Rutten C, Goslings BM, et al. Effects of low-iodide diet on postsurgical radioiodide ablation therapy in patients with differentiated thyroid carcinoma. Clin Endocrinol (Oxf) 2003;58(4):428–435

70. Robbins RJ, Schlumberger MJ. The evolving role of (131)I for the treatment of differentiated thyroid carcinoma. J Nucl Med 2005;46(Suppl 1):28S–37S

71. Van Nostrand D, Atkins F, Yeganeh F, Acio E, Bursaw R, Wartofsky L. Dosimetrically determined doses of radioiodine for the treatment of metastatic thyroid carcinoma. Thyroid 2002;12(2):121–134

72. Hovens GC, Stokkel MP, Kievit J, et al. Associations of serum thyrotropin concentrations with recurrence and death in differentiated thyroid cancer. J Clin Endocrinol Metab 2007;92(7):2610–2615

73. Hollowell JG, Staehling NW, Flanders WD, et al. Serum TSH, T(4), and thyroid antibodies in the United States population (1988 to 1994): National Health and Nutrition Examination Survey (NHANES III). J Clin Endocrinol Metab 2002;87(2):489–499

74. Spencer CA, LoPresti JS, Fatemi S, Nicoloff JT. Detection of residual and recurrent differentiated thyroid carcinoma by serum thyroglobulin measurement. Thyroid 1999;9(5):435–441

75. Preissner CM, Dodge LA, O'Kane DJ, Singh RJ, Grebe SK. Prevalence of heterophilic antibody interference in eight automated tumor marker immunoassays. Clin Chem 2005;51(1):208–210

76. Larson SM, Robbins R. Positron emission tomography in thyroid cancer management. Semin Roentgenol 2002;37(2):169–174

77. Hall TL, Layfield LJ, Philippe A, Rosenthal DL. Sources of diagnostic error in fine needle aspiration of the thyroid. Cancer 1989;63(4):718–725

78. Schaap J, Eustatia-Rutten CF, Stokkel M, et al. Does radioiodine therapy have disadvantageous effects in non-iodine accumulating differentiated thyroid carcinoma? Clin Endocrinol (Oxf) 2002;57(1):117–124

79. Bellantone R, Lombardi CP, Bossola M, et al. Validity of thyroglobulin mRNA assay in peripheral blood of postoperative thyroid carcinoma patients in predicting tumor recurrences varies

according to the histologic type: results of a prospective study. Cancer 2001;92(9):2273–2279

80. Chinnappa P, Taguba L, Arciaga R, et al. Detection of thyrotropin-receptor messenger ribonucleic acid (mRNA) and thyroglobulin mRNA transcripts in peripheral blood of patients with thyroid disease: sensitive and specific markers for thyroid cancer. J Clin Endocrinol Metab 2004;89(8):3705–3709

81. Elisei R, Vivaldi A, Agate L, et al. Low specificity of blood thyroglobulin messenger ribonucleic acid assay prevents its use in the follow-up of differentiated thyroid cancer patients. J Clin Endocrinol Metab 2004;89(1):33–39

82. Grammatopoulos D, Elliott Y, Smith SC, et al. Measurement of thyroglobulin mRNA in peripheral blood as an adjunctive test for monitoring thyroid cancer. Mol Pathol 2003;56(3):162–166

83. Li D, Butt A, Clarke S, Swaminathana R. Real-time quantitative PCR measurement of thyroglobulin mRNA in peripheral blood of thyroid cancer patients and healthy subjects. Ann N Y Acad Sci 2004;1022:147–151

84. Anderson GS, Fish S, Nakhoda K, Zhuang H, Alavi A, Mandel SJ. Comparison of I-123 and I-131 for whole-body imaging after stimulation by recombinant human thyrotropin: a preliminary report. Clin Nucl Med 2003;28(2):93–96

85. Carril JM, Quirce R, Serrano J, et al. Total-body scintigraphy with thallium-201 and iodine-131 in the follow-up of differentiated thyroid cancer. J Nucl Med 1997;38(5):686–692

86. Gerard SK, Cavalieri RR. I-123 diagnostic thyroid tumor whole-body scanning with imaging at 6, 24, and 48 hours. Clin Nucl Med 2002;27(1):1–8

87. Hilditch TE, Dempsey MF, Bolster AA, McMenemin RM, Reed NS. Self-stunning in thyroid ablation: evidence from comparative studies of diagnostic 131I and 123I. Eur J Nucl Med Mol Imaging 2002;29(6):783–788

88. Lassmann M, Luster M, Hänscheid H, Reiners C. Impact of 131I diagnostic activities on the biokinetics of thyroid remnants. J Nucl Med 2004;45(4):619–625

89. Leger AF, Pellan M, Dagousset F, Chevalier A, Keller I, Clerc J. A case of stunning of lung and bone metastases of papillary thyroid cancer after a therapeutic dose (3.7 GBq) of 131I and review of the literature: implications for sequential treatments. Br J Radiol 2005;78(929):428–432

90. Morris LF, Waxman AD, Braunstein GD. The nonimpact of thyroid stunning: remnant ablation rates in 131I-scanned and nonscanned individuals. J Clin Endocrinol Metab 2001;86(8):3507–3511

91. Muratet JP, Giraud P, Daver A, Minier JF, Gamelin E, Larra F. Predicting the efficacy of first iodine-131 treatment in differentiated thyroid carcinoma. J Nucl Med 1997;38(9):1362–1368

92. Park HM, Park YH, Zhou XH. Detection of thyroid remnant/metastasis without stunning: an ongoing dilemma. Thyroid 1997;7(2):277–280

93. Silberstein EB. Comparison of outcomes after (123)I versus (131)I pre-ablation imaging before radioiodine ablation in differentiated thyroid carcinoma. J Nucl Med 2007;48(7):1043–1046

94. Koh JM, Kim ES, Ryu JS, Hong SJ, Kim WB, Shong YK. Effects of therapeutic doses of 131I in thyroid papillary carcinoma patients with elevated thyroglobulin level and negative 131I whole-body scan: comparative study. Clin Endocrinol (Oxf) 2003;58(4):421–427

95. Mazzaferri EL, Robbins RJ, Spencer CA, et al. A consensus report of the role of serum thyroglobulin as a monitoring method for low-risk patients with papillary thyroid carcinoma. J Clin Endocrinol Metab 2003;88(4):1433–1441

96. Schlumberger M, Mancusi F, Baudin E, Pacini F. 131I therapy for elevated thyroglobulin levels. Thyroid 1997;7(2):273–276

97. Dietlein M, Scheidhauer K, Voth E, Theissen P, Schicha H. Fluorine-18 fluorodeoxyglucose positron emission tomography and iodine-131 whole-body scintigraphy in the follow-up of differentiated thyroid cancer. Eur J Nucl Med 1997;24(11):1342–1348

98. Schlüter B, Bohuslavizki KH, Beyer W, Plotkin M, Buchert R, Clausen M. Impact of FDG PET on patients with differentiated thyroid cancer who present with elevated thyroglobulin and negative 131I scan. J Nucl Med 2001;42(1):71–76

99. Palmedo H, Bucerius J, Joe A, et al. Integrated PET/CT in differentiated thyroid cancer: diagnostic accuracy and impact on patient management. J Nucl Med 2006;47(4):616–624

100. Lee YS, Kim SW, Kim SW, et al. Extent of routine central lymph node dissection with small papillary thyroid carcinoma. World J Surg 2007;31(10):1954–1959

5 Medullary Thyroid Carcinoma I

Wojciech M. Wysocki, Andrzej L. Komorowski, Rehan A. Kazi, and Raghav C. Dwivedi

Core Messages

- Medullary thyroid carcinoma (MTC) constitutes 4 to 8% of all thyroid malignancies.

- In general 20% of the MTCs are inherited (mainly in the form of multiple endocrine neoplasia type 2A [MEN2A], MEN2B, and other familial MTC syndromes); the remaining cases are sporadic.

- Clinical appearance of the MTC is similar to differentiated thyroid cancers, but typical tumor location being the upper poles of the thyroid lobes.

- Looking for adrenal abnormalities is mandatory in all patients with a suspected and/or confirmed MTC.

- Surgery (total thyroidectomy with at least bilateral level VI compartmental lymph node dissection) is the only curative treatment for MTC.

- In general 10-year disease-specific survival rate in patients with MTC approaches 75%.

The first description of medullary thyroid carcinoma (MTC) was presented in 1906 by Jaquet; the described case was defined as "malignant goiter with amyloid" having distant metastases.[1] In the second half of the 20th century the MTC was precisely defined as distinct thyroid malignancy (Laskowski in 1958, Hazard et al in 1959, and Williams et al in 1966).[2–4] MTC constitutes 4 to 8% of all thyroid carcinomas; commonest being papillary thyroid carcinoma (60 to 80%) and follicular thyroid carcinoma (10 to 20%).[5,6]

Histogenesis

MTC arises from calcitonin-secreting parafollicular C cells that constitute approximately 1% of all thyroid cells. C cells of the thyroid gland develop from the neural crest and belong to the neuroendocrine family of cells which are spread widely in the human body. The neuroendocrine cell system is called disseminated neuroendocrine system (DNS).[6] Within the thyroid gland neuroendocrine cells are mainly located in the upper portions of both thyroid lobes, and that is why MTC are usually found around the upper poles of the thyroid gland.

The typical microscopic change leading to MTC starts from C-cell hyperplasia (CCH), progresses to early invasive medullary carcinoma, which subsequently turns into an invasive MTC. The presence of CCH within thyroid is typical for inherited form of MTC (i.e., multiple endocrine neoplasia type 2 [MEN2] syndrome).[6]

Histologically MTC is composed of spindle-shaped or rounded cells with numerous fibrous septa and separated by amyloid deposits (amyloid deposits in MTC were described by Jaquet in 1906).[1] The tumor is usually ill defined and nonencapsulated with macroscopic invasion into adjacent tissues. Positive immunohistochemical staining for calcitonin, carcinoembryonic antigen (CEA), and amyloid help establish diagnosis of MTC.

Pearl

- Medullary thyroid carcinoma is usually located in the upper poles of the thyroid lobes because this is where the relative number of parafollicular C cells is the highest.

Genetics

MTC occurs mainly sporadically (70 to 80%), but it could also follow autosomal dominant pattern of inheritance of the disease (i.e., there is a 50% risk for offspring of a carrier to inherit the disease).[6] Inherited variant of MTC presents clinically as MEN2 syndrome. In absolute numbers MEN2 is a rare disease: 1 in 30,000 is affected.[6]

MEN2 virtually always consists of familial appearance of MTC (MTC is a core feature of MEN2) often coexisting with other neoplasms and includes three principal types[5–7]:

1. MEN2A (described in 1961 by Sipple [Sipple syndrome]; approximately 55% of all MEN2 cases)—MTC is found in all cases of the MEN2A type (100% of patients), pheochromocytoma (adrenal locations in 50 to 70% of patients, other locations rare), and hyperparathyroidism (25% of patients).

2. MEN2B (described independently by Wagenmann in 1922 and Froboese in 1923; approximately 5 to 10% of all MEN2 cases)—Again the MTC is found in 100% of patients, multiple mucosal neuromas (100% of patients), pheochromocytoma (adrenal location in 50% of patients, with multiple tumors [often bilateral] in 50% of cases), enteric ganglioneuromatosis (resulting in digestive tract general malfunctioning in 40% of patients), marfanoid appearance (75% of patients).

3. Familial medullary thyroid carcinoma (FMTC; approximately 35 to 40% of all MEN2 cases)—MTC (100% of patients) and—by definition—no pheochromocytoma or other tumors (due to late appearance of pheochromocytoma in MEN2A); this definition is difficult to use in advance, and therefore most families with FMTC are initially managed, observed, and treated as MEN2A families).

In early 1990s *RET* (*REarranged during Transfection*) proto-oncogene germline mutations have been identified in nearly all studied MEN2A, FMTC, and MEN2B patients, however, there are still some families with typical features of MEN syndrome but no identifiable (so far) *RET* mutation. Germline mutations in *RET* gene result in abnormally overactive RET protein in all tissues, in which it is expressed (somatic mutations in *RET* gene are observed in 50% of sporadic MTC cases and are limited to C cells only).

Since the identification of *RET* proto-oncogene mutations, all individuals at risk or suspected of having MEN2A or MEN2B syndrome should ideally have mutational analysis for the *RET* gene as early as possible. Presymptomatic diagnosis based on genetic tests leads to prophylactic surgery (*see* the section on "Surgical Prevention of Medullary Thryoid Carcinoma in Multiple Endocrine Neoplasia Type 2 Syndrome").

Clinical Picture

The clinical appearance of MTC is usually not different from the presentation of patients with differentiated thyroid carcinomas (see Chapter 3, Differentiated Thyroid Carcinomas). If clinically symptomatic, MTC typically presents as solitary, unilateral thyroid nodule, in the upper poles of the thyroid lobe (where the concentration of C-cells is the highest). Sporadic forms of MTC usually develop in the fifth or sixth decade of life. Contrary to that, the hereditary MTC (in MEN2 patients) usually presents at younger age (third or fourth decade of life or even earlier) and presents as multiple, bilateral nodules in the upper poles of the thyroid lobes. Unlike differentiated thyroid cancer, MTC prevalence is almost equal in both the genders.[5,8]

Pearl

- MTC prevalence in men and women is almost equal (unlike differentiated thyroid cancer).

The clinical evaluation of patients with MTC is virtually the same as for patients with differentiated thyroid cancers (*see* Chapter 3 Differentiated Thyroid Carcinomas). The important clinical feature of MTC is that 50 to 75% of patients present initially with metastatic cervical adenopathy. Tumors often grow quickly and presents with compressive symptoms; tracheal compression is seen in approximately 15% of the MTC cases at the time of initial presentation.[3]

Diagnosis and Staging

Fine-needle aspiration biopsy (FNAB) (usually sonographically guided) is generally deemed sufficient to confirm the diagnosis of MTC. FNAB is a cost-effective tool, with low risk of procedure-related complications. There are ambiguities referred to FNAB use in follicular thyroid neoplasms, but in MTC, FNAB provides excellent accuracy (> 90%) with low false-negative outcomes (< 5%). The FNAB can be successfully performed with optimal results for tumors with 1 to 4 cm diameter (< 1 cm it is difficult to sample, and > 4 cm it is uncertain if appropriate portion of the tumor had been sampled).[9] In general, the algorithm for the management of thyroid nodules presented in Chapter 3 is applicable when facing a patient with thyroid nodule and clinical features suggesting MTC.

To diagnose MEN2A (or MEN2B), the only certain way is to confirm *RET* mutation or to identify typical feature of MEN2A (or MEN2B, respectively) also in first-degree relatives of the patient. Alternatively at least two typical clinical features of MEN2A in the individual are required to clinically diagnose MEN2A. For making a clinical diagnosis of MEN2B a preponderance of the classical clinical features of this syndrome in the individual is required. The diagnosis of FMTC requires exclusion of pheochromocytoma in at least two generations of the affected family.[5]

If the MTC is microscopically confirmed, clinical staging should follow. Staging divides patients into prognostic groups to support clinical decisions on optimal treatment strategy. Current tumor-node-metastasis (TNM) staging system (as updated by American Joint Committee on Cancer Staging in 2010) is presented in **Tables 5.1** and **5.2**.

Pearl

- Appropriate clinical staging is a mandatory first step in the assessment of the patient. The initial staging will form the basis for the assessment of treatment outcomes.

- Virtually all MTCs secrete calcitonin, but rarely there may be odd cases with normal calcitonin level.

If MTC is diagnosed by FNAB the recommended management consist of immediate measurement of

Table 5.1   Definitions for Tumor-Node-Metastasis Staging System by American Committee on Cancer Staging (version from 2010)

Primary tumor (T)

- Tx   Primary tumor cannot be assessed
- T0   No evidence of primary tumor
- T1   Tumor 2 cm or less in greatest dimension, limited to the thyroid
- T1a   Tumor 1 cm or less, limited to the thyroid
- T1b   Tumor more than 1 cm but not more than 2 cm in greatest dimension, limited to the thyroid
- T2   Tumor more than 2 cm but not more than 4 cm in greatest dimension, limited to the thyroid
- T3   Tumor more than 4 cm in greatest dimension limited to the thyroid or any tumor with minimal extrathyroid extension (e.g., extension to sternothyroid muscle or perithyroid soft tissues)
- T4a   Moderately advanced disease (tumor of any size extending beyond the thyroid capsule to invade subcutaneous soft tissues, larynx, trachea, esophagus, or recurrent laryngeal nerve)
- T4b   Very advanced disease (tumor invades prevertebral fascia or encases carotid artery or mediastinal vessels)

Regional lymph nodes (N)[a]

- Nx   Regional lymph nodes cannot be assessed
- N0   No regional lymph node metastasis
- N1   Regional lymph node metastasis(-es)
- N1a   Metastasis(-es) to level VI (pretracheal, paratracheal, and prelaryngeal/Delphian lymph nodes)
- N1b   Metastasis(-es) to unilateral, bilateral, or contralateral cervical (levels I, II, III, IV, or V) or retropharyngeal or superior mediastinal lymph nodes (level VII)

Distant metastasis(-es) (M)

- M0   No distant metastasis
- M1   Distant metastasis(-es)

[a]Regional lymph nodes are: central compartment, lateral cervical, upper mediastinal lymph nodes.

Table 5.2   American Joint Committee on Cancer/Tumor-Node-Metastasis Stage Grouping

Stage	T (Tumor)	N (Node)	M (Metastasis)
I	T1	N0	M0
II	T2	N0	M0
	T3	N0	M0
III	T1	N1a	M0
	T2	N1a	M0
	T3	N1a	M0
IVA	T4a	N0	M0
	T4a	N1a	M0
	T1	N1b	M0
	T2	N1b	M0
	T3	N1b	M0
	T4a	N1b	M0
IVB	T4b	Any N	M0
IVC	Any T	Any N	M1

calcitonin level (cut-off value for abnormal level is usually set at 10 or 20 pg/mL),[10] CEA (higher level reflects greater burden of the disease), and calcium in the serum. As previously mentioned, due to the risk of MEN2 syndrome, screening for pheochromocytoma is mandatory (including abdominal computed tomography [CT] and urine methoxy-catecholamine level).[3,5,6]

Pearl

- Looking for adrenal abnormalities is mandatory in all patients with suspected and/or confirmed medullary thyroid carcinoma.

There is a low probability (0.3 to 4.5%) that hypercalcitoninemia results from non-MTC (non-C cells) related causes. Therefore calcitonin-stimulation test is recommended to identify true positive patients: pentagastrin or calcium are used as stimulants; both substances stimulate only C-cells-dependent secretion of calcitonin.[10]

Detailed neck ultrasound should be the next step of initial clinical assessment and staging. Assessment of the vocal cord mobility is a must as for any other thyroid malignancy.

National Comprehensive Cancer Network guidelines recommend genetic counseling and screening for *RET* proto-oncogene mutations (attending physician has to keep in mind that germline mutation should prompt family testing of close relatives [first-degree]).[6]

If nodal metastases (cN1) are clinically present, contrast-enhanced neck and chest/mediastinum CT or magnetic resonance imaging (MRI) is advised. Imaging of neck and chest/mediastinum is also recommended if calcitonin level is over 400 pg/mL.

Treatment

Pearl

- Surgery (total thyroidectomy with at least bilateral level VI compartmental lymph node dissection) is the only curative treatment for MTC and is the standard option for these patients.

Primary Treatment of Medullary Thyroid Carcinoma

If diameter of primary thyroid focus of MTC is ≥ 1 cm the optimal surgical treatment should consist of the following five elements:

1. Total thyroidectomy with bilateral central neck dissection (level VI compartmental dissection).
2. If there are clinically (or on ultrasound) suspected lymph nodes or biopsy-positive lymph nodes—as in point 1—plus modified neck dissection (ipsilateral of bilateral) with therapeutic intention, which includes at least suspected/confirmed levels of the neck lymph node compartments.
3. If there is high-tumor volume of gross disease in adjacent central neck—as in point 1—plus modified neck dissection (ipsilateral) with prophylactic intention.
4. Additionally postoperative radiotherapy could be considered for gross macroscopic extrathyroidal extension (T4a or T4b) with positive margins after resection of all gross disease and following resection of moderate to high-volume disease in the central or lateral neck lymph nodes with extranodal soft tissue extension (this is a controversial issue).

5. In all patients postoperatively levothyroxine should be administered to achieve normalization of thyroid stimulating hormone (TSH) level (as substitution only, contrary to differentiated thyroid carcinoma patients).

If diameter of primary thyroid focus of MTC does not exceed 1 cm the optimal surgical treatment should be total thyroidectomy (additionally one may consider bilateral central neck dissection).[3,5,6,8]

Pearl

- In contrast to differentiated thyroid carcinomas MTC does not uptake iodine and is not sensitive to radioiodine therapy.

Treatment of Initially Advanced Medullary Thyroid Carcinoma

If tracheal lumen is compromised or disease progression initiates pain, bleeding and/or other local symptoms uncontrollable by other means, palliative neck surgery may be an option. However, palliative surgery should be well balanced between benefits (usually short-term and symptomatic only) and risks (often life-threating). If possible, patients should be informed about any respective clinical trials currently enrolling. Nonsurgical palliative measures (radiotherapy, percutaneous interventions, etc.) can also be of use in carefully selected patients.[5,6,8]

Treatment of Recurrent or Residual Medullary Thyroid Carcinoma

If recurrence or residual disease is limited (locoregional), all foci of the disease should be resected, possibly en bloc and postoperative radiotherapy should be considered. Radiotherapy should also be considered if locoregional disease is unresectable or disease quickly progresses.

In patients with distant recurrence, resection or ablation (radiofrequency ablation, thermal ablation, embolization) should be considered, particularly in patients with limited disease burden and/or symptomatic disease. In patients with asymptomatic disease and massive dissemination observation/best supportive care is one of the options, but resection (if possible) or ablation can also be considered. Other options for disseminated patients include: enrollment into clinical trials, radiotherapy for focal symptoms, molecularly targeted therapy (not yet approved outside clinical trials) or dacarbazine-based chemotherapy, best supportive care.[5,6,8]

Surgical Prevention of Medullary Thyroid Carcinoma in Multiple Endocrine Neoplasia Type 2 Syndrome

In patients with MEN2A or FMTC, management algorithm depends on presence or absence of primary hyperparathyroidism (initial diagnostic work-up must include measurement of serum parathyroid hormone and calcium levels). In general, treatment includes total thyroidectomy by the age of 5 years, or at the diagnosis (if after 5 years of age). There are specific mutation-and-risk-dependent recommendations on surgery age available. Therapeutic central (ipsilateral or bilateral) neck dissection should accompany total thyroidectomy always if there are nodal or thyroid abnormalities detected clinically or on palpation, as well as in patients with elevated calcitonin and/or CEA levels. Prophylactic ipsilateral modified neck dissection should be considered in cases with high volume or gross disease in the adjacent central neck compartment. Adjuvant postoperative radiotherapy is seldom used in children, but levothyroxine is always recommended to keep TSH level within normal limits (this is of great importance in children!).

In MEN2A patients with primary hyperparathyroidism: single adenoma of parathyroid should be excised; adenomas/CCH in multiple glands warrants subtotal parathyroidectomy (i.e., leaving functional equivalent of half of the normal parathyroid gland) or total parathyroidectomy with autotransplantation to heterotropic site. Cryopreservation of the parathyroid tissue should also be considered.

In patients with confirmed MEN2B syndrome treatment should be initiated in early childhood—total thyroidectomy should be performed during first year of life or at diagnosis. Surgeon should consider central bilateral neck dissection or more extensive neck dissection if tumor diameter is > 0.5 cm. In children adjuvant radiotherapy is rarely used, but substitutive levothyroxine is administered postoperatively as in adult patients **Tables 5.3** and **5.4**.[3,5,6,8]

Molecular Targeted Therapy in Medullary Thyroid Carcinoma

Identification of *RET* gene lead to RET protein, which is transmembrane receptor belonging to tyrosine kinase superfamily.[11] While surgery remains principal treatment for MTC, research (mainly phase I and II) in the field of molecularly targeted RET tyrosine kinase inhibition in MTC

with sorafenib, sunitinib, and vandetanib among others is currently ongoing.[11] The results so far were disappointing (low rate of partial response, absence of complete response).[8]

Follow-Up

Biochemical cure in MTC is defined as postoperative normalization of calcitonin plasma level (achieved in up to 50% of patients) and that is why this biomarker forms a basis for further follow-up.[3,10]

> **Pearl**
>
> • Postoperative follow-up is based on regular clinical visits (with neck ultrasound) and laboratory measurements of calcitonin and carcinoembryonic antigen.

If basal (i.e., postoperative) calcitonin is undetectable or CEA remains in the reference range (i.e., usually 0 to 6 mg/mL) patient should be observed on a regular basis: annual laboratory measurements (calcitonin, CEA) and neck ultrasound. Additional imaging studies or more frequent testing if calcitonin or CEA levels are significantly increased (no profound testing required if calcitonin/CEA levels are stable). If imaging is negative, observation should follow.[5,6]

If basal calcitonin is detectable or CEA is elevated above upper normal limit neck imaging should be performed as soon as possible (ultrasound is imaging modality of the first choice, with—additionally—bone scan, fluorodeoxy-glucose [FDG]-PET scan, MRI of axial skeleton in patients with evidently elevated calcitonin level [> 150 pg/mL]) and contrast-enhanced neck/chest/abdomen CT/MRI). If no abnormalities are encountered in the imaging, close clinical observation should follow with repeated laboratory measurement every 6 to 12 months. If there is continuous rise in calcitonin/CEA level, the patient should be referred to repeated imaging and—possibly—additional diagnostics tests. No further testing is required if calcitonin/CEA levels are stable. If imaging is negative, observation should follow.[5,6]

Table 5.3 Timing of Prophylactic Total Thyroidectomy in Individuals with Multiple Endocrine Neoplasia Type 2 Syndrome

MEN2 Syndrome Type	Recommended Age for Surgery	Comment
MEN2A	Usually before the age of 5 y	Ideal age is widely disputed; the most common recommendation is to operate before 5 y of age, but strongly depends on mutation type (see **Table 5.4**) and other factors
MEN2B	Usually in the first year of life	MTC in MEN2B is very aggressive and metastasizes early to regional and distant sites
FMTC	In late childhood or adolescence	The precise timing depends on disease onset in the family and mutation type (see **Table 5.4**), as well as rapid increase in calcitonin level (shortened doubling time)

MEN2A, multiple endocrine neoplasia type 2A; y, years; MEN2B, multiple endocrine neoplasia type 2B; MTC, medullary thyroid carcinoma; FMTC, familial medullary thyroid carcinoma.

Table 5.4 Recommended Age of Surgery Depending on RET Proto-Oncogene Mutation Type

Age at Surgery	In the First Year of Life	By the Age of 5	By Age 5–10
Mutation in RET codon	883, 918, 922	611, 618, 620, 634	609, 630, 768, 790, 791, 804, 891
Level of risk	Highest-risk mutations (mainly MEN2B)	Higher-risk mutations (mainly MEN2A)	High-risk mutations (mainly FMTC and MEN2A)

Adapted from references 6 and 7.
RET, REarranged during Transfection; MEN2A, multiple endocrine neoplasia type 2A; MEN2B, multiple endocrine neoplasia type 2B; FMTC, familial medullary thyroid carcinoma.

Pearl

- If calcitonin level increases by more than 20 to 100% of basal measurement, neck ultrasound should be done. If postoperative calcitonin level is > 150 to 200 pg/mL, then the systemic imaging for local/distant failure should be immediately performed.

Prognosis

In general 10-year disease-specific survival rate in patients with MTC approaches 75%. Age at diagnosis greater than 50 years is a strong, independent risk factor for poorer outcomes.[6,9]

A 10-year survival is 90 to 100% if disease at diagnosis was confined to the thyroid (stage I or stage II). In locally advanced (i.e., node positive, stages III and IV) disease the 10-year survival rate for MTC is approximately 60 to 80%, and in initially metastatic settings 10-year survival rate is approximately 20 to 30%, but in oligometastatic group can reach up to 50%.[10]

In MEN2B, prognosis is generally poor: majority (70%) have metastases a diagnosis, and only 40% of therapeutically operated patients survive 5 years from diagnosis.

Clinical Pearls

- Medullary thyroid carcinoma (MTC) represents a minority (4 to 8%) of all thyroid malignancies.

- Looking for adrenal abnormalities is mandatory in all patients with suspected or confirmed MTC, as 20% of MTC cases are inherited as multiple endocrine neoplasia type 2 (MEN2) syndrome (most MEN2 cases include pheochromocytoma).

- Surgery (total thyroidectomy with at least bilateral level VI compartmental lymph node dissection) is the only curative treatment for MTC; radioiodine therapy is of no use in MTC.

- In general 10-year disease-specific survival rate in patients with MTC approaches 75%.

References

1. Jaquet AJ. Ein fall von metastasierenden amyloidtumoren (lymphosarcoma). Virchows Arch 1906;185:251–267
2. Hazard JB, Hawk WA, Crile G Jr. Medullary (solid) carcinoma of the thyroid; a clinicopathologic entity. J Clin Endocrinol Metab 1959;19(1):152–161
3. Jarząb B, Kuzdak K. Nowotwory tarczycy. In Jeziorski A, Szawłowski AW, Towpik E (eds). Chirurgia Onkologiczna. Wydawnictwo Lekarskie PZWL, Warszawa; 2009
4. Williams ED. Histogenesis of medullary carcinoma of the thyroid. J Clin Pathol 1966;19(2):114–118
5. Kloos RT, Eng C, Evans DB, et al; American Thyroid Association Guidelines Task Force. Medullary thyroid cancer: management guidelines of the American Thyroid Association. Thyroid 2009;19(6):565–612
6. Tuttle RM, Kloos RT, Sherman SI, Waguespack SG. (Writing Committee) (2010). Thyroid Carcinoma. NCCN Practice Guidelines in Oncology v.1.2010. www.nccn.org. Accessed 30/10/2012
7. Frank-Raue K, Raue F. Multiple endocrine neoplasia type 2 (MEN 2). Eur J Cancer 2009;45(Suppl 1):267–273
8. Ying AK, Huh W, Bottomley S, Evans DB, Waguespack SG. Thyroid cancer in young adults. Semin Oncol 2009;36(3):258–274
9. Amos K, Habra MA, Perrier ND. Carcinoma of the thyroid and parathyroid glands. In: Feig BW, Berger DH, Fuhrman GM (eds). The M.D. Anderson Surgical Oncology Handbook. 4th ed. Philadelphia:Lippincott Williams & Wilkins;2006
10. van Veelen W, de Groot JW, Acton DS, et al. Medullary thyroid carcinoma and biomarkers: past, present and future. J Intern Med 2009;266(1):126–140
11. Cakir M, Grossman AB. Medullary thyroid cancer: molecular biology and novel molecular therapies. Neuroendocrinology 2009;90(4):323–348

6 Medullary Thyroid Carcinoma II

Jonathan Brett Wallach and Nicholas J. Sanfilippo

Core Messages

- Medullary thyroid carcinoma (MTC) is a neuroendrocrine tumor of the calcitonin-producing thyroid parafollicular C cells and accounts for approximately 4% of thyroid cancers in the United States.

- Approximately 78% of MTC is sporadic, with the rest inherited (familial) and usually part of a multiple endocrine neoplasia type 2 (MEN2) syndrome. There is no age-adjusted difference in survival between sporadic and MEN2A MTC, while the more aggressive MEN2B MTC has shown worse survival rates.

- Diagnostic imaging, which can also examine for locoregional and distant spread, includes radiography, ultrasound or computed tomography (CT) of the neck; radiography or CT of the chest; CT of the upper abdomen; and nuclear medicine scintigraphy or positive emission tomography.

- Confirmatory diagnosis involves pathologic examination of a fine-needle aspiration or surgical specimen.

- Curative treatment always involves at least partial thyroidectomy, with total thyroidectomy usually recommended. Chemotherapy, radiotherapy, and immunoradiotherapy have a role in residual or recurrent disease, while radioiodine therapy is not used.

- Biochemical follow-up involves trending serum calcitonin and carcinoembryonic antigen laboratory values.

- Prognosis depends mostly on the tumor's stage, with age being a controversial factor.

Medullary thyroid carcinoma (MTC) is a neuroendocrine neoplasm of the thyroid parafollicular C cells and accounts for approximately 4% of thyroid cancers, or approximately 1000 cases per year, in the United States.[1] The C cells are located in the upper two-thirds of the thyroid lobes and produce the polypeptide hormone calcitonin, which decreases serum calcium levels. While the thyroid epithelial cells are derived from the embryonic endoderm, the C cells develop from the neural crest, and therefore MTC shares clinical and histological features with other neuroendocrine tumors.

MTC is unique among thyroid neoplasms for its inherited tumor syndromes; approximately 78% of MTCs are sporadic, while the rest appear to be inherited (familial), usually as part of the multiple endocrine neoplasia type 2 (MEN2) syndrome.[2] The malignancy typically presents in the fifth or sixth decade of life for sporadic MTC and in the second or third decade for the inherited type.[2]

Classification

As mentioned earlier, approximately 22% of MTC are inherited (usually as part of MEN2), so MTC is traditionally classified as sporadic versus inherited. As first discovered in 1993, patients with inherited MTC have dominantly acting germline mutations in the *RET* proto-oncogene. The *RET*

protein is a tyrosine kinase receptor that, in conjunction with the accessory molecule glial cell line-derived neurotrophic factor receptor-α, can transduce the glial cell line-derived neurotrophic factor signal via a pathway involving *Ras* and mitogen-activated protein kinase[3,4]; this pathway affects the differentiation, survival, and proliferation of a variety of neuroendocrine cell types. Inherited MTC is subclassified into the following categories:

- MEN2A: MTC and pheochromocytoma + primary parathyroid hyperplasia.
- MEN2B: MTC and pheochromocytoma + mucosal neuromas, intestinal ganglioneuromas, and a marfanoid habitus with a decreased upper/lower body ratio; this subtype has proven to be more aggressive than MEN2A with worse survival rates.[5]
- Familial medullary thyroid carcinoma (FMTC): MTC and no extrathyroidal manifestations.

MEN2A also includes two minor variants: MEN2A with Hirschsprung disease (hypoplasia of the intestinal myenteric plexus) and MEN2A with cutaneous lichen amyloidosis. In addition, approximately 5% of the patients with FMTC have no detectable *RET* mutations and approximately 6% of the patients with sporadic MTC are believed to possess an unknown germline *RET* mutation.[6–10]

Signs and Symptoms

Although MTC can cause symptoms related to hypocalcemia from calcitonin overproduction (such as parasthesias, tetany, carpopedal spasms, petechiae, and hyperactive deep tendon reflexes), approximately 75 to 95% of the patients first present with a solitary thyroid nodule.[2,11,12] Because the C cells are clustered in the upper portion of each thyroid lobe, most nodules are identified there. These nodules may interfere with or become more prominent during swallowing, and for locally advanced or metastatic disease, they may even cause hoarseness, dysphagia, or respiratory difficulty. Cervical lymphadenopathy may be appreciated, indicating locoregional spread.

Patients who present with advanced disease may complain of weight loss, lethargy, bone pain, hemoptysis, or pneumonia symptoms (from aspiration-obstructive or postobstructive pneumonia), while their physical examination may demonstrate abdominal pain, jaundice (from liver metastases), or superior vena cava syndrome. Less commonly, patients with large tumor burdens may present with paraneoplastic syndromes, such as Cushing or carcinoid syndrome, with associated secretory diarrhea and flushing.

Diagnosis and Multiple Endocrine Neoplasia Type 2

Fine-needle aspiration or surgical biopsy with immunostaining for calcitonin is performed for patients presenting with suspicious nodules. MTC pathology reveals enlarged, spindle-shaped, pleomorphic tumor cells with eccentrically displaced nuclei (**Fig. 6.1**); there is no thyroid follicle development because the cells originate from the parafollicular C cells. The cytoplasm may also be slightly granular. However, the biopsy

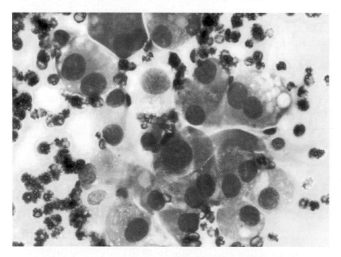

Figure 6.1 Fine-needle aspiration cytology reveals plasmacytoid cells with abundant cytoplasm and eccentric pleomorphic nuclei.

Source: Mehdi G, Maheshwari V, Ansari HA, Sadaf L, Khan MA. FNAC diagnosis of medullary carcinoma thyroid: a report of three cases with review of literature. *J Cytol* 2010;27(2):66–68.

may reveal only C-cell hyperplasia (CCH), not a malignancy. Reactive CCH is caused by stimuli outside the C cell, such as hypercalcemia, hyperparathyroidism, chronic lymphocytic thyroiditis, or thyroid follicular tumors, and is usually not premalignant. By contrast, neoplastic CCH is caused by an intrinsic mutation and is a precursor to MTC.

Various extrathyroidal malignancies can metastasize to the thyroid, including renal cell, breast, melanoma, uterine, and lung carcinoma. If a tumor is suspected to be a metastasis, thyroglobulin staining as well as other markers should be administered to the biopsy specimen to determine the cells' origin.

Diagnostic imaging, which can also examine for locoregional and distant spread, includes radiography, ultrasound, or computed tomography (CT) of the neck; radiography or CT of the chest; CT of the upper abdomen; and nuclear medicine scintigraphy or positron emission tomography (PET). At presentation, spread to local lymph nodes in the neck is common, especially for inherited MTC. Other frequent sites of spread include mediastinal lymph nodes, liver, lung, and bone. An example of PET scan illustrating metastatic MTC is shown in **Fig. 6.2**. Spread to the skin or brain is also seen at presentation but is far less common.

In addition to secreting excessive calcitonin, MTC also produces carcinoembryonic antigen (CEA); therefore, calcitonin and CEA levels are routinely measured to provide more information about the malignancy, its spread, and its activity. The biochemical preoperative analysis provides a baseline for comparison after the thyroidectomy to evaluate the effectiveness of the surgery. While hypercalcitoninemia is usually associated with MTC, this biomarker is not specific for the malignancy[13]; other conditions produce high levels of calcitonin, including hypercalcemia, hypergastrinemia, other neuroendocrine tumors, renal insufficiency, papillary and follicular thyroid carcinomas, and goiter.[13] Indeed, only 10 to 40% of the patients with elevated levels of calcitonin and a thyroid nodule have MTC.[14] However, very high levels of calcitonin (> 100 pg/mL) are essentially pathognomonic for MTC, with a risk approaching 100%, while the risk is approximately 25% for values 50 to 100 pg/mL, 8.3% for values 20 to 50 pg/mL, and with normal risk for values less than 8.5 pg/mL for men and less than 5.0 pg/mL for women.[15]

For patients diagnosed with MTC, it is important to determine whether the malignancy is part of an inherited syndrome. Patients should be asked about a family history of thyroid cancer, especially in first-degree relatives. In addition, a detailed personal and family history should include the presence of pheochromocytoma, hyperparathyroidism, mucosal neuromas, intestinal ganglioneuromas, or any of the other abnormalities associated with MEN2. A 24-hour urinary excretion of metanephrine, catecholamine, and cortisol should be measured to evaluate for pheochromocytoma. Some patients may elect to undergo genetic testing involving polymerase chain reaction amplification of the commonly mutated *RET* exons to determine whether they are at risk for other tumors as part of the MEN2 syndrome. This analysis

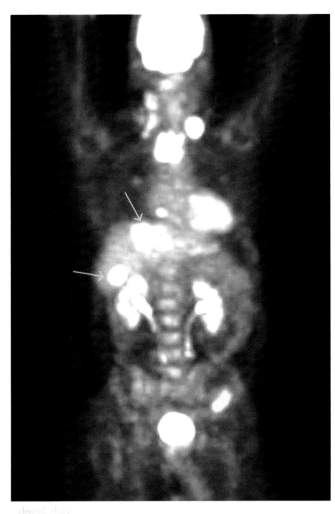

Figure 6.2   Positron emission tomography scan showing extensive uptake in the neck, chest, and liver.

Source: Gorospe EC, Badamas J. Acute liver failure secondary to metastatic medullary thyroid cancer. *Case Reports in Hepatology* 2011 doi:10.1155/2011/603757.

of germline mutations in the *RET* proto-oncogene is the gold standard for determining this risk.[16-18]

Family members of patients with MEN2 may then undergo genetic testing, and if the test is positive, they may decide upon prophylactic thyroidectomy to prevent the development of MTC, as is recommended for most of these patients.[19] Prospective screening for MEN2A has demonstrated improved survival compared with unscreened subjects.[20] Children of these patients who test *RET* positive or who demonstrate elevated basal calcitonin levels in response to pentagastrin (synthetic gastrin) or calcium should undergo a total thyroidectomy and central neck dissection after the age of 5 years.[21]

Staging

At presentation, approximately 30% of the patients with sporadic MTC and nearly all patients with inherited MTC have bilateral or multifocal disease in the thyroid.[2] Furthermore, approximately 40 to 50% of the patients have clinically detectable cervical lymph node involvement, 15% have symptoms of aerodigestive tract invasion such as dysphagia or hoarseness, and 5% have metastatic spread.[2,22,23] Patients whose primary tumor is multifocal are more likely to have nodal spread, especially for sporadic but also for inherited malignancies.[24]

MTC tumor staging is conducted according to the pathologic tumor-node-metathesis criteria, as adopted by the American Joint Committee on Cancer for 2010, and is based on the primary tumor size, the presence or absence of extrathyroidal invasion, local or regional nodal metastases, and distant metastases.[25]

Treatment

MTC can be cured only through complete resection of the primary tumor and all locoregional or distant metastases. Because the primary tumor is bilateral or multifocal in nearly all inherited and many sporadic MTC, total thyroidectomy is the preferred initial treatment. In addition, because about half of the presentations demonstrate primary tumor spread to local lymph nodes, surgical dissection of the adjacent nodal tissue in the central compartment is recommended, from the hyoid bone to the innominate veins and medial to the jugular veins.[24,26] Sampling biopsy should include the lateral jugular and mediastinal lymph nodes, followed by modified neck and/or mediastinal dissections if positive nodes are discovered.[26] Radical neck dissections (which may cause disfiguration) have not been shown to improve prognosis and are not indicated.[26] For all surgeries, the presence or absence of a pheochromocytoma needs to be determined, because this tumor's physiologic effects can cause mortality or substantial morbidity during surgery and should be removed before the thyroidectomy.

Patients should be monitored following surgery for hypoparathyroidism (hypocalcemia) and damage to the superior or recurrent laryngeal nerves. Thyroxine (T4) therapy should be initiated at an initial dose of 75 to 150 μg and adjusted by measuring serum thyroid-stimulating hormone (TSH) levels. Unlike the treatment for other thyroid malignancies, for MTC treatment, suppression of TSH below euthyroidism is not necessary because the C cells are not TSH responsive and radioactive iodine is not used as these tumors do not concentrate iodine.[27]

The serum calcitonin and CEA levels should be measured 6 months after surgery and compared with all earlier values to determine the presence and activity of the malignancy. Patients who are biochemically cured have 10-year survival rate of 98% compared with 70% for patients with persistently elevated calcitonin levels.[28] The prognosis for patients with persistently elevated hypercalcitoninemia depends on the patient's age and malignant spread at surgery[12,28,29]; for patients younger than 20 years, 10-year survival rate is 98% compared with 41% for patients older than 60 years.[29] Patients with very high calcitonin levels should undergo further repeat imaging, including CT and ultrasound of the neck, CT of the chest and abdomen, PET scan, and radionuclide imaging, as well as meticulous microdissection of all locoregional nodal tissue.

If follow-up reveals residual or recurrent disease, additional treatment modalities including chemotherapy, radiotherapy, and/or hormonal therapy are administered. Doxorubicin is the most frequently employed single chemotherapeutic agent, though patients rarely demonstrate a complete response and fewer than 40% demonstrate a partial response.[30,31] However, some patients who have been treated with combination regimens including dacarbazine have shown a complete response.[32] Early external-beam radiotherapy studies have not demonstrated a survival benefit, but this modality may prolong the period until progression or recurrence.[33,34] It can also be used as palliation for painful bone metastases.

Radioimmunotherapy with radiolabeled ^{131}I anti-CEA monoclonal antibodies has been used owing to the expression of CEA by MTC tumor cells. While this modality has demonstrated some promise, it is not yet widely used. One study of patients with metastatic disease compared this treatment for patients with rapid calcitonin doubling times of less than 2 years versus no treatment for 39 patients with contemporaneous untreated MTC with comparable prognostic factors.[35] The report indicated that this modality improved overall survival from 61 months to 110 months.[35]

For patients with flushing as a paraneoplastic effect, subcutaneous octreotide injection has proven effective in reducing the symptoms for sporadic MTC but has no effect or may paradoxically worsen the flushing for inherited MTC.[36] Secretory diarrhea is treated symptomatically with loperamide and diphenoxylate to lengthen transit time in the colon.

Prognosis and Prognostic Factors

As with most cancers, stage is the most important prognostic factor for MTC, with median survival at 4 years being 100% for stage I, 87% for stage II, 44% for stage III, and 0% for stage IV.[12] Sporadic and MEN2A MTC have demonstrated similar survival rates after controlling for age[37,38]; however, MTC associated with MEN2B has shown worse survival.[37]

Age is a controversial prognostic factor for survival, with conflicting results among studies. While one study has demonstrated major differences in disease-free survival among patients older than 40 years compared with patients less than 40 years (95 vs. 65% at 5 years and 75 vs. 50% at 10 years, respectively),[2] another study has shown no differences in survival after adjusting for baseline mortality factors.[39]

Some additional factors that indicate poor prognosis include

- Increased cellular heterogeneity[40]
- Decreased calcitonin on immunostaining[40]
- Increased procalcitonin/calcitonin ratio[41]
- Increased galectin-3 on immunostaining[42]
- Persistent hypercalcitoninemia after thyroidectomy[12]

Future Developments

Currently, a phase II trial of vandetanib, which is a small molecular inhibitor of tyrosine kinases associated with epidermal growth factor receptor, vascular endothelial growth factor, and RET, is being conducted in patients with metastatic familial MTC. Preliminary reports have shown a 50% rate of durable stable disease and a 17% partial response rate.[43] Another ongoing randomized study is comparing vandetanib with placebo in patients with both sporadic and familial MTC. Other studies are combining radioimmunotherapy with cytotoxic chemotherapy.

References

1. Hundahl SA, Cady B, Cunningham MP, et al. Initial results from a prospective cohort study of 5583 cases of thyroid carcinoma treated in the United States during 1996. U.S. and German Thyroid Cancer Study Group. An American College of Surgeons Commission on Cancer Patient Care Evaluation study. Cancer 2000;89(1):202–217

2. Saad MF, Ordonez NG, Rashid RK, et al. Medullary carcinoma of the thyroid. A study of the clinical features and prognostic factors in 161 patients. Medicine (Baltimore) 1984;63(6):319–342

3. Trupp M, Arenas E, Fainzilber M, et al. Functional receptor for GDNF encoded by the *c-ret* proto-oncogene. Nature 1996;381(6585):785–789

4. Robertson K, Mason I. The GDNF-RET signalling partnership. Trends Genet 1997;13(1):1–3

5. Raue F, Frank-Raue K, Grauer A. Multiple endocrine neoplasia type 2. Clinical features and screening. Endocrinol Metab Clin North Am 1994;23(1):137–156

6. Eng C, Clayton D, Schuffenecker I, et al. The relationship between specific RET proto-oncogene mutations and disease phenotype in multiple endocrine neoplasia type 2. International RET mutation consortium analysis. JAMA 1996;276(19):1575–1579

7. Correia-Deur JEM, Toledo RA, Imazawa AT, et al. Sporadic medullary thyroid carcinoma: clinical data from a university hospital. Clinics (Sao Paulo) 2009;64(5):379–386

8. Eng C, Mulligan LM, Smith DP, et al. Low frequency of germline mutations in the RET proto-oncogene in patients with apparently sporadic medullary thyroid carcinoma. Clin Endocrinol (Oxf) 1995;43(1):123–127

9. Wohllk N, Cote GJ, Bugalho MMJ, et al. Relevance of RET proto-oncogene mutations in sporadic medullary thyroid carcinoma. J Clin Endocrinol Metab 1996;81(10):3740–3745

10. Zedenius J, Wallin G, Hamberger B, Nordenskjöld M, Weber G, Larsson C. Somatic and MEN 2A de novo mutations identified in the RET proto-oncogene by screening of sporadic MTC:s. Hum Mol Genet 1994;3(8):1259–1262

11. Dottorini ME, Assi A, Sironi M, Sangalli G, Spreafico G, Colombo L. Multivariate analysis of patients with medullary thyroid carcinoma. Prognostic significance and impact on treatment of clinical and pathologic variables. Cancer 1996;77(8):1556–1565

12. Gagel RF, Hoff AO, Cote GJ. Medullary thyroid carcinoma. In: Braverman LE, Utiger RD, eds. Werner and Ingbar's Thyroid. 9th ed. Philadelphia: Lippincott Williams & Wilkins; 2005:967

13. Toledo SP, Lourenço DM Jr, Santos MA, Tavares MR, Toledo RA, Correia-Deur JE. Hypercalcitoninemia is not pathognomonic of medullary thyroid carcinoma. Clinics (Sao Paulo) 2009;64(7):699–706

14. Borget I, De Pouvourville G, Schlumberger M. Editorial: Calcitonin determination in patients with nodular thyroid disease. J Clin Endocrinol Metab 2007;92(2):425–427

15. Costante G, Meringolo D, Durante C, et al. Predictive value of serum calcitonin levels for preoperative diagnosis of medullary thyroid carcinoma in a cohort of 5817 consecutive patients with thyroid nodules. J Clin Endocrinol Metab 2007;92(2):450–455

16. Decker RA, Peacock ML, Borst MJ, Sweet JD, Thompson NW. Progress in genetic screening of multiple endocrine neoplasia type 2A: is calcitonin testing obsolete? Surgery 1995;118(2):257–263, discussion 263–264

17. Brandi ML, Gagel RF, Angeli A, et al. Guidelines for diagnosis and therapy of MEN type 1 and type 2. J Clin Endocrinol Metab 2001;86(12):5658–5671

18. Gagel RF. Multiple endocrine neoplasia type II and familial medullary thyroid carcinoma. Impact of genetic screening on management. Cancer Treat Res 1997;89:421–441

19. Wells SA Jr, Chi DD, Toshima K, et al. Predictive DNA testing and prophylactic thyroidectomy in patients at risk for multiple endocrine neoplasia type 2A. Ann Surg 1994;220(3):237–247, discussion 247–250

20. Gagel RF, Tashjian AH Jr, Cummings T, et al. The clinical outcome of prospective screening for multiple endocrine neoplasia type 2a. An 18-year experience. N Engl J Med 1988;318(8):478–484

21. Clark OH. Management of medullary carcinoma of the thyroid: surgery. In: Wartofsky L, ed. Thyroid Cancer – A Comprehensive Guide to Clinical Management, Totowa, NJ: Humana Press; 2000:400

22. Bergholm U, Adami HO, Bergström R, et al. Clinical characteristics in sporadic and familial medullary thyroid carcinoma. A nationwide study of 249 patients in Sweden from 1959 through 1981. Cancer 1989;63(6):1196–1204

23. Scollo C, Baudin E, Travagli JP, et al. Rationale for central and bilateral lymph node dissection in sporadic and hereditary medullary thyroid cancer. J Clin Endocrinol Metab 2003;88(5):2070–2075

24. Machens A, Hauptmann S, Dralle H. Increased risk of lymph node metastasis in multifocal hereditary and sporadic medullary thyroid cancer. World J Surg 2007;31(10):1960–1965

25. American Joint Committee on Cancer. In: Greene, FL, Page, DL, Fleming, ID, et al, eds. Cancer Staging Manual. 7th ed. New York: Springer-Verlag; 2010:87–96

26. Fleming JB, Lee JE, Bouvet M, et al. Surgical strategy for the treatment of medullary thyroid carcinoma. Ann Surg 1999;230(5):697–707

27. Saad MF, Guido JJ, Samaan NA. Radioactive iodine in the treatment of medullary carcinoma of the thyroid. J Clin Endocrinol Metab 1983;57(1):124–128

28. Modigliani E, Cohen R, Campos J-M, et al. Prognostic factors for survival and for biochemical cure in medullary thyroid carcinoma: results in 899 patients. The GETC Study Group. Groupe d'étude des tumeurs à calcitonine. Clin Endocrinol (Oxf) 1998;48(3):265–273

29. Scopsi L, Sampietro G, Boracchi P, et al. Multivariate analysis of prognostic factors in sporadic medullary carcinoma of the thyroid. A retrospective study of 109 consecutive patients. Cancer 1996;78(10):2173–2183

30. Porter AT, Ostrowski MJ. Medullary carcinoma of the thyroid treated by low-dose adriamycin. Br J Clin Pract 1990;44(11):517–518

31. Shimaoka K, Schoenfeld DA, DeWys WD, Creech RH, DeConti R. A randomized trial of doxorubicin versus doxorubicin plus cisplatin in patients with advanced thyroid carcinoma. Cancer 1985;56(9):2155–2160

32. Petursson SR. Metastatic medullary thyroid carcinoma. Complete response to combination chemotherapy with dacarbazine and 5-fluorouracil. Cancer 1988;62(9):1899–1903

33. Samaan NA, Schultz PN, Hickey RC. Medullary thyroid carcinoma: prognosis of familial versus sporadic disease and the role of radiotherapy. J Clin Endocrinol Metab 1988;67(4):801–805

34. Brierley J, Tsang R, Simpson WJ, Gospodarowicz M, Sutcliffe S, Panzarella T. Medullary thyroid cancer: analyses of survival and prognostic factors and the role of radiation therapy in local control. Thyroid 1996;6(4):305–310

35. Chatal JF, Campion L, Kraeber-Bodéré F, et al; French Endocrine Tumor Group. Survival improvement in patients with medullary thyroid carcinoma who undergo pretargeted anti-carcinoembryonic-antigen radioimmunotherapy: a collaborative study with the French Endocrine Tumor Group. J Clin Oncol 2006;24(11):1705–1711

36. Modigliani E, Guliana JM, Maroni M, et al. Effects of subcutaneous administration of sandostatin (SMS 201.995) in 18 cases of thyroid medullary cancer. Ann Endocrinol (Paris) 1989;50:484–488

37. O'Riordain DS, O'Brien T, Weaver AL, et al. Medullary thyroid carcinoma in multiple endocrine neoplasia types 2A and 2B. Surgery 1994;116(6):1017–1023

38. Samaan NA, Schultz PN, Hickey RC. Medullary thyroid carcinoma: prognosis of familial versus sporadic disease and the role of radiotherapy. J Clin Endocrinol Metab 1988;67(4):801–805

39. de Groot JW, Plukker JT, Wolffenbuttel BH, Wiggers T, Sluiter WJ, Links TP. Determinants of life expectancy in medullary thyroid cancer: age does not matter. Clin Endocrinol (Oxf) 2006;65(6):729–736

40. Lippman SM, Mendelsohn G, Trump DL, Wells SA Jr, Baylin SB. The prognostic and biological significance of cellular heterogeneity in medullary thyroid carcinoma: a study of calcitonin, l-dopa decarboxylase, and histaminase. J Clin Endocrinol Metab 1982;54(2):233–240

41. Walter MA, Meier C, Radimerski T, et al. Procalcitonin levels predict clinical course and progression-free survival in patients with medullary thyroid cancer. Cancer 2010;116(1):31–40

42. Faggiano A, Talbot M, Lacroix L, et al. Differential expression of galectin-3 in medullary thyroid carcinoma and C-cell hyperplasia. Clin Endocrinol (Oxf) 2002;57(6):813–819

43. Wells SA, Gosnell JE, Gagel RF, et al. Vandetanib in metastatic hereditary medullary thyroid cancer: Follow-up results of an open-label phase II trial. J Clin Oncol 2007;25(Suppl 18):Abstract no. 6018

44. Mehdi G, Maheshwari V, Ansari HA, Sadaf L, Khan MA. FNAC diagnosis of medullary carcinoma thyroid: a report of three cases with review of literature. J Cytol 2010;27(2):66–68

45. Gorospe EC, Badamas J. Acute liver failure secondary to metastatic medullary thyroid cancer. Case Reports in Hepatology 2011 doi:10.1155/2011/603757

7 Anaplastic Carcinoma of the Thyroid

Ilana Doweck and Ohad Ronen

Core Messages

- Anaplastic carcinoma of the thyroid (ACT) is one of the most aggressive human malignancies today and is responsible for a disproportionate number of deaths related to thyroid cancer.

- Data support a transformation pathway of a well-differentiated thyroid cancer into ACT.

- Because of its rare occurrence and rapid fatal outcome, clinical trials that evaluate ACT therapies are particularly challenging to carry out, and thus demonstrate limited results.

- ACT therapy includes surgery, radiotherapy, and chemotherapy and should be managed within a multidisciplinary setting that includes a palliative support team.

- Promising novel molecular-targeted therapies are being investigated.

Fortunately enough anaplastic carcinoma of the thyroid (ACT) is not a very frequent tumor as it is one of the most deadly cancers known. With a median survival period of just a few months from diagnosis,[1] and its rapidly fatal course, ACT has a grim prognosis. Case reports of long-term survivors can be found in the literature, but in every such case the diagnosis should be in doubt.[2] Most patients have either palpable or positive lymph nodes on imaging when diagnosed.[3] Because patients are doomed to die of asphyxiation if left untreated, a tracheotomy is done in all patients along the course of the disease, which provides palliation. In a minority of patients, some form of surgery to remove the tumor can be considered if the tumor is diagnosed at a resectable stage.[4] Radiotherapy (RT) is considered for palliation. Several chemotherapy regimens are being tested, but none has been found to drastically change the course of this fatal disease. Recent investigational and novel therapies will be reviewed.

Epidemiology

An estimated 37,200 new cases of thyroid cancer occur annually in the United States according to the Surveillance, Epidemiology, and End Results (SEER) program 2009 report.[5] Thyroid cancers account for 2.5% of all neoplasms, and ACT accounts for 1 to 2% of all thyroid cancers.[5] Nevertheless, the majority of the 1630 deaths from thyroid cancer expected annually in the United States are related to ACT.[5] It seems that the incidence of thyroid cancer has been increasing while that of ACT has been declining in recent years.[6] One possible explanation for this observed trend can be the increased use of immunohistochemistry (IHC) staining for pathology diagnosis in undifferentiated tumors.[7] Another explanation

is better control of well-differentiated thyroid cancers (WDTCs), which might dedifferentiate into ACT.[8] Also, improvement in socioeconomic status and improvement in the content of iodine in the diet in areas where endemic goiter is common could explain this reduction in ACT incidence.[9]

Clinical Features

ACT is usually diagnosed rather late in life, during the sixth to seventh decade.[1,10] As with other thyroid cancers, women have up to a threefold higher tendency for ACT.[11] A rapidly growing neck mass that is firm and fixed to the surrounding tissues is the most common presenting symptom, is seen in the vast majority of patients,[12] and can even cause superior vena cava syndrome.[13] Pain can result from intralesion hemorrhage and sudden enlargement of the neck mass. The neck mass can span from a small lesion of a few centimeters to an enormous 20-cm mass.[1] Because of its size and its tendency to penetrate and involve surrounding tissues (trachea, larynx, recurrent laryngeal nerves, pharynx, upper esophagus, and strap muscles) in the majority of patients,[12] patients often have related signs and symptoms either at presentation or later during the course of the disease (**Fig. 7.1**). These can be respiratory-related signs and symptoms of dyspnea, hoarseness, stridor, and tachypnea or upper digestive tract-related symptoms of progressive dysphagia, first to solids and then to liquids (**Table 7.1**). Airway management is the most critical issue in patients who present with anaplastic thyroid cancer and initial airway distress.[14] Thirty to 60% of the patients can have metastasis to cervical lymph nodes,[1,15] and nearly half of the patients

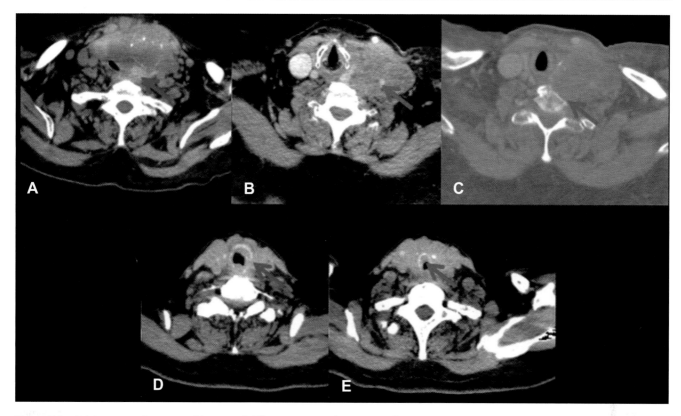

Figure 7.1 Axial computed tomographic scans of different patients showing anaplastic carcinoma of the thyroid arising in the left thyroid lobe, (A) compressing the trachea and invading the esophagus, (B) encasing the carotid artery, (C) eroding the vertebra, and (D) penetrating and destroying the cricoid and (E) the tracheal rings.

will have metastatic spread of disease when diagnosed. Furthermore, during the course of the disease, most patients will develop distant metastasis. The most frequent site for distant metastasis is the lungs, followed by the brain and bones.[1] Thyrotoxicosis is a rare feature of ACT.[16]

Pathology

Before the era of IHC, the diagnosis of ACT was done mainly with the commonly used hematoxylin-eosin stains (**Fig. 7.2**). Based on the patterns of cells seen, several variants of ACT were described—spindle cell, giant cell, squamoid, insular

Table 7.1 Sign and Symptoms of Anaplastic Carcinoma of the Thyroid

Rapidly growing neck mass
Fixed, firm, possibly painful neck mass
Dyspnea
Stridor
Hoarseness
Vocal cord paresis or paralysis
Progressive dysphagia
Lymph node neck metastasis

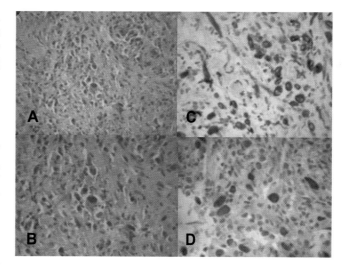

Figure 7.2 Representative images of anaplastic carcinoma of the thyroid are shown at a magnification of (A) ×40 and (B–D) ×100. (A, B) The tumor is composed of highly pleomorphic cells with mitotic figures, apoptotic bodies, and focal necrosis under hematoxylin and eosin stain. (C) The tumor has positive immunohistochemistry (IHC) staining for pankeratin, and (D) it is focally positive for thyroid transcription factor-1 IHC staining. These findings are compatible with anaplastic carcinoma from thyroid origin.

carcinoma, carcinosarcoma, paucicellular, pure squamous cell carcinoma, and small cell. The couple of latter variants carry a poorer prognosis.[17] In all variants, characteristics of rapid proliferation and high grade can be found. Large areas of necrosis, hemorrhage, and invasiveness can be seen under low magnification, and a high mitotic activity, a high tumor proliferative index, and a low apoptotic rate can be seen under higher magnification.[18] During the past few decades, an increased use of IHC techniques has helped more reliably differentiate these tumors from lymphoma, sarcoma, and poorly differentiated medullary thyroid carcinoma.[19] Among the available IHC stains, a battery that includes neuron-specific enolase, chromogranin, calcitonin, vimentin, keratin, α-1 chemotrypsin, desmin, carcinoembryonic antigen, anticytokeratin, and thyroglobulin should be considered. Whenever a patient has a clinical course that is exceeding the expected prognosis, one should question the diagnosis and reanalyze the pathologic examination. The insular variant is thought to derive from a WDTC via a mechanism of *p53* overexpression.[20] Morphologically, solid clusters (insulae) containing a variable number of follicles, high mitotic activity, capsular and vessel invasion, and necrosis lead to the formation of preepitheliomatous patterns, which can be found in 3% of ACT cases.[21] ACT is characterized by markedly reduced lymphocyte/dentritic cell infiltrates, which suggests a protective role of dentritic cells and infiltrating lymphocytes against thyroid tumors.[22] Thyroid cancers are infiltrated with tumor-associated macrophages that may facilitate tumor progression.[23]

Pathogenesis

As described in the previous paragraph, data exist to support a transformation pathway of a WDTC into ACT.[24] Disturbances in the balance between apoptosis and proliferation, in favor of the latter, occur gradually during the progression of malignancy in thyroid tumors.[25] Anaplastic transformation may occur not only in primary tumors but also in metastatic lymph nodes.[26] Most cases, though, might have a de-novo pathogenesis. A history of a known goiter or WDTC that recently grew in an elderly patient should initiate an investigation to rule out anaplastic transformation.[27] There is other evidence that suggests a transformation etiology. The incidence of ACT is higher in areas endemic for goiter and in patients with previously treated WDTC.[28] Furthermore, synchronous diagnosis of WDTC and ACT is common.[29] There are studies that described small islands of WDTC in ACT specimens, and some even reported a transition spectrum of WDTC and ACT on the same slide. Insular and tall cell types of papillary thyroid cancer that are notorious for their aggressive biologic course are more frequently associated with ACT. They can be seen, therefore, as an intermediate form of cells between the well-differentiated papillary carcinoma and the poorly differentiated ACT.[21] Poorly differentiated thyroid carcinomas represent an intermediate entity in the progression of WDTC to ACT.[30]

Review of the literature identified potential new strategies for treating this highly lethal cancer. In studies involving anaplastic cell lines in vitro, it has been shown that the loss of p53 or the presence of abnormal p53 can be responsible for the transformation of WDTC cells to ACT.[31] Knockdown of mutant p53 has been shown to reduce cell viability and exert antitumor activity equivalent to high doses of several chemotherapeutic agents, via the induction of apoptosis.[32] Impairment of p53-mediated repression results in increased GLUT1 and p63 expression, which probably reflects the differential regulation of hypoxia-responsive pathways and basal/stem cell regulatory pathways.[33] In radiation-induced thyroid cancers, the highest frequency of RET amplification-positive cells was observed among patients with ACT with a strong p53 immunoreactivity.[34] FOXA1, a mammalian endodermal transcription factor, may be an important oncogene in thyroid tumorigenesis.[35] In recently published articles, it was shown that an analysis of distinct sets of micro-RNAs (miRNAs) was used as a tool to distinguish poorly differentiated thyroid carcinoma and suggested that a lack of deregulation of some miRNAs may select a subset of WDTC prone to dedifferentiate.[36] BRaf mutations, which belong to the Raf family of serine/threonine kinase, have a central role in the regulation of cell growth, cell division, and cell proliferation and appear to be involved in the tumorigenesis of a subset of ACTs and the majority of lymph node metastases.[37] Sorafenib, a multikinase inhibitor of the BRaf, vascular endothelial growth factor receptor-2, and platelet-derived growth factor receptor-β kinase have been shown to decrease tumor growth and angiogenesis in an orthotopic model of ACT.[38] Anaplastic transformation of thyroid cells is accompanied by the overexpression of a cell proliferation/genetic instability-related gene cluster that includes pololike kinase 1.[39] Apolipoprotein E, known to play a role in cholesterol transport and metabolism, was found to be one of the typical biological characteristics of anaplastic thyroid carcinoma.[40] Results of a recent study demonstrated that gain of chromosome 20 is important in the pathogenesis of ACT and/or progression of differentiated thyroid cancers to ACT in both primary tumors and cell lines.[41] It has been suggested that derangement of the E-cadherin/catenin complex is associated with the transformation of differentiated into anaplastic thyroid carcinoma,[42] as well as ANXA1 expression.[43] An altered expression of serum response factor, a transcription factor of the MADS box family in papillary carcinoma cells, may play an important role in WDTC carcinogenesis and progression.[44] Aberrant tumor suppressor activity and increased proliferative activity were found to be most prevalent in ACT, followed by poorly differentiated thyroid carcinomas and WDTC.[45] Loss of *CBX7* gene expression correlates with a highly malignant phenotype in patients with thyroid cancer.[46] Annexin II and S100A10, a member of the S100 family that forms a heterotetramer with annexin IIH, promote carcinoma invasion and metastasis by plasminogen activation and contribute to the aggressive characteristics of anaplastic carcinoma.[47]

There is evidence to support the observation that estrogen is an important factor in the development of thyroid cancer. The subcellular localization of estrogen receptor α and β may account for the different pathogenesis of thyroid papillary and anaplastic cancers.[48]

The exact mechanisms that are involved in the transformation of WDTC to ACT are not fully understood and need further elucidation. With the recent increased knowledge of the many critical genes and proteins affected in ACT, and the extensive array of targeted therapies being developed for patients with cancer, there are new opportunities to design clinical trials based on tumor molecular profiling and preclinical studies of potentially synergistic combinatorial novel therapies.

Diagnosis

As with other thyroid masses, clinical examination and cytologic specimen acquired through fine-needle aspiration (FNA) are usually the first steps taken and are usually sufficient for diagnosis. A typical clinical presentation, as described above, warrants FNA examination, which can be reliable in nearly 90% of the patients.[49] As mentioned previously, IHC staining must be done to confirm the diagnosis and to suggest other tumors with a curable option.[50] MIB-1 is an antibody against K_i-67, which is a protein expressed in proliferating cells, and is a molecular marker already used in cytological evaluation. MIB-1 index was significantly higher in ACT than in other thyroid cancer types.[51] There is a rare report of implantation of anaplastic thyroid carcinoma along the track of FNA.[52] A large-bore needle biopsy or an open incisional biopsy might be indicated as further IHC staining is needed. In patients with a history of WDTC who develop a rapidly growing mass elsewhere, a possibility of metastatic WDTC with anaplastic transformation must be considered, which can also be diagnosed by FNA biopsy.[53] A preoperative imaging method such as computed tomography scan with intravenous contrast media can be considered to better understand the sometimes difficult anatomy and lack of anatomic and surgical landmarks due to the compressive and invasiveness characteristics of the tumor. In an elderly patient presenting with a large necrotic thyroid mass of low attenuation, anaplastic carcinoma should be included in differential diagnosis.[54] Riedel thyroiditis, a rare thyroid disease characterized by dense fibrous tissues that replace the thyroid gland and invade the adjacent structures, can mimic ACT.[55] In a recently published article, it was reported that ACT demonstrates intense uptake on 18F-fluorodeoxyglucose positron emission tomography (PET) images. In 50% of the patients, the medical records reported a direct impact of PET findings on the management of the patient, relative to other imaging modalities.[56]

A panel of internationally recognized thyroid pathologists held a consensus meeting in Turin, Italy, in 2007. They developed the following consensus diagnostic criteria for poorly differentiated thyroid carcinomas: (1) presence of a solid/trabecular/insular pattern of growth; (2) absence of the conventional nuclear features of papillary carcinoma; and (3) presence of at least one of the following features: convoluted nuclei, mitotic activity ≥ 3 × 10 high power field, and tumor necrosis.[57]

Prognostic Factors and Clinical Course

All ACTs are considered T4 tumors, stratified to T4a, which is intrathyroidal anaplastic carcinoma, and T4b, which is anaplastic carcinoma with gross extrathyroid extension. Therefore, all anaplastic carcinomas are considered Stage IV, in which Stage IVA describes intrathyroidal anaplastic carcinoma, any N, M0; Stage IVB includes anaplastic carcinoma with extrathyroid extension, any N, M0; and stage IVC includes patients with distant metastasis (M1).[58] Although ACT is staged according to the American Joint Committee on Cancer as stage IV, regardless of other prognostic features, several risk factors have been described. Among the favorable prognostic factors are younger age (< 60 or 75 years), female sex (although in several studies it was found to carry an unfavorable prognosis),[59] smaller tumors, no capsular invasion, lack of metastatic disease, and lesser extent of disease.[1,60] The latter defines the tumor as either stage IVA, when the tumor is resectable, or stage IVB, unresectable ACTs. Incidentally detected ACTs are rare, and it is unclear whether they confer a better prognosis.[61] Extensive surgical treatment is recommended for patients with stage IVA tumors, and palliative care is appropriate for patients with stage IVC tumors.[4] For patients with stage IVB, surgical treatment as a primary therapy is appropriate only when curative resection of the tumor is expected.[4] Aneuploidy and high S-phase fraction were shown to be biomarkers of poor clinical outcome in poorly differentiated thyroid carcinoma and ACT.[62] Leukocytosis, hypoalbuminemia, and hypothyroxinemia were reported as poor prognostic indicators.

Management of Anaplastic Carcinoma of the Thyroid

Despite aggressive multimodalty therapy including surgery, radiation, and chemotherapy, there is no effective systemic treatment for ACT. Because of the rarity of the disease, its aggressiveness, and lack of prospective clinical trials, the evidence in the literature emerges from retrospective studies. Treatment options include surgery, RT (external beam), chemotherapy, combined therapy, and investigational clinical trials. Often, a single modality is not effective for ACT. Unfortunately, there are no data to support the efficacy of combined modality treatment to prolong survival or improve the quality of life of patients with ACT, and the outcome is still very poor.

Surgery

Surgical treatment of local disease offers the best opportunity for prolonged survival if the tumor is intrathyroidal.[12]

However, the role of surgery in ACT is controversial. A selected subset of patients with small ACT that is confined to the thyroid gland may benefit from surgical intervention and complete resection of gross disease.[63] When used alone, surgery is seldom adequate to achieve overall control of the disease, but surgery combined with RT or chemotherapy may improve local control. Junor el al[64] found that total or partial thyroidectomy was associated with increased survival. This association was most marked for patients presenting without dyspnea. Betka et al[65] noted that there was no difference in the survival of patients who were treated with primary surgery or primary chemotherapy and/or RT. However, the best results were obtained in patients in whom the tumor was surgically removed after primary chemotherapy and RT. Brignardello et al[4] reported the outcome of 30 patients with ACT. Patients were treated by surgery either before or followed by chemoradiotherapy or chemotherapy alone. Multivariate analysis showed that maximal debulking followed by adjuvant chemoradiotherapy was the only treatment that modified the survival of patients with ACT. Chen et al[60] found that treatment with surgery plus or minus RT was statistically significant as prognostic for survival on multivariate analysis. Swaak-Kragten et al[10] reported that locoregional control was significantly higher in patients who had undergone resection or chemoradiation, with best results for patients who underwent both. However, the survival benefit of patients who had complete response (CR) remained borderline. Three patients survived for more than 5 years; all had undergone surgical resection and chemoradiation. Unfortunately, more than 70% of the patients present with locally aggressive disease in which the tumor infiltrates surrounding tissues such as trachea, esophagus, and larynx and encases major blood vessels,[12] or presents with metastatic disease. The consensus on the surgical treatment of ACT recommends complete surgical resection whenever possible in selected patients,[66] and only if postoperative morbidity is low. Resection of vital structures such as the larynx or the esophagus should be avoided. In this case, there is a high rate of local recurrence despite extensive surgical resection due to the aggressive nature of the tumor,[63] and neither the extent of surgery nor the completeness of resection has a significant effect on survival.[29]

Lateral neck dissection is indicated whenever a complete resection is possible and all gross tumor is removed.

Palliative surgical intervention may be required for patients with ACT who present with airway distress. Usually, resection is not possible and tracheotomy is required to avoid asphyxia. Sometimes, immediate airway control may require debulking of tumor. Cricothyrotomy may be helpful in avoiding acute airway catastrophe.[29] Prophylactic tracheotomy is not indicated because data exist to support that it decreases the survival of patients with ACT because postoperative external RT often could not be administered or was delayed because of local complications of the tracheotomy.[67]

Radiotherapy

RT can be given with a curative or palliative intent, as neoadjuvant or adjuvant therapy to surgery, or in combination with chemotherapeutic drugs. Several studies were able to show statistically significant differences in local control and even in survival between groups who were treated with different radiation protocols, yet the clinical significance of those studies is debatable because no major breakthrough was achieved and median survival improved by only a few months. Nevertheless, because most patients present with a nonresectable disease, due to its tendency to invade neighboring critical structures, RT remains a cornerstone treatment modality in ACT. Because for most patients survival is not altered, when considering RT as a treatment modality in this region and in reviewing studies one should always keep in mind the potential toxicity of radiation, including mucositis of the pharynx, esophagus, trachea, and myelopathy.

Studies examining the timing of RT, the total dose given, the number of fractionation, and modern radiation delivery methods such as three-dimensionally guided radiation therapy (3DRT) and intensity-modulated radiation therapy (IMRT) are described.

Adjuvant RT might be more effective if surgical debulking is achieved.[64] A total radiation dose greater than 30 Gy or even 45 Gy was shown to improve survival.[10,68,69] RT can be given in hyperfractionated doses to address the aggressive doubling time nature of this tumor, yet a recent study described little benefit with the use of this strategy.[70,71] Another study was able to demonstrate improved local control and reduce treatment time.[72] Modern radiation delivery methods try to overcome the limitations caused by the tumor's challenging anatomic location.[73] In an article published by the MD Anderson group in Texas,[74] 53 patients were treated with either 3DRT or IMRT with a median radiation dose of 55 Gy; 74% received concomitant chemotherapy, yet no difference in outcome was achieved compared with historical results.

Chemotherapy

Distant metastasis is very common among patients with ACT at the time of presentation. Kebebew et al[75] reported distant metastasis at the time of presentation in 43% of 516 patients with ACT from SEER analysis. Therefore, systemic chemotherapy was given to patients with ACT; however, it was found that none of the systemic chemotherapy regimens prevented the poor outcome and death of the patients, although the survival period was prolonged for those who responded to treatment, usually by several months.

Doxorubicin has been the most common chemotherapy agent used, either alone or in combination with other antineoplastic agents including cisplatin, bleomycin, vincristine, and melphalan. Doxorubicin, as a single agent, has the most effect on ACT, with 5 to 22% partial response (PR) in several studies.[76-79] Other single agents, such as cisplatin, bleomycin, and etoposide (VP-16), were less effective.[77,80]

Combined chemotherapy showed a slightly improved response. Doxorubicin, 60 mg/m^2 intravenously every 3 weeks, given as a single agent to 21 patients with ACT-induced 5% (1 patient) PR compared with 34% overall response (6 patients, 3 with CR and 3 with PR) for 18 patients treated with a combination of doxorubicin (60 mg/m^2 intravenously every 3 weeks) and cisplatin (40 mg/m^2 every 3 weeks). Two of these patients survived for 41 and 34 months.[79] Combining other antineoplastic agents such as bleomycin[81] to this protocol, protocols including doxorubicin, vincristine, and bleomycin, or other combined chemotherapy regimens did not improve the overall response rate.[13]

Newer protocols with promising results used paclitaxel, given as a single agent either as the only treatment or as induction chemotherapy before surgery and RT. Ain et al[82] reported a total response rate of 53% in 19 patients treated with a 96-hour infusion of paclitaxel every 3 weeks for one to six cycles. However, only one patient had a CR, whereas nine patients had a PR. The median survival for the responder was 32 weeks and for nonresponders was only 7 weeks. Higashiyama et al[83] performed induction chemotherapy by giving paclitaxel on a weekly basis to patients with IVB (nine patients) and IVC (four patients) disease. The response rate was 33% for patients with stage IVB disease and 25% for patients with stage IVC disease. Curative surgery and adjuvant therapy were performed in four of the patients with stage IVB disease, and all four were alive and free of disease 32 months after treatment. Survival of patients with stage IVB disease treated with induction paclitaxel was significantly better compared with historical data of similar patients' group.

Combined Therapy

The lack of effective chemotherapy as well as the failure of each single modality in the management of ACT has led to the application of multimodality regimens, combining surgery, RT, and chemotherapy. Multimodal treatment varied between protocols that applied surgery (when feasible) followed by adjuvant chemoradiotherapy or regimens that consist of neoadjuvant RT combined with chemotherapy (as radiosensitizing agent), followed by surgery (when possible), or chemoradiotherapy for unresectable disease (**Table 7.2**). The most common chemotherapy agent used was doxorubicin, mainly as a radiosensitizer. However, there was no standardized protocol in selecting patients for chemotherapy or RT, and conflicting data exist regarding the results of these protocols.

A 50-year experience of the Mayo Clinic with 134 patients with ACT was reported by McIver et al,[84] in which neither the extent of resection nor postoperative RT or multimodal therapy including surgery, chemotherapy (doxorubicin used for radiosensitization), and RT improved survival.

On the other hand, De Crevoisier et al[85] reported that CR was achieved in 19 of the 30 patients treated with surgery either before or after chemoradiotherapy including twice daily RT 1.25 Gy for a total dose of 40 Gy and six cycles of

doxorubicin. In a median follow-up of 45 months, 7 patients were alive, with 6 of them having complete tumor resection.

Several studies have reported increased survival of patients treated by surgery followed by chemoradiotherapy. Haigh et al[63] found that complete resection of ACT with adjuvant chemotherapy and irradiation was associated with prolonged survival. Agents used for chemotherapy usually were based on doxorubicin, but paclitaxel, cisplatin, carboplatinum, etoposide (VP-16), cyclophosphamide, melphalan, and bleomycin were also used. External beam radiation was administered to the neck or the mediastinum, with the total doses ranging from 45 to 75 Gy. Brignardello et al[4] showed that maximal debulking of ATC followed by adjuvant chemoradiotherapy was the only treatment that improved the survival of patients with ACT compared with chemoradiotherapy followed by surgery or chemotherapy alone. Chang et al[86] found that there was a small improvement in the survival of patients who had complete excision of ACT followed by aggressive multimodality therapy. Heron et al[87] showed in a retrospective study that patients who were treated with surgery and hyperfractionated RT in conjunction with chemotherapy had long-term survival (> 2 years).

On the other hand, there are few studies showing that treatment with chemoradiotherapy before surgery has improved survival. Besic et al[88] reported the treatment results of 79 patients with ACT treated either by primary surgery (26 patients) or by primary chemotherapy and/or RT (53 patients) including 12 patients in whom surgery was performed after chemotherapy or RT. Although the patients in the second group had larger tumors, the best results were obtained in patients whose tumor was surgically removed after primary chemotherapy and RT. Busnardo et al[89] found that only a few patients respond to chemotherapy; however, combined therapy may provide some benefit in patients with ACT, and preoperative chemotherapy and RT may enhance surgical resectability of the primary tumor.

Promising data emerge from newer protocols, including hyperfractionation RT as well as using docetaxel combined with doxorubicin. In the only prospective study using multimodality treatment for ACT, Tennvall et al[72] reported on 55 patients treated with a multimodality regimen consisting of hyperfractionation RT combined with doxorubicin, followed by surgery when feasible. The RT dose varied during the years, from 1 Gy × 2/d until 1988 to 1.3 Gy × 2/d between 1989 and 1992 and 1.6 Gy × 2/d thereafter, to a total dose of 46 Gy. Surgery was possible in 40 patients. Only 13 patients died of local failure. Five patients (9%) survived more than 2 years, and 60% of the patients had no sign of local recurrence, with favorable results in the third group. Foote et al[90] reported enhanced survival in 10 patients with locoregionally confined ACT treated with surgery (where feasible), IMRT, and radiosensitizing + adjuvant chemotherapy including docetaxel and doxorubicin. Five patients (50%) were alive and cancer free at a median follow-up of 44 months (range, 32 to 89 months). Although the protocol improved survival in patients with stage IVA and IVB disease, the benefit in

Table 7.2 Multimodality Therapy for Anaplastic Carcinoma of the Thyroid

Author/Reference	Protocol	No. of Patients	Response Rate	Median Survival	Prolonged Survival
Ain et al[82]	Induction paclitaxel followed by surgery and EBRT	19	10 (1 CR, 9 PR) (53%)	24 wk (responder 32 wk, nonresponder 7 wk)	
McIver et al[84]	Surgery ± EBRT Palliative EBRT or CHT	121		3 mo	10 patients > 1 y (8%)
	Surgery followed by EBRT and doxorubicin	13		3 mo	3 patients > 1 y (23%)
Besic et al[88]	Surgery followed by EBRT and CHT (varied)	26		7 mo	2 patients > 100 mo
	EBRT and CHT or CHT (varied)	53		6 mo	1 patient > 102 mo
	EBRT and CHT followed by surgery	12 out of 53		14.5 mo	1 patient > 31 mo
Haigh et al[63]	Surgery ± EBRT ± CHT (varied)	33		3.8 mo	5 patients > 2 y
Tennvall et al[72]	EBRT (hyperfractionation) + doxorubicin followed by surgery	55	60%	2–4.5 mo	5 patients > 2 y
De Crevoisier et al[85]	Surgery before/after chemoradiotherapy (doxorubicin + hyperfractionation)	30	19 (63%)	10 mo	7 patients > 45 mo
Brignardello et al[4]	Surgery followed by EBRT and CHT (doxorubicin + cisplatin) Adjuvant CHT (doxorubicin + cisplatin)	17	12 (70%)	3.9 mo	5 patients > 1 y
	Nonoperable: EBRT and CHT (doxorubicin + cisplatin) followed by surgery and adjuvant CHT (doxorubicin + cisplatin)	5	1 CR (20%)		1 patient NED at 34 mo
	CHT only	5 patients		3.2 mo	
Higashiyama et al[83]	Induction paclitaxel, surgery and adjuvant therapy ± EBRT	9, stage IVB	3 (1 CR, 2 PR) (33%)	6 mo	4 patients > 32 mo
		4, stage IVC	1 PR (25%)	2 mo	None
Troch et al[91]	EBRT + CHT (docetaxel)	6	4 CR, 2 PR	21.5 mo	5 patients > 21 mo
Foote et al[90]	Surgery, IMRT and CHT (docetaxel + doxorubicin) Adjuvant CHT (docetaxel + doxorubicin)	10, stage IVA and IVB	7 (70%)	44 mo	5 patients > 44 mo

EBRT, external beam radiotherapy; CR, complete response; PR, partial response; wk, weeks; y, year(s); CHT, chemotherapy; mo, months, NED, no evidence of disease; IMRT, intensity-modulated radiation therapy.

patients with metastatic disease remains uncertain. Troch et al[91] treated six patients with ACT with standard external beam radiation of 60 Gy in 30 fractions along with docetaxel 100 mg every 3 weeks for a total of six cycles. With a median follow-up of 21 months, five patients were alive.

Combined modality treatments including surgery and concomitant chemoradiotherapy based on single-institution trials and retrospective reviews from the past decade are presented in **Table 7.2**. As shown, the last few studies indicate, although in highly selected patients, that multimodality treatment including chemotherapy, RT, and surgery, regardless of the sequence of treatment, may further improve the outcome of patients with this dismal disease.

Investigational/Novel Therapies

The poor outcome of patients with current treatment and the new basic science discoveries of the pathogenesis mechanisms of this cancer have led many researchers to investigate new drugs that hopefully will make a breakthrough in curing these patients. It should be stated though that given the rarity of ACT and the number of agents being investigated, patients should be enrolled in a prospective trial. Some of the agents are showing promising results. As explained earlier, the dominant pathogenesis theory is that ACT evolves from WDTC through multiple genetic alterations.[92] This notion is behind the tendency to target multiple pathways with several drugs concomitantly. We will probably have to tailor treatment protocols in a personalized medicine approach in accordance with the precise set of mutations diagnosed for each and every patient.[93]

One very promising group of molecular-targeted agents is the kinase inhibitors (vandetanib, erlotinib, and gefitinib) being investigated in phase I, II, and III clinical trials.[94,95] Another promising group of agents is the antiangiogenic drugs (bevacizumab, sorafanib, and sunitinib), which affect one of the hallmark features of ACT.[96]

As with another notoriously highly resistant malignant melanoma, attacking ACT through the immune system might show good results. The use of dentritic cells or cytotoxic T cells has a relatively low toxicity profile while specifically targeting the cancer cells.[73]

A fascinating research field is reinducing iodine uptake through the expression of the natrium iodide symporter protein. This will hopefully enable clinicians target metastatic disease anywhere in the body as well as primary disease and recurrences with minimal side effects as in WDTC.

A plethora of other agents are available for research and involve the serine/threonine protein kinases, transcription factors such as p53 and NF-κB, and agents that target nucleic acids such as miRNA and viral oncolytic therapy.[97]

Palliative Care

The multidisciplinary team must incorporate early in the treatment of a patient with ACT an overall support for the patient that will include managing symptoms of pain, nausea, anxiety, fatigue, dyspnea, depression, and decreased appetite. Early tracheotomy and/or gastrostomy should be considered to improve swallowing and breathing. The patient and the family should be offered emotional and psychological support in addition to medical support. Ideally, a palliative care team, consisting of medical specialists, nurses, pharmacists, a social worker, physical and occupational therapists, a chaplain, and an ethics consultant, should be available. Given the overall bleak prognosis and extremely short survival time, careful attention to the extent of treatment should be given.

Conclusions

ACT is an aggressive tumor that nearly always has spread systemically by the time of diagnosis or shortly thereafter. ACT probably arises from the dedifferentiation of previous WDTC. On rare occasions, ACT may be diagnosed early when the tumor is small and intrathyroidal and is cured by surgical resection. Patients with ACT should be managed within a multidisciplinary setting, and enrollment in clinical trials is highly encouraged. Patients with inoperable disease at diagnosis should be considered for treatment with combined chemotherapy and RT, providing palliation and minimal survival benefit. Surgical resection should be considered in those who have a good response to treatment. In future, the identification of patients who are likely to benefit from each therapeutic option will be important. There is an ongoing need to develop a new approach to the treatment of patients with ACT with the aim to improve local control while minimizing the impact on quality of life.

Clinical Pearls

- Whenever a patient has a clinical course that is exceeding the expected prognosis, one should question the diagnosis and reanalyze the pathologic examination by using immunohistochemical staining at the least.

- When a patient with well-differentiated thyroid cancer has signs, symptoms, or imaging features of an aggressive characteristic, one should exclude the diagnosis of an anaplastic carcinoma of the thyroid.

- Surgical resection should be considered only in selected patients. Because adjuvant therapy is recommended and the tumor is likely to recur both locally and at distant sites, this modality is used only when the expected morbidity is acceptable.

- Tracheotomy should be done along the course of the disease and should be discussed with the patient as early as possible to avoid the risk of suffocation.

References

1. Kim TY, Kim KW, Jung TS, et al. Prognostic factors for Korean patients with anaplastic thyroid carcinoma. Head Neck 2007;29(8):765–772

2. Pichardo-Lowden A, Durvesh S, Douglas S, Todd W, Bruno M, Goldenberg D. Anaplastic thyroid carcinoma in a young woman: a rare case of survival. Thyroid 2009;19(7):775–779

3. Agrawal S, Rao RS, Parikh DM, Parikh HK, Borges AM, Sampat MB. Histologic trends in thyroid cancer 1969-1993: a clinico-pathologic analysis of the relative proportion of anaplastic carcinoma of the thyroid. J Surg Oncol 1996;63(4):251–255

4. Brignardello E, Gallo M, Baldi I, et al. Anaplastic thyroid carcinoma: clinical outcome of 30 consecutive patients referred to a single institution in the past 5 years. Eur J Endocrinol 2007;156(4):425–430

5. Jemal A, Siegel R, Ward E, Hao Y, Xu J, Thun MJ. Cancer statistics, 2009. CA Cancer J Clin 2009;59(4):225–249

6. Netea-Maier RT, Aben KK, Casparie MK, et al Trends in incidence and mortality of thyroid carcinoma in The Netherlands between 1989 and 2003: correlation with thyroid fine-needle aspiration cytology and thyroid surgery. Int J Cancer 2008;123(7): 1681–1684

7. Tan RK, Finley RK III, Driscoll D, Bakamjian V, Hicks WL Jr, Shedd DP. Anaplastic carcinoma of the thyroid: a 24-year experience. Head Neck 1995;17(1):41–47, discussion 47–48

8. Trimboli P, Ulisse S, Graziano FM, et al. Trend in thyroid carcinoma size, age at diagnosis, and histology in a retrospective study of 500 cases diagnosed over 20 years. Thyroid 2006;16(11):1151–1155

9. Zivaljevic VR, Vlajinac HD, Marinkovic JM, Kalezic NK, Paunovic IR, Diklic AD. Case-control study of anaplastic thyroid cancer: goiter patients as controls. Eur J Cancer Prev 2008;17(2):111–115

10. Swaak-Kragten AT, de Wilt JH, Schmitz PI, Bontenbal M, Levendag PC. Multimodality treatment for anaplastic thyroid carcinoma—treatment outcome in 75 patients. Radiother Oncol 2009;92(1):100–104

11. Gilliland FD, Hunt WC, Morris DM, Key CR. Prognostic factors for thyroid carcinoma: a population-based study of 15,698 cases from the Surveillance, Epidemiology and End Results (SEER) program 1973-1991. Cancer 1997;79(3):564–573

12. Chiacchio S, Lorenzoni A, Boni G, Rubello D, Elisei R, Mariani G. Anaplastic thyroid cancer: prevalence, diagnosis and treatment. Minerva Endocrinol 2008;33(4):341–357

13. Padmanabhan H. Superior vena cava syndrome: a presentation of anaplastic thyroid carcinoma. J Clin Oncol 2010;28(10):e151–e154

14. Shaha AR. Airway management in anaplastic thyroid carcinoma. Laryngoscope 2008;118(7):1195–1198

15. Yau T, Lo CY, Epstein RJ, Lam AK, Wan KY, Lang BH. Treatment outcomes in anaplastic thyroid carcinoma: survival improvement in young patients with localized disease treated by combination of surgery and radiotherapy. Ann Surg Oncol 2008;15(9):2500–2505

16. Phillips JS, Pledger DR, Hilger AW. Rapid thyrotoxicosis in anaplastic thyroid carcinoma. J Laryngol Otol 2007;121(7):695–697

17. Olthof M, Persoon AC, Plukker JT, van der Wal JE, Links TP. Anaplastic thyroid carcinoma with rhabdomyoblastic differentiation: a case report with a good clinical outcome. Endocr Pathol 2008;19(1): 62–65

18. Basolo F, Pollina L, Fontanini G, Fiore L, Pacini F, Baldanzi A. Apoptosis and proliferation in thyroid carcinoma: correlation with bcl-2 and p53 protein expression. Br J Cancer 1997;75(4):537–541

19. Pasieka JL. Anaplastic thyroid cancer. Curr Opin Oncol 2003;15(1):78–83

20. Lam KY, Lo CY, Chan KW, Wan KY. Insular and anaplastic carcinoma of the thyroid: a 45-year comparative study at a single institution and a review of the significance of p53 and p21. Ann Surg 2000;231(3):329–338

21. Albores-Saavedra J, Hernandez M, Sanchez-Sosa S, Simpson K, Angeles A, Henson DE. Histologic variants of papillary and follicular carcinomas associated with anaplastic spindle and giant cell carcinomas of the thyroid: an analysis of rhabdoid and thyroglobulin inclusions. Am J Surg Pathol 2007;31(5):729–736

22. Ugolini C, Basolo F, Proietti A, et al. Lymphocyte and immature dendritic cell infiltrates in differentiated, poorly differentiated, and undifferentiated thyroid carcinoma. Thyroid 2007;17(5):389–393

23. Ryder M, Ghossein RA, Ricarte-Filho JC, Knauf JA, Fagin JA. Increased density of tumor-associated macrophages is associated with decreased survival in advanced thyroid cancer. Endocr Relat Cancer 2008;15(4):1069–1074

24. Takeshita Y, Takamura T, Minato H, et al. Transformation of p53-positive papillary thyroid carcinoma to anaplastic carcinoma of the liver following postoperative radioactive iodine-131 therapy. Intern Med 2008;47(19):1709–1712

25. Xiao GQ, Unger PD, Burstein DE. Immunohistochemical detection of X-linked inhibitor of apoptosis (XIAP) in neoplastic and other thyroid disorders. Ann Diagn Pathol 2007;11(4):235–240

26. Ito Y, Higashiyama T, Hirokawa M, et al. Prognosis of patients with papillary carcinoma showing anaplastic transformation in regional lymph nodes that were curatively resected. Endocr J 2008;55(6):985–989

27. Zhu W, He S, Li Y, et al. Anti-angiogenic activity of triptolide in anaplastic thyroid carcinoma is mediated by targeting vascular endothelial and tumor cells. Vascul Pharmacol 2010;52(1-2):46–54

28. Are C, Shaha AR. Anaplastic thyroid carcinoma: biology, pathogenesis, prognostic factors, and treatment approaches. Ann Surg Oncol 2006;13(4):453–464

29. Aratake Y, Nomura H, Kotani T, et al. Coexistent anaplastic and differentiated thyroid carcinoma. Am J Clin Pathol 2006;125(3):399–406

30. Volante M, Rapa I, Papotti M. Poorly differentiated thyroid carcinoma: diagnostic features and controversial issues. Endocr Pathol 2008;19(3):150–155

31. Lavra L, Ulivieri A, Rinaldo C, et al. Gal-3 is stimulated by gain-of-function p53 mutations and modulates chemoresistance in anaplastic thyroid carcinomas. J Pathol 2009;218(1):66–75

32. Kim TH, Lee SY, Rho JH, et al. Mutant p53 (G199V) gains antiapoptotic function through signal transducer and activator of transcription 3 in anaplastic thyroid cancer cells. Mol Cancer Res 2009;7(10):1645–1654

33. Kim YW, Do IG, Park YK. Expression of the GLUT1 glucose transporter, p63 and p53 in thyroid carcinomas. Pathol Res Pract 2006;202(11):759–765

34. Nakashima M, Takamura N, Namba H, et al. RET oncogene amplification in thyroid cancer: correlations with radiation-associated and high-grade malignancy. Hum Pathol 2007;38(4):621–628

35. Nucera C, Eeckhoute J, Finn S, et al. FOXA1 is a potential oncogene in anaplastic thyroid carcinoma. Clin Cancer Res 2009;15(11):3680–3689

36. Visone R, Pallante P, Vecchione A, et al. Specific microRNAs are downregulated in human thyroid anaplastic carcinomas. Oncogene 2007;26(54):7590–7595

37. Quiros RM, Ding HG, Gattuso P, Prinz RA, Xu X. Evidence that one subset of anaplastic thyroid carcinomas are derived from

papillary carcinomas due to BRAF and p53 mutations. Cancer 2005;103(11):2261–2268

38. Kim S, Yazici YD, Calzada G, et al. Sorafenib inhibits the angiogenesis and growth of orthotopic anaplastic thyroid carcinoma xenografts in nude mice. Mol Cancer Ther 2007;6(6):1785–1792

39. Salvatore G, Nappi TC, Salerno P, et al. A cell proliferation and chromosomal instability signature in anaplastic thyroid carcinoma. Cancer Res 2007;67(21):10148–10158

40. Ito Y, Takano T, Miyauchi A. Apolipoprotein E expression in anaplastic thyroid carcinoma. Oncology 2006;71(5-6):388–393

41. Lee JJ, Foukakis T, Hashemi J, et al. Molecular cytogenetic profiles of novel and established human anaplastic thyroid carcinoma models. Thyroid 2007;17(4):289–301

42. Wiseman SM, Masoudi H, Niblock P, et al. Derangement of the E-cadherin/catenin complex is involved in transformation of differentiated to anaplastic thyroid carcinoma. Am J Surg 2006;191(5):581–587

43. Petrella A, Festa M, Ercolino SF, et al. Annexin-1 downregulation in thyroid cancer correlates to the degree of tumor differentiation. Cancer Biol Ther 2006;5(6):643–647

44. Kim HJ, Kim KR, Park HS, et al. The expression and role of serum response factor in papillary carcinoma of the thyroid. Int J Oncol 2009;35(1):49–55

45. Saltman B, Singh B, Hedvat CV, Wreesmann VB, Ghossein R. Patterns of expression of cell cycle/apoptosis genes along the spectrum of thyroid carcinoma progression. Surgery 2006;140(6):899–905, discussion 905–906

46. Pallante P, Federico A, Berlingieri MT, et al. Loss of the CBX7 gene expression correlates with a highly malignant phenotype in thyroid cancer. Cancer Res 2008;68(16):6770–6778

47. Ito Y, Arai K, Nozawa R, et al. S100A10 expression in thyroid neoplasms originating from the follicular epithelium: contribution to the aggressive characteristic of anaplastic carcinoma. Anticancer Res 2007;27(4C):2679–2683

48. Zeng Q, Chen G, Vlantis A, Tse G, van Hasselt C. The contributions of oestrogen receptor isoforms to the development of papillary and anaplastic thyroid carcinomas. J Pathol 2008;214(4):425–433

49. Malloy KM, Cunnane MF. Pathology and cytologic features of thyroid neoplasms. Surg Oncol Clin N Am 2008;17(1):57–70, viii

50. Daneshbod Y, Omidvari S, Daneshbod K, Negahban S, Dehghani M. Diffuse large B cell lymphoma of thyroid as a masquerader of anaplastic carcinoma of thyroid, diagnosed by FNA: a case report. Cytojournal 2006;3:23

51. Sofiadis A, Tani E, Foukakis T, et al. Diagnostic and prognostic potential of MIB-1 proliferation index in thyroid fine needle aspiration biopsy. Int J Oncol 2009;35(2):369–374

52. Abelardo E, Jaramillo M, Sheffield E, Tierney P. Anaplastic thyroid carcinoma implantation after fine needle aspiration cytology. J Laryngol Otol 2007;121(3):268–270

53. Oktay MH, Smolkin MB, Williams M, Cajigas A. Metastatic anaplastic carcinoma of the thyroid mimicking squamous cell carcinoma: report of a case of a challenging cytologic diagnosis. Acta Cytol 2006;50(2):201–204

54. Lee JW, Yoon DY, Choi CS, et al. Anaplastic thyroid carcinoma: computed tomographic differentiation from other thyroid masses. Acta Radiol 2008;49(3):321–327

55. Won YS, Lee HH, Lee YS, et al. A case of Riedel's thyroiditis associated with benign nodule: mimic of anaplastic transformation. Int J Surg 2008;6(6):e24–e27

56. Bogsrud TV, Karantanis D, Nathan MA, et al. 18F-FDG PET in the management of patients with anaplastic thyroid carcinoma. Thyroid 2008;18(7):713–719

57. Volante M, Collini P, Nikiforov YE, et al. Poorly differentiated thyroid carcinoma: the Turin proposal for the use of uniform diagnostic criteria and an algorithmic diagnostic approach. Am J Surg Pathol 2007;31(8):1256–1264

58. Thyroid. In: Edge SB, Byrd DR, Compton CC, Fritz AG, Greene FI, Trotti A, eds. AJCC Cancer Staging Manual. Chicago, IL: Springer; 2010:88–89

59. Roche B, Larroumets G, Dejax C, et al. Epidemiology, clinical presentation, treatment and prognosis of a regional series of 26 anaplastic thyroid carcinomas (ATC): comparison with the literature. Ann Endocrinol (Paris) 2010;71(1):38–45

60. Chen J, Tward JD, Shrieve DC, Hitchcock YJ. Surgery and radiotherapy improves survival in patients with anaplastic thyroid carcinoma: analysis of the surveillance, epidemiology, and end results 1983-2002. Am J Clin Oncol 2008;31(5):460–464

61. Pacheco-Ojeda LA, Martínez AL, Alvarez M. Anaplastic thyroid carcinoma in Ecuador: analysis of prognostic factors. Int Surg 2001;86(2):117–121

62. Pinto AE, Silva G, Banito A, Leite V, Soares J. Aneuploidy and high S-phase as biomarkers of poor clinical outcome in poorly differentiated and anaplastic thyroid carcinoma. Oncol Rep 2008;20(4):913–919

63. Haigh PI, Ituarte PH, Wu HS, et al. Completely resected anaplastic thyroid carcinoma combined with adjuvant chemotherapy and irradiation is associated with prolonged survival. Cancer 2001;91(12):2335–2342

64. Junor EJ, Paul J, Reed NS. Anaplastic thyroid carcinoma: 91 patients treated by surgery and radiotherapy. Eur J Surg Oncol 1992;18(2):83–88

65. Betka J, Mrzena L, Astl J, et al. Surgical treatment strategy for thyroid gland carcinoma nodal metastases. Eur Arch Otorhinolaryngol 1997;254(Suppl 1):S169–S174

66. Cobin RH, Gharib H, Bergman DA, et al; Thyroid Carcinoma Task Force; American Association of Clinical Endocrinologists. American College of Endocrinology. AACE/AAES medical/surgical guidelines for clinical practice: management of thyroid carcinoma. Endocr Pract 2001;7(3):202–220

67. Hölting T, Meybier H, Buhr H. [Status of tracheotomy in treatment of the respiratory emergency in anaplastic thyroid cancer]. Wien Klin Wochenschr 1990;102(9):264–266

68. Levendag PC, De Porre PM, van Putten WL. Anaplastic carcinoma of the thyroid gland treated by radiation therapy. Int J Radiat Oncol Biol Phys 1993;26(1):125–128

69. Pierie JP, Muzikansky A, Gaz RD, Faquin WC, Ott MJ. The effect of surgery and radiotherapy on outcome of anaplastic thyroid carcinoma. Ann Surg Oncol 2002;9(1):57–64

70. Dandekar P, Harmer C, Barbachano Y, et al. Hyperfractionated accelerated radiotherapy (HART) for anaplastic thyroid carcinoma: toxicity and survival analysis. Int J Radiat Oncol Biol Phys 2009;74(2):518–521

71. Wang Y, Tsang R, Asa S, Dickson B, Arenovich T, Brierley J. Clinical outcome of anaplastic thyroid carcinoma treated with radiotherapy of once- and twice-daily fractionation regimens. Cancer 2006;107(8):1786–1792

72. Tennvall J, Lundell G, Wahlberg P, et al. Anaplastic thyroid carcinoma: three protocols combining doxorubicin, hyperfractionated radiotherapy and surgery. Br J Cancer 2002;86(12):1848–1853

73. Papewalis C, Ehlers M, Schott M. Advances in cellular therapy for the treatment of thyroid cancer. J Oncol 2010;2010:179491

74. Bhatia A, Rao A, Ang KK, et al. Anaplastic thyroid cancer: clinical outcomes with conformal radiotherapy. Head Neck 2010;32(7):829–836

75. Kebebew E, Greenspan FS, Clark OH, Woeber KA, McMillan A. Anaplastic thyroid carcinoma: treatment outcome and prognostic factors. Cancer 2005;103(7):1330–1335

76. Ahuja S, Ernst H. Chemotherapy of thyroid carcinoma. J Endocrinol Invest 1987;10(3):303–310

77. Poster DS, Bruno S, Penta J, Pina K, Catane R. Current status of chemotherapy in the treatment of advanced carcinoma of the thyroid gland. Cancer Clin Trials 1981;4(3):301–307

78. Shimaoka K. Adjunctive management of thyroid cancer: chemotherapy. J Surg Oncol 1980;15(3):283–286

79. Shimaoka K, Schoenfeld DA, DeWys WD, Creech RH, DeConti R. A randomized trial of doxorubicin versus doxorubicin plus cisplatin in patients with advanced thyroid carcinoma. Cancer 1985;56(9):2155–2160

80. Hoskin PJ, Harmer C. Chemotherapy for thyroid cancer. Radiother Oncol 1987;10(3):187–194

81. De Besi P, Busnardo B, Toso S, et al. Combined chemotherapy with bleomycin, adriamycin, and platinum in advanced thyroid cancer. J Endocrinol Invest 1991;14(6):475–480

82. Ain KB, Egorin MJ, DeSimone PA; Collaborative Anaplastic Thyroid Cancer Health Intervention Trials (CATCHIT) Group. Treatment of anaplastic thyroid carcinoma with paclitaxel: phase 2 trial using ninety-six-hour infusion. Thyroid 2000;10(7):587–594

83. Higashiyama T, Ito Y, Hirokawa M, et al. Induction chemotherapy with weekly paclitaxel administration for anaplastic thyroid carcinoma. Thyroid 2010;20(1):7–14

84. McIver B, Hay ID, Giuffrida DF, et al. Anaplastic thyroid carcinoma: a 50-year experience at a single institution.Surgery 2001;130(6):1028–1034

85. De Crevoisier R, Baudin E, Bachelot A, et al. Combined treatment of anaplastic thyroid carcinoma with surgery, chemotherapy, and hyperfractionated accelerated external radiotherapy. Int J Radiat Oncol Biol Phys 2004;60(4):1137–1143

86. Chang HS, Nam KH, Chung WY, Park CS. Anaplastic thyroid carcinoma: a therapeutic dilemma. Yonsei Med J 2005;46(6):759–764

87. Heron DE, Karimpour S, Grigsby PW. Anaplastic thyroid carcinoma: comparison of conventional radiotherapy and hyperfractionation chemoradiotherapy in two groups. Am J Clin Oncol 2002;25(5):442–446

88. Besic N, Auersperg M, Us-Krasovec M, Golouh R, Frkovic-Grazio S, Vodnik A. Effect of primary treatment on survival in anaplastic thyroid carcinoma. Eur J Surg Oncol 2001;27(3):260–264

89. Busnardo B, Daniele O, Pelizzo MR, et al. A multimodality therapeutic approach in anaplastic thyroid carcinoma: study on 39 patients. J Endocrinol Invest 2000;23(11):755–761

90. Foote RL, Molina JR, Kasperbauer JL, et al. Enhanced survival in locoregionally confined anaplastic thyroid carcinoma: a single-institution experience using aggressive multimodal therapy. Thyroid 2011;21(1):25–30

91. Troch M, Koperek O, Scheuba C, et al. High efficacy of concomitant treatment of undifferentiated (anaplastic) thyroid cancer with radiation and docetaxel. J Clin Endocrinol Metab 2010;95(9):E54–E57

92. Stenner F, Liewen H, Zweifel M, et al. Targeted therapeutic approach for an anaplastic thyroid cancer in vitro and in vivo. Cancer Sci 2008;99(9):1847–1852

93. Wiseman SM, Griffith OL, Deen S, et al. Identification of molecular markers altered during transformation of differentiated into anaplastic thyroid carcinoma. Arch Surg 2007;142(8):717–727, discussion 727–729

94. Kurebayashi J, Okubo S, Yamamoto Y, et al. Additive antitumor effects of gefitinib and imatinib on anaplastic thyroid cancer cells. Cancer Chemother Pharmacol 2006;58(4):460–470

95. Landriscina M, Maddalena F, Fabiano A, Piscazzi A, La Macchia O, Cignarelli M. Erlotinib enhances the proapoptotic activity of cytotoxic agents and synergizes with paclitaxel in poorly-differentiated thyroid carcinoma cells. Anticancer Res 2010;30(2):473–480

96. Prichard CN, Kim S, Yazici YD, et al. Concurrent cetuximab and bevacizumab therapy in a murine orthotopic model of anaplastic thyroid carcinoma. Laryngoscope 2007;117(4):674–679

97. Kojic SL, Strugnell SS, Wiseman SM. Anaplastic thyroid cancer: a comprehensive review of novel therapy. Expert Rev Anticancer Ther 2011;11(3):387–402

8 Unusual Tumors of the Thyroid Gland

Derrick T. Lin, Jennifer L. Hunt, and Gregory W. Randolph

Core Messages

- Papillary thyroid cancer (PTC) variants that are more aggressive than typical papillary cancer include tall-cell and diffuse sclerosing variants.

- Follicular variant of PTC is similar in prognosis to PTC overall.

- Cribriform-morular variant may occur in association with familial adenomatous polyposis and requires adenomatous polyposis coli mutational analysis.

- Insular and squamous carcinomas of the thyroid are high-grade lesions with poorer prognosis than typical differentiated thyroid carcinomas.

Variants of Papillary Thyroid Carcinoma

Tall-Cell Variant

Tall-cell variant (TCV) of papillary thyroid carcinoma (PTC) was initially characterized by Hawk and Hazard in 1976.[1] Overall, TCV accounts for approximately 10% of PTCs (**Table 8.1**).

Histologically, TVC is diagnosed by the presence of a papillary tumor whose cells are at least two to three times as high as they are wide.[1–3] Other cytologic features associated with this tumor include distinctive intracytoplasmic borders and eosinophilic cytoplasm (**Fig. 8.1**).

As a group, patients with TCV have both a higher recurrence rate and overall mortality rate than do patients with classical papillary thyroid cancer.[4,5] This finding was initially attributed to the fact that these patients tended to be older and more frequently presented with extrathyroidal extension.[5] Ghossein et al, however, demonstrated that in their series of patients, patients with TCV without extracapsular extension had a higher nodal metastatic rate

than did patients with classical PTC independent of age, gender, and tumor size.[6] In their study, 3 of the 47 patients with TCV without extrathyroidal extension developed distant metastasis, while none of the 62 patients with classical PTC presented with distant metastasis.

Morris et al retrospectively reviewed 278 patients with TCV and 2522 patients with classical PTC at Memorial Sloan Kettering Cancer Center. As in Ghossein et al's study, when compared with patients with classical PTC, patients with TCV presented at an older age, had a higher rate of extracapsular extension, and had a worse 5-year disease-specific survival rate. They concluded that when the major prognostic factors for thyroid cancer were controlled for, tall-cell histology alone remained a significant independent prognostic factor for disease-specific death.[7]

On a molecular level, several studies have shown that TCV tumors have a higher rate of *BRAF* mutations than do classical PTC tumors.[8] Clinical trials are currently under way investigating the use of chemotherapeutic agents targeting *BRAF*.

Currently, there are no studies that have addressed the prognostic implications of cervical lymph node metastasis

Table 8.1 PTC Variants with Clinical Correlations

PTC Variant	Surgical Treatment	Prognosis Relative to Classical PTC
Tall-cell	More aggressive—total thyroid and nodal	Worse than PTC
Diffuse sclerosing	More aggressive—total thyroid and nodal	Worse than PTC
Cribriform-morular	Intermediate	Variable
Follicular	As for classical PTC	Equal to PTC
Columnar cell	Intermediate	Variable

PTC, papillary thyroid carcinoma.

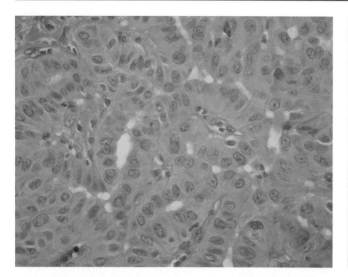

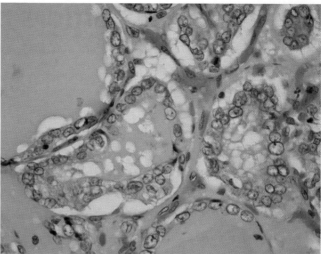

Figure 8.1 Image demonstrating the characteristic features of tall-cell variant of papillary carcinoma. The cells have a tall shape, with the height at least twice the width. The cells also have eosinophilic cytoplasm and distinctive cell borders. Hematoxylin and eosin stain, ×20 original magnification.

Figure 8.2 Image showing the features of follicular variant of papillary carcinoma. The tumor is growing with a pure follicular architecture and demonstrates the nuclear features of papillary carcinoma. Hematoxylin and eosin stain, ×40 original magnification.

in patients with TVC. Given the aggressive nature of TVC, a comprehensive surgical approach is reasonable including total thyroidectomy, elective central nodal exploration, and directed dissection followed by radioactive iodine therapy.

Follicular Variant

Follicular variant (FV) of papillary thyroid cancer, first described in 1977 by Chen and Rosai, is diagnosed histologically by the formation of follicles lined by cells containing nuclear features of papillary carcinoma (**Fig. 8.2**).[9] In 2010, Lin and Bhattacharyya reported an analysis of the national cancer database in the United States reviewing the prevalence and extent of disease characteristics of FV.[10] They found that compared with classical papillary thyroid cancer, age at presentation and sex distribution were similar for FV, the prevalence of lymph node metastasis was lower in FV (14.8 vs. 27.8%), and the mean overall survival of patients with FV was not statistically different from that of patients with classical PTC. These findings have been further supported in other studies.[11,12]

In 1991, Albores-Saavedra et al reported on an unusual entity, the "macrofollicular variant" of PTC, characterized as a well-differentiated carcinoma with large, follicular architecture with nuclear appearance similar to that of PTC.[13] This entity was originally noted to have a low incidence of regional and distant metastasis and an overall good prognosis; however, Cardenas et al reported on two patients with a highly aggressive macrofollicular variant of papillary thyroid cancer.[14]

Given similar survival outcome between FV and PTC, the current recommendations for the management of FV are the same as that for PTC.

Columnar-Cell Variant

Initially described by Evans in 1986, columnar-cell variant (CCV) of PTC is characterized by tall cells with elongated hyperchromatic pseudostratified nuclei (**Fig. 8.3**).[15] To make the diagnosis, a requirement of at least 30% columnar cells is needed. CCV accounts for 0.15 to 0.2% of all papillary carcinomas.[16]

CCV is often associated with an uncertain clinical course. Histologically, small size and encapsulation have been associated with a more favorable prognosis, while large size and extrathyroidal extension have been associated with a worse prognosis.[17] In an analysis of the literature by Chen et al, there were 48 reported cases, 15 men and 33 women with age ranging from 16 to 50 years. In 20 cases, the tumors were clinically indolent, while in 23 cases, the tumors were aggressive. Indolent tumors tended to be smaller (mean 3.6 cm, median 3.8 cm), while clinically aggressive tumors were larger (mean 6.0 cm, median 6.3 cm).[17]

Vickery et al reported on 41 cases of CCV, with 27% having extracapsular spread and 50% having cervical metastasis at presentation.[18] In this study, with a mean follow-up of 43 months, 33% had locoregional recurrence, 36% developed distant metastasis, and there was a 29% disease-specific mortality rate. The authors concluded that prognosis was poor if the tumor showed extracapsular extension; however, CCV itself did not predict a poor outcome. Chen et al reported similar results in nine patients with CCV.[17] The four indolent neoplasms in this study were small (mean 2.1 cm), encapsulated, well circumscribed, and affected younger and predominantly female patients. The five aggressive neoplasms were large (mean 6.7 cm), diffusely infiltrative with extrathyroidal extension, and affected older and predominantly male patients.

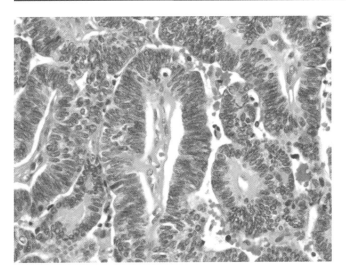

Figure 8.3 Image showing the features of columnar-cell variant of papillary carcinoma. The cells show nuclei with condensed, dark chromatin that are pseudostratified. Hematoxylin and eosin stain, ×20 original magnification.

The treatment for CCV, therefore, should be based on clinical and histologic evaluation. Appropriately aggressive therapy, total thyroidectomy, central neck dissection, and adjuvant radioactive iodine should be considered in patients demonstrating extracapsular extension. External beam radiation may be considered in patients in whom complete surgical resection has not been achieved.

Diffuse Sclerosing Variant

Diffuse sclerosing variant (DSV) of PTC is uncommon. To date, approximately 150 cases have been reported in the literature.[18–53] Vickery et al was the first to describe this new variant of PTC in 1985.[18] Histologically, DSV is characterized by diffuse involvement of both lobes of the thyroid gland with dense fibrosis, lymphatic infiltrate, multiple foci of squamous metaplastic changes, and numerous psammoma bodies.[18]

Clinically, patients with DSV tend to be younger than patients with classical papillary thyroid cancer.[18–53] The mean age of patients with DSV ranges from 19.5 to 34.7 years. In a 35-year comparative study by Lam and Lo of 15 patients with DSV, the mean age of patients with DSV was 29 versus 46 years for patients with classical PTC.[53] Furthermore, compared with patients with classical papillary thyroid cancer, patients with DSV had larger tumors (mean diameter, 3.6 vs. 2.2 cm), had a higher incidence of lymph node metastasis (80 vs. 43%), and frequent disease recurrence.

Because survival data for DSV are derived from case reports and small series, the overall clinical behavior remains controversial.[18–54] In the previously mentioned study by Lam and Lo, the 10-year survival rate of patients with classical papillary thyroid cancer was 92% while the 10-year survival rate of patients with DSV was 93%.[53] However, in this study, the treatment protocol for patients with DSV was more

aggressive. This included initial "radical surgery" followed by radioactive treatment. An active search for suspicious lymph nodes at the initial operation is recommended because of the higher risk of nodal metastasis.

Cribriform-Morular Variant

First described by Harach et al in 1994, cribriform-morular variant (CMV) of papillary thyroid cancer is characterized by the papillary growth of tall columnar cells, cribriform pattern, solid and spindle cells, squamoid morules, and peculiar nuclear clearing (**Fig. 8.4**).[55] CMV can be either sporadic or familial. Familial CMV is associated with familial adenomatous polyposis where adenomatous polyposis coli (*APC*) mutations may play an important role.[56–58] Familial CMV is usually multifocal and occurs more often in women.[59] Sporadic tumors, on the other hand, usually present as solitary nodules and are not associated with colonic polyps.[56,57,60,61] Because of these distinct characteristics, total thyroidectomy is generally recommended for familial CMV while a lobectomy may be considered in the sporadic form. Interestingly, Plail et al reported that because up to 30% of thyroid carcinomas may be diagnosed 4 to 12 years before the development of colonic polyps, colonoscopy and *APC* gene analysis are recommended in these patients.[62]

Insular Carcinoma

Insular carcinoma was described by Carcangiu et al in 1984 as the presence of histologically well-defined nests of tumor cells with round, dark, and monomorphic nuclei and scant cytoplasm (*see* **Table 8.2**).[63] Insular cell carcinomas tend to be large, greater than 4 cm, and often exhibit extracapsular spread. Sywak et al evaluated 213 patients with insular thyroid cancer, reporting a predominance of female patients

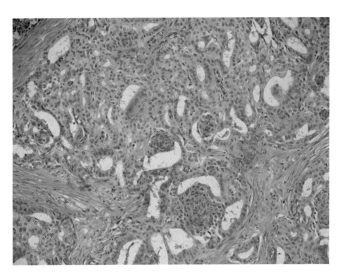

Figure 8.4 Image demonstrating a cribriform-morular variant of papillary carcinoma. There are papillary formations, cribriform growth, and one morular formation. Hematoxylin and eosin stain, ×10 original magnification.

Table 8.2 Unusual Thyroid Tumors and Their Prognosis

Tumor Type	Key Point	Prognosis
Cribriform-morular variant	Total if familial, APC mutation testing required	Fair-poor
Insular carcinoma	High-grade lesion	Poor
Metastases to the thyroid gland	May be PET+, generally with known history of primary tumor	Poor
Squamous cell carcinoma of the thyroid	High-grade lesion, rule out nonthyroid squamous lesion and squamoid anaplastic	Poor
Mucoepidermoid carcinoma (and SMECE)	Solitary lesion arising from ultimobranchial/lateral thyroid anlagen	Poor
CASTLE	Solitary lesion, arising from ultimobranchial/lateral thyroid anlagen	Fair
SETTLE	Solitary lesion, thymic differentiation, rule out sarcoma	Good

PET, positron emission tomography; SMECE, sclerosing mucoepidermoid carcinoma with eosinophilia; CASTLE, carcinoma showing thymic-like differentiation; APC, adenomatous polyposis coli; SETTLE, spindle epithelial tumor with thymic-like differentiation.

and mean tumor size of 5.5 cm, with 44% exhibiting extracapsular extension and 51% with clinically apparent cervical metastasis.[64] Locoregional recurrence or distant metastasis was seen in 64% with a disease-specific mortality of 32%. The insular variant meets many of the criteria of poorly differentiated carcinoma, and many experts believe that it may be a precursor to anaplastic thyroid carcinoma.[65]

Aggressive surgical management, total thyroidectomy, and central neck dissection followed by radioactive iodine or external beam radiation in the setting of incomplete resection is recommended.

Metastases to the Thyroid Gland

It is uncommon for tumors from other organ systems to metastasize to the thyroid gland. The most common tumor to demonstrate metastases to the thyroid is renal cell carcinoma.[66–68] Other tumors in the literature that have been reported as metastatic disease appear in isolated case reports and include breast carcinoma, Merkel cell carcinoma, pancreatic adenocarcinoma, lung and colon carcinoma, and other rare tumors.[66,69–72]

The clinical presentation of metastases to the thyroid gland varies, depending on the site of origin from the tumor. An extensive literature about the radiologic presentation does not exist, but case reports have identified that renal cell carcinoma (RCC) may be positive on positron emission tomography scanning.[73] In many of these cases of metastasis to the thyroid gland, the patient will present with a clinical history of the tumor and with widespread metastatic disease. But with RCC in particular, patients may have only a distant history of thveir primary tumor.[74,75] Some patients will present with their thyroid lesion as a first manifestation of their primary malignancy.[70]

Diagnosing metastatic disease preoperatively may be nearly impossible, as fine-needle aspiration cytology will rarely be definitive. There are several case reports of the cytopathologic features of metastatic tumors in thyroid, from which it is clear that metastatic tumors will often mimic primary thyroid tumorson on cytology.[70] On occasion, a tumor from another organ may also metastasize to a primary thyroid tumor, such as a follicular adenoma or a papillary carcinoma.[66] In this scenario, it becomes even more challenging to make a preoperative diagnosis from the cytologic features.

Grossly, these tumors are usually clinical, somewhat nonspecific, and present as mass lesions or diffuse infiltration of the thyroid gland. The exception is metastatic RCC, which almost always has a striking yellow appearance, due to the lipid content within the cytoplasm of the tumor cells (**Fig. 8.5**).

Histologically, the metastatic tumor may have specific or nonspecific cellular features. Again, RCC is one of the most striking, with characteristic nested growth and an extensive vascular network in the background. In RCC, the metastatic tumor cells often have low-grade, monomorphic nuclei with clear, vacuolated cytoplasm. At the immunohistochemistry

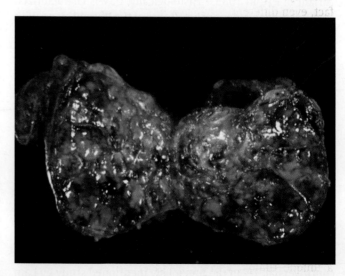

Figure 8.5 A gross image of a metastatic renal cell carcinoma of the thyroid. The tumor has a yellow appearance and has massive hemorrhage, which are characteristic gross features of metastatic renal cell carcinoma.

level, metastases are invariably negative for thyroglobulin and for thyroid transcription factor 1 (TTF-1) markers.[68] Other markers that are associated with the organ of the primary tumor may be used to further subclassify these tumors. For example, metastatic RCC will commonly be positive for vimentin, PAX8, CD10, EMA, and RCC antigen. Some caution is required in using isolated immunohistochemical stains without the panel approach. This can easily be illustrated by the fact that PAX8 also can stain primary thyroid tumors.[68]

Other tumors can also present with metastases to the thyroid, and the immunohistochemical staining patterns are variably sensitive and specific. The most reliable markers to indicate nonthyroid origin will be the absence of TTF and thyroglobulin. Other markers that will be used will depend entirely on the tumor of origin.

Many metastatic tumors are surgically excised because of the suspicion of a primary thyroid tumor rather than as treatment for metastatic disease. Although local control of this metastatic disease is possible, most patients have widespread distant metastatic disease.[76]

Squamous Cell Carcinoma of the Thyroid

Pure primary squamous cell carcinoma (SCC) of the thyroid is exceedingly rare, though there are many other tumors and entities in the thyroid that may have squamous differentiation.[77] In fact, both benign and malignant primary thyroid entities can be in the differential diagnosis because of overlapping histologic features. These include squamous metaplasia, hyperplastic ultimobranchial body rests, mucoepidermoid carcinoma (MEC), papillary carcinoma with squamous metaplasia, and anaplastic thyroid carcinoma.[78–80]

As SCC usually presents with a mass lesion, patients may undergo fine-needle aspiration biopsy preoperatively. These cytologic preparations can be quite challenging and, in fact, even differentiating between the various entities with squamous differentiation on final pathology may be difficult and may require special studies.

In the largest series of primary SCC in the thyroid literature, most patients presented with a rapidly enlarging thyroid mass lesion.[77,81] The tumors demonstrated typical squamous morphology, with epithelioid cells demonstrating intracellular bridges and keratin pearl formation. Varying degrees of differentiation have been noted, though most of these malignancies will be on the poorly differentiated end of the spectrum. Special stains can be used to demonstrate the epithelial nature of the cells, with positive staining for cytokeratin markers and p63, which is a marker of squamous differentiation. These tumors are also usually positive for TTF-1.[77,81]

It remains unclear whether SCC of the thyroid is truly a unique tumor type or whether it simply represents a variant morphology of undifferentiated (anaplastic) thyroid carcinoma. The behavior of these tumors is quite similar to that of undifferentiated carcinoma. In most cases reported in the literature, primary SCC of the thyroid behaves in a

very aggressive fashion, with most patients dying from their disease within a year of diagnosis.[77,81–83] SCC of the thyroid can also occur in conjunction with better differentiated primary thyroid tumors (**Fig. 8.6**). Perhaps the most common entity to have squamous metaplasia is TCV of papillary carcinoma. Even when present as a minor component, squamous differentiation in these tumors may portend a more aggressive disease.[79,84]

Mucoepidermoid Carcinoma and Sclerosing Mucoepidermoid Carcinoma with Eosinophilia

Tumors with both glandular and squamoid differentiation in the thyroid gland were first identified in the 1970s and were grouped under the terminology MEC.[85] A second type of tumor was later identified with slightly different morphology and was called sclerosing MEC with eosinophilia (SMECE). These tumors are relatively rare in comparison to other well-differentiated thyroid carcinomas. The etiology of MEC and SMECE has been distributed in the literature, especially in reference to the cell of origin. Most of the literature suggests that the origin of MEC and SMECE arises from ultimobranchial body rests, which are remnants of the lateral thyroid anlage.[86–89]

MEC and SMECE generally present as solitary thyroid mass lesions. Patients may be slightly younger, with more male patients being affected with them than with typical well-differentiated PTCs.[90] Preoperative cytopathology will often be performed, but the cytologic features may be somewhat nonspecific and reveal only features of poorly differentiated carcinoma.[91,92]

With MEC and SMECE, there is characteristically moderate to severe chronic lymphocytic thyroiditis, which may be associated with autoantibodies (Hashimoto thyroiditis).[87,93] Histologically, these tumors demonstrate an

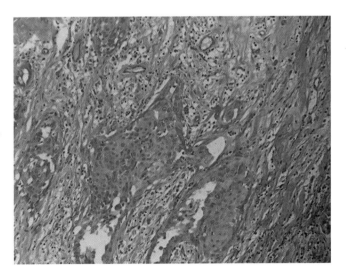

Figure 8.6 Image demonstrating a squamous cell carcinoma of the thyroid. The tumor is an infiltrative malignancy with squamous differentiation. Hematoxylin and eosin stain, ×20 original magnification.

invasive growth pattern with islands of malignant cells that show both squamoid and glandular-type differentiation (**Fig. 8.7**). The glandular formations can be identified by positive mucicarmine staining. Along with the MEC islands, some tumors also exhibit extensive sclerosis and inflammatory cell infiltrates that are rich in eosinophils. These latter tumors have been subclassified as SMECE. Both types of MEC are generally strongly and diffusely positive for p63, which is associated with squamous differentiation in all organ sites. p63 is also positive in tumor branchial body rests, which suggests that MEC may be related to these embryological remnants. The tumors are often negative for thyroglobulin and may also be negative for TTF-1.[94] Occasionally, MEC and SMECE may also arise in conjunction with a conventional PTC.[93]

MEC and SMECE are generally treated surgically with either lobectomy or total thyroidectomy. However, given the lack of expression of thyroglobulin and the proposed etiology from nonfollicular-derived embryological remnants, radioactive iodine may not be identical.[95]

Carcinoma Showing Thymic-Like Differentiation

Carcinoma showing thymic-like differentiation (CASTLE) is another extremely rare primary thyroid tumor that has been reported only in isolated case reports and very small series. This tumor has also been referred to as intrathyroidal epithelial thymoma.[96] The etiology of this lesion has been controversial in the literature. Although classically this tumor was initially thought to arise from thymic remnants, studies suggest that it may arise from ultimobranchial body rests with thymic-like differentiation.[96–98]

CASTLE typically presents as a solitary mass lesion in the thyroid. Grossly, the lesions are often fleshy and have a

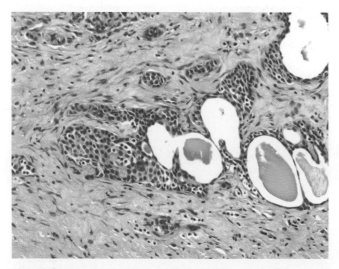

Figure 8.7 Image showing the morphologic features of a mucoepidermoid carcinoma of the thyroid. The tumor cells are growing in sheets and have both squamoid and glandular features. Hematoxylin and eosin stain, ×10 original magnification.

lobulated cut surface. Histologically, CASTLE demonstrates a lobular type of infiltrative growth and is frequently associated with lymphoplasmacytic inflammatory cell infiltrates. Cytologically, the tumor cells can show diverse appearances, including spindled, squamoid, or vesicular type cells. Special stains for this tumor are somewhat nonspecific, with the exception of CD5.[96,99] Nearly all these tumors will stain positive for CD5, which is a marker of thymic derivation.[99]

The cytologic and histologic features of CASTLE have been likened to those seen in undifferentiated squamous carcinoma of the nasopharynx (nasopharyngeal carcinoma), which is associated with Epstein-Barr virus (EBV) in endemic regions. Importantly, EBV has not been identified as a causal factor in CASTLE.[99] Along with the histologic similarities, preoperative fine-needle aspiration of CASTLE can also show similarities with the features of undifferentiated nasopharyngeal carcinoma.[100]

In the literature, most cases of CASTLE have been treated with a surgical approach, including total or subtotal thyroidectomy, or a simple lobectomy.[96] Patients may also be treated with postoperative radiation therapy and/or chemotherapy.[101,102] The prognosis for these patients is somewhat variable, with recurrence in about one-third of patients.[96] Five- and 10-year disease-specific survival rates are high in patients without nodal metastases but are between 50 and 75% when lymph node metastases were identified at presentation.[96,103]

Spindle Epithelial Tumor with Thymic-Like Differentiation

Another rare thyroid tumor associated with thymic differentiation, termed spindle epithelial tumor with thymic-like differentiation (SETTLE), was first described in 1991 by Chan and Rosai.[104] This tumor occurs in a relatively unique population, with a strong propensity for children and young adults.[105–107]

Preoperative diagnosis of SETTLE is extremely challenging due to overlapping and somewhat nonspecific cytologic features.[108,109] SETTLE is often mistaken for a sarcoma on the preoperative fine-needle aspiration, given the spindle cell nature of the tumor.[110] Grossly, these tumors are usually solitary mass lesions that have a firm white tan cut surface. On histologic examination, SETTLE shows highly cellular lesion composed of spindle cells, growing in a whorled, storiform, or intersecting pattern (**Fig. 8.8**).[110,111] In addition to the spindle cell elements, there is usually an identifiable epithelial component.[111] This epithelial component usually shows some type of glandular differentiation with cyst-like structures that can be lined by a variety of epithelial subtypes, including columnar cells, goblet cells, and rarely even pseudostratified-ciliated epithelium.[110,112]

On immunohistochemical staining, the glandular cell component of SETTLE is positive for cytokeratin.[110] The spindle cell component may also be positive for cytokeratins but is usually also positive for smooth muscle actin.[111,112]

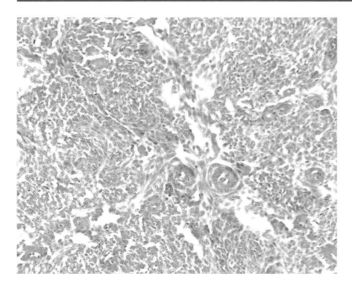

Figure 8.8 Image showing the morphologic features of a spindle epithelial tumor with thymic-like differentiation. The tumor is composed of cellular spindle cells, with rare glandular formations. Hematoxylin and eosin stain, ×20 original magnification.

Rare cases of SETTLE have been studied with molecular assays. The most important use for a molecular assay is to differentiate SETTLE from synovial sarcoma, which is the main entity in differential diagnosis.[112] The assay utilized is generally a fluorescent in situ hybridization analysis for the translocation present in synovial sarcoma. Although cases of translocation-positive synovial sarcoma can rarely occur as either primary or metastatic tumors of the thyroid gland, SETTLE should be definitively negative for the translocation.[112]

SETTLE is usually treated with primary surgery. These tumors are generally thought to be relatively indolent and to have a good overall prognosis.[113] Some cases of SETTLE, however, will metastasize, and rare patients will die from their disease (*see* **Table 8.2**).[107,112,113]

References

1. Hawk WA, Hazard JB. The many appearances of papillary carcinoma of the thyroid. Cleve Clin Q 1976;43(4):207–215
2. Johnson TL, Lloyd RV, Thompson NW, Beierwaltes WH, Sisson JC. Prognostic implications of the tall cell variant of papillary thyroid carcinoma. Am J Surg Pathol 1988;12(1):22–27
3. DeLellis RA, Lloyd RV, Heitz PU, Eng C, eds. World Health Organization Classification of Tumours: Pathology and Genetics of Tumours of Endocrine Organs. Lyon: IARC; 2004
4. Ghossein R, Livolsi VA. Papillary thyroid carcinoma tall cell variant. Thyroid 2008;18(11):1179–1181
5. Michels JJ, Jacques M, Henry-Amar M, Bardet S. Prevalence and prognostic significance of tall cell variant of papillary thyroid carcinoma. Hum Pathol 2007;38(2):212–219
6. Ghossein RA, Leboeuf R, Patel KN, et al. Tall cell variant of papillary thyroid carcinoma without extrathyroid extension: biologic behavior and clinical implications. Thyroid 2007;17(7):655–661
7. Morris LG, Shaha AR, Tuttle RM, Sikora AG, Ganly I. Tall-cell variant of papillary thyroid carcinoma: a matched-pair analysis of survival. Thyroid 2010;20(2):153–158
8. Adeniran AJ, Zhu Z, Gandhi M, et al. Correlation between genetic alterations and microscopic features, clinical manifestations, and prognostic characteristics of thyroid papillary carcinomas. Am J Surg Pathol 2006;30(2):216–222
9. Chem KT, Rosai J. Follicular variant of thyroid papillary carcinoma: a clinicopathologic study of six cases. Am J Surg Pathol 1977;1(2):123–130
10. Lin HW, Bhattacharyya N. Clinical behavior of follicular variant of papillary thyroid carcinoma: presentation and survival. Laryngoscope 2010;120(4):712–716
11. Chang HY, Lin JD, Chou SC, Chao TC, Hsueh C. Clinical presentations and outcomes of surgical treatment of follicular variant of the papillary thyroid carcinomas. Jpn J Clin Oncol 2006;36(11):688–693
12. Lang BH, Lo CY, Chan WF, Lam AK, Wan KY. Classical and follicular variant of papillary thyroid carcinoma: a comparative study on clinicopathologic features and long-term outcome. World J Surg 2006;30(5):752–758
13. Albores-Saavedra J, Gould E, Vardaman C, Vuitch F. The macrofollicular variant of papillary thyroid carcinoma: a study of 17 cases. Hum Pathol 1991;22(12):1195–1205
14. Cardenas MG, Kini S, Wisgerhof M. Two patients with highly aggressive macrofollicular variant of papillary thyroid carcinoma. Thyroid 2009;19(4):413–416
15. Evans HL. Columnar-cell carcinoma of the thyroid: a report of two cases of an aggressive variant of thyroid carcinoma. Am J Clin Pathol 1986;85(1):77–80
16. Wenig BM, Thompson LD, Adair CF, Shmookler B, Heffess CS. Thyroid papillary carcinoma of columnar cell type: a clinicopathologic study of 16 cases. Cancer 1998;82(4):740–753
17. Chen JH, Faquin WC, Lloyd RV, Nosé V. Clinicopathological and molecular characterization of nine cases of columnar cell variant of papillary thyroid carcinoma. Mod Pathol 2011;24(5):739–749
18. Vickery AL Jr, Carcangiu ML, Johannessen JV, Sobrinho-Simoes M. Papillary carcinoma. Semin Diagn Pathol 1985;2(2):90–100
19. Matias-Guiu X, Esquius J. Aberrant expression of HLA-DR antigen in diffuse sclerosing variant of papillary carcinoma of thyroid. J Clin Pathol 1989;42(12):1309
20. Carcangiu ML, Bianchi S. Diffuse sclerosing variant of papillary thyroid carcinoma: clinicopathologic study of 15 cases. Am J Surg Pathol 1989;13(12):1041–1049
21. Wu PS, Leslie PJ, McLaren KM, Toft AD. Diffuse sclerosing papillary carcinoma of thyroid: a wolf in sheep's clothing. Clin Endocrinol (Oxf) 1989;31(5):535–540
22. Soares J, Limbert E, Sobrinho-Simões M. Diffuse sclerosing variant of papillary thyroid carcinoma: a clinicopathologic study of 10 cases. Pathol Res Pract 1989;185(2):200–206
23. Caruso G, Tabarri B, Lucchi I, Tison V. Fine needle aspiration cytology in a case of diffuse sclerosing carcinoma of the thyroid. Acta Cytol 1990;34(3):352–354
24. Chan JK. Papillary carcinoma of thyroid: classical and variants. Histol Histopathol 1990;5(2):241–257
25. Fujimoto Y, Obara T, Ito Y, Kodama T, Aiba M, Yamaguchi K. Diffuse sclerosing variant of papillary carcinoma of the thyroid: clinical importance, surgical treatment, and follow-up study. Cancer 1990;66(11):2306–2312
26. Mizukami Y, Nonomura A, Michigishi T, et al. Diffuse sclerosing variant of papillary carcinoma of the thyroid: report of three cases. Acta Pathol Jpn 1990;40(9):676–682
27. Hayashi Y, Sasao T, Takeichi N, Kuma K, Katayama S. Diffuse sclerosing variant of papillary carcinoma of the thyroid: a histopathological study of four cases. Acta Pathol Jpn 1990;40(3):193–198

28. Schröder S, Bay V, Dumke K, et al. Diffuse sclerosing variant of papillary thyroid carcinoma: S-100 protein immunocytochemistry and prognosis. Virchows Arch A Pathol Anat Histopathol 1990;416(4):367–371

29. Gómez-Morales M, Alvaro T, Muñoz M, et al. Diffuse sclerosing papillary carcinoma of the thyroid gland: immunohistochemical analysis of the local host immune response. Histopathology 1991;18(5):427–433

30. Alejo M, Peiro G, Oliva E, Matias-Guiu X. Leu-M 1 immunoreactivity in papillary carcinomas of the thyroid gland: microcarcinoma, encapsulated, conventional and diffuse sclerosing subtypes. Virchows Arch A Pathol Anat Histopathol 1991;419(5):447–448

31. Macák J, Michal M. Diffuse sclerosing variant of papillary thyroid carcinoma. Cesk Patol 1993;29(1):6–8

32. Moreno Egea A, Rodriguez Gonzalez JM, Sola Perez J, Soria T, Parrilla Paricio P. Clinicopathological study of the diffuse sclerosing variety of papillary cancer of the thyroid: presentation of 4 new cases and review of the literature. Eur J Surg Oncol 1994;20(1):7–11

33. Nikiforov Y, Gnepp DR. Pediatric thyroid cancer after the Chernobyl disaster: pathomorphologic study of 84 cases (1991-1992) from the Republic of Belarus. Cancer 1994;74(2):748–766

34. Damiani S, Dina R, Eusebi V. Cytologic grading of aggressive and nonaggressive variants of papillary thyroid carcinoma. Am J Clin Pathol 1994;101(5):651–655

35. Scott GC, Meier DA, Dickinson CZ. Cervical lymph node metastasis of thyroid papillary carcinoma imaged with fluorine-18-FDG, technetium-99m-pertechnetate and iodine-131-sodium iodide. J Nucl Med 1995;36(10):1843–1845

36. Caplan RH, Wester S, Kisken AW. Diffuse sclerosing variant of papillary thyroid carcinoma: case report and review of the literature. Endocr Pract 1997;3(5):287–292

37. Lloyd RV, Ferreiro JA, Jin L, Sebo TJ. TGFB, TGFB receptors, Ki-67, and p27(Kip)l expression in papillary thyroid carcinomas. Endocr Pathol 1997;8(4):293–300

38. Martín-Pérez E, Larrañaga E, Serrano P. Diffuse sclerosing variant of papillary carcinoma of the thyroid. Eur J Surg 1998;164(9):713–715

39. Kumarasinghe MP. Cytomorphologic features of diffuse sclerosing variant of papillary carcinoma of the thyroid: a report of two cases in children. Acta Cytol 1998;42(4):983–986

40. Albareda M, Puig-Domingo M, Wengrowicz S, et al. Clinical forms of presentation and evolution of diffuse sclerosing variant of papillary carcinoma and insular variant of follicular carcinoma of the thyroid. Thyroid 1998;8(5):385–391

41. Khan AR, Abu-Eshy SA. Variants of papillary carcinoma of the thyroid: experience at Asir Central Hospital. J R Coll Surg Edinb 1998;43(1):20–25

42. Trovato M, Villari D, Bartolone L, et al. Expression of the hepatocyte growth factor and c-met in normal thyroid, non-neoplastic, and neoplastic nodules. Thyroid 1998;8(2):125–131

43. Muzaffar M, Nigar E, Mushtaq S, Mamoon N; Armed Forces Institute of Pathology. The morphological variants of papillary carcinoma of the thyroid: a clinico-pathological study—AFIP experience. J Pak Med Assoc 1998;48(5):133–137

44. Ohori NP, Schoedel KE. Cytopathology of high-grade papillary thyroid carcinomas: tall-cell variant, diffuse sclerosing variant, and poorly differentiated papillary carcinoma. Diagn Cytopathol 1999;20(1):19–23

45. Imamura Y, Kasahara Y, Fukuda M. Multiple brain metastases from a diffuse sclerosing variant of papillary carcinoma of the thyroid. Endocr Pathol 2000;11(1):97–108

46. Santoro M, Thomas GA, Vecchio G, et al. Gene rearrangement and Chernobyl related thyroid cancers. Br J Cancer 2000;82(2):315–322

47. Kebapci N, Efe B, Kabukcuoglu S, Akalin A, Kebapci M. Diffuse sclerosing variant of papillary thyroid carcinoma with primary squamous cell carcinoma. J Endocrinol Invest 2002;25(8):730–734

48. Marchesi M, Biffoni M, Biancari F, Berni A, Campana FP. Predictors of outcome for patients with differentiated and aggressive thyroid carcinoma. Eur J Surg Suppl 2003;588(588):46–50

49. Triggiani V, Ciampolillo A, Maiorano E. Papillary thyroid carcinoma, diffuse sclerosing variant, with abundant psammoma bodies. Acta Cytol 2003;47(6):1141–1143

50. Chow SM, Chan JK, Law SC, et al. Diffuse sclerosing variant of papillary thyroid carcinoma—clinical features and outcome. Eur J Surg Oncol 2003;29(5):446–449

51. Borson-Chazot F, Causeret S, Lifante JC, Augros M, Berger N, Peix JL. Predictive factors for recurrence from a series of 74 children and adolescents with differentiated thyroid cancer. World J Surg 2004;28(11):1088–1092

52. Hirokawa M, Kuma S, Miyauchi A, et al. Morules in cribriform-morular variant of papillary thyroid carcinoma: immunohistochemical characteristics and distinction from squamous metaplasia. APMIS 2004;112(4-5):275–282

53. Lam AK, Lo CY. Diffuse sclerosing variant of papillary carcinoma of the thyroid: a 35-year comparative study at a single institution. Ann Surg Oncol 2006;13(2):176–181

54. LiVolsi VA, Albores-Saavedra J, Asa SL, et al. Papillary carcinoma. In: DeLellis RA, Llyod RV, Heitz PU, Eng C, eds. World Health Organization Classification of Tumours: Pathology and Genetics—Tumors of Endocrine Organs. Lyon: International Agency for Research on Cancer; 2004:57–66</edb>

55. Harach HR, Williams GT, Williams ED. Familial adenomatous polyposis associated thyroid carcinoma: a distinct type of follicular cell neoplasm. Histopathology 1994;25(6):549–561

56. Cameselle-Teijeiro J, Chan JK. Cribriform-morular variant of papillary carcinoma: a distinctive variant representing the sporadic counterpart of familial adenomatous polyposis-associated thyroid carcinoma? Mod Pathol 1999;12(4):400–411

57. Tomoda C, Miyauchi A, Uruno T, et al. Cribriform-morular variant of papillary thyroid carcinoma: clue to early detection of familial adenomatous polyposis-associated colon cancer. World J Surg 2004;28(9):886–889

58. Uchino S, Noguchi S, Yamashita H, et al. Mutational analysis of the APC gene in cribriform-morula variant of papillary thyroid carcinoma. World J Surg 2006;30(5):775–779

59. Hirokawa M, Maekawa M, Kuma S, Miyauchi A. Cribriform-morular variant of papillary thyroid carcinoma—cytological and immunocytochemical findings of 18 cases. Diagn Cytopathol 2010;38(12):890–896

60. Ng SB, Sittampalam K, Goh YH, Eu KW. Cribriform-morular variant of papillary carcinoma: the sporadic counterpart of familial adenomatous polyposis-associated thyroid carcinoma. A case report with clinical and molecular genetic correlation. Pathology 2003;35(1):42–46

61. Xu B, Yoshimoto K, Miyauchi A, et al. Cribriform-morular variant of papillary thyroid carcinoma: a pathological and molecular genetic study with evidence of frequent somatic mutations in exon 3 of the beta-catenin gene. J Pathol 2003;199(1):58–67

62. Plail RO, Bussey HJ, Glazer G, Thomson JP. Adenomatous polyposis: an association with carcinoma of the thyroid. Br J Surg 1987;74(5):377–380

63. Carcangiu ML, Zampi G, Rosai J. Poorly differentiated ("insular") thyroid carcinoma: a reinterpretation of Langhans' "wuchernde Struma." Am J Surg Pathol 1984;8(9):655–668

64. Sywak M, Pasieka JL, Ogilvie T. A review of thyroid cancer with intermediate differentiation. J Surg Oncol 2004;86(1):44–54

65. Silver CE, Owen RP, Rodrigo JP, Rinaldo A, Devaney KO, Ferlito A. Aggressive variants of papillary thyroid carcinoma. Head Neck 2011;33(7):1052–1059

66. Stevens TM, Richards AT, Bewtra C, Sharma P. Tumors metastatic to thyroid neoplasms: a case report and review of the literature. Patholog Res Int 2011;art no 238693

67. Chin CJ, Franklin JH, Moussa M, Chin JL. Metastasis from renal cell carcinoma to the thyroid 12 years after nephrectomy. CMAJ 2011;183(12):1398–1399

68. Cimino-Mathews A, Sharma R, Netto GJ. Diagnostic use of PAX8, CAIX, TTF-1, and TGB in metastatic renal cell carcinoma of the thyroid. Am J Surg Pathol 2011;35(5):757–761

69. Kelly ME, Kinsella J, d'Adhemar C, Swan N, Ridgway PF. A rare case of thyroid metastasis from pancreatic adenocarcinoma. JOP 2011;12(1):37–39

70. Skowrońska-Jóźwiak E, Krawczyk-Rusiecka K, Adamczewski Z, et al. Metastases of breast cancer to the thyroid gland in two patients—a case report. Endokrynol Pol 2010;61(5):512–515

71. Stoll L, Mudali S, Ali SZ. Merkel cell carcinoma metastatic to the thyroid gland: aspiration findings and differential diagnosis. Diagn Cytopathol 2010;38(10):754–757

72. Cherk MH, Moore M, Serpell J, Swain S, Topliss DJ. Metastatic colorectal cancer to a primary thyroid cancer. World J Surg Oncol 2008;6:122

73. Kaushik A, Ho L. Thyroid metastasis from primary renal cell cancer on FDG PET/CT. Clin Nucl Med 2011;36(1):56–58

74. Manohar K, Mittal BR, Kashyap R, Bhattacharya A, Singh B. Renal cell carcinoma presenting as isolated thyroid metastasis 13 years after radical nephrectomy, detected on F-18 FDG PET/CT. Clin Nucl Med 2010;35(10):818–819

75. Sindoni A, Rizzo M, Tuccari G, et al. Thyroid metastases from clear cell renal carcinoma 18 years after nephrectomy. Ann Endocrinol (Paris) 2010;71(2):127–130

76. NixonI J, Whitcher M, Glick J, et al. Surgical management of metastases to the thyroid gland. Ann Surg Oncol 2011;18(3): 800–804

77. Booya F, Sebo TJ, Kasperbauer JL, Fatourechi V. Primary squamous cell carcinoma of the thyroid: report of ten cases. Thyroid 2006;16(1):89–93

78. Ryska A, Ludvíková M, Rydlová M, Cáp J, Zalud R. Massive squamous metaplasia of the thyroid gland—report of three cases. Pathol Res Pract 2006;202(2):99–106

79. Ashraf MJ, Azarpira N, Khademi B, Peiravi M. Squamous cell carcinoma associated with tall cell variant of papillary carcinoma of the thyroid. Indian J Pathol Microbiol 2010;53(3):548–550

80. Musso-Lassalle S, Butori C, Bailleux S, Santini J, Franc B, Hofman P. A diagnostic pitfall: nodular tumor-like squamous metaplasia with Hashimoto's thyroiditis mimicking a sclerosing mucoepidermoid carcinoma with eosinophilia. Pathol Res Pract 2006;202(5):379–383

81. Lam KY, Lo CY, Liu MC. Primary squamous cell carcinoma of the thyroid gland: an entity with aggressive clinical behaviour and distinctive cytokeratin expression profiles. Histopathology 2001;39(3):279–286

82. Zimmer PW, Wilson D, Bell N. Primary squamous cell carcinoma of the thyroid gland. Mil Med 2003;168(2):124–125

83. Bronner MP, LiVolsi VA. Spindle cell squamous carcinoma of the thyroid: an unusual anaplastic tumor associated with tall cell papillary cancer. Mod Pathol 1991;4(5):637–643

84. Kleer CG, Giordano TJ, Merino MJ. Squamous cell carcinoma of the thyroid: an aggressive tumor associated with tall cell variant of papillary thyroid carcinoma. Mod Pathol 2000;13(7):742–746

85. Rhatigan RM, Roque JL, Bucher RL. Mucoepidermoid carcinoma of the thyroid gland. Cancer 1977;39(1):210–214

86. Hunt JL, LiVolsi VA, Barnes EL. p63 expression in sclerosing mucoepidermoid carcinomas with eosinophilia arising in the thyroid. Mod Pathol 2004;17(5):526–529

87. Chan JK, Albores-Saavedra J, Battifora H, Carcangiu ML, Rosai J. Sclerosing mucoepidermoid thyroid carcinoma with eosinophilia: a distinctive low-grade malignancy arising from the metaplastic follicles of Hashimoto's thyroiditis. Am J Surg Pathol 1991;15(5):438–448

88. Harach HR. A study on the relationship between solid cell nests and mucoepidermoid carcinoma of the thyroid. Histopathology 1985;9(2):195–207

89. Viciana MJ, Galera-Davidson H, Martín-Lacave I, Segura DI, Loizaga JM. Papillary carcinoma of the thyroid with mucoepidermoid differentiation. Arch Pathol Lab Med 1996;120(4):397–398

90. Moreno Egea A, Rodriguez Gonzalez JM, Sola Perez J, Soria T, Parrilla Paricio P. Clinicopathological study of the diffuse sclerosing variety of papillary cancer of the thyroid: presentation of 4 new cases and review of the literature. Eur J Surg Oncol 1994;20(1):7–11

91. Geisinger KR, Steffee CH, McGee RS, Woodruff RD, Buss DH. The cytomorphologic features of sclerosing mucoepidermoid carcinoma of the thyroid gland with eosinophilia. Am J Clin Pathol 1998;109(3):294–301

92. Bondeson L, Bondeson AG. Cytologic features in fine-needle aspirates from a sclerosing mucoepidermoid thyroid carcinoma with eosinophilia. Diagn Cytopathol 1996;15(4):301–305

93. Baloch ZW, Solomon AC, LiVolsi VA. Primary mucoepidermoid carcinoma and sclerosing mucoepidermoid carcinoma with eosinophilia of the thyroid gland: a report of nine cases. Mod Pathol 2000;13(7):802–807

94. Albores-Saavedra J, Gu X, Luna MA. Clear cells and thyroid transcription factor I reactivity in sclerosing mucoepidermoid carcinoma of the thyroid gland. Ann Diagn Pathol 2003;7(6): 348–353

95. Frazier WD, Patel NP, Sullivan CA. Pathology quiz case 1: sclerosing mucoepidermoid carcinoma with eosinophilia (SMECE). Arch Otolaryngol Head Neck Surg 2008;134(3):333–335, 335

96. Ito Y, Miyauchi A, Nakamura Y, Miya A, Kobayashi K, Kakudo K. Clinicopathologic significance of intrathyroidal epithelial thymoma/carcinoma showing thymus-like differentiation: a collaborative study with Member Institutes of The Japanese Society of Thyroid Surgery. Am J Clin Pathol 2007;127(2):230–236

97. Reimann JD, Dorfman DM, Nosé V. Carcinoma showing thymus-like differentiation of the thyroid (CASTLE): a comparative study: evidence of thymic differentiation and solid cell nest origin. Am J Surg Pathol 2006;30(8):994–1001

98. Dorfman DM, Shahsafaei A, Miyauchi A. Intrathyroidal epithelial thymoma (ITET)/carcinoma showing thymus-like differentiation (CASTLE) exhibits CD5 immunoreactivity: new evidence for thymic differentiation. Histopathology 1998;32(2):104–109

99. Shek TW, Luk IS, Ng IO, Lo CY. Lymphoepithelioma-like carcinoma of the thyroid gland: lack of evidence of association with Epstein-Barr virus. Hum Pathol 1996;27(8):851–853

100. Ng WK, Collins RJ, Shek WH, Ng IO. Cytologic diagnosis of "CASTLE" of thyroid gland: report of a case with histologic correlation. Diagn Cytopathol 1996;15(3):224–227

101. Chow SM, Chan JK, Tse LL, Tang DL, Ho CM, Law SC. Carcinoma showing thymus-like element (CASTLE) of thyroid: combined modality treatment in 3 patients with locally advanced disease. Eur J Surg Oncol 2007;33(1):83–85

102. Roka S, Kornek G, Schüller J, Ortmann E, Feichtinger J, Armbruster C. Carcinoma showing thymic-like elements—a rare malignancy of the thyroid gland. Br J Surg 2004;91(2):142–145

103. Cappelli C, Tironi A, Marchetti GP, et al. Aggressive thyroid carcinoma showing thymic-like differentiation (CASTLE): case report and review of the literature. Endocr J 2008;55(4):685–690

104. Chan JK, Rosai J. Tumors of the neck showing thymic or related branchial pouch differentiation: a unifying concept. Hum Pathol 1991;22(4):349–367

105. Casco F, Illanes Moreno M, González Cámpora R, Moreno A, Galera Ruiz H. Spindle epithelial tumor with thymuslike differentiation in a 2-year-old boy: a case report. Anal Quant Cytol Histol 2010;32(1):53–57

106. Ajmi S, Trimeche S, Nouira M, Sfar R, Trabelsi A, Essabbah H. Spindle epithelial tumor with thymus-like differentiation of the thyroid. Clin Nucl Med 2008;33(12):887–888

107. Cheuk W, Jacobson AA, Chan JK. Spindle epithelial tumor with thymus-like differentiation (SETTLE): a distinctive malignant thyroid neoplasm with significant metastatic potential. Mod Pathol 2000;13(10):1150–1155

108. Kloboves-Prevodnik V, Jazbec J, Us-Krasovec M, Lamovec J. Thyroid spindle epithelial tumor with thymus-like differentiation (SETTLE): is cytopathological diagnosis possible? Diagn Cytopathol 2002;26(5):314–319

109. Tong GX, Hamele-Bena D, Wei XJ, O'Toole K. Fine-needle aspiration biopsy of monophasic variant of spindle epithelial tumor with thymus-like differentiation of the thyroid: report of one case and review of the literature. Diagn Cytopathol 2007;35(2):113–119

110. Su L, Beals T, Bernacki EG, Giordano TJ. Spindle epithelial tumor with thymus-like differentiation: a case report with cytologic, histologic, immunohistologic, and ultrastructural findings. Mod Pathol 1997;10(5):510–514

111. Chetty R, Goetsch S, Nayler S, Cooper K. Spindle epithelial tumour with thymus-like element (SETTLE): the predominantly monophasic variant. Histopathology 1998;33(1):71–74

112. Folpe AL, Lloyd RV, Bacchi CE, Rosai J. Spindle epithelial tumor with thymus-like differentiation: a morphologic, immunohistochemical, and molecular genetic study of 11 cases. Am J Surg Pathol 2009;33(8):1179–1186

113. Erickson ML, Tapia B, Moreno ER, McKee MA, Kowalski DP, Reyes-Múgica M. Early metastasizing spindle epithelial tumor with thymus-like differentiation (SETTLE) of the thyroid. Pediatr Dev Pathol 2005;8(5):599–606

9 Paragangliomas of the Head and Neck

David Myssiorek

Core Messages

- Paragangliomas are slow-growing neuroendocrine tumors that can exhibit multicentricity, rare biochemical activity, uncommon malignancy, and may be genetically transmitted.

- About 10 to 50% are familial paragangliomas.

- Only 3% of paragangliomas are biochemically active so testing for catecholamines should be reserved for patients with hypertension, tachycardia, or flushing.

- Multicentricity may be seen in up to 20% of sporadic cases compared with 50% of familial paragangliomas.

- On imaging, carotid paragangliomas can be distinguished from vagal paragangliomas by posterior and anterior displacement of the internal carotid artery.

- Excision of paragangliomas exceeding 3 cm probably benefits from embolization.

- Somatostatin-receptor scintigraphy allows for confirmation of paraganglioma location, identifying multiple tumors, and screening for familial paraganglioma and recurrence.

- A team approach to the management of these tumors is strongly recommended.

- Factors included in determining the best management of a paraganglioma include age, comorbidity, size of the mass, and existing cranial neuropathies.

- Lymph nodes encountered during paraganglioma resection should be sent to pathology to rule out evidence of metastasis.

- When laryngeal paraganglioma is suspected, a contrast computed tomography scan is recommended and transmucosal biopsy should be avoided to prevent excessive bleeding and mucosal scarring.

Paraganglionic tissue was first described by Von Haller in 1743, but it was not until 1862 that the first carotid paraganglioma was described.[1] Scudder excised the first carotid paraganglioma in 1903. These tumors are classically described as slow growing. They have the potential for multicentricity, hereditary transmission, biochemical activity, and malignancy.

Paraganglionic cells are neural crest-derived cells that can be found from the base of the skull to the pelvis. These cells are part of the diffuse neuroendocrine system and are associated with nerves that have sympathetic systems. In the head and neck, paragangliomas are found along major vessels and the vagus nerve. Specific paraganglion cell sites are the carotid body, jugular bulb, Jacobsen's tympanic plexus, vagus nerve, and supraglottic and infraglottic sites. The anatomic location of these slow-growing tumors gives rise to their more modern names (carotid paraganglioma, vagal paraganglioma, and jugular paraganglioma). The aforementioned were previously called carotid body tumors, glomus vagale, and glomus jugulare. Glomus tumors are of blood vessel origin, not neural crest derivation, and therefore the term *glomus* is a misnomer and is misleading.

Paragangliomas have features that make them fascinating and determine their management. Anywhere from 10 to 50% are familially inherited, depending on where the study was performed.[1] They are generally benign and slow growing and uncommonly are biochemically active. Multicentricity is more common in the familial variety. Management may be observation, surgical, or radiotherapeutical.

The prevalence of paragangliomas is higher in communities living at high altitudes.[2,3] Persons living at altitudes higher than 2000 m have been found to have an increased incidence of paraganglioma.[3] Jech et al found no succinate dehydrogenase subunit B (*SDHB*) or SDH subunit D (*SDHD*) mutation in a small series of high-altitude paragangliomas.[4] A similar increase in prevalence of paragangliomas in the Alps has not been observed.[5] Some centers see more familial paraganglioma patients, increasing the number of patients seen and the percentage of familial patients evaluated. The most common paraganglioma is the carotid paraganglioma followed by the jugulotympanic paraganglioma.

Natural Course of Disease

Tumor growth has been estimated to be 1.0 mm per year for actively growing tumors.[6] In the same study including 48 tumors at three sites (carotid paraganglioma, vagal paraganglioma, and jugulotympanic paragangliomas), the doubling times for these sites were 7.13, 8.89, and 13.8 years, respectively. Forty percent of the tumors had no growth while being observed, and 81% of the tumors had a doubling time of greater than 3 years. Symptoms of paragangliomas are directly dependent on the site of the tumor, size of the tumor, and biochemical activity, if any. Therefore, tumor progression is uncommon, and observation in asymptomatic patients may be a reasonable treatment plan.

Grossly, paragangliomas are rubbery vascular masses, usually densely adherent to surrounding structures, especially larger tumors. Carotid paragangliomas splay the internal and external carotid arteries, but they arise from the carotid body, which is located on the deep side of the bifurcation. The vagal paraganglions are found on the deep surface of the internal carotid artery, intermittently involving the vagus nerve. The tumors vary from gray to dark red.

Microscopically, the hallmark of paraganglioma is Zellballen (**Fig. 9.1**). Chief cells and sustentacular cells are arranged in balls of cells. The central cells of the cell ball are polygonal. The surrounding cells are eosinophilic with occasional basophilic sustentacular cells. The chief cells are the active cells of the paraganglioma containing intracytoplasmic dense core granules. Immunostaining with chromogranin, synaptophysin, neuron-specific enolase, and neurofilament stain is usually positive, whereas immunostaining with mucicarmine, periodic acid-Schiff, and argentaffin stains is negative.

Biological activity is present in less than 3% of the patients with head and neck paragangliomas.[7] The paraganglioma chief cells lack *N*-methyl transferase and cannot convert norepinephrine to epinephrine, making these tumors chemically inactive. A fivefold increase in catecholamine levels is required for patients to experience palpitations, headache, sweating, and flushing. Patients with biochemically active tumors will have hypertension, and

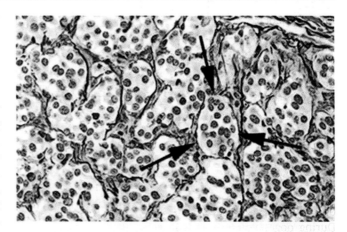

Figure 9.1   A micrograph of Zellballen, the organoid arrangement of chief cells and sustentacular cells that make up paraganglionic tissue.

they should have a 24-hour urine test for vanillyl mandelic acid and metanephrines. In addition, further studies should be carried out to rule out associated pheochromocytomas.

Multicentricity has been estimated to be present in 10 to 20% of sporadic cases.[8] In a review of 1000 carotid paragangliomas, 31% of the cases were found to be bilateral if the patients had familial paragangliomas as opposed to 4% in sporadic cases.[9] Multicentricity is estimated to be present in 10 to 50% of familial cases.[9,10] In a study by Netterville et al on vagal paragangliomas, 80% of the cases were multicentric.[11] Multiple paragangliomas should prompt a search for a familial origin in these tumors. It is possible that the variation in these numbers depends on the prevalence of familial paragangliomas in the study performed because multicentricity is a feature of familial tumors.

Hereditary Paragangliomas

Head and neck paragangliomas may present as sporadic or familial varieties (**Table 9.1**). Familial forms should be sought for several reasons. The hallmarks of a familial paraganglioma are known family member with a paraganglioma, multiple paragangliomas, younger age at onset/detection, male sex, and vagal paragangliomas.[12] If a patient has the familial form, he or she is at risk for multiple tumors, which changes the treatment strategy. It promotes genetic screening for family members, allowing for earlier detection and treatment. One genetic variant (SDHB *vide infra*) is associated with a higher

Table 9.1   Familial versus Sporadic Head and Neck Paraganglioma

Factor	Sporadic	Familial	References
Parent/sibling with PGL	No	Yes	
Multicentricity	10–20%	10–50%	1
Age at detection	Older	Younger	1
SDH mutation	30%	100%	13
Vagal PGL	Less likely	More likely	12
Male sex	Less likely	More likely	12

PGL, paraganglioma; SDH, succinyl dehydrogenase.

rate of pheochromocytomas and an increased incidence of malignant paragangliomas.

Some paragangliomas have been associated with other tumor syndromes. MEN 2, von Hippel-Lindau disease, and neurofibromatosis type 1 have been linked to an increased risk of pheochromocytoma development.[13]

The gene(s) for the familial variety of paraganglioma has been localized to chromosome 11q23.[14] Alterations in the SDH subunits (A, B, C, and D) result in tumor generation. The most common alteration is in SDHD for *PGL1*.[15] *PGL1* is inherited in a Mendelian fashion with genomic imprinting. In this instance, the paternally activated gene, if passed on, will give rise to a phenotypically positive offspring. During oogenesis, the gene is inactivated, resulting in no phenotypically positive children. However, a male carrier of an inactivated *PGL1* gene will pass this gene on in a classic Mendelian fashion. The second most common PGL syndrome is the *SDHB* mutation. These cases have no parent-of-origin heritage and are more prone to malignancy.[16] Germline mutations of *SDHB*, *SDHC*, and *SDHD* have been found in 30% of the sporadic cases.[13] Despite the lack of familial characteristics, this suggests that all patients with paragangliomas should be screened for paraganglioma syndromes.

History and Physical Examination

Typically, the patient with a head and neck paraganglioma presents with a slow-growing, painless neck mass. Because paragangliomas are relatively rare, they are often not suspected in the initial evaluation of the patient with a neck mass. Unless very large or biochemically active, these tumors do not produce symptoms; therefore, a high index of suspicion is required to diagnose these lesions. The average duration from first detection to correct diagnosis is commonly quoted at 4 years. Probably the most common presentation in patients with sporadic paragangliomas is either a positive computed tomography (CT) scan obtained for the evaluation of the neck mass or an incidental finding in patients getting duplex Doppler scans to evaluate carotid stenosis (**Fig. 9.2**).

Notation about the sex of the patient and age at onset may be helpful in determining whether the patient has a familial paraganglioma. A family history of paraganglioma should be sought. An earlier treatment for a paraganglioma or multiple tumors strongly suggests a familial tumor. Keep in mind that a history of pheochromocytoma is also strongly suggestive of one of the paraganglioma syndromes. The patient's place of origin (endemic areas or high-altitude dwelling) must be considered.[17]

Symptoms of hearing loss, tinnitus, cranial neuropathy, Horner syndrome, dysphagia, and dysphonia need to be elicited. They may be subtle with moderate-sized tumors. Headaches, palpitations, flushing, and sweating may be signs of biochemical activity. A history of elevated heart rate and hypertension must be obtained in every patient.

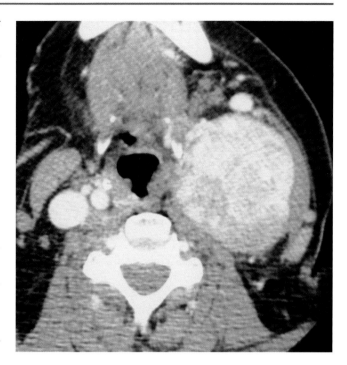

Figure 9.2   Typical appearance of a carotid paraganglioma.

Physical examination of all regions of the head and neck should be performed. Tympanic paragangliomas will present with a red mass behind the tympanic membrane (**Fig. 9.3**). Brown sign is a blanching of the tympanic paraganglioma when pneumotoscopic pressure is placed on the tympanic membrane. With carotid paraganglioma, the mass can be moved in the anterior/posterior plane but not in the craniocaudad plane. These authors find bruits to be uncommon, but the carotid pulse is transmitted through the

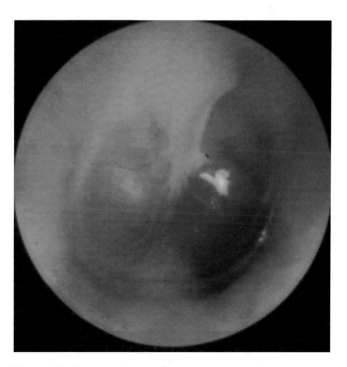

Figure 9.3   Tympanic paraganglioma.

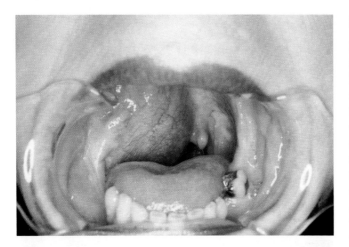

Figure 9.4 Soft palatal bulging secondary to a large right carotid paraganglioma.

mass. When larger, carotid paragangliomas have findings similar to those of parapharyngeal space tumors: unilateral serous otitis, snoring, and bulging of the soft palate (**Fig. 9.4**).

The nonotologic head and neck paragangliomas can all give rise to cranial nerve damage. Cranial nerve involvement is a late sign (cranial nerves IX through XII). Dysphagia and/ or hoarseness can occur with larger carotid tumors. The larger the paraganglioma, the more likely pretreatment neuropathy will be present. Dysphagia can be subtle and due to neural involvement or mass effect. Vagal tumors arise higher in the parapharyngeal space and frequently involve cranial nerves at the time of presentation (**Fig. 9.5**).

In vagal paragangliomas, the vagus nerve is involved early and the site of involvement can be determined by physical examination. Masses at the nodose ganglion will paralyze the vocal fold and spare the soft palate.

After getting the history and physical examination, imaging should be obtained. The goals of imaging are to determine the size, location, relationship to the carotid artery, discover multiple paragangliomas, and reveal local invasion/destruction, especially at the skull base.

Imaging

Imaging plays a critical role in the diagnosis, management, and surveillance of these tumors. The patient suspected of having a paraganglioma may be evaluated by CT, magnetic resonance imaging (MRI), and/or the angiographic equivalent of these modalities. CT scanning can provide critical information about size, location, multicentricity, and local tissue involvement (**Fig. 9.6**). It is probably not as sensitive as MRI at the skull base and with regard to local tissue involvement. CT scanning with contrast can reveal an enhancing mass splaying the internal and external carotid arteries in carotid paragangliomas. The vagal paragangliomas will displace the internal carotid artery anteriorly, while the carotid paragangliomas will displace it posteriorly (**Fig. 9.7A, B**). CT scanning of the temporal bone demonstrates the bony anatomy of the middle ear and jugular foramen.[18] Tympanic paragangliomas appear as soft-tissue masses on the cochlear promontory. Ossicular destruction is evident as these tumors grow. Jugular paragangliomas destroy by erosion, expanding the jugular fossa. Larger tumors erode into the eustachian tube, carotid canal, and neuroforamina (**Fig. 9.8**). Very large lesions will destroy the jugular spine and the hypoglossal canal, and finally will invade the cranial contents.

Flow voids within paragangliomas create the classic "salt and pepper" appearance on MRI (**Fig. 9.9**). Dural involvement and skull base involvement are best detected with gadolinium-enhanced MRI.

If a lesion is detected, further confirmation can be obtained with [111]Indium pentetreotide (octreotide) imaging (**Fig. 9.10**). Octreotide is a radiolabeled somatostatin analog that targets receptor-rich cells. It differs from positron emission tomography (PET) imaging in that it is a measure

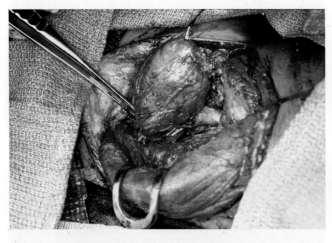

Figure 9.5 Right vagal paraganglioma. Note the position of the underlying carotid artery.

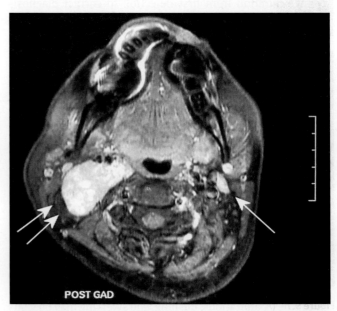

POST GAD

Figure 9.6 Magnetic resonance imaging of a right carotid paraganglioma.

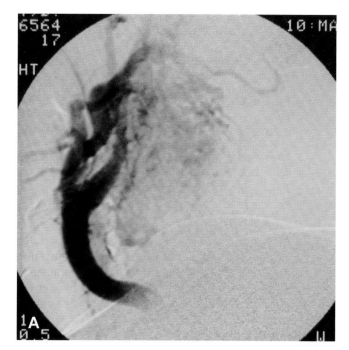

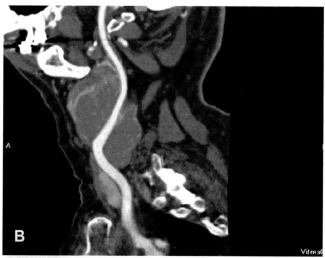

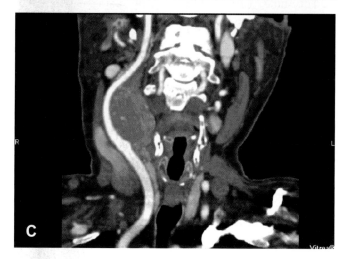

Figure 9.7   (A) This carotid paraganglioma has displaced the internal carotid artery posteriorly. (B, C) These vagal paragangliomas have displaced the internal carotid artery anteriorly.

of receptor density rather than cell activity. Published sensitivity of this scan is in excess of 90%.[19] It is also beneficial in determining multifocal tumors, metastases from malignant paragangliomas, and has been used as a screening method for familial paragangliomas.[20,21] The latter has been supplanted by genetic testing. 18-Fluorine L-3, 4-dihydroxyphenylalanine (^{18}F-DOPA) PET has been shown to be an even more sensitive modality than octreotide. It is more extensive as well. Imaging of neuroendocrine tumors with ^{18}F-DOPA PET has an accuracy of 90%.[22] Hoegerle et al studied paragangliomas with ^{18}F-DOPA PET.[23] They demonstrated the superiority of ^{18}F-DOPA PET scanning in detecting small paragangliomas that could be missed on MRI. Both these modalities have replaced metaiodobenzylguanidine (MIBG) imaging for paragangliomas.

The role of arteriography, critical in the past, has been limited (**Fig. 9.11A to C**). CT angiography and MR angiography have been able to determine the relationship of the tumor to the carotid arteries. They can also determine occlusion and potential feeder vessels. In patients with a large paraganglioma, four-vessel angiography can determine feeding vessels, flow dynamics of the tumor, tumor location, and multicentricity.[24] Its most important role is allowing embolization of large tumors in which resection will be performed. Persky et al determined that presurgical embolization decreases intraoperative blood loss.[24] Most head and neck paragangliomas derive some vascularization from the ascending pharyngeal artery. Other arteries from the external carotid artery, the internal maxillary artery, the vertebral artery, and even the internal carotid artery may supply these tumors depending on the location. Embolization is safe when experienced angiographers perform it. Tikkakoski et al recommended embolization for paragangliomas greater than 3 cm.[25] Netterville et al recommended embolization for carotid paragangliomas to reduce blood loss and improve the ability to excise these tumors by providing a bloodless operative field.[26] Blood loss after embolization of carotid paragangliomas was decreased by 1 to 200 mL. It is also recommended for vagal paragangliomas in patients with tumors greater than 3 cm.[27] Smaller tumors can be managed by experienced teams of surgeons without embolization. **Fig. 9.12A, B** shows an angiogram and intraoperative exposure of a small carotid paraganglioma.

Complications of embolization include stroke and cranial neuropathy. Stroke is caused by reflux of embolic material from the external carotid artery into the internal carotid artery or flow of embolization particles through anastomotic channels into the central nervous system's blood supply.

Malignant Paragangliomas

Malignant paragangliomas are not typical malignancies because their diagnosis is dependent on behavior rather than abnormal histology.[28] The benign lesion is indistinguishable from the malignant variant under the microscope. Malignancy is defined by regional or distant metastases.

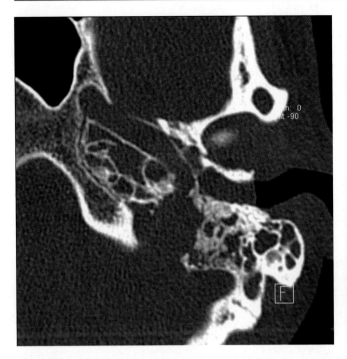

Figure 9.8 A computed tomography scan of the left temporal bone revealing a widened jugular foramen and filling of the middle ear by tumor.

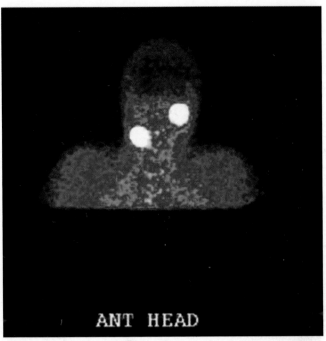

Figure 9.10 [111]Indium pentetreotide (octreotide) image of a patient with bilateral paragangliomas.

Less than 5% of paragangliomas are cancerous.[29] Locally aggressive behavior is not a determinant of malignancy either, except in sinonasal paragangliomas, which are rare.

In the head and neck, vagal paragangliomas have the highest rate of malignancy. In a review by Druck et al, 19% of the vagal paragangliomas were considered cancerous.[30] Sniezek et al found a rate of 10%.[27] The common sites for metastases included cervical lymph nodes, lung, and bone. The malignant potential is genetically driven. In a report by Boedeker et al, 34% of the patients with *SDHB* mutations were found to have malignancies.[16]

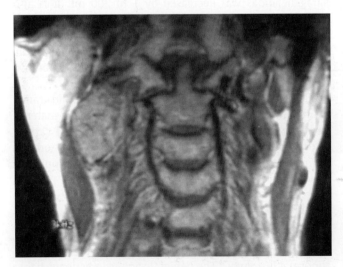

Figure 9.9 The "salt and pepper" appearance of a carotid paraganglioma in a coronal magnetic resonance image.

Carotid paragangliomas are uncommonly malignant. van der Mey et al cited an incidence of 1.4%.[31] Laryngeal paragangliomas rarely present as malignancies, with one bona fide case reported.[32]

During excision, lymph nodes are invariably in the dissection field and should be removed. This maneuver provides first echelon information about potential malignancy and makes the operative field clearer.[29]

Currently, the treatment for malignant paragangliomas remains surgical followed by radiation therapy. No chemotherapy regimens have helped at the time of this writing.

Fifty-nine cases of malignant paragangliomas of the head and neck extracted from the National Cancer Database diagnosed between 1985 and 1996 revealed 51 cases of malignant paragangliomas in which the location of metastasis was recorded.[33] Most of the paragangliomas (68.6%) were confined to regional lymph nodes, and 31.4% of the patients had distant disease. The overall 5-year survival rate was 60%. Regional invasion was associated with a survival rate of 77% versus 12% if distant sites were involved.

If possible, surgical excision of local disease offers the best chance of cure. Treatment of primary and metastatic disease usually involves radiation to affected sites. Chemotherapy with vincristine, cyclophosphamide, and dacarbazine resulted in partial or complete responses in 55% of the patients in one study.[34] Unfortunately, combining radiation and chemotherapy has provided little improvement in outcome.[35] Mesna, ifosfamide, doxorubicin, dacarbazine, gemcitabine, paclitaxel, and etoposide-cisplatin have been advocated, but toxicities are high.[36,37]

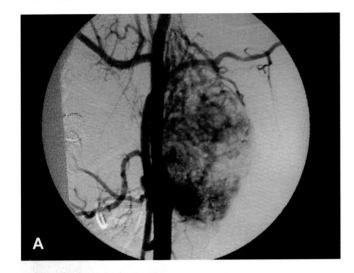

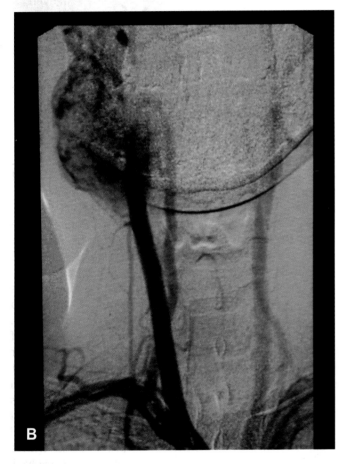

Figure 9.11 (A) Right carotid angiogram of a vagal paraganglioma. Note the lack of splaying of the internal and external carotid arteries. (B) Four-vessel angiography of a right vagal paraganglioma showing location at the skull base.

[131]I MIBG is taken up by paraganglioma cells in neurosecretory granules. In a study by Scholz et al, administration of ^{131}I MIBG to patients with malignant paragangliomas or pheochromocytomas resulted in a 30% radiographic response.[38] A positive response was associated with a median survival period of 22 months. High-dose [131]I

MIBG resulted in a 5-year survival rate of 75% in 19 patients with paraganglioma.[39] Similarly, radiolabeled somatostatin analogs such as octreotide have not resulted in lasting responses.[40]

Treatment of paragangliomas at all locations is usually surgical. The goal of surgery is complete resection of the tumor. One must consider the slow growth of these tumors, possible biochemical activity, and increased incidence of complications with larger tumors (cranial neuropathies and cerebrovascular accidents) before undertaking an operation. Extremes of age, poor medical condition, and preexistent contralateral cranial neuropathy would promote a nonsurgical approach. A team approach is always recommended. All radiology studies require review by the team preoperatively. The interventional radiologist may provide information on the vascular anatomy of the tumor. Embolization, if selected, should be performed 24 hours before surgery. In many instances, the surgical team consists of the head and neck surgeon and a vascular surgeon.

Patients with biochemically active paragangliomas require preoperative α and β adrenergic blockade.[41] Alpha adrenergic blockade should commence before β blockade. Unopposed α stimulation may result in hypertensive crisis. Alpha blockade should start 10 days before surgery. Goals for this blockade should be a systolic blood pressure of less than 120 mm Hg. After successful blockade, β blockers should be started slowly. Despite blockade, acute crises have been reported and should be treated like a pheochromocytoma.

The most common paraganglioma is the carotid paraganglioma. In a study by van der Mey et al, patients were managed by observation.[42] With a 32-year follow-up of 108 patients, no survival advantage was found in patients treated surgically or radiotherapeutically or by observation. This must be considered when deciding to operate on carotid paragangliomas. Arterial disruption should be anticipated, and vascular surgical expertise is frequently necessary. The risk of cerebrovascular accidents has not been a major one because of the immediate vascular repair, but the risk of cranial neuropathy increases with increased tumor size.[43-45]

Bilateral carotid paragangliomas present a particular challenge and are the most common combination of multiple paragangliomas. Attempts at simultaneous bilateral surgical excision are not recommended. In this case if one carotid paraganglioma has caused a cranial neuropathy, then that lesion should be resected first. The second lesion may be resected at a later date to avoid the labile blood pressure that occurs after the resection of bilateral baroreceptor function. If there are no symptoms preoperatively, then the smaller carotid paraganglioma should be resected first. The larger lesion is more likely to be associated with postoperative vagal or hypoglossal nerve injury.

Older patients deserve special consideration. Older patients do not rebound well following surgically induced mono or multiple cranial neuropathies. The growth rate of these tumors is slow, and unless the tumor has caused

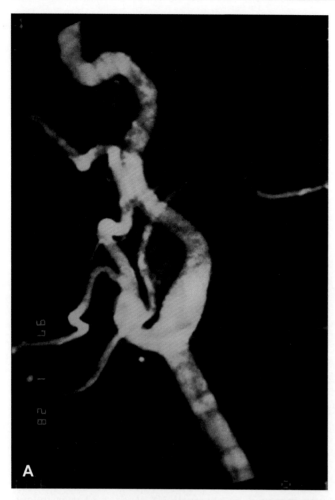

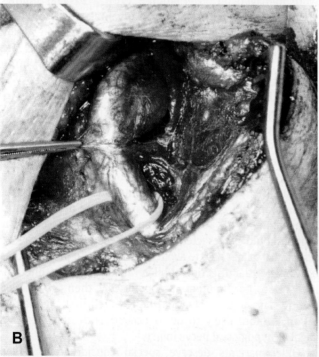

Figure 9.12 (A) An angiogram of a small carotid paraganglioma. (B) Intraoperative exposure of a small carotid paraganglioma. Small paragangliomas do not require embolization.

a cranial neuropathy it is extremely unlikely to affect that patient in his or her lifetime. For similar reasons, surgery on infirm patients should be avoided if possible.

The technique of removal starts with having the imaging available in the operating room, positioning the patient with the neck in extension facing away from the lesion. Two different incisions have generally been used: the horizontal and the incision along the anterior border of the sternocleidomastoid muscle. Vascular surgeons tend to be more familiar with the latter incision, which is used frequently in carotid endarterectomy. The advantages of this incision are rapid access, good healing, and minimal flap elevation. The horizontal incision allows excellent access, very good healing, and a more cosmetic outcome.

Meticulous dissection is required for all steps of carotid paraganglioma excision. Upon reflecting the sternocleidomastoid muscle, lymph nodes are frequently encountered. Because vagal paragangliomas have a higher risk of malignancy, dissection of lymph nodes during the extirpation is advised. Levels II and III are in the operative field and easily accessible. They should be removed to provide clear access and potential information about malignancy. The next step is dissection of the lower cranial nerves (cranial nerves IX through XII). Approximately 20% of the cases result in permanent lower cranial neuropathy.[31] The tenth cranial nerve should be identified and traced superiorly (**Fig. 9.13**). The ninth cranial nerve is harder to define in this surgery. Vascular control of the common carotid artery, internal carotid artery, and external carotid artery with vascular loops should be performed at the outset of the procedure. Not only does this step afford control of the arterial system, but it also allows manipulation of the tumor. If the superior artery can be identified, the superior laryngeal nerve may be discovered coming medially from behind the carotid artery. The carotid body is on the posterior surface of the carotid bifurcation in the adventitia of the artery. Therefore, the tumor is located posterior to the artery. The plane of dissection ideally is periadventitial, but not always accessible because of tumor vessel recruitment. Sutures and clips can be used to decrease blood loss, but most surgeons prefer a fine-tipped bipolar cautery to aid in this step of the dissection. Some surgeons dissect proximally along the external carotid artery to the ascending pharyngeal artery, which is frequently a dominant arterial supply to the tumor if the ligation decreases blood loss. Other surgeons dissect the internal carotid artery off the tumor to the bifurcation. It is not necessary to resect the external carotid artery. During dissection of the bifurcation, low-dose heparin (50 IU/kg body weight) can be given during temporary occlusion of the carotid artery, if necessary. In the event of damage, the patient needs to be heparinized as the vessel is bypassed or repaired. Internal carotid artery ligation results in cerebrovascular accident in approximately two-thirds of the patients.

Other options include radiation therapy or observation. Radiation is felt to arrest tumor growth; however, as

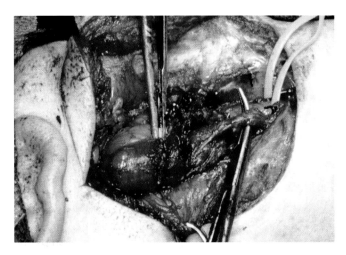

Figure 9.13 The tenth cranial nerve isolated from the carotid paraganglioma during resection.

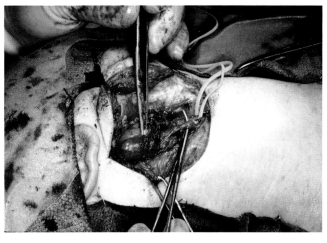

Figure 9.14   The vagal nerve inseparable from a vagal paraganglioma.

shown earlier, tumor growth may be immeasurable over many years. If radiation is elected, 45 Gy in 25 fractions is suggested.[46] Vagal paragangliomas differ from carotid paragangliomas in many ways. They are usually located superiorly to the carotid body and tend to push the internal and external carotid arteries anteromedially. The vagal paraganglioma may involve the jugular foramen or invade the middle cranial fossa. During growth, the lesion is more likely to present orally as a bulge in the soft palate. However, the lesion may grow through the jugular foramen resulting in the so-called dumbbell tumor. Virtually every vagal paraganglioma is associated with the vagus nerve, and excision rarely spares the vagus nerve and its attendant neuropathy (**Fig. 9.14**). Miller et al reported 2 of 16 vagal paragangliomas with normal vocal fold activity/swallowing after excision.[47] Woods et al found vagal neuropathy in 21 of 24 (87%) resected vagal paragangliomas.[48] Netterville et al's series reported 100% vagal neuropathy in a series of 46 tumors.[11] Other lower cranial nerves have been involved/damaged secondarily to vagal paragangliomas or their surgery.

In Netterville et al's series,[11] 17% of the patients had hypoglossal neuropathy at presentation. Other nerves included glossopharyngeal (11%), spinal accessory (11%), facial (6%), and vagus (28%). Miller et al determined that a combination of cranial nerves X and XII damage resulted in the greatest risk of aspiration postoperatively.[47] These facts must be taken into account when considering an operation for vagal paragangliomas.

Less Common Paragangliomas

Paraganglion cells can be found along the major vasculature and parasympathetic nervous system of the neck.[49] Considering that 0.01 to 0.6% of head and neck tumors are paragangliomas and that the bulk of these are carotid, jugulotympanic, and vagal paragangliomas, other locations are rare.

Laryngeal Paragangliomas

Paraganglion cells can be found in the superior paraglottic space (supraglottic paraganglioma) lateral to the quadrangular membrane and laterally in the infraglottic space. It is possible that some of the thyroidal paragangliomas reported were actually infraglottic paragangliomas. Supraglottic paragangliomas are far more common than infraglottic paragangliomas. Approximately 14% of laryngeal paragangliomas are infraglottic.[32]

These patients present with hoarseness and sore throat. If the tumor is very large, it can obstruct the airway. Physical examination will reveal a submucosal bulge in the false vocal fold on laryngeal examination (**Fig. 9.15**). There has been one report of a malignancy in the larynx,[32] and lymphadenopathy has not been reported. Laryngeal paragangliomas have not been associated with hereditary paraganglioma syndromes.

The diagnosis can be made preoperatively without a biopsy, but most patients get biopsied through the mucosa, because the index of suspicion for this tumor is low. This results in brisk bleeding from this very vascular tumor. Tracheotomy and/or packing of the larynx are frequently necessary. If a submucosal laryngeal mass is detected, CT scanning with contrast or MR imaging will disclose a very vascular tumor (**Fig. 9.16**). CT scanning with contrast should reveal a vascular tumor, and its relationship to the thyroid and cricoid cartilages, size, and degree of airway compromise can be evaluated. Octreotide imaging can distinguish between lymphoma, neurilemmoma, and paraganglioma. A negative or weakly positive study argues against paraganglioma. The differential diagnosis of solid submucosal lesions in the larynx includes lymphoma carcinoid, minor salivary gland cancers, cartilaginous tumors, and adenocarcinoma.[50]

The treatment of laryngeal paragangliomas is surgical. Embolization is not necessary because the blood supply is invariably through the laryngeal branch of the superior

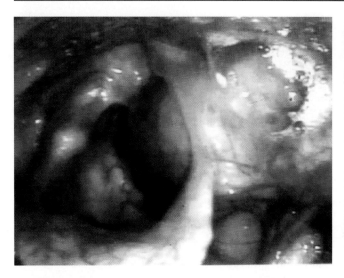

Figure 9.15 A left supraglottic paraganglioma found submucosally in the false vocal fold.

Printed with permission from: John Wiley and Sons. Brown SM, Myssiorek D. Lateral thyrotomy for excision of laryngeal paragangliomas. *Laryngoscope* 2006;116(1):157–159.

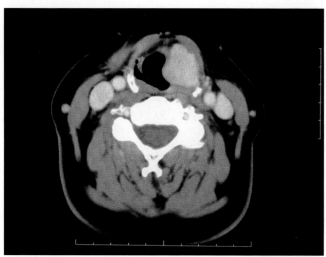

Figure 9.16 Computed tomography scan of a supraglottic paraganglioma. It is submucosal and hypervascular.

Printed with permission from: John Wiley and Sons. Brown SM, Myssiorek D. Lateral thyrotomy for excision of laryngeal paragangliomas. *Laryngoscope* 2006;116(1):157–159.

thyroid artery. The tumor can be removed via a lateral laryngotomy.[51] The artery is identified and ligated, taking care to avoid the internal branch of the superior laryngeal nerve, as it enters the thyrohyoid membrane. The thyrohyoid membrane is incised, and the lesion is easily identified. Blunt and sharp dissection along the capsule is usually easy, and the tumor can be resected while sparing mucosa as long as a preoperative deep biopsy was not performed. The thyroid cartilage's superior edge can be taken down to improve exposure. Closure can be performed by reapproximation of the thyrohyoid membrane or oversewing the strap muscles. A drain decreases the chances of the fistula postoperatively.

Infraglottic paragangliomas are derived from the vagal paraganglionic tissue. The symptoms associated with infraglottic paragangliomas are hoarseness and obstruction, but hemoptysis is also reported. The treatment of these tumors is surgical. Total laryngectomy is not necessary. Again, a lateral approach or laryngofissure is the best approach to these tumors.[52] No treatment of the neck is necessary. Lymphadenopathy should raise the suspicion of other neuroendocrine cancers or epithelial cancers. Endoscopic complete removal has been reported with lasting success.

Sinonasal Paragangliomas

These are very rare tumors[52] and are assumed to originate from the paraganglionic tissue in the pterygopalatine fossa.[53] They are more common in women and tend to arise in the ethmoidal region, but have been reported in all the paranasal sinuses. They present as expansile nasal lesions, with the most common symptoms being congestion, obstruction, rhinorrhea, and epistaxis. They are rarely biochemically active.[49] These masses are encapsulated, pulsatile, and polypoid. The differential diagnoses include esthesioneuroblastoma, glioma, angiofibroma, rhabdomyosarcoma, meningioma, angiosarcoma, and hemangiopericytoma. Tumors from the jugular, orbital, and vagal paragangliomas may present in the sinonasal region.[54] Although they are usually benign, the sinonasal paragangliomas are the most likely to be malignant of all the paragangliomas.[25] Approximately 24% are malignant.[55] This may be partially because of the criterion used to evaluate malignancy. Local invasion into brain or other nonneuroendocrine tissue is considered a malignant marker.

Complete excision is the treatment for sinonasal paragangliomas. Classically open techniques such as medial maxillectomy via lateral rhinotomy or facial degloving have been used. Successful endoscopic removal has also been reported with good follow-up.[54]

References

1. Myssiorek D. Head and neck paragangliomas: an overview. Otolaryngol Clin North Am 2001;34(5):829–836, v
2. Pacheco-Ojeda L, Durango E, Rodriquez C, Vivar N. Carotid body tumors at high altitudes: Quito, Ecuador, 1987. World J Surg 1988;12(6):856–860
3. Rodríguez-Cuevas S, López-Garza J, Labastida-Almendaro S. Carotid body tumors in inhabitants of altitudes higher than 2000 meters above sea level. Head Neck 1998;20(5):374–378
4. Jech M, Alvarado-Cabrero I, Albores-Saavedra J, Dahia PL, Tischler AS. Genetic analysis of high altitude paragangliomas. Endocr Pathol 2006;17(2):201–202

5. Baysal BE. Genomic imprinting and environment in hereditary paraganglioma. Am J Med Genet C Semin Med Genet 2004;129C(1):85–90

6. Jansen JC, van den Berg R, Kuiper A, van der Mey AG, Zwinderman AH, Cornelisse CJ. Estimation of growth rate in patients with head and neck paragangliomas influences the treatment proposal. Cancer 2000;88(12):2811–2816

7. Lawson W. Glomus bodies and tumors. N Y State J Med 1980;80(10):1567–1575

8. Balatsouras DG, Eliopoulos PN, Economou CN. Multiple glomus tumours. J Laryngol Otol 1992;106(6):538–543

9. Grufferman S, Gillman MW, Pasternak LR, Peterson CL, Young WG Jr. Familial carotid body tumors: case report and epidemiologic review. Cancer 1980;46(9):2116–2122

10. Gardner P, Dalsing M, Weisberger E, Sawchuk A, Miyamoto R. Carotid body tumors, inheritance, and a high incidence of associated cervical paragangliomas. Am J Surg 1996;172(2):196–199

11. Netterville JL, Jackson CG, Miller FR, Wanamaker JR, Glasscock ME. Vagal paraganglioma: a review of 46 patients treated during a 20-year period. Arch Otolaryngol Head Neck Surg 1998;124(10): 1133–1140

12. Neumann HP, Erlic Z, Boedeker CC, et al. Clinical predictors for germline mutations in head and neck paraganglioma patients: cost reduction strategy in genetic diagnostic process as fall-out. Cancer Res 2009;69(8):3650–3656

13. Boedeker CC, Neumann HP, Offergeld C, et al. Clinical features of paraganglioma syndromes. Skull Base 2009;19(1):17–25

14. Baysal BE, Ferrell RE, Willett-Brozick JE, et al. Mutations in SDHD, a mitochondrial complex II gene, in hereditary paraganglioma. Science 2000;287(5454):848–851

15. Neumann HP, Pawlu C, Peczkowska M, et al; European-American Paraganglioma Study Group. Distinct clinical features of paraganglioma syndromes associated with SDHB and SDHD gene mutations. JAMA 2004;292(8):943–951

16. Boedeker CC, Neumann HP, Maier W, Bausch B, Schipper J, Ridder GJ. Malignant head and neck paragangliomas in SDHB mutation carriers. Otolaryngol Head Neck Surg 2007;137(1):126–129

17. Neumann HP, Eng C. The approach to the patient with paraganglioma. J Clin Endocrinol Metab 2009;94(8):2677–2683

18. Lustrin ES, Palestro C, Vaheesan K. Radiographic evaluation and assessment of paragangliomas. Otolaryngol Clin North Am 2001;34(5):881–906, vi

19. Kwekkeboom DJ, van Urk H, Pauw BK, et al. Octreotide scintigraphy for the detection of paragangliomas. J Nucl Med 1993;34(6): 873–878

20. Telischi FF, Bustillo A, Whiteman ML, et al. Octreotide scintigraphy for the detection of paragangliomas. Otolaryngol Head Neck Surg 2000;122(3):358–362

21. Myssiorek D, Palestro CJ. [111]Indium pentetreotide scan detection of familial paragangliomas. Laryngoscope 1998;108(2):228–231

22. Kauhanen S, Seppänen M, Ovaska J, et al. The clinical value of [18F] fluoro-dihydroxyphenylalanine positron emission tomography in primary diagnosis, staging, and restaging of neuroendocrine tumors. Endocr Relat Cancer 2009;16(1):255–265

23. Hoegerle S, Ghanem N, Altehoefer C, et al. 18F-DOPA positron emission tomography for the detection of glomus tumours. Eur J Nucl Med Mol Imaging 2003;30(5):689–694

24. Persky MS, Setton A, Niimi Y, Hartman J, Frank D, Berenstein A. Combined endovascular and surgical treatment of head and n eck paragangliomas—a team approach. Head Neck 2002;24(5): 423–431

25. Tikkakoski T, Luotonen J, Leinonen S, et al. Preoperative embolization in the management of neck paragangliomas. Laryngoscope 1997;107(6):821–826

26. Netterville JL, Reilly KM, Robertson D, Reiber ME, Armstrong WB, Childs P. Carotid body tumors: a review of 30 patients with 46 tumors. Laryngoscope 1995;105(2):115–126

27. Sniezek JC, Netterville JL, Sabri AN. Vagal paragangliomas. Otolaryngol Clin North Am 2001;34(5):925–939, vi

28. Walsh RM, Leen EJ, Gleeson MJ, Shaheen OH. Malignant vagal paraganglioma. J Laryngol Otol 1997;111(1):83–88

29. Rinaldo A, Myssiorek D, Devaney KO, Ferlito A. Which paragangliomas of the head and neck have a higher rate of malignancy? Oral Oncol 2004;40(5):458–460

30. Druck NS, Spector GJ, Ciralsky RH, Ogura JH. Malignant glomus vagale: report of a case and review of the literature. Arch Otolaryngol 1976;102(10):534–536

31. van der Mey AG, Jansen JC, van Baalen JM. Management of carotid body tumors. Otolaryngol Clin North Am 2001;34(5):907–924, vi

32. Barnes L. Paragangliomas of the larynx. J Laryngol Otol 1993;107(7):664, author reply 665–666

33. Lee JH, Barich F, Karnell LH, et al; American College of Surgeons Commission on Cancer; American Cancer Society. National Cancer Data Base report on malignant paragangliomas of the head and neck. Cancer 2002;94(3):730–737

34. Huang H, Abraham J, Hung E, et al. Treatment of malignant pheochromocytoma/paraganglioma with cyclophosphamide, vincristine, and dacarbazine: recommendation from a 22-year follow-up of 18 patients. Cancer 2008;113(8):2020–2028

35. Sisson JC, Shapiro B, Shulkin BL, Urba S, Zempel S, Spaulding S. Treatment of malignant pheochromocytomas with [131]-I metaiodobenzylguanidine and chemotherapy. Am J Clin Oncol 1999;22(4):364–370

36. Bravo EL, Kalmadi SR, Gill I. Clinical utility of temozolomide in the treatment of malignant paraganglioma: a preliminary report. Horm Metab Res 2009;41(9):703–706

37. Mora J, Cruz O, Parareda A, Sola T, de Torres C. Treatment of disseminated paraganglioma with gemcitabine and docetaxel. Pediatr Blood Cancer 2009;53(4):663–665

38. Scholz T, Eisenhofer G, Pacak K, Dralle H, Lehnert H. Clinical review: current treatment of malignant pheochromocytoma. J Clin Endocrinol Metab 2007;92(4):1217–1225

39. Fitzgerald PA, Goldsby RE, Huberty JP, et al. Malignant pheochromocytomas and paragangliomas: a phase II study of therapy with high-dose ^{131}I-metaiodobenzylguanidine (^{131}I-MIBG). Ann N Y Acad Sci 2006;1073:465–490

40. Kau R, Arnold W. Somatostatin receptor scintigraphy and therapy of neuroendocrine (APUD) tumors of the head and neck. Acta Otolaryngol 1996;116(2):345–349

41. Joynt KE, Moslehi JJ, Baughman KL. Paragangliomas: etiology, presentation, and management. Cardiol Rev 2009;17(4):159–164

42. van der Mey AG, Frijns JH, Cornelisse CJ, et al. Does intervention improve the natural course of glomus tumors? A series of 108 patients seen in a 32-year period. Ann Otol Rhinol Laryngol 1992;101(8):635–642

43. Hallett JW Jr, Nora JD, Hollier LH, Cherry KJ Jr, Pairolero PC. Trends in neurovascular complications of surgical management for carotid body and cervical paragangliomas: a fifty-year experience with 153 tumors. J Vasc Surg 1988;7(2):284–291

44. Evenson LJ, Mendenhall WM, Parsons JT, Cassisi NJ. Radiotherapy in the management of chemodectomas of the carotid body and glomus vagale. Head Neck 1998;20(7):609–613

45. Weed DT, Netterville JL, O'Malley BB. Paragangliomas of the head and neck. In: Harrison LB, Sessions RB, Hong WK, eds. Head and Neck Cancer: A Multidisciplinary Approach. Philadelphia, PA: Lippincott-Raven; 1999:777–798

46. Mendenhall WM, Hinerman RW, Amdur RJ, et al. Treatment of paragangliomas with radiation therapy. Otolaryngol Clin North Am 2001;34(5):1007–1020, vii–viii

47. Miller RB, Boon MS, Atkins JP, Lowry LD. Vagal paraganglioma: the Jefferson experience. Otolaryngol Head Neck Surg 2000;122(4):482–487

48. Woods CI, Strasnick B, Jackson CG. Surgery for glomus tumors: the Otology Group experience. Laryngoscope 1993;103 (11, Pt 2, Suppl 60):65–70

49. Pellitteri PK, Rinaldo A, Myssiorek D, et al. Paragangliomas of the head and neck. Oral Oncol 2004;40(6):563–575

50. Ferlito A, Barnes L, Wenig BM. Identification, classification, treatment, and prognosis of laryngeal paraganglioma: review of the literature and eight new cases. Ann Otol Rhinol Laryngol 1994;103(7):525–536

51. Brown SM, Myssiorek D. Lateral thyrotomy for excision of laryngeal paragangliomas. Laryngoscope 2006;116(1):157–159

52. Myssiorek D, Halaas Y, Silver CE. Laryngeal and sinonasal paragangliomas. Otolaryngol Clin North Am 2001;34(5):971–982, vii

53. Mauren PR, Andrea MC, Vanessa SM, et al. Nasal paraganglioma: a case report. Rev Bras Otorrinolaringol (Engl Ed) 2005;71:237–240

54. Mouadeb DA, Chandra RK, Kennedy DW, Feldman M. Sinonasal paraganglioma: endoscopic resection with a 4-year follow-up. Head Neck 2003;25(12):1077–1081

55. Lecanu JB, Arkwright S, Halimi PH, Trotoux J, Bonfils P. Multifocal malignant paraganglioma of the paranasal sinuses: a case report. Otolaryngol Head Neck Surg 2002;126(4):445–447

B. Aerodigestive Neoplasms of the Head and Neck

10 Cancers of the Lip and Oral Cavity

Suhail I. Sayed and A. K. D'Cruz

Core Messages

- Cancers of the lip and oral cavity are unique and occur with the highest frequency in Southeast Asia due to the unique habit of tobacco chewing.

- Numerous subsites within the oral cavity have distinct biological features. Proper assessment of the epicenter of the lesions is hence imperative.

- There are well-defined premalignant lesions of the lip and oral cavity.

- Early stage tumors are usually treated with single modality, with surgery being indicated in the majority.

- Locally advanced tumors are treated with combined modality, the treatment being surgery followed by adjuvant radiotherapy/chemoradiation.

- The majority of the cancer patients present late and hence emphasis for treatment should be on early detection.

- Similarly, treatment outcomes should be improved by providing the modality giving the best possible health-related quality of life.

Cancers of the lip and oral cavity rank tenth in the list of cancers prevalent in the world population. Globally, oral cancers account for approximately 405,000 new cases diagnosed each year with two-thirds of them occurring in developing countries (Sri Lanka, India, Pakistan, and Bangladesh).[1] In these countries, lip and oral cavity cancer is most commonly seen in men and accounts for 30% of all new cancer cases diagnosed annually. In India, the incidence rate seen in men is 4.5 to 6.1/100,000 but may be as high as 13.9/100,000 in certain regions such as Bhopal.[2,3] Oral cancers in the Indian population usually occur a decade earlier compared to the western population, with 60 to 80% of them presenting in an advanced stage (III/IV).[4] Cosmesis and important functions such as speech and swallowing are therefore affected both by the disease itself and treatment. Emphasis therefore should be on prevention and early detection to avoid significant impact on health-related quality of life.

Relevant Anatomy and Distinctive Features

The oral cavity extends anterior from the skin–vermilion junction of the lips to the junction of the hard and soft palate and the line of circumvallate papillae. It is further subdivided into various subsites, each with a distinct International Classification of Diseases code (**Fig. 10.1**). Epidemiologically too, oral cavity cancers differ in their prevalence according to the geographical areas with varying patterns of tobacco use. It is imperative for a clinician to identify the epicenter of origin of the cancer as each subsite has a distinct biological behavior and impact for treatment.

Lip (C00.0 to C00.9)

Extent: The lip begins at the junction of the vermilion border with the skin and includes only the vermilion surface or that portion of the lip that comes into contact with the opposing lip. It is well defined into an upper and lower lip joined at the commissures of the mouth.

Lymphatic drainage: *Upper lip*—Buccal, parotid→prevascular facial nodes→submandibular nodes→upper deep cervical nodes. *Lower lip*—Submandibular nodes→upper deep cervical nodes.

Distinctive features: Cancers of the lip are commonly seen in pipe and cigar smokers. Also, people chronically exposed to harmful ultraviolet rays such as farmers can develop these cancers. These tumors are predominantly treated by surgical excision and require complex reconstruction to provide adequate cosmesis.

Buccal Mucosa (C06.0 to C06.2, C06.7, and C06.8)

Extent: Buccal mucosa includes all the membrane lining of the inner surface of the cheeks and lips from the line of contact of the opposing lips to the line of attachment

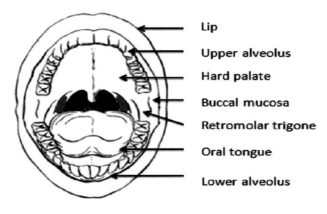

Figure 10.1   Anatomic subsites of the oral cavity.

of the mucosa to the alveolar ridge (upper and lower) and pterygomandibular raphe. The membranous lining overlying the ascending ramus of the mandible behind the third molar to the maxillary tuberosity at the apex is known as the "retromolar trigone" and is important oncologically as the tumors involving this region have a propensity for early spread to the infratemporal fossa rendering them unamenable for surgery.

Lymphatic drainage: Parotid, submental, submandibular→ upper deep cervical nodes.

Distinctive features: In India, buccal mucosa cancers outnumber cancers at all other sites. Gingivobuccal cancers are also known as *Indian oral cancer*, and constitute 60% of all oral cancers in the country. The site of this cancer is distinctive in view of the placement of the betel quid.

Lower Alveolar Ridge (C03.1)

Extent: Lower alveolar ridge refers to the mucosa overlying the alveolar process of the mandible which extends from the line of attachment of mucosa in the buccal gutter to the line of free mucosa of the floor of the mouth. It extends to the ascending ramus of the mandible posteriorly. In view of their proximity to the bone, these tumors exhibit early bone erosion and have a higher propensity for early nodal metastasis.

Lymphatic drainage: Submental (Ia) and submandibular (Ib).

Distinctive features: Gingivobuccal cancers behave differently compared with other subsites of the oral cavity with respect to stage at presentation, propensity for neck metastasis, and recurrence patterns (**Table 10.1**).

Upper Alveolar Ridge (C03.0)

Extent: Upper alveolar ridge refers to the mucosa overlying the alveolar process of the maxilla which extends from the line of attachment of the mucosa in the upper gingival buccal gutter to the junction of the hard palate. Its posterior margin is the upper end of the pterygopalatine arch.

Lymphatic drainage: Submental (Ia), submandibular (Ib), and retropharyngeal nodes.

Table 10.1   Biological Disparity in Oral Cavity Cancers

Parameters	Gingivobuccal Cancers	Tongue/Floor of Mouth Cancers
Stage at presentation	I and II (13%) III (15%) IV (72%)	I and II (40%) III (33%) IV (27%)
Propensity for neck metastasis	Low	High
Metastatic rates	N0: 55–60% N+: 40–45%	N0: 25–30% N+: 70–75%
First echelon node	Level Ib (submandibular)	Level II (upper jugular) and III (mid jugular)
Patterns of failure	Predominantly local	Predominantly regional
Reconstruction	Difficult Composite (mucosa + skin + bone)	Easier Bone and skin rarely involved

Adapted from reference 5.

Retromolar Gingiva (Retromolar Trigone, C06.2)

Extent: Retromolar gingiva is the attached mucosa overlying the ascending ramus of the mandible from the level of the posterior surface of the last molar teeth to the apex superiorly, adjacent to the tuberosity of the maxilla.

Lymphatic drainage: Submental (Ia) and submandibular (Ib).

Distinctive features: The tumors of this region have a high propensity for nodal metastasis as well as early spread to infratemporal fossa.

Floor of the Mouth (C04.0, C04.1, C04.8, and C04.9)

Extent: This is a semilunar space over the mylohyoid and hyoglossus muscles, extending from the inner surface of the lower alveolar ridge to the undersurface of the tongue. Its posterior boundary is the base of the anterior pillar of the tonsil. It is divided into two sides by the frenulum of the tongue and contains the ostia of the submaxillary and sublingual salivary glands. The mylohyoid muscles attached to the mylohyoid line on the inner surface of the mandible act as a diaphragm between the oral cavity and neck, and serve as an important landmark in therapeutic decision making.

Lymphatic drainage: Submental (Ia) and submandibular nodes (Ib).

Distinctive feature: Floor of the mouth cancers have high propensity for early nodal metastasis (unilateral and contralateral).

Hard Palate (C05.0)

Extent: Hard palate is the semilunar area between the upper alveolar ridge and the mucous membrane covering the palatine process of the maxillary palatine bones. It extends from the inner surface of the superior alveolar ridge to the posterior edge of the palatine bone.

Lymphatic drainage: Retropharyngeal nodes→deep cervical nodes.

Distinctive features: The mucosa overlying the hard palate closely adheres to the underlying periosteum by regularly arranged Sharpey fibers. This mucosa also contains numerous minor salivary glands which may give rise to minor salivary gland tumors. The hard palate is the most common site for the occurrence of adenoid cystic carcinomas.

Anterior Two-Thirds of the Tongue (Oral Tongue, C02.0 to C02.3, C02.8, and C02.9)

Extent: The anterior two-thirds of the tongue is the freely mobile portion of the tongue that extends anteriorly from the line of the circumvallate papillae to its undersurface at the junction of the floor of the mouth. It is composed of four areas: the tip, the lateral borders, the dorsum, and the undersurface (nonvillous ventral surface of the tongue). The undersurface of the tongue is considered a separate category by the World Health Organization (WHO).

Lymphatic drainage: Tip—submental nodes (Ia), rest of the tongue: submandibular nodes (Ib).

Distinctive features: Anterior two-thirds of the tongue plays an important part in the functions of speech and swallowing (Phases I and II). Hence, any surgery involving excision of the tongue musculature has a direct bearing on the functional outcomes for the patient. Tongue cancers have a higher propensity for nodal metastasis (ipsilateral and contralateral) in view of the abundant vascularity of the organ. The surgery of these tumors usually encompasses a bilateral neck dissection to improve locoregional control. Also, a higher incidence of occult metastasis is seen in tongue cancers ranging from 20 to 40%.[4]

Epidemiology

Globally, oral cancers account for approximately 405,000 new cases diagnosed each year with two-thirds of them occurring in developing countries (Sri Lanka, India, Pakistan, and Bangladesh).[5] In these countries oral cancer is the most common cancer in men and accounts for 30% of all new cancer cases annually (**Fig. 10.2**).

Etiological Factors

The oral cavity by virtue of its function is exposed to a variety of carcinogenic or potentially carcinogenic substances. The

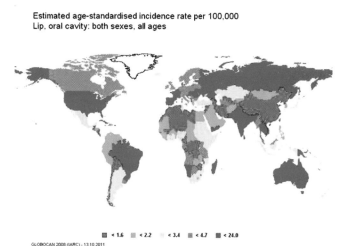

Estimated age-standardised incidence rate per 100,000
Lip, oral cavity: both sexes, all ages

■ < 1.6   ■ < 2.2   < 3.4   ■ < 4.7   ■ < 24.0

GLOBOCAN 2008 (IARC) - 13.10.2011

Figure 10.2   World age-standardized incidence rates of men for lip and oral cavity cancers (2008 estimates).

Source: http://globocan.iarc.fr/map.

most common etiological agents are depicted in **Fig. 10.3** and briefly described below.

Tobacco and Tobacco Products

Tobacco is the single most important factor implicated in the etiology of oral cancers. Globally, tobacco is responsible for the death of 1 in 10 adults (5 million deaths per year) with 2.41 (1.80 to 3.15) million deaths in the developing countries and 2.43 (2.13 to 2.78) million deaths in the developed countries. Evidence from the population-based registry in India has shown that tobacco is responsible for 50% of the cancers seen

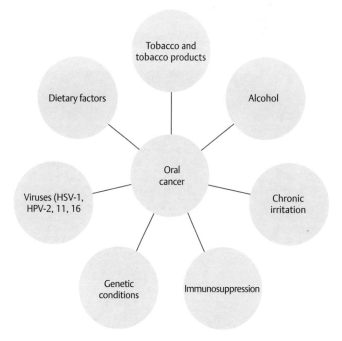

Figure 10.3   Common etiological agents for oral cavity cancer. HPV, human papillomavirus; HSV, herpes simplex virus.

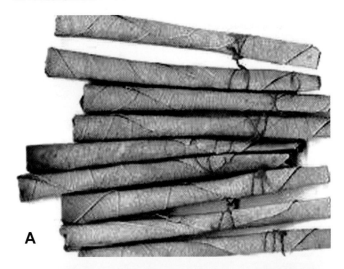

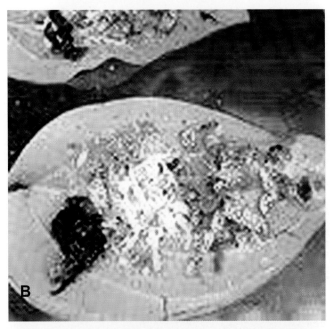

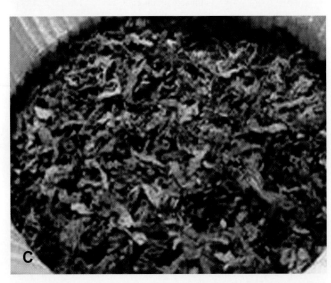

Figure 10.4 Tobacco and tobacco-related products commonly consumed in India.

in the Indian population. Tobacco is a mixture of carcinogenic compounds such as polycyclic aromatic hydrocarbons and nitrosamines. Tobacco is consumed in different forms, viz., tobacco smoking and smokeless forms (**Fig. 10.4** and **Table 10.2**). The oral use of smokeless tobacco is widely prevalent in India; its different methods of consumption include chewing, sucking, and applying tobacco preparations to the teeth and gums. Smokeless tobacco products are often made at home but are also manufactured. Tobacco carcinogenesis is a multistep process[6] and is depicted in **Fig. 10.5**.

Alcohol

In the work of McCoy and Wynder, strong evidence exists to support the concept of synergistic activity of alcohol with tobacco.[7] The proposed mechanisms for alcohol cocarcinogenesis are shown in **Fig. 10.5** and **Table 10.3**.

Dietary Factors

Although there has been no conclusive study to correlate dietary deficiency with carcinogenicity, a few studies have shown a protective function of vitamin A in preventing cancer.[8]

Chronic Irritation

Various studies have analyzed the role of chronic irritation in carcinogenesis. Factors which have been implicated to date include poor oral and dental hygiene, sharp tooth, ill-fitting dentures, syphilis, chronic mouthwash usage, and marijuana consumption.[9–11]

Viruses

Viruses such as herpes simplex virus and human papillomavirus (HPV)-2, 11, and 16 have been suspected to cause oral cancers; but to date no definite proof has been found.[12,13]

Immunosuppression

HIV-infected patients are more prone to develop Kaposi sarcoma and non-Hodgkin lymphoma (NHL) in the oral

Table 10.2 Different Forms of Tobacco Consumption

Smokeless	Tobacco Smoking
Paan (betel quid) with tobacco	Beedis
Paan masala	Cigarette
Mainpuri tobacco	Cigar
Mawa	Cheroot
Tobacco and slaked lime (khaini)	Chuttas (reverse smoking)
Chewing tobacco	Dhumtis
	Pipe
	Hookah
	Hooklis
	Chillum

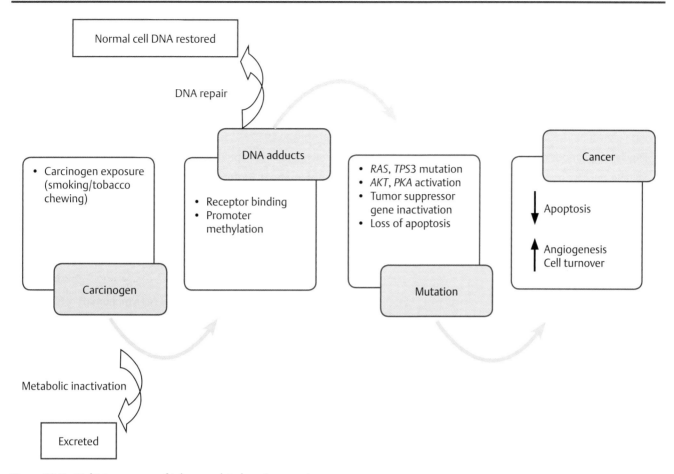

Figure 10.5 Multistep process of tobacco-related carcinogenesis.

cavity. Kaposi sarcoma is associated with human herpesvirus 8 while NHL is with Epstein-Barr virus.[14] Similarly, immunosuppression associated with kidney transplantation and bone marrow transplant has been implicated in the development of oral cancer.[15]

Genetic Factors

Patients having genetic mutations which affect the process of deoxyribonucleic acid repair, viz, xeroderma pigmentosum, Fanconi anemia, and ataxia telangiectasia are more prone to develop oral cancers.[16]

Pathology

The oral cavity is involved with a variety of pathologies, both benign and malignant. Among the malignant lesions described by the WHO, 95% are squamous cell carcinomas (SCCs) (**Table 10.4**).

Potentially Malignant Lesions of the Lip and Oral Cavity

The WHO in 2005 modified the terminology, definitions, and classification of oral lesions with a predisposition to malignant transformation and proposed the

term "potentially malignant" for "premalignant" or "precancerous" lesions.[17] Also, it recommended abandoning the traditional distinction between potentially malignant lesions and potentially malignant conditions and using the term "potentially malignant disorders" instead.[17] The potentially malignant lesions of the oral cavity include leukoplakia, erythroleukoplakia, and submucous fibrosis (SMF).

Table 10.3 Proposed Mechanism of Alcohol Co-Carcinogenesis

Local Effects	Systemic Effects
Solvent for potential carcinogens	Alcohol metabolism—acetaldehyde
Mucosa injury-aids carcinogen uptake	Production of other free radicals
Acetaldehyde production by oral bacteria	Chronic alcoholics • CYP2E1 enzyme induction • Nutritional deficiencies
Carcinogenic impurities Chronic alcoholics • Poor salivary flow • Gastroesophageal reflux	Altered retinoid metabolism • Reduced immune surveillance

Table 10.4   World Health Organization Classification for Oral Cavity Lesions

A. Epithelial Tumors		C. Soft Tissue Tumors	
Malignant epithelial tumors		Kaposi sarcoma	9140/3
a. Squamous cell carcinoma		Lymphangioma	9170/0
• Verrucous carcinoma		Ectomesenchymal chondromyxoid tumor	
• Basaloid squamous cell carcinoma		Focal oral mucinosis	
• Papillary squamous cell carcinoma		Congenital granular cell epulis	
• Spindle cell carcinoma		**D. Hematolymphoid Tumors**	
• Acantholytic squamous cell carcinoma		DLBCL	9680/3m
• Adenosquamous carcinoma		Mantle-cell lymphoma	9673/3
• Carcinoma cuniculatum		Follicular lymphoma	9690/3
Epithelial precursor lesions		Extranodal marginal zone B-cell lymphoma of MALT type	9699/3
Benign epithelial tumors		Burkitt lymphoma	9687/3
a. Papillomas		T-cell lymphoma (including anaplastic large cell lymphoma)	9714/3
• Squamous cell papilloma and verruca vulgaris		Extramedullary plasmacytoma	9734/3
• Condyloma acuminatum		Langerhans cell histiocytosis	9751/1
• Focal epithelial hyperplasia		Extramedullary myeloid sarcoma	9930/3
b. Granular cell tumor		Follicular dendritic-cell sarcoma/tumor	9758/3
c. Keratoacanthoma		**E. Mucosal Malignant Melanoma**	
B. Salivary Gland Tumors		**F. Tumors of Bone**	
a. Salivary gland carcinomas	8050/0	Odontogenic carcinomas	
• Acinic cell carcinoma	8550/3	• Metastasizing (malignant) ameloblastoma	9310/3
• Mucoepidermoid carcinoma	8430/3	• Ameloblastic carcinoma—primary type	9270/3
• Adenoid cystic carcinoma	8200/3	• Ameloblastic carcinoma—secondary type (dedifferentiated),	9270/3
• Polymorphous low-grade adenocarcinoma	8525/3	• Intraosseous	
• Basal cell adenocarcinoma	8147/3	• Ameloblastic carcinoma—secondary type (dedifferentiated),	9270/3
• Epithelial–myoepithelial carcinoma	8562/3	• Peripheral	
• Clear cell carcinoma, not otherwise specified	8310/3	• Primary intraosseous squamous cell carcinoma – solid	9270/3
• Cystadenocarcinoma	8450/3	• Type	
• Mucinous adenocarcinoma	8480/3	• Primary intraosseous squamous cell carcinoma derived from keratocystic odontogenic tumor	9270/3
• Oncocytic carcinoma	8290/3		
• Salivary duct carcinoma	8500/3	• Primary intraosseous squamous cell carcinoma derived from odontogenic cysts	9270/3
• Myoepithelial carcinoma	8982/3		
• Carcinoma ex pleomorphic adenoma	8941/3	• Clear cell odontogenic carcinoma	9341/3
b. Salivary gland adenomas	8050/0	• Ghost cell odontogenic carcinoma	9302/3
• Pleomorphic adenoma	8940/0	• Odontogenic sarcomas	
• Myoepithelioma	8982/0	• Ameloblastoma fibrosarcoma	9330/3
• Basal cell adenoma	8147/0	• Ameloblastic fibrodentino and fibro-odontosarcoma	9290/3
• Canalicular adenoma	8149/0	**G. Secondary Tumors**	
• Duct papilloma	8503/0		
• Cystadenoma			

DLBCL, diffuse large B-cell lymphoma; MALT, mucosa-associated lymphoid tissue.

Leukoplakia

Leukoplakia is defined as "a white plaque of questionable risk having excluded (other) known diseases or disorders that carry no increased risk for cancer" (**Fig. 10.6**).[17] Globally, the estimated reported prevalence of oral leukoplakia

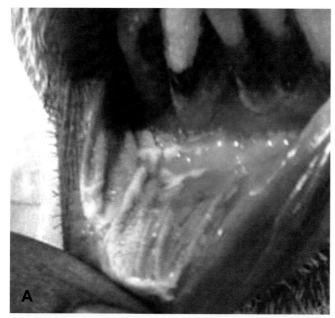

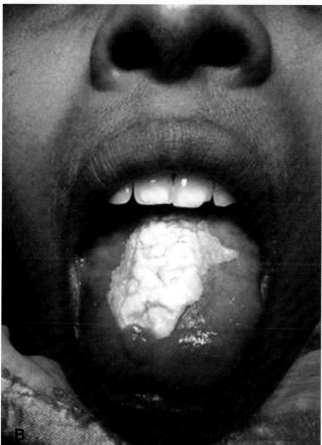

Figure 10.6   Leukoplakia seen on the (A) buccal mucosa and (B) tongue.

is approximately 2%.[18] Whereas, the annual malignant transformation rate is 1%, resulting in development of oral cancer in 20 per 100,000 people per year. Leukoplakia is six times more common among smokers compared with nonsmokers.[19] Alcohol is an independent risk factor, regardless of beverage type or drinking pattern.[20] The role of HPV is still being explored.[20–22]

Clinically, leukoplakia is divided into two types.

1. Homogeneous type (flat, thin, uniform white in color)
2. Nonhomogeneous type

The nonhomogeneous type has been defined as a white and red lesion ("erythroleukoplakia"), that may be either irregularly flat (speckled) or nodular. Verrucous leukoplakia is yet another type of nonhomogeneous leukoplakia. Although verrucous leukoplakia usually has a uniform white appearance, its verrucous texture distinguishes it from homogeneous (flat) leukoplakia. Verrucous leukoplakia is clinically difficult to distinguish from verrucous carcinoma. Proliferative verrucous leukoplakia (PVL) is another subtype of verrucous leukoplakia, characterized by multifocal presentation, resistance to treatment and a high rate of malignant transformation.[17,18,20] PVL is more prevalent in elderly women and there may be no history of tobacco use. The risk factors associated with an increased rate of malignant transformation are represented in **Table 10.5**. Clinical and histological classification is shown in **Tables 10.6** and **10.7**.[23]

Biopsy or excision is preferable for the diagnosis and prevention of malignant transformation. The management algorithm for leukoplakia is shown in **Fig. 10.7**.[24]

Erythroplakia

Erythroplakia is defined as a "bright red velvety patch that cannot be characterized clinically or pathologically as being caused by any other condition." Histologically, erythroplakia exhibits some degree of dysplasia and may even have foci of carcinoma in situ. Higher rates (68%) of aneuploidy are seen in erythroplakic lesions and serve as a surrogate marker for

Table 10.5   High Risk Factors for Malignant Transformation

Females
Long duration of leukoplakia
Location on the tongue or floor of mouth[17]
Leukoplakia in nonsmokers
Size greater than 2 cm[17,20]
Nonhomogeneous (speckled/nodular) type
Presence of dysplastic changes
Presence of *Candida albicans*
Molecular markers (loss of heterozygosity at loci 3p14 and 9p21, expression of a novel molecule podoplanin, suprabasal expression of p53, presence of high-risk HPV 16, immunohistochemistry pattern of cyclin D1, p27 and p63, and the expression of cytokeratin 8.[66–70]

HPV, human papillomavirus.

Table 10.6 World Health Organization Histological Classification that Histologically Categorizes Precursor and Related Lesions

WHO Classification	SIN	Ljubljana Classification of SIN
Squamous cell hyperplasia		Squamous cell (simple) hyperplasia
Mild dysplasia	SIN 1	Basal/parabasal cell hyperplasia
Moderate dysplasia	SIN 2	Atypical hyperplasia
Severe dysplasia	SIN 3c	Atypical hyperplasia
Carcinoma in situ	SIN 3c	Carcinoma in situ

Adapted from reference 23.
WHO, World Health Organization; SIN, squamous intraepithelial neoplasia.

Table 10.7 Classification and Staging System for Oral Leukoplakias (OL-System)

L (size of leukoplakia)

- Lx: Size not specified
- L1: Single/multiple (< 2 cm)
- L2: Single/multiple (2–4 cm)
- L3: Single/multiple (> 4 cm)

P (pathologic features)

- Px: Absence/presence of epithelial dysplasia not reported
- P0: No epithelial dysplasia
- P1: Mild/moderate dysplasia
- P2: Severe dysplasia

OL-staging system

- Stage I: L1P0
- Stage II: L2P0
- Stage III: L3P0 or L1/2P1
- Stage IV: L3P1 or any L P2

malignant transformation. Surgical excision is the treatment of choice for this pathology.

Lichen Planus

Lichen planus clinically presents as lacy white lines on a violaceous background on the buccal mucosa, often accompanied by symptoms of pain and burning sensations (**Fig. 10.8**). Histologically, it is characterized by band-like subepithelial mononuclear infiltrate of T cells and histiocytes and degenerating basal keratinocytes that form colloid bodies. This pathology has an annual malignant transformation rate of 1%.[25]

Oral Submucous Fibrosis

Oral submucous fibrosis (OSMF) is caused by chronic exposure to betel nut and tobacco. This pathology is characterized by a generalized dense scarring of the oral soft tissue resulting in trismus. Histological findings vary according to the stage of the disease and include subepithelial fibrosis, chronic inflammation, hyalinization, and loss of vascularity. The annual malignant transformation rate is approximately 0.5%.[26]

Natural History of Oral Squamous Cell Carcinoma (Genetic Progression Model)

Oral carcinogenesis is a multistep process that involves biomolecular changes brought by carcinogens leading to premalignant changes which in turn lead to malignancy. It was Slaughter who first described the concept of "field cancerization" wherein multiple carcinogenic insults to the mucosa of the upper aerodigestive tract lead to alteration in the molecular milieu of the lining cells.[27,28] These mutations result in development of a progeny that has the ability of uncontrolled cell division, eventually developing into malignancy. This theory also provides insight into the development of second primaries in this region. Development of a second primary is the main cause of mortality in early-stage oral cancers. The genetic model of carcinogenesis is depicted in **Fig. 10.9**.

Site Distribution

The site distribution of oral cavity cancer is in direct correlation with the regions that are maximally exposed to carcinogens, for example, gingivobuccal sulcus.[4] It is these areas where salivary stagnation occurs exposing the mucosa to tremendous carcinogenic insults.[29] Great disparity exists in the distribution of oral cancer sites among developing and developed countries, and the answer lies in the difference in habits peculiar to the population, i.e. chewing vs. smoking tobacco, (**Fig. 10.10**).

Regional Metastasis

Cervical lymph node metastasis is considered the single most important prognostic factor in oral cavity SCC. The 5-year survival reduces to approximately 50% after development of nodal metastasis.[30] The site of nodal metastasis depends on the primary subsite, T stage, and histopathological features. Lymphatic spread from a tumor follows a step-wise orderly pattern. The nodal metastasis seen at different sites is depicted in **Table 10.8** and **Figs. 10.11.1** to **10.11.4**.

Diagnosis

Clinical Evaluation

A detailed clinical history should be obtained from the patient presenting with an oral cavity lesion. The patient should be inquired regarding his addictions (tobacco, alcohol, etc.) with the aim of identifying the possible risk factors. Similarly, a detailed family history should be elicited to rule out any genetic susceptibility conditions. Patients having comorbid (such as conditions (diabetes, cardiac problems, or asthma) should be evaluated with regard to the current

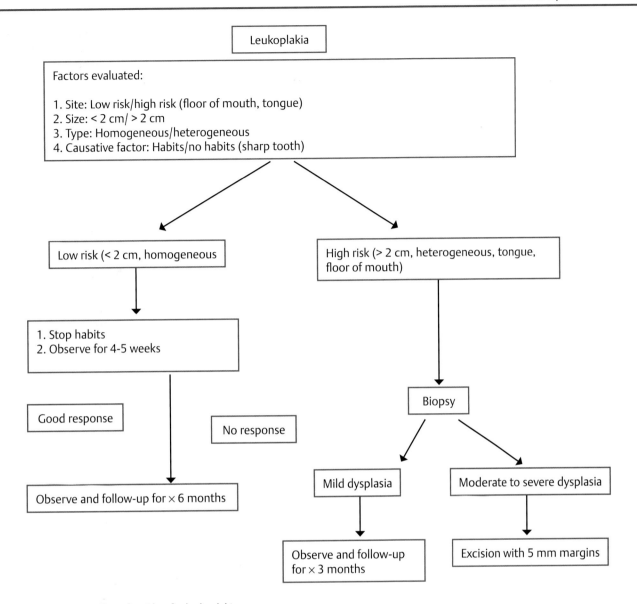

Figure 10.7   Management algorithm for leukoplakia.

Adapted from reference 24.

disease status and a physician referral should be obtained in case of derangements. The clinical examination should also include, apart from the oral cavity, 90 degree Hopkins telescopy to rule out a second primary and document vocal cord status along with a detailed evaluation of the neck to detect neck metastasis. Patients presenting with trismus and advanced disease who are not amenable for routine clinical evaluation should be examined under anesthesia to map the tumor extent and plan the required therapeutic approach. The symptomatology of each subsite of the oral cavity is unique and is briefly described in **Table 10.9.**

Investigations

Laboratory work-up should be ordered to rule out any underlying comorbid conditions which are likely to affect therapeutic management of the cancer patient. A formal

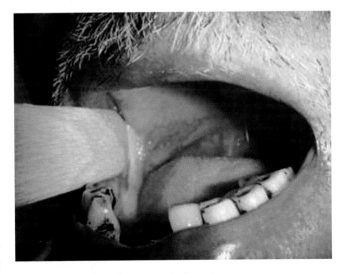

Figure 10.8   Lichen planus over the buccal mucosa.

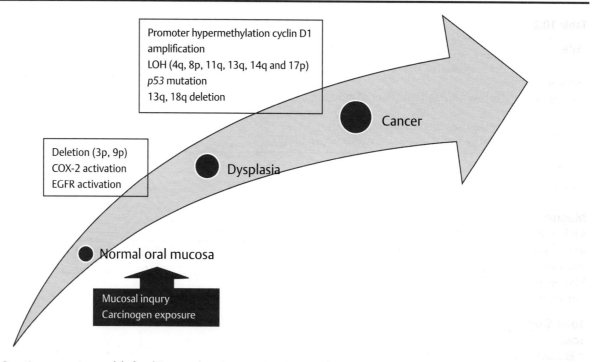

Figure 10.9 Genetic progression model of multistep oral carcinogenesis. COX-2, cyclooxygenase-2; EGFR, epidermal growth factor receptor.

biopsy (punch, knife, or fine-needle aspiration) should be done for primary diagnosis of the tumor. Patients presenting with a neck node with no detectable primary should be subjected for a fine-needle aspiration cytology (FNAC) for primary diagnosis. For inaccessible lesions/trismus the biopsy should be obtained under general anesthesia.

Radiological investigations comprise a variety of options (chest X-ray, orthopantomogram [OPG], computed tomography [CT] scan, magnetic resonance imaging [MRI] scan, Dentascan, positron emission tomography [PET] scan) which should be ordered judiciously to get an idea of the disease status, extent, staging, as well as therapeutic planning.

Primary Disease

The main aim is to assess the extent of soft tissue involvement and bone involvement (**Table 10.10**).

Orthopantomogram (OPG)

OPG has a high specificity (93%) to detect bone erosion, but requires at least 30% of the bone to be eroded to detect it. Hence not routinely used, but can be employed in patients having a clinically visible bone involvement.

Computed Tomography Scan

It is the most common modality employed in oral cancers. Its advantages include good soft tissue discrimination, vessel identification, and assessment of bone involvement. The "puffed-cheek" method provides an adequate delineation of the tumor extent. This helps to assess the involvement of that surface of the mucosa which is normally apposed, such as the cheeks, gingiva, lips, and buccal vestibule. It also predicts the extension of the disease into the buccinator space and retromolar trigone. Dentascans are special coronal

reconstruction of the mandible that is useful in assessing mandibular invasion. Its disadvantages include radiation exposure, possible contrast sensitivity, and dental amalgam interference.

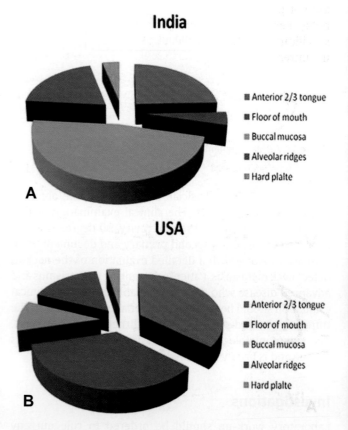

Figure 10.10 Disparity in the site distribution of oral cavity cancers. *Adapted from* references 16 and 78.

Table 10.8 Incidence of Nodal Metastasis Seen in Oral Cavity Cancers

Site	Primary Echelon	Incidence of Nodal Metastasis	Occult Metastasis	Bilateral Metastasis	Only Contralateral Metastasis
Anterior tongue	Level II	15–75%	25%	25%	3%
Buccal mucosa	Level I, II	10%	5% (depending of tumor thickness)	–	–
Alveolar ridges	Level I, II, V (6%)	30% (T4–70%)	–	–	–
Floor of mouth	Level I, II	47–53%	12–30%	10%	–

Adapted from references 71 to 76.

Magnetic Resonance Imaging Scan

MRI scan offers better soft tissue discrimination and medullary cavity involvement, and predicts perineural invasions. It is preferred in patients with dental amalgam. MRI is mainly used in scanning of tongue and base of tongue lesions.

Bone Single-Photon Emission Computed Tomography Scan

It is usually done in patients with negative CT or MRI scan. Negative bone single-photon emission computed tomography scan rules out mandibular invasion (100% sensitivity).[31]

Neck

Ultrasonography (USG) is used to screen nodal diseases that are not palpable clinically in view of < 1 cm nodes/thick bulky necks/postradiotherapy neck. USG-guided FNAC is specific in predicting nodal metastasis. USG is used to follow-up untreated node-negative neck in oral cancers.

Distant Metastasis

PET scan is currently employed to rule out distant metastasis in patients with advanced disease, patients with bulky level III and IV nodes; second primary; postchemoradiation neck to rule out residual disease, and in recurrent tumor setting.

Preoperative Dental and Prosthetic Counseling

Patients who are planned for surgery requiring reconstruction (pedicle/free flap) should be evaluated by a speech swallowing pathologist, a prosthodontist to design the obturators for bone defects, dental scaling, and planning osseointegrated implants, and a plastic surgeon to provide the patient with adequate knowledge of the reconstructive procedure and give him a choice as per his requirements.

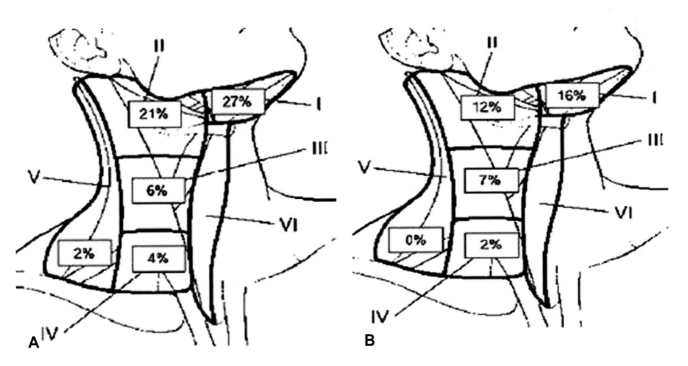

Figure 10.11.1 (A) Node-negative neck—Incidence of occult lymph node metastasis in the clinically node-negative patient with carcinoma alveolar ridge. (B) Node-positive neck—Incidence of lymph node metastasis in the clinically node-positive patient.

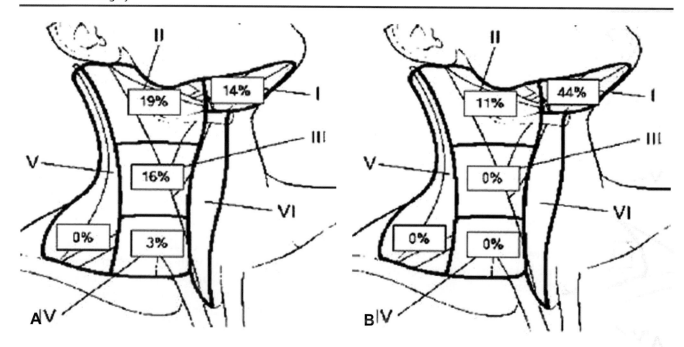

Figure 10.11.2 (A) Node-negative neck—Incidence of occult lymph node metastasis in the clinically node-negative patient with carcinoma at the floor of the mouth. (B) Node-positive neck—Incidence of lymph node metastasis in the clinically node-positive patient.

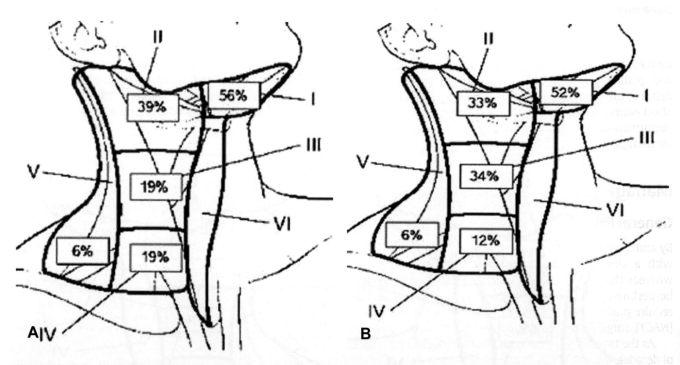

Figure 10.11.3 (A) Node-negative neck—Incidence of occult lymph node metastasis in the clinically node-negative patient with carcinoma floor oral tongue. (B) Node-positive neck—Incidence of lymph node metastasis in the clinically node-positive patient.

TNM Staging

After undergoing a complete clinico-radiological evaluation, the patient's tumor is staged based on the primary tumor characteristics (T), nodal disease (N), and distant metastasis (M). Based on the TNM grouping the patient's disease status is staged according to the TNM stage grouping. Recently, the American Joint Committee on Cancer has published a new 7th edition with some modifications (**Tables 10.11** and **10.12**).

Although TNM staging is globally used as a standard form of communication among the treating clinicians, the system has caveats that need to be addressed to make the current TNM staging robust in its applicability. The TNM staging though serving as a prognostic indicator in oral

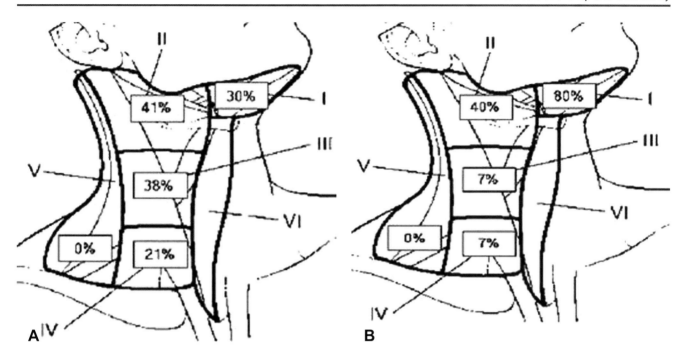

Figure 10.11.4 (A) Node-negative neck—Incidence of occult lymph node metastasis in the clinically node-negative patient with carcinoma buccal mucosa. (B) Node-positive neck—Incidence of lymph node metastasis in the clinically node-positive patient.

cavity cancers does not take into consideration host factors and pathologic features, for example, tumor thickness/depth of invasion/lymphovascular spread that are known to affect patient survival and outcomes. Medical comorbidities, performance, and nutritional status are equally important for therapeutic management.[32]

Management of Oral Cavity Cancers

General Principles

By and large, patients with an early-stage tumor are treated with a single modality approach (surgery/radiotherapy) whereas those with an advanced stage of disease who are borderline-operable or those with unresectable disease may require multimodality therapy (neoadjuvant chemotherapy [NACT], surgery, chemoradiation, and targeted therapy).

As the treatment options have increased in the past couple of decades, it is still imperative to plan the best form of initial therapy for delivering best possible outcomes. A multidisciplinary approach should be employed in treating patients to provide adequate tumor control, survival, and maintenance of quality of life. The following factors should be considered before embarking on a therapeutic procedure (**Fig. 10.12**).

The planning of the treatment should be performed in a joint clinical session comprising the surgeon, radiation oncologist, medical oncologist, plastic surgeon, and a speech–language pathologist. The clinician should explain the diagnosis and treatment plan, likely complications, and the need for postoperative adjuvant therapy (radiotherapy/

chemoradiation) to the patient and his relatives in detail, taking into consideration the requirements of the patient. The chances of failure of the therapeutic procedures, likely disability, and various forms of rehabilitation also need to be explained. The patients should be urged to stop any addictions if they were still using them.

Patients who present in an advanced stage and are not amenable to routine treatment modalities are counseled on the available options, viz., clinical trial participation, supportive care, or palliative care.

Surgical Management

Lip and oral cavity cancers are best treated with surgery. This modality allows a one-stage locoregional clearance of the disease and provides the clinician with useful information regarding the histological characteristics and margins status of the tumor, both having a prognostic importance.

Lip

Functional and cosmetic considerations are of paramount importance when planning the repair of a lip defect. The lip serves various important functions such as retaining oral contents, phonation, and allowing passage of objects into the oral cavity, such as dentures. Microstomia is an important complication of lip repair that can hinder oral hygiene and the use of dentures, and so should be avoided during lip repair. Adequate clinical margins of the resection of lip SCC should be 5 to 10 mm. The neck is usually observed when clinically negative, but for large T3/T4 and those with clinically positive neck, an ipsilateral neck dissection is

Table 10.9 Clinical Features of an Oral Cavity Cancer

Subsites	Symptoms
Anterior 2/3 tongue	Early lesions • Granular nodule, nonhealing ulcer Advanced tumors • Exophytic/ulcerative lesion • Ankyloglossia (Floor of mouth/hypoglossal nerve involvement) • Trismus • Fetor oris
Alveolar ridge	Odynophagia Loose tooth Bleeding gums Ill-fitting dentures Trismus (signifies extension to infratemporal fossa, involving pterygoid muscles) Altered sensation over lip (signifies involvement of the mandibular canal and inferior alveolar nerve)
Buccal mucosa	Early • Painless nonhealing ulcer (mostly exophytic) • Surrounding leukoplakia Advanced • Trismus • Skin involvement Orocutaneous fistula
Floor of mouth	Painful, infiltrative lesions Excessive salivation Ankyloglossia Early involvement of the mandible

performed. For T3/T4 lesions crossing midline an ipsilateral selective neck dissection (SND) I–III should be combined with a contralateral SND I–III. The various forms of lip defects and reconstructive modalities offered are briefly illustrated in **Figs. 10.13** and **10.14**.

Floor of the Mouth and Oral Tongue
The floor of the mouth and anterior two-thirds of the tongue are considered together in view of their common ablative and reconstructive principles.

Early T1/T2 Lesions
For early T1/T2 lesions a wide excision with 1 cm tumor-free margins confirmed grossly on frozen section when available is the standard treatment (**Fig. 10.15**). Small tongue excisions (< 1/3) can be closed primarily. Neck management is discussed in detail in the section on neck metastasis.

T3 and T4 Lesions
Patients with larger T3 and T4 disease need to be evaluated for extent and route of surgical resection after proper

Table 10.10 Comparative Evaluation of Imaging Modalities Used for Oral Cancer Evaluation

Modality	Sensitivity	Specificity
CT	58.1	95.7
MRI	62.6	100
Bone SPECT	100	56.5

CT, computed tomography; MRI, magnetic resonance imaging; SPECT, single-photon emission computed tomography.

preoperative evaluation (**Fig. 10.16**). For lesions located posteriorly and for patients having trismus, an anterior labiomandibulotomy or a lateral mandibulotomy for access to the floor of the mouth, lingual gutter, and tongue can be done. Similarly, a mandibular lingual release (pull through), dropping the floor of the mouth and tongue into the neck can also be attempted.[33] A median mandibulotomy is associated with a facial incision and some damage to the anatomic structures in the floor of the mouth, but it preserves the inferior alveolar neurovascular bundle. On the other hand, midline and paramedian incisions give good cosmetic outcomes.[34] There are proponents of the step-like mandibulotomy but, nowadays with advancements in reconstructive methods, this technique is losing its sheen. After mandibulotomy, if the bone is found to be involved by the tumor, segmental mandibulectomy is done and reconstructed with a free fibula osteocutaneous flap.

In developing countries many patients present in an advanced stage of disease involving multiple subsites requiring massive resection and posing a challenge for reconstruction. Lesions involving the lateral border tongue encroaching the floor of the mouth but sparing the mandible can be reconstructed using a thin, pliable, reconstruction such as the radial forearm free flap or lateral upper arm free flap.[35] Due to its pliability this flap helps in the mobility of the remnant tongue and provides functional speech and swallowing. Reinnervated radial forearm free flaps are also employed for tongue reconstruction.[36] For massive tongue and floor-of-mouth defects, bulkier pedicled flaps (such as a large pectoralis) and free flaps (rectus, subscapular, and anterolateral thigh) are usually used as they provide bulk and assist in swallowing. Sometimes palatal prostheses are added to occlude this oral cavity dead space further and aid in swallowing. For floor-of-mouth lesions abutting the mandible but not involving it radiologically, an oblique marginal mandibulectomy excising the lingual plate can be done to get an adequate lateral margin.

Patients with involvement of the disease extending to the hyoid or involving the laryngeal framework (preepiglottic space) are treated with a palliative intent. A brief overview of tongue reconstruction is shown in **Fig. 10.17**.

Buccal Mucosa

Early T1/T2 Lesions
Small buccal mucosa lesions can be excised per orally, but large lesions extending to upper/lower gingivobuccal

Table 10.11 TNM Staging of the Lip and Oral Cavity according to AJCC, 7th Edition

Primary tumor (T)

- Tx: Primary tumor cannot be assessed
- T0: No evidence of primary tumor
- Tis: Carcinoma in situ
- T1: Tumor 2 cm or less in greatest dimension
- T2: Tumor more than 2 cm but not more than 4 cm in greatest dimension
- T3: Tumor more than 4 cm in greatest dimension
- T4a: Moderately advance local disease
- (Lip) Tumor invades through cortical bone, inferior alveolar nerve, floor of mouth, or skin of face, i.e., chin or nose
- (Oral cavity) Tumor invades adjacent structures only (e.g., through cortical bone, [mandible or maxilla] into deep [extrinsic] muscle of tongue [genioglossus, hyoglossus, palatoglossus, and styloglossus], maxillary sinus, skin of face)
- T4b: Very advance local disease
- Tumor invades masticator space, pterygoid plates, or skull base, and/or encases internal carotid artery

(Note: Superficial erosion alone of bone/tooth socket by gingival primary is not sufficient to classify a tumor as T4)

Regional lymph nodes (N)

- Nx: Regional lymph nodes cannot be assessed
- N0: No regional lymph node metastasis
- N1: Metastasis in a single ipsilateral lymph node, 3 cm or less in greatest dimension
- N2: Metastasis in a single ipsilateral lymph node, more than 3 cm but not more than 6 cm in greatest dimension; or in multiple ipsilateral lymph nodes, none more than 6 cm in greatest dimension; or in bilateral or contralateral lymph nodes, none more than 6 cm in greatest dimension
- N2a: Metastasis in single ipsilateral lymph node more than 3 cm but not more than 6 cm in greatest dimension
- N2b: Metastasis in multiple ipsilateral lymph node, none more than 6 cm in greatest dimension
- N2c: Metastasis in bilateral or contralateral lymph nodes, none more than 6 cm in greatest dimension
- M3: Metastasis in a lymph node more than 6 cm in greatest dimension

Adapted from reference 77.

TNM, tumor-node-metastasis; AJCC, American Joint Committee on Cancer.

Table 10.12 Stage Grouping according to TNM Staging

Distant metastasis (M)

- M0: No distant metastasis (no pathologic M0; use clinical M to complete stage group)
- M1: Distant metastasis

Staging

- Stage 0: Tis N0 M0
- Stage I: T1 N0 M0
- Stage II: T2 N0 M0
- Stage III: T3 N0 M0/ T1 N1 M0/ T2 N1 M0/ T3 N1 M0
- Stage IVA: T4a N0 M0/ T4a N1 M0/ T1 N2 M0/ T2 N2 M0/ T3 N2 M0/ T4a N2 M0
- Stage T4A: Any T N2 M0
- Stage IVB: Any T N3 M0/ T4b any N M0
- Stage IVC: Any T any N M1

Stage unknown

Adapted from reference 77.

TNM, tumor-node-metastasis.

sulcus will warrant raising a cheek flap for adequate tumor excision. These lesions can be excised surgically or by a carbon dioxide (CO_2) laser. Small lesions of the buccal mucosa can be excised and either be kept raw for healing by secondary intention or closed primarily, or if large, covered using a split thickness skin graft. Also, for deeper defects temporalis muscle/temporoparietal fascial flap can be used.[37,38] For tumors of the buccal mucosa extending to the gingivobuccal sulcus but not involving the mandible, a marginal mandibulectomy (buccal plate excision) can be attempted to provide adequate medial margins (**Fig. 10.18**).[39]

Carbon Dioxide Laser

The CO_2 laser has proved to be an important asset in the management of early-stage oral cavity cancers. It is particularly effective in superficial and easily accessible oral lesions (premalignant and malignant), a specific indication being a lesion with imperceptible margins with adjacent premalignant changes.

T3 and T4 Operable Lesions

In developing countries around 50 to 60% of patients present in an advanced stage and among these approximately half

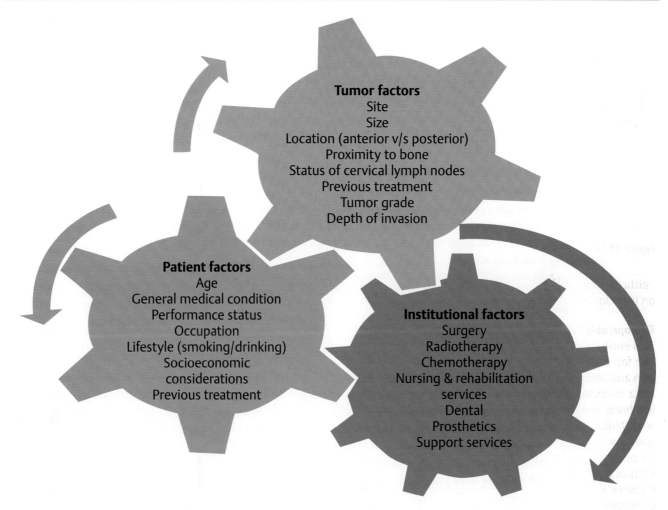

Figure 10.12   Factors to be considered before planning treatment.

are deemed operable. Hence proper case selection is needed to expect adequate locoregional control.

The choice of treatment primarily is surgical which is to be followed by adjuvant therapy depending on histopathological factors. In this scenario, offering radiotherapy as the primary treatment results in poor treatment outcomes and poor survival. In an adjuvant setting radiotherapy can be offered to patients with verrucous carcinoma, a gingivobuccal sulcus lesion with superficial bone erosion and no soft tissue infiltration or lymph node metastasis; well-differentiated superficial exophytic lesions with no soft tissue or lymph node involvement. Patients with more aggressive histology and histopathological features of positive/close surgical cut margins and perinodal extension should be offered concomitant chemoradiation.

For defects only involving the buccal mucosa and the mandible with an intact overlying skin, reconstruction is offered by free fibula osteocutaneous free flap (FFOCF) or pectoralis major myocutaneous flap (**Fig. 10.19**). If the mandible is sacrificed, and there is a through-and-through full thickness cheek defect, then reconstruction can be done using FFOCF or deltopectoral-PMMC flap.

For larger tumor defects involving the cheek skin, folded free radial artery forearm flap or a temporalis muscle flap can be used to provide the inner lining and the external coverage should be provided with a cervicofacial advancement flap. For larger defects, a pedicled flap option would be a pectoralis myocutaneous flap with the skin paddle rotated either internally in combination with a deltopectoral flap/externally (spiral)/folded (bipaddle).[40] The microvascular flaps that can be tried are a radial forearm flap with a de-

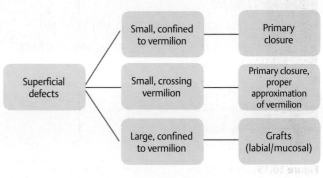

Figure 10.13   Repair of superficial lip defects.

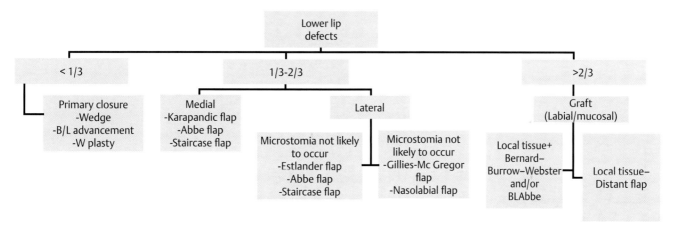

Figure 10.14 Repair of lower lip defects.

epithelialized portion that would allow the flap to be folded on itself for internal and external lining.[41]

T4 Inoperable Lesions

This entity is a common occurrence in developing countries. The features which deem a tumor inoperable are extensive skin and soft tissue involvement, extension to infratemporal fossa involving pterygoid musculature, and fixed N3 node involving the carotids and prevertebral muscles. Patients with bulky nodes presenting at levels IV and V often do poorly with treatment and frequently fail distantly. Also, an ominous symptom of early onset trismus in a patient with oral cavity cancer should be dealt with caution as it signifies involvement of the pterygoid musculature. Once categorized as "inoperable" these patients should be offered the best supportive care in the form of adequate pain relief, feeding for nutritional support, and local wound care in case of fungating growth. Palliative treatment in the form of radiotherapy/chemotherapy or chemoradiation in a select group of patients with no gross bony involvement can be tried. Metronomic chemotherapy which includes frequent administration of antiangiogenic agents (celecoxib, methotrexate) can also be offered to patients.

Upper Alveolar Ridge and Hard Palate

Lesions involving the upper alveolar ridge require an upper lip split incision which can be extended as a lateral rhinotomy incision for adequate exposure. The upper alveolar ridge and hard palate are also considered together in view of the cancers in these subsites that usually involve both. In view

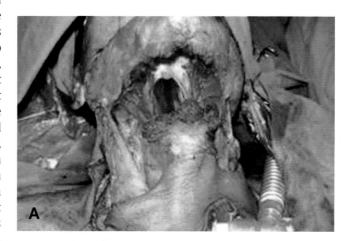

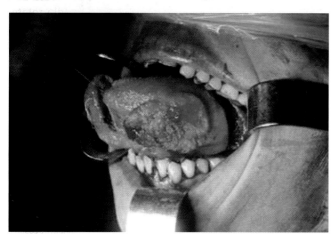

Figure 10.15 T2 lesion involving left lateral border tongue.

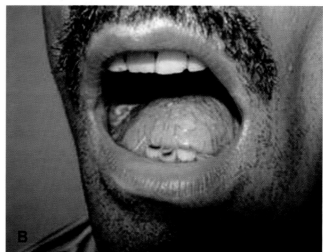

Figure 10.16 T4 tongue lesion requiring total glossectomy and reconstructed with anterolateral thigh flap.

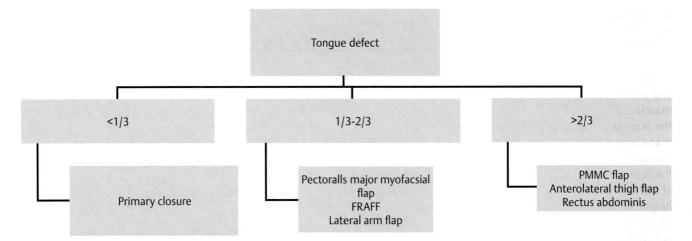

Figure 10.17 Reconstructive options for tongue cancers. FRAFF, free radial artery forearm flap; PMMC, pectoralis major myocutaneous.

of the dense adherent mucosa in this region, tumors tend to involve the bone even in early stages. Hence surgical ablation of this region always encompasses bony resection.

For smaller defects local mucosal rotation flaps, temporalis flaps, and palatal island flaps can be used. Upper alveolectomy per se can be covered with a split thickness skin graft and can be given obturators, which provides adequate functional outcome. Larger defects involving the complete hard palate along with facial skin need to be reconstructed using a bulky flap (anterolateral thigh/rectus abdominis).

Management of the Mandible

The buccal mucosa carcinoma has a propensity to spread to involve the mandible. The growth overlying the mandible, adherent to mandible, or growth with large area of abutment mandates detailed examination and imaging to assess mandibular involvement. The buccal mucosa growth involves the mandible through multiple mechanisms, through the occlusal surface, neural foramina, periodontal membrane, or at the point of abutment. Studies have proved that the

tumor spreads to involve the mandible through the point of abutment. Multiple small cortical defects representing the attachment of Sharpeys fibers binding the attached mucosa to

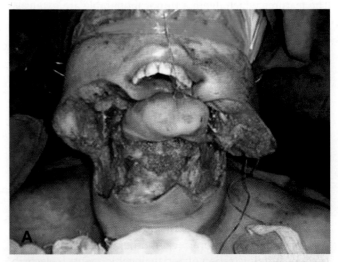

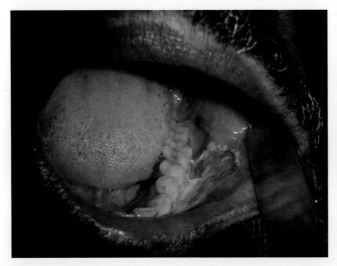

Figure 10.18 Buccal mucosa lesion requiring a marginal mandibulectomy.

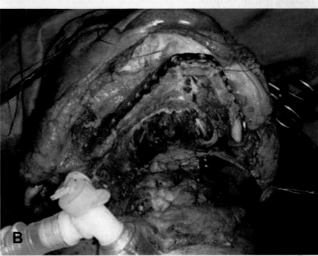

Figure 10.19 T4 lesion lower alveolus reconstructed with a free fibula osteocutaneous flap.

the bone are the weak points through which the tumor gains entry.[42–44]

Any involvement of the mandible requires surgery to be planned depending on the extent of the involvement. Tumors lying close to the mandible with absence of adequate margin and presence of superficial erosion of the mandible require marginal mandibulectomy. It is necessary to preserve 1 cm of the bony strut to have a functional mandible after marginal mandibulectomy (**Fig. 10.20**). Failure to preserve the adequate strut predisposes to the spontaneous postsurgical fracture. In edentulous and atrophic mandible the feasibility of the marginal mandibulectomy depends on the vertical height of the mandible. Marginal mandibulectomy should be performed cautiously in irradiated mandibles as there are high chances of pathologic fracture. Following are the indications for marginal mandibulectomy:

- Tumor-abutting mandible
- Minimal cortical erosion
- Minimal involvement of the dentate segment

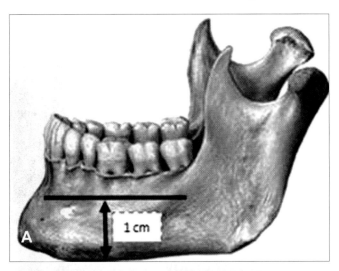

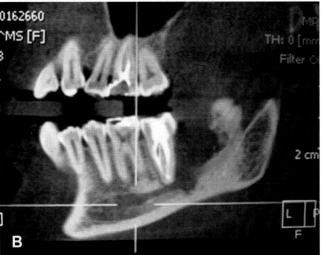

Figure 10.20 Prerequisite for marginal mandibulectomy (computed tomographic scan showing bone erosion with involvement of the alveolar neurovascular canal).

The marginal mandibulectomy should be smooth "canoe-shaped" and should not have any sharp angles at the ends, which have a high propensity for pathologic fractures under stress.

Segmental mandibulectomy should be performed whenever there is extension of the disease to involve the cancellous bone of the mandible or the inferior alveolar nerve. Segmental mandibulectomy is also required in cases where there is extensive soft tissue paramandibular disease. The indications for segmental mandibulectomy are as follows:

- Gross bony erosion
- Gross paramandibular spread
- Involvement of the medullary cavity and inferior alveolar nerve
- Edentulous patient ("pipestem"; cannot preserve 1 cm mandible)
- Postradiotherapy mandible (periosteal barrier is deficient)

Management of the Neck

As discussed previously, it is a known fact that around 30% patients with oral squamous cell carcinoma (OSCC) can harbor occult nodal metastasis. Nodal metastasis reduces the overall survival by 50% and serves as a useful prognostic indicator. Hence, adequate management of neck is of utmost importance in the management of an OSCC patient. Management of a clinically node-negative patient is controversial with still no consensus yet reached between elective versus wait and watch policy.[45] Tumors of the oral cavity follow an orderly, predictable metastatic pattern which is from level I to III. Hence a SND removing levels I to III would prove adequate in clinically node-negative patients. Tumors of the tongue and floor of the mouth have a higher incidence of nodal metastasis and hence these patients need to undergo a neck dissection. The following factors are considered to be high risk and predict a higher chance of neck metastasis (**Table 10.13**). The treatment algorithm for managing a node-negative neck is shown in **Fig. 10.21**.

Sentinel Node Biopsy

Management of oral cavity cancers presenting with clinically node-negative neck still remains controversial with no consensus reached. Literature suggests an occult nodal metastatic rate of > 30% in oral cavity SCC depending on the size and site of the primary and the diagnostic methods used.[46,47] It has been a major challenge for clinicians to detect the

Table 10.13 High Risk Factors for Nodal Metastasis

Tongue and floor of mouth cancers
T3–T4 lesions
> 6 mm thick
High-grade tumor
Infiltrative pattern of growth
Adverse histopathological features (lymphovascular emboli, perineural invasion)

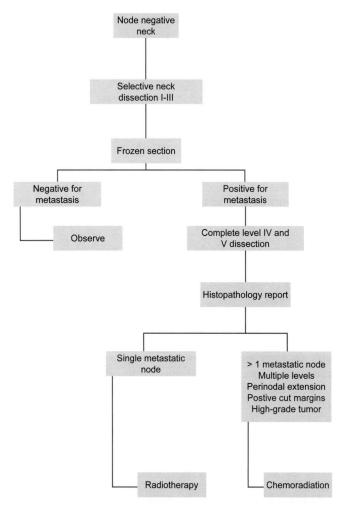

Figure 10.21 Treatment algorithm for a clinically node-negative neck.

subset of patients who do not harbor micrometastasis in the neck nodes. Doing this will eventually avoid unnecessary neck dissections and prevent resultant morbidity, viz., shoulder dysfunction, scarring, etc. To fix this problem, the technique of sentinel node biopsy (SNB) has been propounded. This diagnostic technique has already been employed in breast cancer and melanoma but it still remains to be validated in head and neck cancers (HNCs). The word "sentinel" literally means "first area of contact"; in neck metastasis it means the "first drainage site." The concept of SNB is based on the fact that lymphatic spread occurs in an orderly pattern with the sentinel node receiving the first metastatic tumor cells, and hence if the sentinel node is free of tumor metastasis then other more distal nodes should also be considered as disease free. Hence a negative SNB will act as a surrogate marker of an node-negative neck.

To perform a sentinel lymph node biopsy, the physician performs a lymphoscintigraphy, whereby a low-activity radioactive substance is injected near the tumor. The injected substance, filtered sulfur colloid, is tagged with the radionuclide technetium-99m. The injection protocols differ from doctor to doctor but the most common is a 500-μCi dose divided among five tuberculin syringes with half-inch,

24-gauge needles. The sulfur colloid is slightly acidic and causes minor stinging. A gentle massage of the injection sites spreads the sulfur colloid, relieving the pain and speeding up the lymph uptake. Scintigraphic imaging is usually started within 5 minutes of injection and the node appears from 5 minutes to 1 hour. This is usually done several hours before the actual biopsy. About 15 minutes before the biopsy the physician injects a blue dye in the same manner. Then, during the biopsy, the physician visually inspects the lymph nodes for staining and uses a gamma probe or a Geiger counter to assess which lymph nodes have taken up the radionuclide. One or several nodes may take up the dye and radioactive tracer, and these nodes are designated the *sentinel lymph nodes*. The surgeon then removes these lymph nodes and sends them to a pathologist for rapid examination under a microscope to look for the presence of cancer.

A frozen section procedure is commonly employed (which takes less than 20 minutes), so if neoplasia is detected in the lymph node a further lymph node dissection may be performed. In the case of malignant melanoma, many pathologists eschew frozen sections for more accurate "permanent" specimen preparation due to the increased instances of false-negative results with melanocytic staining.

Early applications of this technique in HNCs have found a success rate of around 50 to 60% in identifying the sentinel node using lymphoscintigraphy and intraoperative probes.[48] Stoekli et al in a 5-year follow-up study of 134 patients found an identification rate of 95% with a sensitivity of 91% and a negative predictive value of 95%. They also reported an identification rate of 98% and a negative predictive value of 94% in the largest single-institution trial of 51 patients.[49] Alkureishi et al have given the current best practice guidelines for the provision of SNB in patients with early oral cancer.[50]

Radiotherapy and Concomitant Chemoradiotherapy

Radiotherapy

Radiotherapy in the oral cavity is used commonly in an adjuvant setting. In view of the high morbidity and poor results compared with surgery in oral cancers, radiotherapy is rarely used primarily, though comparable results have been obtained when brachytherapy is used in place of external radiation for the treatment of early oral cancers.[51] In an adjuvant setting radiotherapy is given in a dose of 66 Gy and is indicated in the situations[52,53] given in **Table 10.14**.

It is imperative to complete the radiotherapy course with the "package time" which is arbitrary 100 days for better locoregional control.[54]

Adjuvant Chemoradiation

In patients having histological findings of positive resection margins and/or perinodal spread, the concomitant administration of intravenous cisplatin (100 mg/m^2, days

Table 10.14 Indications for Adjuvant Radiotherapy

Tumor factors
- T3–T4 tumors
- Bone involvement
- High-grade tumor
- Positive margins
- Lymphovascular and perineural invasion

Nodal factors
- > 2 metastatic nodes
- > 1 lymph node level
- N2/3
- Perinodal extension

1, 22, and 43) and radiotherapy (66 to 70 Gy) has provided an improvement in locoregional control and survival.[52,53] Nevertheless, this form of treatment is toxic to the patients, with only 70% completing the total course duration. Patients not fit for chemotherapy can be given targeted therapy (cetuximab) along with radiotherapy for better locoregional control.[55]

Neoadjuvant Chemotherapy

This form of chemotherapy regime is used in borderline operable patients with an aim to convert inoperable tumors to operable tumors. Licitra et al in a randomized controlled trial have shown that in patients who received NACT, mandible preservation rates were higher (31 vs. 52%) compared with the control group and there was a decreased requirement for radiotherapy in the NACT group (33 vs. 46%). However, no survival benefit was seen.[56] In India many patients present at an advanced stage with soft tissue disease reaching the masticator space. These patients would never come for surgery per primum and hence are given two/three cycles of cisplatin and 5-fluorouracil and after a response evaluation these patients are evaluated for surgery. To date there is no level I evidence for the use of NACT in locally advanced OSCC and trials are being conducted to provide conclusive evidence.

Photodynamic Therapy

In cases of oral premalignant lesions, photodynamic therapy has been proposed as an alternative to surgery. The methods involve systemic administration of a photosensitizing agent (5-aminolevulinic acid) which on activation by an external light source converts to a cytotoxic drug destroying the region which is illuminated. Once activated by light at wavelengths matching their specific absorption, these photosensitizers produce singlet oxygen that is then capable of killing cells directly, sublethal mutagenesis, and induction of apoptosis. Photosensitizers may be administered systemically, or in the case of skin lesions, topically. PDT is especially suitable for small, localized, and superficial tumors. In oral lesions it provides less scarring and can be used in patients presenting with multiple primary tumors for which surgery would prove mutilating. Copper et al

reported on 27 patients with 42 second or multiple primary head and neck tumors treated by photodynamic therapy and reported that 28 out of 42 tumors were cured (67%) with cure rates for stage I or in situ disease being 85 versus 38% for stage II/III disease.[57]

Chemoprevention of Oral Cancers

Chemoprevention has been defined as "the use of natural or synthetic agents to reverse, suppress or prevent progression to invasive cancer without killing healthy cells."[58] Due to "field carcinogenesis" the entire lining of the oral cavity mucosa develops molecular changes which exhibit in the form of cancer at different stages. This process needs to be reversed to prevent the occurrence of malignancy and in this lies the role of chemoprevention. To date various agents have been evaluated for their chemopreventive efficacy. The list includes the following:

- Retinoids: all-trans retinoic acid (ATRA), 13-*cis* retinoic acid (13cRA), 9-*cis* retinoic acid (9cRA), retinyl palmitate, and fenretinide.
- Alpha-tocopherol
- Soybean (Bowman-Birk inhibitor)
- *N*-acetylcysteine
- Green tea extracts
- Pomegranate juice
- Curcumin analogs
- Celecoxib (COX-2 antagonist)

Retinoids

Among these, retinoids are the agents most commonly studied. These vitamin A analogs are responsible for modulation of epithelial differentiation and proliferation by acting on the specific retinoic acid receptors as shown in the figure.

The first trial to use retinoids was by Hong et al in 1986.[59] The salient features of the trial are given below:

- 3-month placebo-controlled, double-blinded trial
- High-dose 13cRA (2 mg/kg/d)
- 44 patients with oral leukoplakia
- Complete/partial response (PR) in 67% of patients in the treatment group
- 10% PR in the placebo group

Drawbacks of this study were as follows:

- Significant dose-related, reversible toxicity was encountered
- Cheilitis and dry skin (88%)
- Conjunctivitis (76%)
- Dose reduction to 1 mg/kg/d was in 47%; a corresponding lower remission rate in this group was observed.
- Also, within 3 months more than half of all treated patients developed new lesions.

This was followed by a study by Lippman et al in 1993[60]

- Randomized, placebo-controlled trial.
- Patients with dysplastic or symptomatic hyperplastic lesions.
- 3-month *induction course* of high-dose 13cRA (1.5 mg/kg/d) → 9-month *maintenance course* with low-dose 13cRA (0.5 mg/kg/d) or B-carotene (30 mg/d) *provided there was a clear response during the induction phase.*
- Induction phase: 55% response rate.
- Maintenance phase: 8% of the 13 cRA progressed compared with 55% of the B-carotene group.
- Progression to SCC occurred in seven patients receiving B-carotene and in only one patient who received 13cRA.
- No patients discontinued therapy due to toxicity.
- 10-year follow-up of this trial showed that the two treatment groups had no discernible difference in cancer rates.

In preventing the occurrence of second primaries, Khuri et al[61] conducted a trial with the following features:

- Randomized phase III trial.
- 1191 patients (stage I and II HNC).
- Isotretinoin (30 mg/d) versus placebo × 3 years → evaluation for SPT × 4 years.

The results of this trial are summarized below:

- Primary tumors recurred in 97 patients at an annual rate of 2.8%.
- No significant difference in overall survival, SPT reduction, or recurrence-free survival (the annual rate of SPT being 4.7% in both groups).

Another trial led by van Zandwijk et al (EUROSCAN)[62] had the following features:

- 2592 patients: head and neck (60%) or lung cancer (40%)
- Retinyl palmitate and *N*-acetylcysteine
- Retinyl palmitate (300,000 IU daily for 1 year followed by 150,000 IU for the second year)
- *N*-acetylcysteine (600 mg daily for 2 years)

The EUROPEAN trial should:

- No statistically significant difference in overall survival or event-free survival.
- No benefit for *N*-acetylcysteine.

COX-2 Inhibitors

There are two isoforms of cyclooxygenase (COX). The COX-1 isoform is related to normal cell activity, but COX-2 plays a key role in inflammation. Celecoxib is one of the newly developed inhibitors that specifically targets COX-2. The study by Wang et al provided the first evidence that celecoxib is highly effective and safe for the inhibition of oral carcinoma cells in a nude mouse model.[63] It suggests its preventive efficacy in oral cancer. Antiangiogenic activity of celecoxib is thought to be a major cause of its efficacy in the early treatment of carcinoma. Recently, it has been shown that aneuploid oral dysplastic lesions, which are lesions at the greatest risk of cancer progression, have selective upregulation of COX-2.[64]

Epidermal Growth Factor Receptor Inhibitors

Premalignant and malignant lesions of the oral cavity express epidermal growth factor inhibitors (EGFR) to an extent of 80 to 100%.[65] Activation of EGFR occurs by phosphorylation through tobacco and this form of phosphorylated EGFR has been found in 50% of dysplastic oral lesions and 100% of carcinomas. Hence, there exists a possibility of using EGFR inhibitors for chemoprevention.

Rehabilitation

Rehabilitation is an important constituent in the management of a cancer patient. The various physical, emotional, and psychosocial changes resulting from ablative surgery makes the patient vulnerable to psychological problems such as depression. The process of rehabilitation should begin as soon as the patient is diagnosed with the disease and should take into account functional aspects of the oral cavity, dental and prosthetic rehabilitation, and social readjustments. This process involves a close liaison between the patient, his caretakers, and the medical staff.

References

1. GLOBOCAN. 2008. Cancer incidence, mortality and prevalence Worldwide IARC. Cancer Base No.5 (computer program) version 2.0. Lyon: IARC Press; 2008
2. Pathak KA, Nason RW, Talole SD, Abdoh AA. Are buccal cancers in India and Canada any different? J Surg Oncol 2008;97(6):529–532
3. Warnakulasuriya S. Global epidemiology of oral and oropharyngeal cancer. Oral Oncol 2009;45(4-5):309–316
4. Fakih AR, Rao RS, Borges AM, Patel AR. Elective versus therapeutic neck dissection in early carcinoma of the oral tongue. Am J Surg 1989;158(4):309–313
5. Walvekar RR, Chaukar DA, Deshpande MS, et al. Squamous cell carcinoma of the gingivobuccal complex: predictors of locoregional failure in stage III-IV cancers. Oral Oncol 2009;45(2):135–140
6. Khariwala SS, Hatsukami D, Hecht SS. Tobacco carcinogen metabolites and DNA adducts as biomarkers in head and neck cancer: potential screening tools and prognostic indicators. Head Neck 2012;34(3):441–447
7. McCoy GD, Wynder EL. Etiological and preventive implications in alcohol carcinogenesis. Cancer Res 1979;39(7 Pt 2):2844–2850
8. McLaughlin JK, Gridley G, Block G, et al. Dietary factors in oral and pharyngeal cancer. J Natl Cancer Inst 1988;80(15):1237–1243
9. Axell T, Holmstrup P, Kramer IRH, et al. International seminar on oral leukoplakia and associated lesions to tobacco habits. Community Dent Oral Epidemiol 1984;12:145–154
10. Wynder EL, Kabat G, Rosenberg S, Levenstein M. Oral cancer and mouthwash use. J Natl Cancer Inst 1983;70(2):255–260
11. Donald PJ. Marijuana smoking—possible cause of head and neck carcinoma in young patients. Otolaryngol Head Neck Surg 1986;94(4):517–521

12. Shillitoe EJ, Greenspan D, Greenspan JS, Silverman S Jr. Immunoglobulin class of antibody to herpes simplex virus in patients with oral cancer. Cancer 1983;51(1):65–71

13. Watts SL, Brewer EE, Fry TL. Human papillomavirus DNA types in squamous cell carcinomas of the head and neck. Oral Surg Oral Med Oral Pathol 1991;71(6):701–707

14. Fortner JG, Shiu MH. Organ transplantation and cancer. Surg Clin North Am 1974;54(4):871–876

15. Ficarra G, Eversole LE. HIV-related tumors of the oral cavity. Crit Rev Oral Biol Med 1994;5(2):159–185

16. Schantz SP, Hsu TC. Head and neck cancer patients express increased clastogen-induced chromosome fragility. Head Neck 1989;11:337–343

17. Warnakulasuriya S, Johnson NW, van der Waal I. Nomenclature and classification of potentially malignant disorders of the oral mucosa. J Oral Pathol Med 2007;36(10):575–580

18. Petti S. Pooled estimate of world leukoplakia prevalence: a systematic review. Oral Oncol 2003;39(8):770–780

19. Baric JM, Alman JE, Feldman RS, Chauncey HH. Influence of cigarette, pipe, and cigar smoking, removable partial dentures, and age on oral leukoplakia. Oral Surg Oral Med Oral Pathol 1982;54(4):424–429

20. Bagan JV, Jimenez Y, Murillo J, et al. Lack of association between proliferative verrucous leukoplakia and human papillomavirus infection. J Oral Maxillofac Surg 2007;65(1):46–49

21. Campisi G, Giovannelli L, Aricò P, et al. HPV DNA in clinically different variants of oral leukoplakia and lichen planus. Oral Surg Oral Med Oral Pathol Oral Radiol Endod 2004;98(6):705–711

22. Fornatora M, Jones AC, Kerpel S, Freedman P. Human papillomavirus-associated oral epithelial dysplasia (koilocytic dysplasia): an entity of unknown biologic potential. Oral Surg Oral Med Oral Pathol Oral Radiol Endod 1996;82(1):47–56

23. Barnes L, Eveson JW, Reichart PA, Sidransky D. World Health Organization classification of tumors. Pathology and genetics. Head and neck tumors. World Health Organization; 2005

24. van der Waal I. Potentially malignant disorders of the oral and oropharyngeal mucosa; present concepts of management. Oral Oncol 2010;46(6):423–425

25. Gandolfo S, Richiardi L, Carrozzo M, et al. Risk of oral squamous cell carcinoma in 402 patients with oral lichen planus: a follow-up study in an Italian population. Oral Oncol 2004;40(1):77–83

26. Murti PR, Bhonsle RB, Pindborg JJ, Daftary DK, Gupta PC, Mehta FS. Malignant transformation rate in oral submucous fibrosis over a 17-year period. Community Dent Oral Epidemiol 1985;13(6):340–341

27. Slaughter DP, Southwick HW, Smejkal W. Field cancerization in oral stratified squamous epithelium; clinical implications of multicentric origin. Cancer 1953;6(5):963–968

28. Lippman SM, Sudbø J, Hong WK. Oral cancer prevention and the evolution of molecular-targeted drug development. J Clin Oncol 2005;23(2):346–356

29. Lederman M. The anatomy of cancer. With special reference to tumours of the upper air and food passages. J Laryngol Otol 1964;78:181–208

30. Shah JP. Patterns of cervical lymph node metastasis from squamous carcinomas of the upper aerodigestive tract. Am J Surg 1990;160(4):405–409

31. Van Cann EM, Koole R, Oyen WJG, et al. Assessment of mandibular invasion of squamous cell carcinoma by various modes of imaging: constructing a diagnostic algorithm. Int J Oral Maxillofac Surg 2008;37(6):535–541

32. Manikantan K, Sayed SI, Syrigos KN, et al. Challenges for the future modifications of the TNM staging system for head and neck

cancer: case for a new computational model? Cancer Treat Rev 2009;35(7):639–644

33. Devine JC, Rogers SN, McNally D, Brown JS, Vaughan ED. A comparison of aesthetic, functional and patient subjective outcomes following lip-split mandibulotomy and mandibular lingual releasing access procedures. Int J Oral Maxillofac Surg 2001;30(3):199–204

34. Dubner S, Spiro RH. Median mandibulotomy: a critical assessment. Head Neck 1991;13(5):389–393

35. Hara I, Gellrich NC, Duker J, et al. Swallowing and speech function after intraoral soft tissue reconstruction with lateral upper arm free flap and radial forearm free flap. Br J Oral Maxillofac Surg 2003;41(3):161–169

36. Netscher D, Armenta AH, Meade RA, Alford EL. Sensory recovery of innervated and non-innervated radial forearm free flaps: functional implications. J Reconstr Microsurg 2000;16(3):179–185

37. Wong TY, Chung CH, Huang JS, Chen HA. The inverted temporalis muscle flap for intraoral reconstruction: its rationale and the results of its application. J Oral Maxillofac Surg 2004;62(6):667–675

38. Alonso del Hoyo J, Fernandez Sanroman J, Gil-Diez JL, Diaz Gonzalez FJ. The temporalis muscle flap: an evaluation and review of 38 cases. J Oral Maxillofac Surg 1994;52(2):143–147, discussion 147–148

39. Pathak KA, Deshpande MS, Mathur N, et al. Buccal plate excision for buccal paramandibular spread. J Surg Oncol 2006;94(3):257–259

40. Vartanian JG, Carvalho AL, Carvalho SM, Mizobe L, Magrin J, Kowalski LP. Pectoralis major and other myofascial/myocutaneous flaps in head and neck cancer reconstruction: experience with 437 cases at a single institution. Head Neck 2004;26(12):1018–1023

41. Disa JJ, Liew S, Cordeiro PG. Soft-Tissue reconstruction of the face using the folded/multiple skin island radial forearm free flap. Ann Plast Surg 2001;47(6):612–619

42. McGregor AD, MacDonald DG. Routes of entry of squamous cell carcinoma to the mandible. Head Neck Surg 1988;10(5):294–301

43. McGregor AD, MacDonald DG. Patterns of spread of squamous cell carcinoma within the mandible. Head Neck 1989;11(5):457–461

44. Marchetta FC, Sako K, Murphy JB. The periosteum of the mandible and intraoral carcinoma. Am J Surg 1971;122(6):711–713

45. D'Cruz AK, Dandekar MR. Elective versus therapeutic neck dissection in the clinically node negative neck in early oral cavity cancers: do we have the answer yet? Oral Oncol 2011;47(9):780–782

46. Byers RM, El-Naggar AK, Lee YY, et al. Can we detect or predict the presence of occult nodal metastases in patients with squamous carcinoma of the oral tongue? Head Neck 1998;20(2):138–144

47. Po Wing Yuen A, Lam KY, Lam LK, et al. Prognostic factors of clinically stage I and II oral tongue carcinoma-A comparative study of stage, thickness, shape, growth pattern, invasive front malignancy grading, Martinez-Gimeno score, and pathologic features. Head Neck 2002;24(6):513–520

48. Paleri V, Rees G, Arullendran P, Shoaib T, Krishman S. Sentinel node biopsy in squamous cell cancer of the oral cavity and oral pharynx: a diagnostic meta-analysis. Head Neck 2005;27(9):739–747

49. Stoeckli SJ, Alkureishi LW, Ross GL. Sentinel node biopsy for early oral and oropharyngeal squamous cell carcinoma. Eur Arch Otorhinolaryngol 2009;266(6):787–793

50. Alkureishi LW, Burak Z, Alvarez JA, et al; European Association of Nuclear Medicine Oncology Committee; European Sentinel Node Biopsy Trial Committee. Joint practice guidelines for radionuclide lymphoscintigraphy for sentinel node localization in oral/oropharyngeal squamous cell carcinoma. Ann Surg Oncol 2009;16(11):3190–3210

51. Wallner PE, Hanks GE, Kramer S, McLean CJ. Patterns of Care Study. Analysis of outcome survey data-anterior two-thirds of tongue and floor of mouth. Am J Clin Oncol 1986;9(1):50–57

52. Bernier J, Domenge C, Ozsahin M, et al; European Organization for Research and Treatment of Cancer Trial 22931. Postoperative irradiation with or without concomitant chemotherapy for locally advanced head and neck cancer. N Engl J Med 2004;350(19):1945–1952

53. Cooper JS, Pajak TF, Forastiere AA, et al; Radiation Therapy Oncology Group 9501/Intergroup. Postoperative concurrent radiotherapy and chemotherapy for high-risk squamous-cell carcinoma of the head and neck. N Engl J Med 2004;350(19):1937–1944

54. Rosenthal DI, Liu L, Lee JH, et al. Importance of the treatment package time in surgery and postoperative radiation therapy for squamous carcinoma of the head and neck. Head Neck 2002;24(2):115–126

55. Bonner JA, Harari PM, Giralt J, et al. Radiotherapy plus cetuximab for squamous-cell carcinoma of the head and neck. N Engl J Med 2006;354(6):567–578

56. Licitra L, Grandi C, Guzzo M, et al. Primary chemotherapy in resectable oral cavity squamous cell cancer: a randomized controlled trial. J Clin Oncol 2003;21(2):327–333

57. Copper MP, Triesscheijn M, Tan IB, Ruevekamp MC, Stewart FA. Photodynamic therapy in the treatment of multiple primary tumours in the head and neck, located to the oral cavity and oropharynx. Clin Otolaryngol 2007;32(3):185–189

58. Sporn MB. Dichotomies in cancer research: some suggestions for a new synthesis. Nat Clin Pract Oncol 2006;3:364–373

59. Hong WK, Endicott J, Itri LM, et al. 13-cis-retinoic acid in the treatment of oral leukoplakia. N Engl J Med 1986;315(24):1501–1505

60. Lippman SM, Batsakis JG, Toth BB, et al. Comparison of low-dose isotretinoin with beta carotene to prevent oral carcinogenesis. N Engl J Med 1993;328(1):15–20

61. Khuri FR, Lee JJ, Lippman SM, et al. Isotretinoin effects on head and neck cancer recurrence and second primary tumors. Proc Am Soc Clin Oncol 2003;22:359a

62. van Zandwijk N, Dalesio O, Postorino, et al. EUROSCAN, a randomized trial of vitamin A and N-acetylcysteine in patients with head and neck cancer or lung cancer. J Natl Cancer Inst 2000;92(12):977–986

63. Wang Z, Fuentes CF, Shapshay SM. Antiangiogenic and chemopreventive activities of celecoxib in oral carcinoma cell. Laryngoscope 2002;112(5):839–843

64. Subdø J, Ristimaki A, Sondeesen JE, et al. Cyclooxygenase-2 (Cox-2) expression in high-risk premalignant oral lesions. Oral Oncol 2003;39(5):497–505

65. Grandis JR, Tweardy DJ. Elevated levels of transforming growth factor alpha and epidermal growth factor receptor messenger RNA are early markers of carcinogenesis in head and neck cancer. Cancer Res 1993;53(15):3579–3584

66. Kawaguchi H, El-Naggar AK, Papadimitrakopoulou V, et al. Podoplanin: a novel marker for oral cancer risk in patients with oral premalignancy. J Clin Oncol 2008;26(3):354–360

67. Vora HH, Trivedi TI, Shukla SN, Shah NG, Goswami JV, Shah PM. p53 expression in leukoplakia and carcinoma of the tongue. Int J Biol Markers 2006;21(2):74–80

68. Luo CW, Roan CH, Liu CJ. Human papillomaviruses in oral squamous cell carcinoma and pre-cancerous lesions detected by PCR-based gene-chip array. Int J Oral Maxillofac Surg 2007;36(2):153–158

69. Kövesi G, Szende B. Prognostic value of cyclin D1, p27, and p63 in oral leukoplakia. J Oral Pathol Med 2006;35(5):274–277

70. Gires O, Mack B, Rauch J, Matthias C. CK8 correlates with malignancy in leukoplakia and carcinomas of the head and neck. Biochem Biophys Res Commun 2006;343(1):252–259

71. Byers RM, Newman R, Russell N, Yue A. Results of treatment for squamous carcinoma of the lower gum. Cancer 1981;47(9):2236–2238

72. Willén R, Nathanson A. Squamous cell carcinoma of the gingiva. Histological classification and grading of malignancy. Acta Otolaryngol 1973;75(4):299–300

73. Spiro RH, Huvos AG, Wong GY, Spiro JD, Gnecco CA, Strong EW. Predictive value of tumor thickness in squamous carcinoma confined to the tongue and floor of the mouth. Am J Surg 1986;152(4):345–350

74. Lindberg R. Distribution of cervical lymph node metastases from squamous cell carcinoma of the upper respiratory and digestive tracts. Cancer 1972;29(6):1446–1449

75. Strong EW. Carcinoma of the tongue. Otolaryngol Clin North Am 1979;12(1):107–114

76. Fakih AR, Rao RS, Borges AM, Patel AR. Elective versus therapeutic neck dissection in early carcinoma of the oral tongue. Am J Surg 1989;158(4):309–313

77. Greene F, Page D, Fleming I, et al. AJCC Cancer Staging Manual. 7th ed. New York, NY: Springer-Verlag; 2010

78. Mehta FS, Gupta PC, Daftary DK, Pindborg JJ, Choksi SK. An epidemiologic study of oral cancer and precancerous conditions among 101,761 villagers in Maharashtra, India. Int J Cancer 1972;10(1):134–141

11 Oropharynx Cancer

M. Boyd Gillespie

Core Messages

- Oropharyngeal squamous cell carcinoma (SCC) is increasing in incidence in the United States compared with other head and neck cancer sites.

- High-risk human papillomavirus strains have been confirmed as a major etiologic factor in oropharyngeal SCC and are the principal cause of the rising incidence of the disease.

- There is controversy concerning the best method of treatment for oropharyngeal SCC. However, there are several guidelines that a managing physician can follow to optimize oncologic and functional outcomes.

- Minimally invasive surgical methods including transoral laser microsurgery and transoral robotic surgery are increasingly being viewed as viable treatment options for oropharyngeal SCC.

Oropharyngeal squamous cell carcinoma (SCC) is a highly lethal and debilitating disease that is increasing in incidence compared with other head and neck cancer (HNC) sites. The critical location of this cancer creates a burden of disease which is greater than the numbers would indicate because of high treatment-related morbidity, including difficulties with speech and swallowing, malnourishment, tooth loss, chronic pain, reduced shoulder mobility, reduced quality of life, and altered physical appearance.

These morbidities often require ongoing medical treatment long after the cancer is treated to preserve health and quality of life. Current trends in the management of oropharyngeal SCC are focused on determining whether patients with certain subsets of disease can undergo less-intensive therapy while providing adequate oncologic control and minimizing long-term morbidity.

Anatomy

The oropharynx is an anatomically distinct region with a cancer pathophysiology, presentation, and treatment that differentiates it from the more anterior oral cavity. Many nonhead and neck trained specialists and researchers and many large cancer databases fail to take this distinction into account and unfortunately combine oropharyngeal and oral cavity SCC cases, thereby weakening the conclusions that can be drawn from the data. It is therefore critical for head and neck specialists to train others in the relevant anatomy of the oropharynx to allow proper staging and disease reporting.

The oropharynx is the posterior throat and consists of four subsites: the soft palate, lateral pharyngeal wall, posterior pharyngeal wall, and base of tongue. The soft palate is the superior margin of the oropharynx and extends from the posterior border of the bony palate to the posterior edge of the uvula. The lateral pharyngeal wall consists of the anterior tonsillar pillars (anterior pharyngeal arches), the palatine tonsils or tonsillar fossae, and the posterior tonsillar pillars (posterior pharyngeal arches). The posterior pharyngeal wall is contiguous with the posterior wall of the nasopharynx and hypopharynx and extends from the level of the soft palate superiorly to the cricoid cartilage inferiorly. The base of the tongue is the posterior one-third of the tongue extending from the anterior tonsillar pillar and circumvallate papillae anteriorly to the vallecula posteriorly. The base of the tongue often has lingual tonsils on its superior surface, which form the base of Waldeyer ring of pharyngeal lymphoid tissue.

The oropharynx is bordered by two clinically relevant spaces that have treatment implications.[1] The parapharyngeal space is lateral to the lateral oropharyngeal wall and consists of the parapharyngeal fat pad, pterygoid musculature, and branches of the internal maxillary artery and trigeminal nerve. Tumor invasion of this space may result in trismus, indicating late stage disease requiring multimodality therapy. The retropharyngeal space is located behind the pharyngeal constrictor muscles that make up the posterior pharyngeal wall. The retropharyngeal space consists of loose areolar connective tissue and lymph nodes that may be the first echelon of spread of tumors of the posterior tonsillar pillar and posterior pharyngeal wall. The retropharyngeal nodes may be difficult to access and remove with a standard neck dissection and may provide a conduit for spread to additional nodes in the cervical lymphatic chain contralateral to the primary tumor.[2]

The oropharynx plays a critical role in swallowing function with contributions from 20 paired muscle groups and 5 cranial nerves. The main swallowing function of the oropharynx is the safe transfer of the liquid or food bolus from the oral cavity to the upper esophagus in a rapid (< 500 ms) fashion that protects the airway from bolus penetration or aspiration. Oropharynx cancer and its treatment may result in the reduced swallowing function and safety.

Epidemiology

Approximately 5000 new cases of oropharyngeal SCC occur in the United States each year, of which 90% are SCCs.[2] Like other HNC sites, traditional risk factors for oropharyngeal SCC include tobacco (all forms), marijuana, and alcohol. Unlike other HNC sites that are decreasing in incidence with the reduction in the prevalence of cigarette smoking, oropharyngeal SCC is increasing in incidence each year, especially in people younger than 45 years in Western societies.

Recent evidence has confirmed that certain high-risk strains of human papillomavirus (HPV) are responsible for the increasing incidence of oropharyngeal SCC of the tonsil and tongue observed over the past 30 years. HPV subtype 16 is estimated to be responsible for up to 60% of SCCs of the tonsil and base of the tongue.[3] HPV-related oropharyngeal SCC appears to be a unique molecular, epidemiological, and clinical entity (**Table 11.1**).

HPV-related SCC appears to follow a distinct molecular pathway distinguishing it from traditional non-HPV SCC. Repeated tobacco and alcohol exposure cause mutational loss of the *p16* and *p53* genes as early neoplastic events in up to 80% of SCCs.[4] In most cases of HPV-related head and neck squamous cell carcinoma (HNSCC), unmutated wild-type *p53* is present, but degraded by the E6 protein, and

p16 is overexpressed on tissue immunohistochemistry.[5,6] Therefore, it has been suggested that HPV is the likely cause of HNSCC if the cancer demonstrates normal *p53* without mutations, overexpression of *p16*, in-situ hybridization of HPV DNA, and/or the presence of HPV E6 and E7 RNA in microdissected tumor by quantitative reverse transcription-polymerase chain reaction in ratios of > 1 copy number per 100 tumor cells.[5]

Although more research is needed to ascertain the mode of transmission, high-risk HPV is a known cause of cervical cancer in women, and it is therefore assumed that HPV spreads to the throat through sexual contact. The commercially available vaccines can reduce infection by HPV strains most responsible for genital warts and cancer if given before the initiation of sexual activity. Presently, the vaccine is only being widely offered and covered by insurance for preadolescent and adolescent girls despite the fact that men also develop genital warts, are purveyors and reservoirs for the virus, and may develop HPV-related HNSCC. In fact, based on Surveillance Epidemiology and End Results data, there are more cancers of the tonsil and tongue regions each year in the United States, 60% of which are thought to be due to HPV, than there are cancers of the uterine cervix. Therefore, clinicians who treat these diseases hope that both boys and girls will have greater access to these HPV-prevention vaccines in the future.

The difference in the prognosis in HPV-positive oropharyngeal SCC compared with HPV-negative oropharyngeal SCC provides the strongest argument for the increased use of HPV testing of oropharyngeal tumors.

Table 11.1 Differences between HPV-Negative and HPV-Positive HNSCC

Factor	HPV-Negative HNSCC	HPV-Positive HNSCC
Molecular factors	*p53* mutational loss common Rb upregulated p16 underexpression D cyclin overexpression No HPV DNA/RNA	*p53* wild-type present Rb downregulated p16 overexpression D cyclin underexpression HPV DNA (type 16 in > 85% of the cases) HPV E6 and E7 RNA
Epidemiological factors	Heavy smoking Heavy alcohol use Low marijuana exposure Poor dentition Low oral sex exposure Older age (> 50 y) Lower socioeconomic status African race Deceasing incidence	No smoking at all Mild/moderate alcohol use High marijuana exposure Intact dentition High oral sex exposure Younger age (< 45 y) Higher socioeconomic status Caucasian race Increasing incidence
Clinical factors	All head and neck sites Worse survival Radiation response unpredictable	Predominantly oropharynx (tonsil and tongue base) Better survival More radiosensitive

HPV, human papilloma virus; HNSCC, head and neck squamous cell carcinoma; y, year(s).

A growing body of evidence has shown that patients who are HPV-positive have a better prognosis compared with patients who are HPV-negative regardless of the treatment method.[7,8] A meta-analysis of 23 studies analyzing survival in 1747 patients with HNC stratified for HPV status found a hazard ratio of 0.72 (95% CI, 0.5–1.0) for overall survival in patients with HPV-positive oropharyngeal cancer and a hazard ratio of 0.51 (95% CI, 0.4–0.7) for disease-free survival in patients with HPV-negative oropharyngeal cancer.[9] A study that assessed the HPV status of patients with oropharyngeal SCC undergoing a randomized trial of concurrent chemoradiation therapy found a significant 58% reduction in the risk of death 3 years after the treatment in the HPV-positive cohort while controlling for age, race, stage, tobacco exposure, and treatment received.[10] Therefore, it is estimated that HPV-positive status in oropharyngeal SCC may lower the risk of overall mortality by 28 to 58%.

Differences in HPV rates have been proposed as a possible explanation for the higher death rate from HNC observed in blacks compared with whites. A retrospective review of a clinical trial of induction chemotherapy followed by concurrent chemoradiation therapy found significant racial differences in HPV positivity with 35% of the white patients having HPV-positive tumors compared with only 4% of the black patients.[11] The lower median overall survival observed for blacks (20.9 months) compared with whites (70.6 months) was present only when HPV-positive cases were considered because whites with HPV-negative tumors had an equally poor survival compared with blacks.

Clinical Presentation

Oropharyngeal SCC is typically asymptomatic in its earliest stages. Therefore, a complete examination should be performed routinely by all general health care providers and oral health specialists as part of the routine physical examination. The soft palate, tonsillar region, and posterior pharyngeal wall can usually be adequately visualized with a tongue blade or retractor and light source. Visual inspection of the base of the tongue requires either a mirror or a fiberoptic scope; however, digital palpation for a firm or raised mass with a gloved finger can substitute if these are not readily available. Early lesions may appear as white or erythematous lesions with ulceration or exophytic growth. HPV-related lesions often have a exophytic, papillomatous, strawberry-like appearance as opposed to HPV-negative lesions that are often ulcerative (**Fig. 11.1A, B**). If the lesion can be sufficiently visualized, biopsy can be performed in the office with cupped forceps after applying a topical anesthetic spray. Lesions that are less accessible due to anatomy or patient cooperation may require directed laryngoscopy and biopsy in the operating suite.

Early symptoms of oropharyngeal tumors include chronic sore throat, odynophagia, and dysphagia, whereas late symptoms include neck mass, trismus, tongue or chin numbness, and weight loss. A thorough fiberoptic examination of the oropharynx is a necessary measure for any patient with persistent sore throat or swallowing difficulty lasting more than 2 weeks because most infectious causes should have resolved in that time frame. Patients with unilateral otalgia without ear pathology require a thorough oropharyngeal examination.

Regional nodal adenopathy is present in more than 50% of the patients with oropharyngeal SCC at presentation. In fact, an enlarged neck node is often the presenting sign of the disease. Therefore, a thorough oropharyngeal examination is the standard of care for any patient with enlarged cervical adenopathy. Radiographic imaging (e.g., computed tomography (CT) of neck with intravenous contrast) and fine-needle aspiration with cytological analysis is recommended for any large or suspicious lymph node that has failed to respond to an appropriate course of antibiotics or other conservative therapy. The presence of a cystic node on imaging strongly suggests an oropharyngeal primary tumor in cases of occult primary tumor (**Fig. 11.2**).

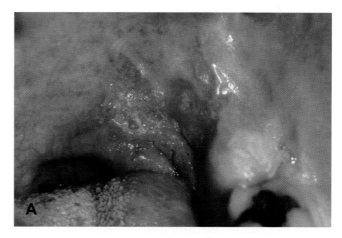

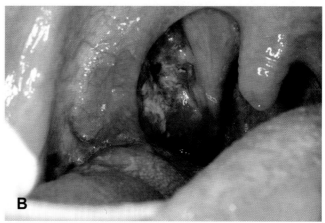

Figure 11.1 (A) Human papillomavirus (HPV)-associated oropharyngeal tumors may have a papillomatous, strawberry-like gross appearance, whereas (B) HPV-negative tumors are often endophytic and ulcerative.

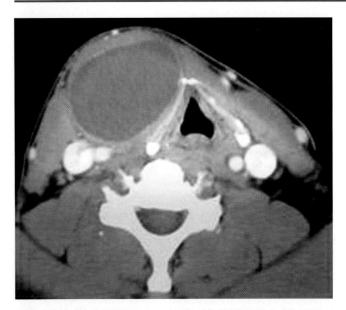

Figure 11.2 A cystic neck mass requires a thorough inspection, biopsy, and tonsillectomy to rule out occult oropharyngeal cancer.

Staging

Accurate clinical staging is the first step in formulating a treatment plan for a lesion of the oropharynx that is confirmed to be SCC on histopathological examination (**Table 11.2**). Clinical staging requires three components: (1) comprehensive head and neck examination, (2) upper airway endoscopy (fiberoptic and/or operative), and (3) radiographic imaging. On the basis of these three components—tumor, node, metastasis—group staging criteria established by the American Joint Commission on Cancer (AJCC) should be documented in the patient's permanent medical record before the treatment initiation (www.cancerstaging.org).

A comprehensive head and neck examination notes the physical characteristics of the tumor and surrounding tissues (e.g., tumor site, size, palpable neck nodes, deep muscle or bone invasion, trismus, vocal cord mobility, and cranial nerve function). Office-based fiberoptic endoscopy is indicated to characterize the extent of the tumor, evaluate the status of the airway, and assess for second primary tumors, which may be present in up to 5% of

the cases. Operative endoscopy under general anesthesia may be required to better assess and obtain biopsies of tumors of the sinonasal cavity, nasopharynx, larynx, and hypopharynx. In cases of neck metastasis of unknown primary, tongue base biopsy and bilateral tonsillectomy should be considered.[12]

Radiographic evaluation of the upper aerodigestive tract and neck is necessary for accurate staging, but the optimal type of imaging to obtain varies on the basis of tumor site, stage, availability, patient tolerance, renal function, and allergy history (**Table 11.2**). Radiographic assessment of the lungs is necessary to assess for distant metastasis and second primaries in patients not receiving positron emission tomography -computed tomography (PET-CT), and it may consist of plain AP and lateral chest films in nonsmokers or chest CT scans in smokers and patients with underlying pulmonary disease.

Fluoro-2-deoxy-D-glucose PET-CT is a highly sensitive functional imaging modality that takes advantage of the higher glucose metabolism of cancer cells to concentrate a glucose analogue radiotracer within the tumor that can be imaged and superimposed on the anatomic image of a CT scan. PET-CT has superior positive and negative predictive values compared with CT and magnetic resonance imaging (MRI) when evaluating SCC. In addition, PET-CT can assess for the presence of distant metastases that have reached sufficient detection thresholds (mean 4 mm greatest diameter).[13,14] However, PET-CT is costly and subject to both false-negative results and false-positive results and should therefore be used in accordance with the findings of numerous clinical studies. PET-CT is indicated in the following scenarios: (1) before treatment with combined chemoradiation therapy because it provides a baseline study to use as comparison when later assessing treatment response; (2) the evaluation of late-stage tumors (stage IVa), low neck disease (level IV or V), poor performance status/anorexia, or suspicious pulmonary nodules because detection of distant metastasis may allow the morbidity of a major surgery to be avoided unless otherwise indicated for palliative reasons; or (3) the evaluation of unknown primary tumors with nodal neck disease because it has greater sensitivity for small and submucosal tumors compared with conventional imaging. In general, PET-CT is not indicated for detecting occult neck disease in the clinical and radiographically negative

Table 11.2 Preferred Radiographic Methods for Certain Clinical Scenarios

Tumor Site	Tumor Subsite	Tumor Stage	Preferred Test
Oropharynx	Tonsil	I, II, III	CT or PET-CT
	Base of tongue	I, II, III	CT, MRI, or PET-CT
	Posterior wall	I, II, III	MRI or PET-CT
	Any	IVa, IVb, IVc	PET-CT
	Low neck disease (level 4 or 5)	Any	PET-CT
Unknown primary	Unknown	Any	PET-CT

CT, computed tomography; PET-CT, positron emission tomography-computed tomography; MRI, magnetic resonance imaging.

neck because of the lack of sensitivity in the detection of micrometastases.

Because of the complexity of the disease and the multiple treatment options available, patients with oropharyngeal SCC benefit from the discussion of their history and plan of care at a multidisciplinary tumor board. At a minimum, the multidisciplinary tumor board should include the ENT/head and neck surgeon, a radiation oncologist, a medical oncologist, a surgical pathologist, and a diagnostic radiologist. In addition, comprehensive tumor boards greatly benefit from the input of other care providers such as reconstructive surgeons, dentists, cancer nurses, speech–language pathologists, physical therapists, occupational therapists, social workers, cancer scientists, and clinical trial coordinators. Tumor board review of the plan of care is helpful in all cases but should be mandatory for all advanced (stages III and IV), complex, or recurrent cases. Patients with advanced, complex, and/or recurrent disease may therefore benefit from a consultation with, or referral to, a comprehensive tertiary care center that has fellowship-trained HNC specialists.

Ancillary Interventions

The treatment of later stage III and IV SCCs of the oropharynx may result in a period of significant dysphagia that may last for 6 months or more. Pretreatment evaluation by a speech-language pathologist is therefore of benefit. A modified barium swallow or fiberoptic evaluation of swallow may identify patients who are at risk for aspiration pneumonia or suggest swallowing maneuvers that can help the patient maintain an oral diet during therapy. A percutaneous gastrostomy tube should be considered before treatment in patients with large tumors or tumor-related cachexia to maintain nutritional support and hydration. Patients should be encouraged to continue even minimal levels of daily oral intake during combined chemoradiation therapy to maintain the patency of the pharyngeal and esophageal lumen and to reduce the long-term risk of radiation fibrosis of the pharyngeal musculature. Tracheotomy and/or conservative tumor debulking should be performed to establish a patent airway in patients with advanced oropharyngeal cancer who present with significant airway obstruction.

Treatment

Early stage I and II oropharyngeal SCCs can be treated with either surgery or radiation alone, whereas more advanced stage III and IV cancers require surgery and radiation with or without chemotherapy or combined chemoradiation with surgical salvage as indicated. The best treatment for a particular tumor is largely a function of the tumor site, stage, and availability of cancer treatment resources. Selecting the most appropriate treatment can be challenging because clinical trial data demonstrate relative equivalency in survival of patients treated with surgery and radiation compared with those treated with combined chemoradiation. Because of the lack of a survival benefit of one particular regimen compared with another, the preferences of patients and their families should be given serious consideration. A treatment table (**Table 11.3**) was developed after literature review by the members of the Medical University of South Carolina Head and Neck Tumor Program to serve as a ready reference for physicians and patients who most decide between competing treatment options. Physicians can help patients make the best decision for themselves by educating patients and their families about the disease and by arranging consultations with various treating specialists. A review of the National Comprehensive Cancer Network (NCCN) guidelines on HNSCC should be performed annually because of ongoing advancements in oncologic care. These guidelines are offered free of charge with registration on the Web site of the NCCN (www.nccn.org).

Stage I or II Disease—Oropharynx

Radiation is often preferred as a single modality because of its ability to effectively treat both the primary tumor and the draining lymph node basin, which will contain occult metastases in at least 30% of the cases. Intensity-modulated radiation therapy should be considered when feasible because of reduced morbidity on surrounding normal tissues. Surgery will less often result in single modality treatment because of the frequent need for adjuvant radiation for close or positive margins, high-risk histopathological features, and findings of multiple positive nodes on selective neck dissection. In addition, surgery alone will often fail to address retropharyngeal nodal groups that may be at risk. Surgery should usually be reserved for patients who refuse to undergo a radiation protocol, who have early (T in situ, T1, or T2) disease, or for cases who need excisional biopsy to establish a diagnosis. Minimally invasive surgical techniques such as transoral laser microsurgery and transoral robotic surgery can be considered in T1 or T2 oropharyngeal tumors if the tumor can be excised transorally with negative margins. Surgery can be repeated as necessary to obtain negative margins, and survival is not affected as long as negative margin status is ultimately achieved.[15] Transoral resection by microscopic laser techniques with or without robotic assistance results in few complications with excellent

Table 11.3 Treatment Options for Oropharyngeal Cancer

Stage	Treatment Option(s)
I and II	S or RT
III and IVa	CRT (concurrent) ± S salvage or S + RT (CRT if unfavorable path)
IVb and IVc	CRT
Recurrent	S ± CRT or clinical trial or hospice care

S, surgery; RT, radiotherapy; CRT, chemoradiotherapy.

functional and disease outcomes at experienced centers of care.[16,17] Adjuvant radiation or chemoradiation can be given after surgical resection without compromising survival in patients whose surgical pathology demonstrates high-risk features such as close (≤ 2 mm) margins, lymphovascular invasion, perineural invasion, multiple involved lymph nodes, or extracapsular lymph node extension.[16]

Stage III or IVa Disease—Oropharynx

Therapeutic options for advanced (III or IV) stage oropharyngeal cancer include chemotherapy with radiation with or without surgical salvage or surgery with radiation with or without chemotherapy. Selecting the most appropriate treatment for a given individual is challenging because clinical trial data demonstrate relative equivalency in survival of patients treated with surgery and radiation compared with those treated with combined chemoradiation.[18]

Combined chemotherapy with radiation for advanced oropharyngeal cancer requires less patient selection than surgical approaches and can be used in most cases of advanced disease. The chemotherapy and radiation should be given concurrently (simultaneous fashion) when feasible for better locoregional control.[19] Concurrent chemoradiation therapy will be generally preferred over surgery if primary surgery would require a mandibulotomy or need for free-tissue flap reconstruction. Three to five cycles of induction chemotherapy followed by concurrent chemoradiation may be appropriate in patients at high risk for distant metastasis (e.g., N3 or level IV/V neck disease) or in patients with large volume disease who require rapid cytoreduction for symptom palliation.[20] The currently preferred chemotherapeutic approach uses dual drug therapy consisting of a platinum-based drug (e.g., cisplatinum and carboplatinum) and 5-flurouracil or taxol analog.

The use of newer targeted small molecule biologic therapy is likely to increase in the future. Targeted therapy uses antibodies or small molecules to disrupt oncogenic pathways within tumors in ways that are tumor specific and less toxic than traditional therapies. Several clinical trials are investigating whether the addition of these agents to standard chemoradiation regimens results in improved locoregional control and disease-free survival. The anti-epidermal growth factor receptor (anti-EGFR) antibody cetuximab (Erbitux) is currently indicated for use with radiation therapy in patients who cannot tolerate platinum-based chemotherapy.[21,22]

Patients should undergo repeat neck CT with intravenous contrast, or other appropriate imaging, and comprehensive head and neck examination within 6 weeks of treatment completion. Patients with suspected persistent disease at the primary site should be restaged with biopsy and offered surgical salvage if positive in the absence of locally unresectable or distant metastatic disease. Salvage surgery for persistent disease at the primary site should be radical and will likely require microvascular flap reconstruction. Salvage neck dissection with rebiopsy of the primary site should be performed if there are clinically palpable or radiographically suspicious nodes but no detectable tumor at the primary site.

Patients with an initially complete clinical and radiographic response should be followed by monthly physical examinations with a follow-up PET-CT at ≥ 10-week posttherapy. PET-CT is helpful in evaluating the tumor site that is often difficult to follow clinically because of surrounding tissue edema and fibrosis. Follow-up PET-CTs performed before 10 weeks are subject to high rates of false-positives because of ongoing treatment-related inflammation at the tumor site. Positive findings on PET-CT should be followed with a biopsy, whereas a negative scan has a high negative predictive value (> 95%), can help avoid unnecessary biopsies, and likely indicates complete therapeutic response.[13]

Surgery followed by radiation may be indicated in select cases of advanced oropharyngeal cancer. Primary surgery is most effective for T1 or T2, or select T3 tumors with limited N1 or N2b (mobile) neck disease if the primary tumor can be fully excised transorally with negative margins without the need for mandibulotomy.[23] Surgery should be strongly considered as a primary modality in patients with contraindications to platinum-based chemotherapy, such as significant sensorineural hearing loss or renal failure. The best functional outcomes are achieved with tonsillar tumors with minimal soft palate and tongue base extension because the tonsil has a natural capsule that makes radical excision beyond the tumor more feasible. Local flaps from the remaining uvula or soft palate tissue can be easily rotated into the pharyngectomy defect to promote rapid healing and velopharyngeal competence (**Fig. 11.3**).[24] Ipsilateral neck dissection of levels 2 to 4 should be performed during the same surgery in most cases as long as there is no significant communication between the oropharynx and the neck, which would result in a salivary fistula. In one large series, the overall 5-year survival and disease-specific survival rate was 88 and 92%, respectively, in a series of 84 patients with AJCC stage III or IV oropharyngeal cancer undergoing transoral laser microsurgery.[16]

Adjuvant radiation is indicated after surgical resection of all patients with AJCC stage III or IV oropharyngeal cancer. The radiation should be delivered within 5 to 6 weeks of surgery to reduce the risk of locoregional recurrence. An advantage of surgical resection is the potential for reducing total radiation dosages to the primary site and therefore potentially reducing the long-term morbidity of radiation therapy. If the primary tumor is excised to clear margins, a radiation dose of 60 to 62 Gy is sufficient compared with the higher dosages of 66 to 70 Gy used in most primary chemoradiation protocols.[25,26] Concurrent chemotherapy should be added in cases of close or positive surgical margins, low (level 4) cervical lymph nodes, and/or extracapsular nodal disease.

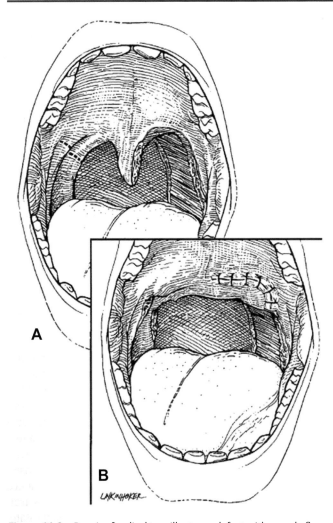

Figure 11.3 Repair of radical tonsillectomy defect with a uvula flap.

Surveillance and Follow-Up

Patients with oropharyngeal cancer, like other head and neck sites, are at the highest risk for recurrent disease within the first 2 years after treatment. Close clinical follow-up is therefore indicated within the first 2 years and should consist of visits to various care providers (e.g., head and neck surgeon, radiation oncologist, and medical oncologist) on an every-other-month basis. After 2 years, patients can be seen every 4 to 6 months followed by yearly visits after 5 years.

Patient weight and oral intake should be assessed at follow-up visits. Patients with dysphagia should be evaluated with a modified barium swallow to determine whether they would benefit from swallowing therapy or dilation of fibrotic segments of the upper esophagus. Chronic neck and shoulder pain is common after neck dissection and should be addressed with referral to a licensed physical therapist. Patients with chronic pain requiring analgesics may benefit from a consultation with a chronic pain clinic. Routine surveillance imaging of the head and neck (e.g., CT, MRI, and PET-CT) in the absence of signs and symptoms has low yield and may result in needless follow-up tests

(e.g., biopsies) with added costs and potential for complications. A posterioranterior and a lateral chest film once a year provide screening for lung metastasis. Thyroid function testing should be performed yearly because of the high rate of hypothyroidism after head and neck irradiation.

Recurrent Oropharyngeal Cancer

Even with adherence to best practice guidelines of the NCCN, up to 50% of the patients with advanced stage oropharyngeal cancer who undergo appropriate therapy will present with locoregional disease recurrence or distant metastasis within 2 years of diagnosis. Currently, there is no accepted standard of care to guide physicians and patients facing this difficult situation. Repeat imaging with PET-CT is indicated to determine whether the disease is localized and therefore amendable to surgical salvage for potential cure.

Surgical salvage often requires radical excision with complex microvascular reconstruction; therefore, most of these patients will benefit from referral to a center performing comprehensive HNSCC care (**Fig. 11.4**). Small recurrences may be amendable to transoral laser microsurgery techniques in select cases.[27] Because of the high failure rates and potential morbidity, surgical salvage should be reserved for highly motivated patients of higher functional capacity who are otherwise fairly healthy, have strong social support, and are likely to benefit from maintenance of quality of life and improved pain control and hygiene.

Reirradiation protocols have recently been used to provide local tumor palliation for patients who are far removed from the initial radiation therapy.[28] Reirradiation regimens are complex and have the potential for severe complications (e.g., carotid blowout) and therefore should only be offered at centers offering comprehensive head and neck care. Palliative chemotherapy may reduce tumor

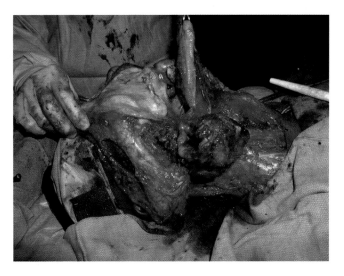

Figure 11.4 Mandibulotomy and free tissue transfer is usually required to salvage local recurrence of oropharyngeal cancer.

burden and improve pain and function. The anti-EGFR antibody cetuximab is approved by the U.S. Food and Drug Administration for unresectable and/or metastatic HNSCC previously treated with a platinum-based regimen.

Patients and physicians facing recurrent and/or metastatic HNSCC are strongly encouraged to investigate whether there is an option for participation in a clinical trial. A full list of HNSCC clinical trials can be found at the up-to-date government Web site www.clinicaltrials.gov. Participation in a clinical trial can give patients and families the satisfaction of fighting the cancer while generating new knowledge that may help future cancer sufferers and may provide some coverage for the cost of care by leading cancer experts.

The benefits of hospice care should be discussed with patients who are too ill or who decide to forgo further active treatment. Hospice provides comprehensive end-of-life care, including pain control, hygiene, nutritional, social, and spiritual support, which can help patients die with dignity in their own homes.

References

1. Cohan DM, Popat S, Kaplan SE, Rigual N, Loree T, Hicks WL Jr. Oropharyngeal cancer: current understanding and management. Curr Opin Otolaryngol Head Neck Surg 2009;17(2):88–94

2. Lin DT, Cohen SM, Coppit GL, Burkey BB. Squamous cell carcinoma of the oropharynx and hypopharynx. Otolaryngol Clin North Am 2005;38(1):59–74, viii

3. Hammarstedt L, Lindquist D, Dahlstrand H, et al. Human papillomavirus as a risk factor for the increase in incidence of tonsillar cancer. Int J Cancer 2006;119(11):2620–2623

4. Califano J, van der Riet P, Westra W, et al. Genetic progression model for head and neck cancer: implications for field cancerization. Cancer Res 1996;56(11):2488–2492

5. Weinberger PM, Yu Z, Haffty BG, et al. Molecular classification identifies a subset of human papillomavirus–associated oropharyngeal cancers with favorable prognosis. J Clin Oncol 2006;24(5):736–747

6. Rose BR, Li W, O'Brien CJ. Human papillomavirus: a cause of some head and neck cancers? Med J Aust 2004;181(8):415–416

7. Fakhry C, Westra WH, Li S, et al. Improved survival of patients with human papillomavirus-positive head and neck squamous cell carcinoma in a prospective clinical trial. J Natl Cancer Inst 2008;100(4):261–269

8. Nichols AC, Faquin WC, Westra WH, et al. HPV-16 infection predicts treatment outcome in oropharyngeal squamous cell carcinoma. Otolaryngol Head Neck Surg 2009;140(2):228–234

9. Ragin CCR, Taioli E. Survival of squamous cell carcinoma of the head and neck in relation to human papillomavirus infection: review and meta-analysis. Int J Cancer 2007;121(8):1813–1820

10. Ang KK, Harris J, Wheeler R, et al. Human papillomavirus and survival of patients with oropharyngeal cancer. N Engl J Med 2010;363(1):24–35

11. Settle K, Posner MR, Schumaker LM, et al. Racial survival disparity in head and neck cancer results from low prevalence of human papillomavirus infection in black oropharyngeal cancer patients. Cancer Prev Res (Phila) 2009;2(9):776–781

12. McQuone SJ, Eisele DW, Lee DJ, Westra WH, Koch WM. Occult tonsillar carcinoma in the unknown primary. Laryngoscope 1998;108(11 Pt 1):1605–1610

13. Kutler DI, Wong RJ, Schoder H, Kraus DH. The current status of positron-emission tomography scanning in the evaluation and follow-up of patients with head and neck cancer. Curr Opin Otolaryngol Head Neck Surg 2006;14(2):73–81

14. Emonts P, Bourgeois P, Lemort M, Flamen P. Functional imaging of head and neck cancers. Curr Opin Oncol 2009;21(3):212–217

15. Jäckel MC, Ambrosch P, Martin A, Steiner W. Impact of re-resection for inadequate margins on the prognosis of upper aerodigestive tract cancer treated by laser microsurgery. Laryngoscope 2007;117(2):350–356

16. Rich JT, Milov S, Lewis JS Jr, Thorstad WL, Adkins DR, Haughey BH. Transoral laser microsurgery (TLM) +/– adjuvant therapy for advanced stage oropharyngeal cancer: outcomes and prognostic factors. Laryngoscope 2009;119(9):1709–1719

17. Moore EJ, Olsen KD, Kasperbauer JL. Transoral robotic surgery for oropharyngeal squamous cell carcinoma: a prospective study of feasibility and functional outcomes. Laryngoscope 2009;119(11):2156–2164

18. Calais G, Alfonsi M, Bardet E, et al. Randomized trial of radiation therapy versus concomitant chemotherapy and radiation therapy for advanced-stage oropharynx carcinoma. J Natl Cancer Inst 1999;91(24):2081–2086

19. Pignon JP, Bourhis J, Domenge C, Designé L, on behalf of the MACH-NC Collaborative Group. Chemotherapy added to locoregional treatment for head and neck squamous-cell carcinoma: three meta-analyses of updated individual data. Lancet 2000;355(9208):949–955

20. Haddad RI, Tishler RB, Norris C, et al. Phase I study of C-TPF in patients with locally advanced squamous cell carcinoma of the head and neck. J Clin Oncol 2009;27(27):4448–4453

21. Gold KA, Lee HY, Kim ES. Targeted therapies in squamous cell carcinoma of the head and neck. Cancer 2009;115(5):922–935

22. Langer CJ. Targeted therapy in head and neck cancer: state of the art 2007 and review of clinical applications. Cancer 2008;112(12):2635–2645

23. Walvekar RR, Li RJ, Gooding WE, et al. Role of surgery in limited (T1-2, N0-1) cancers of the oropharynx. Laryngoscope 2008;118(12):2129–2134

24. Gillespie MB, Eisele DW. The uvulopalatal flap for reconstruction of the soft palate. Laryngoscope 2000;110(4):612–615

25. Pradier O, Christiansen H, Schmidberger H, et al. Adjuvant radiotherapy after transoral laser microsurgery for advanced squamous carcinoma of the head and neck. Int J Radiat Oncol Biol Phys 2005;63(5):1368–1377

26. Rieger JM, Zalmanowitz JG, Wolfaardt JF. Functional outcomes after organ preservation treatment in head and neck cancer: a critical review of the literature. Int J Oral Maxillofac Surg 2006;35(7):581–587

27. Grant DG, Salassa JR, Hinni ML, Pearson BW, Hayden RE, Perry WC. Transoral laser microsurgery for recurrent laryngeal and pharyngeal cancer. Otolaryngol Head Neck Surg 2008;138(5):606–613

28. Lee N, Chan K, Bekelman JE, et al. Salvage re-irradiation for recurrent head and neck cancer. Int J Radiat Oncol Biol Phys 2007;68(3):731–740

12 Cancer of the Nasopharynx

Tanya Fancy and Eric J. Lentsch

Core Messages

- Nasopharyngeal carcinoma comprises the majority of nasopharyngeal malignancies.

- Multiple environmental and genetic factors play a role in the pathogenesis of this disease.

- The mainstay of treatment is radiation alone or radiation combined with chemotherapy for more advanced disease.

- Research into the optimum timing and duration of chemotherapy is still ongoing.

- Surgery has a greater role to play in the event of recurrent or persistent disease (in the neck and/or the nasopharynx) after the failure of primary treatment.

Tumors of the nasopharynx are classified by the World Health Organization (WHO) into several categories based on histology.[1] These include epithelial tumors, soft tissue tumors, bone and cartilage tumors, malignant lymphomas, tumorlike lesions, secondary tumors, and unclassified tumors. This chapter focuses on nasopharyngeal carcinoma (NPC), a malignant epithelial tumor that constitutes 75 to 95% of nasopharyngeal malignancies in low-risk populations and virtually all nasopharyngeal cancers in high-risk populations.[2]

Nasopharyngeal Carcinoma

NPC is an uncommon tumor in western Europe and North America, occurring sporadically, with an age-adjusted incidence of less than 1 per 100,000 population for both sexes.[3] This neoplasm occurs with greater frequency in Southeast Asia, and especially in the Guangdong Province of southern China, where reported incidences range from 15 to 80 per 100,000 population.[4] Intermediate incidence rates have been reported in North Africa, in the Mediterranean basin, and among the Alaskan Eskimo population.[4-6] Men are affected three times more often than women,[7] and 80% of these tumors occur in people aged 45 to 85 years.[8] Although NPC is rare in the pediatric population, a bimodal age distribution has been described specific to low-risk areas,[9] with the first peak occurring from 15 to 24 years and the second from 65 to 79 years. Globally, the mean age of occurrence in high-risk populations is 40 to 50 years[5] and this bimodal distribution is not appreciated. Children, therefore, comprise a greater proportion (up to 16%) of the patients with NPC in nonendemic areas than in endemic areas such as China (0.1%).[10]

Epidemiology

The pathogenesis of this disease reflects complex interactions between genetic susceptibility, dietary factors, population migration patterns, and environmental exposures (including viral agents such as Epstein-Barr virus [EBV]). This multifactorial etiology is supported by the fact that the incidence of NPC is lower among first-generation Chinese who migrate to low-incidence areas in the West. However, Chinese born in North America still have a seven times higher incidence of NPC than do Caucasians.[11] There is also a trend toward decreasing incidence the further the population has immigrated.[12] Within at-risk Asian populations, NPC is more often of the nonkeratinizing or undifferentiated type, tends to present at a more advanced stage, and more likely to appear at an earlier age than in low-incidence populations.[5,6] However, Chinese ethnicity itself is an independent and favorable prognosticator for survival in NPC.[13]

Chromosomal abnormalities in chromosomes 1, 3, 4, 6, 9, 11–17, and X have been described in its pathogenesis.[14] Human leukocyte antigen associations reported in the literature include B17, B18, BW46, and A2. Dietary factors that have been linked to the development of NPC include the consumption of salted fish and preserved vegetables.[2,15,16] Diets lacking in fresh fruits, fiber, and carotene have also been implicated.[16] Increased intake of oranges and tangerines has been shown to cause a reduction in the risk of development of NPC.[15] As yet, no clear association has been established between NPC and tobacco or alcohol use,[17,18] although exposure to domestic wood fires is an independent risk factor for NPC.[19]

EBV is a DNA virus from the herpes virus group. The virus is ubiquitous and is usually acquired in early childhood. Once a person is infected with the virus, he or she develops immunity but the virus remains within specific circulating B lymphocytes or is shed through saliva for the rest of the individual's life.[20] EBV is consistently detected in NPC, regardless of geographic region or extent of tumor differentiation. Most individuals infected with the virus do not develop NPC, and so it is believed that EBV is not the initiating event in NPC, but a second event after the initial transformation of epithelial cells of the nasopharynx. The presence of a single form of viral DNA suggests that these tumors are clonal proliferations of a single cell that was initially infected with EBV.[21]

Specific latent viral genes are expressed on NPC cells and in early dysplastic lesions. These genes encode for Epstein-Barr nuclear antigen (EBNA) 1 to 6; latent membrane protein types 1, 2A, and 2B; and EBV-encoded RNA (EBER) 1 and 2. These EBV antigens and EBERs are not expressed by normal nasopharyngeal cells. Their oncogenic products block apoptosis and senescence and alter cellular gene expression and growth to cause rapid proliferation and invasion by tumor cells.[21]

The typical serological profile in NPC consists of an increase in immunoglobulin G (IgG) and immunoglobulin A (IgA) against viral capsid antigen (VCA) and early antigen (EA) and in IgG anti-EBNA.[5] This profile differs in patients without NPC who are infected with EBV, in whom there are elevated levels of immunoglobulin M and IgG against EA and VCA antigens on EBV (but not IgA).

Anatomy

The nasopharynx extends from the skull base to the level of the soft palate and is continuous with the nasal cavity via the choanae anteriorly. It is a tubular passage with a sloping roof, its posterior wall being formed by the basisphenoid, the basiocciput, and the first cervical vertebra. The Eustachian tube orifices are located in the lateral wall of the nasopharynx, just medial to the medial pterygoid plate. The opening to each forms a comma-shaped elevation known as the torus tubarius. The nasopharynx constitutes part of Waldeyer ring.

The primary tumor generally arises from the lateral nasopharynx, most commonly at the pharyngeal recess (fossa of Rosenmüller) medial to the medial crus of the Eustachian tube, and is characterized by a rich submucosal lymphatic plexus, resulting in the early development of cervical nodal metastases.

Presentation and Diagnosis

The symptoms related to early disease are subtle and nonspecific, and thus many patients with primary NPC are diagnosed once the tumor has progressed to an advanced stage. Almost 80% of nasopharyngeal tumors are T2 or T3 at the initial presentation.[7] Less than 1% of the patients are diagnosed incidentally and are asymptomatic at the time of diagnosis.

Cervical lymphadenopathy is the most common presenting symptom and is found in up to 90% of the patients,[7,22] with bilateral neck involvement occurring in as many as 50% of the cases.[17,22] Lymphatic involvement of the first echelon nodes, the retropharyngeal nodes, is often detected only radiologically. Occasionally, they may be appreciated as a nodular submucosal swelling in the posterior pharynx on physical examination. Lymphatic spread tends to occur to the jugulodigastric and upper jugular nodes first and then subsequently to the lower jugular and supraclavicular nodal groups. Involvement of that latter group has been shown to have prognostic significance, as reflected in the nodal staging system.

Other presenting symptoms relate to the presence of tumor in the nasopharynx (nasal discharge, obstruction, and epistaxis), Eustachian tube dysfunction (tinnitus and hearing loss), or cranial nerve and skull base involvement with tumor (diplopia, headache, facial pain, and anesthesia). Cranial nerve involvement is present in up to 20% of the patients at diagnosis. The most commonly affected cranial nerve is the fifth, specifically the maxillary division.[7] Also commonly involved are the sixth, twelfth, and third cranial nerves.[7,22–24] The level of recovery of cranial nerve involvement in response to treatment has been shown to be an independent factor affecting prognosis.[25] NPC has a propensity to invade adjacent anatomic regions fairly early, spreading into the nasal cavity (20%) or via the pharyngeal muscles into the oropharynx (15%).[26] Parapharyngeal space invasion occurs in more than 80% of the patients.[26] Involvement of the skull base occurs in 25 to 35% of the patients,[5] and intracranial involvement is not uncommon.[26,27] The classic clinical triad of neck mass, nasal obstruction, and serous otitis media or conductive hearing loss is relatively infrequent.[5]

More than 250 cases of paraneoplastic syndrome associated with NPC have been reported in the literature. These syndromes may be divided into six categories: dermatologic, rheumatoid, endocrinologic, hematologic, neurologic, and ocular. Dermatomyositis is the most common cutaneous manifestation; while syndrome of inappropriate antidiuretic hormone secretion and Cushing syndrome are the more common endocrinologic manifestations.[28] Other features include clubbing of the fingers and toes, tumor fever, polyneuropathy, and optic neuritis. The paraneoplastic syndrome may appear before the tumor itself manifests. Most often, the paraneoplastic syndrome resolves in parallel with the primary tumor and may prove useful in monitoring for tumor response or recurrence.[28]

Distant dissemination of NPC is found in approximately 10% of the patients[5,7,26,27,29] at presentation and commonly involves the bones (70 to 80% of the patients with distant disease), lungs, liver, and extra-regional nodes.[5,7] The initial work-up generally includes a chest radiograph, bone scans, and ultrasound of the liver, the objective being to rule out distant disease. Alternatively, computed tomography (CT) of the chest and abdomen may be performed, and, more recently, whole-body positron emission tomography (PET) scans are being used as part of the initial staging work-up.

Definitive diagnosis is made by endoscopic-guided biopsy of the primary nasopharyngeal tumor, usually under local anesthesia. General anesthesia may be indicated after multiple negative biopsies in patients with a strong clinical suspicion of disease or when submucosal disease exists that would require deep biopsies. The mucosa around the fossa of Rosenmüller yields the highest positive biopsy rate when direct examination or imaging does not reveal macroscopic tumor but NPC is strongly suspected.[5]

CT and magnetic resonance imaging (MRI) are well established as complementary imaging modalities in the initial staging of NPC. CT is useful in assessing cervical lymph node status and skull base invasion, while MRI is more accurate in detecting the primary tumor, the presence of parapharyngeal extension, retropharyngeal lymphadenopathy, and cranial nerve involvement.[30] Tumor volume calculated from imaging studies is also a reliable indicator (in addition to the T classification of the tumor) for predicting tumor response to radiotherapy.[31,32]

PET is widely used for evaluating squamous cell carcinomas (SCCs) in other sites of the head and neck. Fused PET/CT images provide more accurate interpretations of the overall tumor-node-metastasis (TNM) system stage than standalone PET or CT.[33,34] Studies suggest that PET/CT may be more accurate than conventional imaging in the evaluation of early treatment response and in the detection of recurrent and residual NPC.[35,36] Its role in the initial staging and treatment planning is less clear, and currently, its utility at the time of diagnosis is confined to the detection of distant metastases in patients with advanced locoregional disease and as a baseline study for comparison with future scans used to assess treatment response and detect residual disease after treatment.[35,37] Studies have demonstrated discordance between ^{18}F-fluorodeoxy-D-glucose PET/CT and MRI when evaluating for invasion into the skull base, cavernous sinus, brain, and orbit, where it is thought that PET may undermap the extent of tumor.[35] However, cadaveric studies by Daisne et al reveal that although the volume of primary cancers is smaller on PET (than on CT or MRI), PET provides the most accurate assessment of gross tumor volume.[38]

Laboratory tests that complement the work-up include complete blood counts, serum chemistries, lactate dehydrogenase level, erythrocyte sedimentation rate, and EBV serological profile. Baseline audiogram is also recommended because hearing is likely to worsen with radiation and with the use of certain ototoxic chemotherapeutic agents, such as cisplatin.

Staging

The stage of disease at the time of diagnosis is the most important prognosticator. The most recent TNM staging system for NPC proposed by the American Joint Committee on Cancer (AJCC) is given in **Tables 12.1** and **12.2**. Alternative

systems that are used more commonly in Asia include Ho's 1978 system and the 1992 Chinese Staging System.

Pathology

NPC arises from the epithelial cells that line the surface of the nasopharynx. The malignant cells are polygonal, with nuclei that are round or oval with scant chromatin and prominent nucleoli. The cells are frequently intermingled with lymphoid cells in the nasopharynx, giving rise to the term lymphoepithelioma.[21,39] Electron microscopy studies have determined that these tumor cells are of squamous origin and that the undifferentiated type is a form of SCC.[21]

The WHO classification (1978) recognizes three histopathological types: (1) keratinizing SCC (similar to other sites in the upper aerodigestive tract), (2) nonkeratinizing carcinoma, and (3) undifferentiated carcinoma. In the 1991 WHO classification, the keratinizing SCC subtype was retained while the last two subtypes were combined under the category of "nonkeratinizing carcinoma." This new category was further divided into differentiated and undifferentiated types. Lymphoepithelioma-like carcinoma was considered a variant of undifferentiated carcinoma.[40] The current WHO classification maintains this terminology with the addition of the category "basaloid SCC" (**Table 12.3**).

The vast majority of patients in endemic regions display the nonkeratinizing undifferentiated pattern, while the keratinizing SCC is the pattern more commonly seen in low-incidence areas. In general, nonkeratinizing carcinomas have a stronger relationship with EBV and tend to be more radiosensitive, with better locoregional control rates (resulting in improved 5-year survival), despite a higher rate of distant metastases than the keratinizing type.[41-43] The Chinese ethnicity survival advantage is demonstrated among patients with keratinizing nasopharyngeal SCC as well.[42]

A hypothesis describing the stepwise progression of the histological features that occur as a result of underlying genetic events in the development of NPC has been described.[4] Patches of dysplasia occur initially and are associated with allelic losses on the short arms of chromosomes 3 and 9,[4] possibly in response to environmental carcinogens. This in turn causes inactivation of tumor suppressor genes *p14*, *p15*, and *p16*.[4] It is believed that these initial areas of dysplasia are the sources of the tumor but on their own they are unlikely to progress further. Latent EBV infection is critical in the progression to severe dysplasia. Allelic losses on chromosomes 11q, 13q, and 16q and gains on chromosome 12 eventually lead to invasive carcinoma.[44] The aberrant expression of cadherins and mutations in p53 contributes to the development of metastases.[4]

Management

Radiation therapy is the mainstay of the treatment of NPC. As a single modality, its use is restricted to small tumors limited

Table 12.1 TNM Staging of Nasopharyngeal Carcinoma

Primary tumor (T)

- Tx   Primary tumor cannot be assessed
- T0   No evidence of primary tumor
- Tis   Carcinoma in-situ
- T1   Tumor confined to the nasopharynx, or tumor extends to oropharynx and/or nasal cavity without parapharyngeal extension[a]
- T2   Tumor with parapharyngeal extension[a]
- T3   Tumor involves bony structures of skull base and/or paranasal sinuses
- T4   Tumor with intracranial extension and/or involvement of cranial nerves, hypopharynx, orbit or with extension to the infratemporal fossa/masticator space

Regional lymph nodes (N)

- Nx   Regional lymph nodes cannot be assessed
- N0   No regional lymph node metastasis
- N1   Unilateral metastasis in cervical lymph node(s), 6 cm or less in greatest dimension, above the supraclavicular fossa, and/or unilateral or bilateral, retropharyngeal lymph nodes, 6 cm or less, in greatest dimension[b]
- N2   Bilateral metastasis in cervical lymph node(s), 6 cm or less in greatest dimension, above the supraclavicular fossa[b]
- N3   Metastasis in a lymph node(s)[b] > 6 cm and/or to supraclavicular fossa[b]
- N3a   Greater than 6 cm in dimension
- N3b   Extension to the supraclavicular fossa[c]

Distant metastasis (M)

- M0   No distant metastasis
- M1   Distant metastasis

Used with the permission of American Joint Committee on Cancer (AJCC), Chicago, Illinois. Pharynx. In: Edge SB, Byrd DR, Compton CC et al, eds. *AJCC Cancer Staging Manual,* 7th ed. New York, NY: Springer; 2010: 41–56.

[a]Parapharyngeal extension denotes posterolateral infiltration of tumor.

[b]Midline nodes are considered ipsilateral nodes.

[c]Supraclavicular zone or fossa is relevant to the staging of nasopharyngeal carcinoma and is the triangular region originally described by Ho. It is defined by three points: (1) the superior margin of the sternal end of the clavicle, (2) the superior margin of the lateral end of the clavicle, and (3) the point where the neck meets the shoulder. Note that this would include caudal portions of levels IV and VB. All cases with lymph nodes (whole or part) in the fossa are considered N3b.

to the primary site. Combination with systemic therapy is indicated as soon as early lymph node involvement occurs.[30]

Early Stage Disease

This group (stage I disease) comprises the minority of patients with NPC and may be effectively treated with radiation therapy alone to the primary site and elective neck irradiation.[45] Clinical trials have demonstrated no survival advantage with the addition of chemotherapy to radiation therapy in this patient population. Patients in this group generally have a favorable outcome, with 5-year local

control rates ranging from 80 to 95%.[45] Although radiation therapy alone was previously thought to be appropriate in addressing patients with T2 (parapharyngeal extension) and N1 disease, it is now known that these patients have a worse outcome with single modality therapy and should be treated with concomitant chemoradiotherapy.[45]

Locally Advanced Disease

The majority of patients with NPC belong to this group (stage II and higher), but despite advances in its delivery techniques, radiation therapy alone has yielded disappointing results.

Table 12.2 Anatomic Stage/Prognostic Groups of Nasopharyngeal Carcinoma

Stage	Definition		
	Tumor	**Node**	**Metastasis**
Stage 0	Tis	N0	M0
Stage I	T1	N0	M0
Stage II	T1	N1	M0
	T2	N0	M0
	T2	N1	M0
Stage III	T1	N2	M0
	T2	N2	M0
	T3	N0	M0
	T3	N1	M0
	T3	N2	M0
Stage IVA	T4	N0	M0
	T4	N1	M0
	T4	N2	M0
Stage IVB	Any T	N3	M0
Stage IVC	Any T	Any N	M1

Used with permission of the American Joint Committee on Cancer (AJCC), Chicago, Illinois. Pharynx. In: Edge SB, Byrd DR, Compton CC et al, eds. *AJCC Cancer Staging Manual*, 7th ed. New York, NY: Springer 2010:41–56.

Table 12.3 Histological Classification of Nasopharyngeal Carcinoma

Keratinizing squamous cell carcinoma

Nonkeratinizing squamous cell carcinoma
- Undifferentiated
- Differentiated

Basaloid squamous cell carcinoma

The surrounding dose-limiting structures (including the spinal cord, brainstem, eyes, temporal lobes, pituitary-hypothalamic axis, parotid glands, and middle and inner ears) complicate the delivery of high-dose radiation, making local control in this patient group challenging.[17] Numerous trials have added chemotherapy, be it neoadjuvant, concomitant, or adjuvant, to improve on the treatment response achieved with radiation therapy alone. Data suggest that chemotherapy improves the effect of radiation by tumor volume reduction, increase in radiosensitization, and reduction in the number of micrometastases, thus improving overall survival and reducing the development of distant metastases.[46] The addition of chemotherapy does bring with it a higher incidence of acute hematologic and mucosal toxicities as well as the associated health care costs. Evidence exists that multidrug regimens are superior to single agents, with cisplastin-based combinations being the most active.[17,47]

The 1997 Intergroup Study was the first to demonstrate improved overall survival with the use of concurrent chemotherapy and radiotherapy compared with radiotherapy alone in patients with stage III and IV NPC.[48] The drawbacks of this study, however, were poor compliance with the adjuvant chemotherapy and questions about its applicability to endemic regions (where nonkeratinizing NPC is more prevalent). Several subsequent clinical trials in Asian patients confirmed these findings by demonstrating a definite treatment advantage (improved survival and improved control of distant metastasis) with the application of concurrent chemoradiotherapy (**Table 12.4**).[48–54]

A meta-analysis of 2450 patients with NPC included randomized trials in which patients were assigned to radiation therapy alone or radiotherapy combined with chemotherapy.[55] All the trials included patients with biopsy-proven NPC without distant metastases. Their data showed that the addition of chemotherapy resulted in a significant reduction in the risk of locoregional recurrence and distant metastasis as well as improved overall survival. However, adjuvant chemotherapy did not show benefit for any of the end points evaluated in their analysis. A meta-analysis by Yang et al demonstrated an increase in overall survival by 11% at 5 years after treatment with chemoradiotherapy when compared with radiotherapy alone.[56] In addition, the distant metastatic rate was reduced by 12% with the use of chemoradiotherapy. The major benefit from chemotherapy has been found only in those studies that administered concomitant chemoradiotherapy with or without

Table 12.4 Randomized Phase III Trials in Patients with Locoregionally Advanced Nasopharyngeal Carcinoma, Comparing Concomitant Chemoradiotherapy with Radiotherapy Alone

Trial	n	Protocol	Parameter	Results	Stage
Al-Sarraf et al (1998)[48]	147	3 cycles concurrent cDDP followed by 3 cycles adjuvant cDDP-5-FU vs. RT alone	3-y OS 3-y PFS	S (p = 0.005) S (p = 0.001)	AJCC stage III–IV
Lin et al (2003)[49]	284	2 cycles concurrent cDDP-5-FU vs. RT alone	5-y OS 5-y PFS	S (p = 0.0022) S (p = 0.0012)	AJCC stage III–IV
Chan et al (2005)[50]	350	6 cycles concurrent cDDP vs. RT alone	5-y OS	S (p = 0.049)	Ho's N3, N2, or N1 ≥ 4 cm
Wee et al (2005)[51]	221	3 cycles concurrent cDDP followed by 3 cycles adjuvant cDDP-5-FU vs. RT alone	3-y OS	S (p = 0.0061)	AJCC stage III–IV
Zhang et al (2008)[52]	115	6 cycles concurrent oxaliplatin (weekly) vs. RT alone	2-y OS 2-y MFS 2-y RFS	S (p = 0.01) S (p = 0.02) S (p = 0.02)	AJCC stage III–IV
Chen (2008)[53]	316	7 cycles concurrent cDDP followed by 3 cycles adjuvant cDDP-5-FU vs. RT alone	2-y OS 2-y RFS 2-y MFS	S (p = 0.003) S (p = 0.007) S (p = 0.024)	
Lee et al (2010)[54]	348	3 cycles concurrent cDDP followed by 3 cycles adjuvant cDDP-5-FU vs. RT alone	5-y FFR 5-y PFS	S (p = 0.014) S (p = 0.035)	AJCC T1 4N2 3M0

n, number of patients enrolled; cDDP, cisplatin; 5-FU, 5-fluorouracil; RT, radiation therapy; y, year; AJCC, American Joint Committee on Cancer; MFS, metastasis-free survival; RFS, recurrence-free survival; OS, overall survival; FFR, failure-free rate; PFS, progression-free survival.

adjuvant chemotherapy, and not for induction or adjuvant chemotherapy alone.[56–58]

Similarly, another meta-analysis of 1528 patients from six randomized trials showed that the addition of chemotherapy to radiation therapy increased disease-free/progression-free survival by 37% at 2 years, 40% at 3 years, and 34% at 4 years after treatment.[17] The greatest improvement in these parameters as well as in overall survival was shown in the U.S. Intergroup Trial using concurrent cisplatin and radiation followed by postradiation cisplatin and 5-flurouracil (5-FU).[48]

The role of adjuvant chemotherapy, however, is still controversial because the existing randomized trials compare concurrent chemoradiotherapy followed by adjuvant chemotherapy to radiation therapy alone, without a concurrent chemoradiation-only arm for comparison.[48,53] A randomized multicenter trial by Rossi et al compared adjuvant chemotherapy with radiation therapy alone and failed to show benefit from the administration of vincristine, cyclophosphamide, and adriamycin after curative radiotherapy.[57]

The role of neoadjuvant chemotherapy also has yet to be defined. Ma et al conducted a randomized trial comparing patients with locoregionally advanced NPC who received neoadjuvant cisplatin, bleomycin, and 5-FU with patients receiving radiation therapy alone.[59] Their data did not reveal significant survival benefit with the addition of chemotherapy. Since then, however, several phase II trials have shown promising results with neoadjuvant regimens, including improved 3-year overall survival for patients receiving neoadjuvant chemotherapy followed by concurrent chemoradiation when compared with patients receiving chemoradiation alone.[60] Follow-up with a phase III trial is therefore warranted.

Sequelae of Therapy

Patients undergoing treatment for NPC generally experience salivary, dental, and dystrophic complications in the same pattern and frequency as noted in other head and neck carcinomas. Survivors can experience several late sequelae, which result from the effects of radiation on adjacent dose-limiting organs, including neuroendocrine and auditory complications, radiation-induced fibrosis, and carotid artery stenosis.[61] Trismus as a result of pterygoid muscle fibrosis is quite common. Hypothyroidism may occur as a result of radiation effects to the neck or the hypothalamus. Neurological sequelae, however, although rare, are the most debilitating and account for nearly every treatment-related death.[5] These include temporal lobe necrosis, disorders of the pituitary-hypothalamic axis, cranial nerve palsies, and cognitive and neuropsychological dysfunctions.[62]

Metastatic Disease

In metastatic NPC, chemotherapy may be considered in patients with adequate performance status, and although generally palliative in intent, some long-term disease-free survivors have been reported.[5,63] Combination regimens with platinum and 5-FU are generally used as first-line therapy, with response rates of 66 to 76% reported.[64] Other chemotherapeutic agents that may be used either in multidrug combinations or as single agents include docetaxel, ifosfamide, gemcitabine, capecitabine, irinotecan, doxorubicin, oxaliplatin, vinorelbine, and paclitaxel.[65] The combination of gemcitabine and cisplatin has been shown to be effective and well tolerated in patients with recurrent and metastatic NPC.[66] Targeted therapy with tyrosine kinase inhibitors such as gefitinib and sorafenib is also being investigated.

Recurrent Disease

The treatment of recurrent disease is tailored to individual patients, and decisions are based on the location, volume, and extent of the tumor recurrence. Depending on the type of failure, various treatment options are available.

Surgery has a limited role in the management of the primary tumor, but it becomes an important modality in the management of persistent or recurrent neck disease after radiation therapy.[17] For NPC, the incidence reported in the literature for isolated recurrence in the neck after combined chemoradiation is low. This incidence increases in patients who present initially with advanced nodal disease. Failure of regression of neck nodes after completion of combined modality treatment, clinical progression in lymph node size, and reappearance of lymph nodes are all suspicious for recurrent or residual disease. Pathologic confirmation using fine-needle aspiration cytology is often difficult to obtain due to radiation-induced fibrosis within the nodes. When the neck is the only site with residual disease, surgical salvage with radical neck dissection has yielded the most favorable results.[67] In the presence of extranodal spread, brachytherapy can be applied in addition to surgical excision.[21] If surgical salvage is not an option, a second course of radiation therapy may be applied, taking into consideration the toxicity associated with reirradiation.

Small tumors localized to the nasopharynx without bony invasion may be treated with stereotactic radiation, brachytherapy, or nasopharyngectomy. Stereotactic radiation therapy has achieved response rates up to 66%,[68–70] but it is a fairly new technology without long-term follow-up. Higher local control rates are obtained when the total equivalent dose is greater than 55 Gy.[70] Brachytherapy, most commonly using radioactive gold grains, may be implanted transnasally or via a transpalatal approach. Intracavitary brachytherapy has also been used in NPC, and results in the literature are promising.[71] For recurrences at the primary site that are more invasive or advanced, a second course of external beam radiation (at a greater dosage than the initial treatment) is required. The introduction of intensity-modulated radiotherapy (IMRT) has significantly reduced the incidence of radiation-related complications, including a significant improvement in xerostomia-related variables of quality of life.[72] IMRT modulates the radiation beams so that the dose delivered to critical organs is limited without compromising tumor coverage.

The challenge of salvage surgery for recurrent disease at the primary site is to obtain negative margins while preserving important neurovascular structures and anatomic barriers. The more popular of the anterior surgical approaches—the maxillary swing approach and the midface degloving approach—are generally used for recurrent T1 or T2 disease, with evidence to support improved survival with the maxillary swing approach.[73] Margin status is an important predictor for local control, while dural or brain involvement affects survival.[74] The more recent literature describes endoscopic nasopharyngectomy as a minimally invasive, safe, and oncological modality for the en bloc resection of selected recurrent NPC.[75] A 2-year overall survival rate of 84.2% and a progression-free survival of 82.6% have been reported with this technique, but these numbers represent a highly selective group of patients and long-term results are pending.

Novel Techniques

The association between EBV and NPC provides opportunity for investigation into newer treatment strategies. Two immunotherapy modalities have been developed: viral vector-introduced peptides and dendritic cell vaccination. Dendritic cells are antigen-presenting cells that are able to activate naive CD4+ and CD8+ T cells.[45] A clinical trial by Lin et al used dendritic cells in patients with NPC and was able to demonstrate a substantial immune response with the generation of EBV epitope-specific cytotoxic T cells in the peripheral blood.[76] However, 14 of 16 patients developed disease progression. A phase I study using EBV-specific cytotoxic T cells in patients with refractory NPC has also shown encouraging results.[77] Gene therapy with viral vectors is still an experimental approach.

Molecular therapies targeting vascular endothelial growth factor receptors and epidermal growth factor receptors in patients with NPC are under evaluation.[78]

Follow-Up

Documentation of remission both at the primary site and in the neck is essential. A thorough physical examination including endoscopic examination with or without biopsy is a necessary part of follow-up, but treatment-induced changes may impair visualization. Radiologic imaging can be helpful in differentiating radiation-induced fibrosis from tumor recurrence, and MRI is generally superior to CT in this regard.[5,79,80] It is especially challenging to differentiate between residual tumor and slowly regressing tumor. Follow-up every 4 to 6 months for the first 3 to 5 years is recommended because locoregional relapses, if detected early, are amenable to radical salvage treatment.[21,81] Evaluation of thyroid function should be performed periodically in patients who underwent radiation to the neck.

After remission has been achieved, EBV serology may be helpful, as elevated anti-VCA, anti-EA IgG, and IgA are often indicative of clinical relapse.[82] Post-therapeutic EBV DNA also appears to correlate strongly with progression-free and overall survival and accurately reflects the residual tumor load.[30]

Adenoid Cystic Carcinoma

Nasopharyngeal adenoid cystic carcinoma (NACC) is a rare malignancy, representing less than 5% of nasopharyngeal cancers.[83] The tumor is locally invasive, with a tendency to perineural invasion but has a lower incidence (3 to 15%) of regional lymphatic metastasis than does NPC.[83,84] EBV infection has not been shown to have a significant role in the development of NACC. Because of its low radiosensitivity, the management of adenoid cystic carcinoma of the nasopharynx is primarily surgical, with the addition of adjuvant radiation therapy for patients with advanced tumors or incomplete resection. The addition of chemotherapy has not been shown to improve survival.

References

1. Shanmugaratnam K, Sobin LH. The World Health Organization histological classification of tumours of the upper respiratory tract and ear. A commentary on the second edition. Cancer 1993;71(8):2689–2697
2. Yu MC. Diet and nasopharyngeal carcinoma. Prog Clin Biol Res 1990;346:93–105
3. Parkin DM, Whelan SL, Ferlay J, Raymond L, Young J, eds. Cancer Incidence in Five Continents. Vol 7. IARC Scientific Publications No 143. Lyon: IARC Press; 1997;:814–815
4. Chan AT, Teo PML, Johnson PJ. Nasopharyngeal carcinoma. Ann Oncol 2002;13(7):1007–1015
5. Fandi A, Altun M, Azli N, Armand JP, Cvitkovic E. Nasopharyngeal cancer: epidemiology, staging, and treatment. Semin Oncol 1994;21(3):382–397
6. Ho JH. An epidemiologic and clinical study of nasopharyngeal carcinoma. Int J Radiat Oncol Biol Phys 1978;4(3):183–198
7. Skinner DW, Van Hasselt CA, Tsao SY. Nasopharyngeal carcinoma: modes of presentation. Ann Otol Rhinol Laryngol 1991;100(7):544–551
8. Mittra ES, Iagaru A, Quon A, Fischbein N. PET imaging of skull base neoplasms. PET Clin 2007;2(4):489–510
9. Bray F, Haugen M, Moger TA, Tretli S, Aalen OO, Grotmol T. Age-incidence curves of nasopharyngeal carcinoma worldwide: bimodality in low-risk populations and aetiologic implications. Cancer Epidemiol Biomarkers Prev 2008;17(9):2356–2365
10. Huang TB. Cancer of the nasopharynx in childhood. Cancer 1990;66(5):968–971
11. Dickson RI. Nasopharyngeal carcinoma: an evaluation of 209 patients. Laryngoscope 1981;91(3):333–354
12. Yu WM, Hussain SS. Incidence of nasopharyngeal carcinoma in Chinese immigrants, compared with Chinese in China and South East Asia: review. J Laryngol Otol 2009;123(10):1067–1074
13. Ou SH, Zell JA, Ziogas A, Anton-Culver H. Epidemiology of nasopharyngeal carcinoma in the United States: improved survival of Chinese patients within the keratinizing squamous cell carcinoma histology. Ann Oncol 2007;18(1):29–35
14. Li X, Wang E, Zhao YD, et al. Chromosomal imbalances in nasopharyngeal carcinoma: a meta-analysis of comparative genomic hybridization results. J Transl Med 2006;4:4
15. Yuan JM, Wang XL, Xiang YB, Gao YT, Ross RK, Yu MC. Preserved foods in relation to risk of nasopharyngeal carcinoma in Shanghai, China. Int J Cancer 2000;85(3):358–363
16. Jia WH, Luo XY, Feng BJ, et al. Traditional Cantonese diet and nasopharyngeal carcinoma risk: a large scale case control study in Guangdong, China. BMC Cancer 2010;10(446):1–7
17. Huncharek M, Kupelnick B. Combined chemoradiation versus radiation therapy alone in locally advanced nasopharyngeal carcinoma: results of a meta-analysis of 1,528 patients from six randomized trials. Am J Clin Oncol 2002;25(3):219–223
18. Ali H, al-Sarraf M. Nasopharyngeal cancer. Hematol Oncol Clin North Am 1999;13(4):837–847
19. Zheng YM, Tuppin P, Hubert A, et al. Environmental and dietary risk factors for nasopharyngeal carcinoma: a case-control study in Zangwu County, Guangxi, China. Br J Cancer 1994;69(3):508–514
20. Klein E, Kis LL, Klein G. Epstein-Barr virus infection in humans: from harmless to life endangering virus-lymphocyte interactions. Oncogene 2007;26(9):1297–1305
21. Wei WI, Sham JS. Nasopharyngeal carcinoma. Lancet 2005;365(9476):2041–2054
22. Lee AW, Foo W, Law SC, et al. Nasopharyngeal carcinoma: presenting symptoms and duration before diagnosis. Hong Kong Med J 1997;3(4):355–361
23. Ozyar E, Atahan IL, Akyol FH, Gürkaynak M, Zorlu AF. Cranial nerve involvement in nasopharyngeal carcinoma: its prognostic role and response to radiotherapy. Radiat Med 1994;12(2):65–68
24. Hoppe RT, Goffinet DR, Bagshaw MA. Carcinoma of the nasopharynx. Eighteen years' experience with megavoltage radiation therapy. Cancer 1976;37(6):2605–2612
25. Huang W, Mo H, Deng M, et al. [Relationship between cranial nerve involvement in nasopharyngeal carcinoma and the prognosis]. Lin Chung Er Bi Yan Hou Tou Jing Wai Ke Za Zhi 2009;23(21):964–967
26. Sham JST, Choy D. Prognostic value of paranasopharyngeal extension of nasopharyngeal carcinoma on local control and short-term survival. Head Neck 1991;13(4):298–310
27. Teo P, Leung SF, Yu P, Lee WY, Shiu W. A retrospective comparison between different stage classifications for nasopharyngeal carcinoma. Br J Radiol 1991;64(766):901–908
28. Toro C, Rinaldo A, Silver CE, Politi M, Ferlito A. Paraneoplastic syndromes in patients with nasopharyngeal cancer. Auris Nasus Larynx 2009;36(5):513–520

29. Tang SGJ, Lin FJ, Chen MS, Liaw CC, Leung WM, Hong JH. Prognostic factors of nasopharyngeal carcinoma: a multivariate analysis. Int J Radiat Oncol Biol Phys 1990;19(5):1143–1149

30. Faivre S, Janot F, Armand JP. Optimal management of nasopharyngeal carcinoma. Curr Opin Oncol 2004;16(3):231–235

31. Shen C, Lu JJ, Gu Y, Zhu G, Hu C, He S. Prognostic impact of primary tumor volume in patients with nasopharyngeal carcinoma treated by definitive radiation therapy. Laryngoscope 2008;118(7): 1206–1210

32. Chu ST, Wu PH, Chou P, Lee CC. Primary tumor volume of nasopharyngeal carcinoma: prognostic significance for recurrence and survival rate. Eur Arch Otorhinolaryngol 2008;265(Suppl 1): S115–S120

33. Chen YK, Su CT, Ding HJ, et al. Clinical usefulness of fused PET/CT compared with PET alone or CT alone in nasopharyngeal carcinoma patients. Anticancer Res 2006;26(2B):1471–1477

34. Gordin A, Golz A, Daitzchman M, et al. Fluorine-18 fluorodeoxyglucose positron emission tomography/computed tomography imaging in patients with carcinoma of the nasopharynx: diagnostic accuracy and impact on clinical management. Int J Radiat Oncol Biol Phys 2007;68(2):370–376

35. King AD, Ma BB, Yau YY, et al. The impact of 18F-FDG PET/CT on assessment of nasopharyngeal carcinoma at diagnosis. Br J Radiol 2008;81(964):291–298

36. Yen RF, Hong RL, Tzen KY, Pan MH, Chen THH. Whole-body 18F-FDG PET in recurrent or metastatic nasopharyngeal carcinoma. J Nucl Med 2005;46(5):770–774

37. Chua ML, Ong SC, Wee JT, et al. Comparison of 4 modalities for distant metastasis staging in endemic nasopharyngeal carcinoma. Head Neck 2009;31(3):346–354

38. Daisne JF, Duprez T, Weynand B, et al. Tumor volume in pharyngolaryngeal squamous cell carcinoma: comparison at CT, MR imaging, and FDG PET and validation with surgical specimen. Radiology 2004;233(1):93–100

39. Godtfredsen E. On the histopathology of malignant nasopharyngeal tumors. Acta Pathol Microbiol Scand 1944;55(Suppl):38–319

40. Barnes L, Eveson JW, Reichart P, Sidransky D, eds. Pathology and Genetics of Head and Neck Tumours (IARC WHO Classification of Tumours). Lyon: IARC Press; 2005:81–98

41. Gokce T, Unlu I, Akcay C. Evaluation of overall survival of nasopharyngeal carcinoma patients treated in ten years at a single institution. J BUON 2010;15(1):36–42

42. Marks JE, Phillips JL, Menck HR. The National Cancer Data Base report on the relationship of race and national origin to the histology of nasopharyngeal carcinoma. Cancer 1998;83(3):582–588

43. Reddy SP, Raslan WF, Gooneratne S, Kathuria S, Marks JE. Prognostic significance of keratinization in nasopharyngeal carcinoma. Am J Otolaryngol 1995;16(2):103–108

44. Hui AB, Lo KW, Leung SF, et al. Detection of recurrent chromosomal gains and losses in primary nasopharyngeal carcinoma by comparative genomic hybridisation. Int J Cancer 1999;82(4): 498–503

45. Caponigro F, Longo F, Ionna F, Perri F. Treatment approaches to nasopharyngeal carcinoma: a review. Anticancer Drugs 2010;21(5):471–477

46. Afqir S, Ismaili N, Errihani H. Concurrent chemoradiotherapy in the management of advanced nasopharyngeal carcinoma: current status. J Cancer Res Ther 2009;5(1):3–7

47. Chan ATC, Teo PML, Ngan RKC, et al. A phase III randomized trial comparing concurrent chemotherapy-radiotherapy with radiotherapy alone in locoreginally advanced nasopharyngeal carcinoma [abstract]. Proc Am Soc Clin Oncol 2000;19:415a

48. Al-Sarraf M, LeBlanc M, Giri PGS, et al. Chemoradiotherapy versus radiotherapy in patients with advanced nasopharyngeal cancer: phase III randomized Intergroup study 0099. J Clin Oncol 1998;16(4):1310–1317

49. Lin JC, Jan JS, Hsu CY, Liang WM, Jiang RS, Wang WY. Phase III study of concurrent chemoradiotherapy versus radiotherapy alone for advanced nasopharyngeal carcinoma: positive effect on overall and progression-free survival. J Clin Oncol 2003;21(4):631–637

50. Chan AT, Leung SF, Ngan RK, et al. Overall survival after concurrent cisplatin-radiotherapy compared with radiotherapy alone in locoregionally advanced nasopharyngeal carcinoma. J Natl Cancer Inst 2005;97(7):536–539

51. Wee J, Tan EH, Tai BC, et al. Randomized trial of radiotherapy versus concurrent chemoradiotherapy followed by adjuvant chemotherapy in patients with American Joint Committee on Cancer/International Union against cancer stage III and IV nasopharyngeal cancer of the endemic variety. J Clin Oncol 2005;23(27):6730–6738

52. Zhang L, Zhao C, Peng PJ, et al. Phase III study comparing standard radiotherapy with or without weekly oxaliplatin in treatment of locoregionally advanced nasopharyngeal carcinoma: preliminary results. J Clin Oncol 2005;23(33):8461–8468

53. Chen Y, Liu MZ, Liang SB, et al. Preliminary results of a prospective randomized trial comparing concurrent chemoradiotherapy plus adjuvant chemotherapy with radiotherapy alone in patients with locoregionally advanced nasopharyngeal carcinoma in endemic regions of china. Int J Radiat Oncol Biol Phys 2008;71(5):1356–1364

54. Lee AW, Tung SY, Chua DT, et al. Randomized trial of radiotherapy plus concurrent-adjuvant chemotherapy vs radiotherapy alone for regionally advanced nasopharyngeal carcinoma. J Natl Cancer Inst 2010;102(15):1188–1198

55. Langendijk JA, Leemans CR, Buter J, Berkhof J, Slotman BJ. The additional value of chemotherapy to radiotherapy in locally advanced nasopharyngeal carcinoma: a meta-analysis of the published literature. J Clin Oncol 2004;22(22):4604–4612

56. Yang AK, Liu TR, Guo X, et al. [Concurrent chemoradiotherapy versus radiotherapy alone for locoregionally advanced nasopharyngeal carcinoma: a meta-analysis]. Zhonghua Er Bi Yan Hou Tou Jing Wai Ke Za Zhi 2008;43(3):218–223

57. Rossi A, Molinari R, Boracchi P, et al. Adjuvant chemotherapy with vincristine, cyclophosphamide, and doxorubicin after radiotherapy in local-regional nasopharyngeal cancer: results of a 4-year multicenter randomized study. J Clin Oncol 1988;6(9):1401–1410

58. Baujat B, Audry H, Bourhis J, et al; MAC-NPC Collaborative Group. Chemotherapy in locally advanced nasopharyngeal carcinoma: an individual patient data meta-analysis of eight randomized trials and 1753 patients. Int J Radiat Oncol Biol Phys 2006;64(1): 47–56

59. Ma J, Mai HQ, Hong MH, et al. Results of a prospective randomized trial comparing neoadjuvant chemotherapy plus radiotherapy with radiotherapy alone in patients with locoregionally advanced nasopharyngeal carcinoma. J Clin Oncol 2001;19(5):1350–1357

60. Hui EP, Ma BB, Leung SF, et al. Randomized phase II trial of concurrent cisplatin-radiotherapy with or without neoadjuvant docetaxel and cisplatin in advanced nasopharyngeal carcinoma. J Clin Oncol 2009;27(2):242–249

61. Cheng SW, Ting AC, Lam LK, Wei WI. Carotid stenosis after radiotherapy for nasopharyngeal carcinoma. Arch Otolaryngol Head Neck Surg 2000;126(4):517–521

62. Nasr Ben Ammar C, Chaari N, Kochbati L, et al. [Brain radionecrosis in patients irradiated for nasopharyngeal carcinoma: about nine cases]. Cancer Radiother 2007;11(5):234–240

63. Cheng LC, Sham JS, Chiu CS, Fu KH, Lee JW, Mok CK. Surgical resection of pulmonary metastases from nasopharyngeal carcinoma. Aust N Z J Surg 1996;66(2):71–73

64. Wang TL, Tan YO. Cisplatin and 5-fluorouracil continuous infusion for metastatic nasopharyngeal carcinoma. Ann Acad Med Singapore 1991;20(5):601–603

65. Chan ATC, Felip E; ESMO Guidelines Working Group. Nasopharyngeal cancer: ESMO clinical recommendations for diagnosis, treatment and follow-up. Ann Oncol 2009;20(Suppl 4):123–125

66. Wang J, Li J, Hong X, et al. Retrospective case series of gemcitabine plus cisplatin in the treatment of recurrent and metastatic nasopharyngeal carcinoma. Oral Oncol 2008;44(5):464–470

67. Wei WI, Mok VWK. The management of neck metastases in nasopharyngeal cancer. Curr Opin Otolaryngol Head Neck Surg 2007;15(2):99–102

68. Seo Y, Yoo H, Yoo S, et al. Robotic system-based fractionated stereotactic radiotherapy in locally recurrent nasopharyngeal carcinoma. Radiother Oncol 2009;93(3):570–574

69. Wu SX, Chua DT, Deng ML, et al. Outcome of fractionated stereotactic radiotherapy for 90 patients with locally persistent and recurrent nasopharyngeal carcinoma. Int J Radiat Oncol Biol Phys 2007;69(3):761–769

70. Leung TW, Wong VY, Tung SY. Stereotactic radiotherapy for locally recurrent nasopharyngeal carcinoma. Int J Radiat Oncol Biol Phys 2009;75(3):734–741

71. Maalej M, Ben Ammar CN, Kochbati L, et al. Brachytherapy for primary and recurrent nasopharyngeal carcinoma: treatment techniques and results. Cancer Radiother 2007;11(3):117–121

72. Veldeman L, Madani I, Hulstaert F, De Meerleer G, Mareel M, De Neve W. Evidence behind use of intensity-modulated radiotherapy: a systematic review of comparative clinical studies. Lancet Oncol 2008;9(4):367–375

73. Vlantis AC, Yu BK, Kam MK, et al. Nasopharyngectomy: does the approach to the nasopharynx influence survival? Otolaryngol Head Neck Surg 2008;139(1):40–46

74. Hao SP, Tsang NM, Chang KP, Hsu YS, Chen CK, Fang KH. Nasopharyngectomy for recurrent nasopharyngeal carcinoma: a review of 53 patients and prognostic factors. Acta Otolaryngol 2008;128(4):473–481

75. Chen MY, Wen WP, Guo X, et al. Endoscopic nasopharyngectomy for locally recurrent nasopharyngeal carcinoma. Laryngoscope 2009;119(3):516–522

76. Lin CL, Lo WF, Lee TH, et al. Immunization with Epstein-Barr Virus (EBV) peptide-pulsed dendritic cells induces functional CD8+ T-cell immunity and may lead to tumor regression in patients with EBV-positive nasopharyngeal carcinoma. Cancer Res 2002;62(23): 6952–6958

77. Straathof KC, Bollard CM, Popat U, et al. Treatment of nasopharyngeal carcinoma with Epstein-Barr virus–specific T lymphocytes. Blood 2005;105(5):1898–1904

78. Chan AT, Hsu MM, Goh BC, et al. Multicenter Phase II study of cetuximab in combination with carboplatin in patients with recurrent or metastatic nasopharyngeal carcinoma. J Clin Oncol 2005;23(30):7757–7758

79. Comoretto M, Balestreri L, Borsatti E, Cimitan M, Franchin G, Lise M. Detection and restaging of residual and/or recurrent nasopharyngeal carcinoma after chemotherapy and radiation therapy: comparison of MR imaging and FDG PET/CT. Radiology 2008;249(1):203–211

80. Chong VF, Mukherji SK, Ng SH, et al. Nasopharyngeal carcinoma: review of how imaging affects staging. J Comput Assist Tomogr 1999;23(6):984–993

81. Chiesa F, De Paoli F. Distant metastases from nasopharyngeal cancer. ORL J Otorhinolaryngol Relat Spec 2001;63(4):214–216

82. de-Vathaire F, Sancho-Garnier H, de-Thé H, et al. Prognostic value of EBV markers in the clinical management of nasopharyngeal carcinoma (NPC): a multicenter follow-up study. Int J Cancer 1988;42(2):176–181

83. Liu TR, Yang AK, Guo X, et al. Adenoid cystic carcinoma of the nasopharynx: 27-year experience. Laryngoscope 2008; 118(11):1981–1988

84. Wang CC, See LC, Hong JH, Tang SG. Nasopharyngeal adenoid cystic carcinoma: five new cases and a literature review. J Otolaryngol 1996;25(6):399–403

13 Management of Hypopharynx Cancer

Nicholas J. Sanfilippo and Ariel E. Marciscano

Core Messages

- A multidisciplinary approach is necessary to devise an appropriate therapeutic algorithm.

- Prognosis of cancer of the hypopharynx is associated with less favorable survival outcomes than that of other head and neck malignancies because of high incidence of submucosal involvement and cervical lymphatic spread at the time of presentation.

- Computed tomography, magnetic resonance imaging, and positron emission tomography are the recommended imaging modalities in the diagnostic and preoperative work-up. In addition, they are indicated for the detection of locoregional recurrence and persistent disease and the assessment of treatment response.

- Clinical staging generally guides treatment. Preservation of function, quality of life, and toxicities of treatment should all be considered when selecting an optimal treatment regimen. Surgery, radiation therapy, and chemotherapy all have an important role in management.

- Biological agents such as cetuximab show promise as an adjunctive treatment of hypopharyngeal squamous cell carcinomas. Randomized prospective clinical trials demonstrating efficacy in comparison to standard chemoradiotherapy regimens are necessary to further define a potential role for cetuximab.

Management of hypopharyngeal cancer poses a unique and difficult challenge to physicians. Because of the central location of the hypopharynx, its relation to several critical anatomic structures, and its integral role in swallowing, speech, and phonation, the management of hypopharyngeal cancer demands special attention. A collaborative effort between head and neck surgery, radiation, and medical oncology is often necessary to maximize both survival and quality of life. Furthermore, great care must be taken in the planning, management, and follow-up of these patients, as there are formidable reconstructive and functional challenges posed by surgical intervention and other treatment-related morbidities and impairments.

Carcinomas of the hypopharynx are rare in comparison to other head and neck cancers (HNCs), comprising only 4.3% of all head and neck malignancies.[1] Roughly, 2500 new cases of hypopharyngeal cancer are diagnosed in the United States each year.[2] Moreover, the incidence of laryngeal cancer is four to five times higher than that of hypopharyngeal cancer. The overwhelming majority of hypopharyngeal malignancies are of epithelial origin. Approximately 95% are squamous cell carcinomas (SCCs), and thus they are the primary focus of this discussion. There is a clear gender difference, as men are more likely to develop hypopharyngeal cancer, particularly those of African American descent. In fact, a 3:1 male-to-female ratio has been demonstrated in the United States. However, there exists a subset of female patients with Plummer-Vinson

syndrome who are more susceptible than men to develop hypopharyngeal cancers—specifically of the postcricoid area.[3] Epidemiologic studies have also demonstrated a correlation between increased age and increased incidence of malignancy. The mean age of presentation is 65 years. As with other SCCs of the head and neck, hypopharyngeal cancers have a strong association with both chronic alcohol and tobacco use. Recently, seropositivity for human papillomavirus subtype 16 has been identified as an independent risk factor for head and neck SCCs.[4] It should also be noted that very rarely (< 5%) hypopharyngeal cancers present as adenocarcinomas, lipomas, melanomas, or lymphoproliferative malignancies such as angiocentric T-cell lymphoma, non-Hodgkin lymphoma, and mucosa-associated lymphoid tissue. Other rare types of hypopharyngeal carcinomas include basaloid squamoid carcinomas, spindle cell carcinomas, small cell carcinomas, nasopharyngeal-type undifferentiated carcinomas, and carcinomas of the minor salivary glands.[5]

Cancer of the hypopharynx is often a devastating disease with a poor prognosis. Although these cancers are generally aggressive and poorly differentiated, the early stages of disease are often clinically silent. At the time of presentation, most patients already have extensive submucosal spread and a high incidence of cervical lymph node metastasis: roughly 70 to 80% of the patients initially present with stage III or IV disease.[1,6] The overall 5-year survival rate is approximately 30% for patients with carcinoma of the hypopharynx.[1]

Anatomy

The anatomic boundaries of the hypopharynx can be conceptualized as the region between the oropharynx and the esophageal introitus (**Fig. 13.1**). More precisely, the hyoid bone constitutes the superior border of the hypopharynx, which extends inferiorly to the cricoid cartilage at the most inferior aspect. The cricopharyngeus delineates the transition point of the pharynx to the cervical esophagus. Of note, the hypopharyngeal region excludes the larynx. Indeed, the anterior wall of the hypopharynx is bounded by the posterior surface of the larynx while the retropharyngeal space denotes the posterior border of the hypopharynx. Because of the anatomic proximity of the larynx and the hypopharynx, the larynx is vulnerable to invasion by neoplastic processes of the hypopharynx.[7] Furthermore, this anatomic distinction between the larynx and the hypopharynx offers clinical relevance. Although only millimeters apart, the low metastatic potential and high curability of laryngeal cancers dramatically contrast the early dissemination and poor prognosis of stage-matched hypopharyngeal cancers.[8]

Conceptually and clinically, the hypopharynx anatomy is subdivided into three distinct regions: pyriform sinuses, postcricoid area, and the posterior pharyngeal wall. Approximately, 65 to 85% of hypopharyngeal cancers arise from the pyriform sinus, 10 to 20% from the posterior pharyngeal wall, and 5 to 15% from the postcricoid area.[9,10] The pyriform sinuses are bilateral recesses on each side of the larynx bounded superiorly by the pharyngoepiglottic folds and inferiorly by the cricoid cartilage. These anatomic boundaries form an inverted pyramidal-shaped space. Deep

to the mucosa of the pyriform sinus lie both the recurrent laryngeal nerve and the internal laryngeal nerve, which is a branch of the superior laryngeal nerve. Laryngeal invasion has been noted with tumors of the pyriform sinus with medial extension.[11] The posterior pharyngeal wall extends from the level of the hyoid bone superiorly to the uppermost aspect of the cricopharyngeus inferiorly. Tumors of this hypopharyngeal sublocale may extend into the prevertebral tissue, as this area is only posteriorly confined by a potential retropharyngeal space before abutting the vertebral and paravertebral anatomy.[12] The postcricoid region forms the anterior wall of the hypopharynx and extends from the posterior surface of the arytenoid cartilages superiorly to the cricoid cartilage inferiorly. The postcricoid area connects the paired pyriform sinuses. Although a rare location for hypopharyngeal carcinoma, tumors of the postcricoid region have a tendency to involve the recurrent laryngeal nerve, paratracheal nodes, and thyroid because of a close anatomic relationship with the medially situated tracheoesophageal groove.[12]

The hypopharynx has an extensive lymphatic drainage network that exits superiorly via the thyrohyoid membrane and drains primarily into the jugulodigastric and mid-jugular (level III) lymph node chains. There is an additional drainage from the spinal accessory, retropharyngeal, paratracheal lymph nodes as well as the paraesophageal lymph nodes within the supraclavicular fossa. Different regions of the hypopharyngeal anatomy receive different lymphatic drainage, thus influencing the different yet characteristic patterns of dissemination of metastatic disease for each sublocale. At presentation, bilateral paratracheal lymphadenopathy is commonly found among patients with

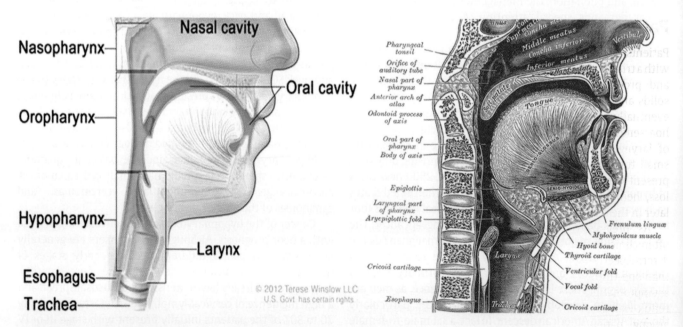

Figure 13.1 Anatomy of the hypopharynx—sagittal view.

Adapted from: PDQ® Hypopharyngeal Cancer Treatment, Bethesda, MD, National Cancer Institute (left) and 20th U.S. edition of Gray's Anatomy of the Human Body (right). http://cancer.gov/cancertopics/pdq/treatment/hypopharyngeal/HealthProfessional.

metastatic disease. In general, the pyriform sinus primarily drains to the upper (level II) and mid (level III) jugular chains, posterior cervical nodes, and retropharyngeal nodes. The posterior hypopharyngeal wall receives similar drainage to the mid-jugular and retropharyngeal nodes. Finally, the mid and lower jugular chains as well as the paratracheal lymph nodes receive lymph flow from the postcricoid area.[13]

The act of deglutition is a key function of the hypopharynx and is coordinated by both sensory and motor input of the glossopharyngeal and vagus nerves that contribute to the pharyngeal plexus. The motor innervation of the hypopharynx is predominantly vagal. The superior and middle pharyngeal constrictors receive motor input via the superior pharyngeal nerve and the pharyngeal branches of the vagus, while the inferior pharyngeal constrictor receives innervation from the external and recurrent branches of the vagus nerve. With regard to sensory innervation, the internal laryngeal branch of the superior laryngeal nerve traverses the lateral wall of the pyriform sinus and the thyrohyoid membrane, where it merges with the vagus nerve.[5,12] Of note, the phenomenon of referred otalgia that comprises part of the classic symptom triad (*see* the section on Patient Evaluation) for patients with hypopharyngeal cancer results from cross-innervation at a common point of synapse. The sensory portions of the internal laryngeal branch of the superior laryngeal nerve synapse on the jugular ganglion along with sensory nerves of the external auditory canal (Arnold nerve, a division of the vagus), leading to symptoms of referred otalgia. The superior thyroid arteries form the main arterial supply of the hypopharynx with collateral supply via the lingual and ascending pharyngeal arteries. The venous drainage follows that of the arterial supply.[5,12]

Patient Evaluation

Patients with cancer of the hypopharynx classically present with a triad of symptoms: chronic throat pain, referred otalgia, and progressive dysphagia. Dysphagia often starts with solids and progresses to inability to tolerate liquids, which eventually results in malnourishment. Symptomatology of hoarseness and airway obstruction are generally indicative of laryngeal nerve involvement or paralysis. Specifically, small tumors of the postcricoid area have been known to present with a foreign body sensation in the throat. Weight loss, hemoptysis, and laryngeal stridor generally present later in the disease course.

As previously mentioned, hypopharyngeal cancer is often clinically silent until more advanced stages of disease. A retrospective study by Hoffman et al reported that more than one-third of the patients with stage I or II disease were asymptomatic at presentation. In addition, gastroesophageal reflux was the second most common presenting symptoms among patients with stage I or II disease.[14] Among symptomatic patients with stage III or IV disease, the most common presenting symptom was an asymptomatic neck mass. Palpable lymphadenopathy was present in up to 70%

of the patients with pyriform sinus lesions upon initial presentation. Of note, a large majority (62.7%) of patients with advanced disease also presented asymptomatically. It should be noted that the prevalence of distant metastases among patients with hypopharyngeal cancers is among the highest for all HNCs. It has been reported that up to 60% of hypopharyngeal SCCs have spread to regional nodes at the time of diagnosis and as many as 17% may be associated with distant metastases when clinically diagnosed.[15,16]

An extensive work-up is requisite for a patient presenting with suspected hypopharyngeal cancer. The initial evaluation should involve a thorough history and physical examination, with emphasis on the head and neck examination. The neurologic examination and assessment of palpable cervical and supraclavicular lymphadenopathy should also be key components of the physical examination. The next step is visualization of the lesion. Currently, flexible laryngoscopy is the modality of choice for visualization of the mucosal anatomy and airway. The assessment of the integrity of the vocal cords for signs of fixation or impaired mobility is important because vocal cord involvement is part of the clinical staging work-up; furthermore, recognizing signs impending airway compromise can be lifesaving. Indirect laryngoscopy or indirect mirror examination are viable alternatives. Triple endoscopy (nasopharyngolaryngoscopy, esophagoscopy, and bronchoscopy) with biopsy under anesthesia should be performed for definitive tissue diagnosis. With cancers of unknown primary site, directed biopsies of the nasopharynx, the hypopharynx, and the base of the tongue, as well as ipsilateral or bilateral tonsillectomy, should be performed.[17] However, fine-needle aspiration should be the first diagnostic step if neck lymphadenopathy is present. In general, core biopsy is contraindicated, as it may be detrimental to later therapeutic surgical intervention. The use of the barium swallow study as a diagnostic test has decreased in popularity, but it may still be used if the lesion prevents endoscopic examination. In addition, it is used postoperatively to examine residual deglutition function as well as to assess for gross anatomic defects such as strictures and fistulae.

Subsequent to the establishment of a biopsy-proved diagnosis, the pretreatment work-up ensues to define local and regional extent of the disease. Cancer of the hypopharynx is staged clinically. Standard imaging involves chest X-ray, computed tomography (CT) with contrast, and/or magnetic resonance imaging (MRI) with contrast of the primary tumor, oral cavity, and neck. CT and MRI both offer unique advantages and the study of choice is based on clinician preferences. CT is superior in the assessment of cartilage and bone invasion, while MRI is a better study to assess soft-tissue involvement (**Fig. 13.2**). In addition, those patients with suspected or proven advanced stage III or IV disease should be considered for positron emission tomography-computed tomography (PET-CT) imaging. PET scanning is also a useful imaging modality for the evaluation of unknown primaries as well as treatment response and when MRI or CT yields equivocal

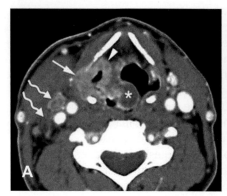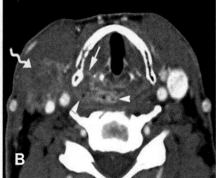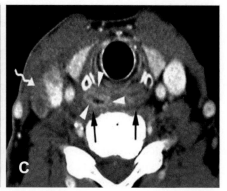

Figure 13.2 Axial contrast-enhanced computed tomography image of a T4aN2b pyriform sinus lesion. (A) Supraglottic level. The soft tissue mass invades the paraglottic space and extends through the thyrohyoid membrane into the extralaryngeal tissues. Asterisk denotes thickened right aryepiglottic fold. (B) Glottic level. Between the thyroid and the arytenoid cartilage, tumor extends into the true vocal cord (arrow). Bulky disease in the apex of the pyriform sinus showing midline extension (arrowheads). (C) Subglottic level. Retrocricoidal tumor extension (arrowheads). Curved arrows denote adenopathy.

Adapted from: Hermans R. Staging of laryngeal and hyperharyngeal cancer: value of imaging studies. *Cancer Imaging* 2008;8:S94–S107.

results. The metastatic work-up is completed with relevant laboratory studies (complete blood count, liver function tests [LFTs], blood urea nitrogen-to-creatinine ratio, prothrombin time/partial thromboplastin time, basic metabolic profile, thyroid stimulating hormone [TSH]) and additional imaging based on clinical suspicion. Finally, the patient should undergo pretreatment anesthesia studies and surgical clearance. In addition, nutrition, speech and swallowing evaluation, and pulmonary function testing should be sought as indicated, as well as a formal dental evaluation, which is mandatory before the initiation of radiotherapy. Planning for posttreatment morbidities must be anticipated. The majority of patients undergoing chemoradiotherapy should have prophylactic placement of a feeding tube or consideration for a percutaneous gastrostomy tube. The patient population presenting with cancers of the hypopharynx generally have significant morbidities related to chronic alcohol and tobacco use. Extensive work-up of comorbidities such as cardiovascular disease, chronic obstructive pulmonary disease, liver dysfunction, and malnutrition should be done preoperatively to determine whether a patient is a surgical candidate. Therefore, great care should be taken during preoperative assessment and optimization to reduce perioperative and postoperative complications and morbidities.

Staging

Current clinical staging guidelines are based on recommendations of the American Joint Committee on Cancer (AJCC) as reported in the seventh edition of the *AJCC Cancer Staging Manual*.[18] Clinical and radiographic findings are used to prognosticate outcomes of hypopharyngeal carcinoma. In general, clinical stage determines the treatment plan and management.

As per TNM (tumor-node-metastasis) classification, T1 tumors are limited to a single subsite of the hypopharynx

and/or are 2 cm or greater in greatest dimension. Tumors that invade more than one subsite of the hypopharynx or an adjacent site are considered T2 tumors. With regard to size, T2 tumors are greater than 2 cm but do not exceed 4 cm and are without fixation of the hemilarynx. T3 tumors are greater than 4 cm or with fixation of the hemilarynx or extension to the esophagus. T4a tumors represent moderately advanced local disease and demonstrate involvement of the thyroid/cricoid cartilage, hyoid bone, thyroid gland, or central compartment soft tissue. Finally, T4b tumors constitute very advanced local disease in which there is invasion of the prevertebral fascia, encasement of the carotid artery, or mediastinal involvement. With regard to nodal staging, N0 disease demonstrates no regional lymph node metastasis. N1 disease is metastasis in a single ipsilateral lymph node that is 3 cm or less in greatest dimension. A single ipsilateral lymph node greater than 3 cm but less than 6 cm is considered N2a disease. If there are multiple ipsilateral lymph nodes involved all measuring less than 6 cm, the patient is staged as N2b. Locoregional metastases in bilateral or contralateral lymph node are N2c disease. Similar to N2a and N2b disease, N2c nodal disease cannot exceed 6 cm in greatest dimension. N3 disease is bulky disease, in which lymph nodes measure greater than 6 cm. Finally, there are no distant metastases in M0 disease, while M1 disease signifies distantly disseminated disease.

Furthermore, anatomic staging can be used to prognosticate patients. Both stage I and stage II disease are characterized by lack of nodal involvement. They are differentiated by tumor size and degree of invasion; stage I (T1N0M0) disease consists of smaller, less invasive T1 tumors, while stage II (T2N0M0) disease comprises larger or more invasive T2 tumors. Importantly, this distinction between stage I and stage II disease carries prognostic significance as the 5-year disease-specific survival rate is 63.1 and 57.5%, respectively. stage III disease has a 5-year disease-specific survival rate of 41.8% and comprises both T3N0M0 disease and T1-T3N1M0 disease, signifying that locoregional spread to a single small ipsilateral lymph node influences prognosis even among smaller and/or less invasive tumors. Any T4a tumor is considered stage IVa regardless of nodal involvement (T4aN0-N2M0). Furthermore, any T1 to T3 tumor with N2 nodal disease (T1-T3N2M0) is also stage IVa. stage IVb (T4bN0-N3M0 or T1-T4bN3M0) disease consists of any T4b tumor regardless of nodal involvement or any N3 nodal disease regardless of tumor size or degree of local invasion/extension. Finally, stage IVc disease is distantly metastasized. Collectively, stage IV disease has the worst overall prognosis with a 5-year disease-specific survival rate of 22%.[14]

Overview of Treatment

The management of hypopharyngeal carcinoma is complex, and there is no universal standard of care for this disease. When reviewing the treatment options for hypopharyngeal cancer, there are two ways that one should conceptualize management. First, the concept of early versus advanced disease is used when determining the most appropriate treatment regimen. Second, the principle of organ preservation is important to the management of this disease; if a patient can achieve similar treatment outcome with lesser functional deficits, this route should always be pursued.

Treatment by Clinical Stage

The key clinical distinction that must first be made is whether it is a resectable or nonresectable lesion. A simplistic classification of hypopharynx cancer management is as follows: (1) early resectable not requiring total laryngectomy (T1/N0 and favorable T2/N0), (2) advanced resectable requiring total laryngectomy (T1/N+, T2 to T4a with any N), and (3) nonresectable disease. Although a disease may indeed be resectable, it does not necessitate resection as the primary therapeutic intervention.

Early resectable hypopharyngeal cancers are considered as those that do not require total laryngectomy. In general, lesions amenable to this conservative management have no nodal disease and are T1 or select T2 lesions with favorable features (exophytic, nonapex/limited to medial wall of pyriform sinus, low volume on CT). For T1/N0 and select T2/N0 disease, both definitive radiotherapy and surgical management are viable options. Radiotherapy is generally preferred to surgery for the management of early resectable lesions because of similar outcomes but superior retention of function. Definitive radiotherapy may be followed by salvage surgery if residual tumor is identified. With regard to the surgical management of early resectable disease, partial laryngopharyngectomy via endoscopy or open approaches with simultaneous neck dissection is feasible even though less popular. If adverse features (extracapsular extension, perineural invasion) or positive margins are present, re-excision or adjuvant radiotherapy/chemoradiotherapy may be indicated.

Advanced resectable hypopharyngeal cancers generally require total laryngectomy. Lesions that require total laryngectomy are any node-positive T1 to T3 lesions or T4a lesions with nodal involvement. The treatment algorithm is less clearly defined for lesions of this extent, and various surgical and nonsurgical approaches are under investigation. T4a lesions generally warrant surgical management initially, while the less advanced T1 to T3 lesions are more amenable to nonoperative approaches.

For T1/N+ and T2 or T3/any N lesions, combined chemotherapy and radiotherapy is the current mainstay of the management.[19] A surgical option involves laryngopharyngectomy and neck dissection (including level VI nodes) with subsequent radiotherapy or chemoradiotherapy if highly adverse features are present.[20] The optimal combination and schedule of radiation and chemotherapy is evolving, but recent data may suggest a change in paradigm, regarding induction chemotherapy versus concurrent chemoradiotherapy.[21-23]

For more advanced yet still resectable T4a lesions with any nodal disease, the preferred management is surgery with neck dissection followed with adjuvant chemoradiotherapy. For unresectable lesions, the preferred management is enrollment in clinical trials. In general, management is based on performance status and various combinations of chemotherapy and radiation can be used.

Surgery

The surgical management of hypopharynx cancers is based on the ability to spare the larynx while achieving appropriate surgical margins and minimizing functional loss. Because of the high incidence of occult submucosal extension, the minimal resection margins recommended as 1.5 cm superiorly, 3 cm inferiorly, and 2 cm laterally are required. These margins are extended for patients with history of irradiation to 2 cm superiorly, 4 cm inferiorly, and 3 cm laterally.[24] Lesions not requiring total laryngectomy are considered conservative surgical approaches, while those requiring total laryngectomy warrant radical surgical approaches. The specific surgical technique chosen for each hypopharyngeal lesion is dependent not only on clinical staging but also on surgeon preference and location of the lesion. Locally advanced stage III and IV tumors undergo postoperative radiotherapy or postoperative chemoradiotherapy if high-risk features are present.

Among the options for conservative surgery are partial pharyngectomy, partial laryngopharyngectomy, and supracricoid hemilaryngectomy. Partial pharyngectomy is indicated for T1 and T2 lesions that are confined to the posterior or lateral wall of the pyriform sinus without involvement of the pyriform apex or larynx. Because of the minimal amount of critical tissue loss involved in partial pharyngectomy, retention of swallowing function is usually possible.[5,12] T1, T2, and T3 lesions of the medial pyriform wall may be resected with partial laryngopharyngectomy. Partial laryngopharyngectomy involves hemilaryngectomy and partial pharyngectomy. Retention of a part of the larynx may often help preserve speech and deglutition function. Again, the tumor must not involve the apex of the pyriform sinus and vocal cord mobility must be unimpaired.[25] Supracricoid hemilaryngectomy is an extension of the partial laryngopharyngectomy to remove the supracricoid hemilarynx along with the pyriform sinus, ispsilateral thyroid lobe, and true and false vocal cords (**Fig. 13.3**). A musculoperichondrial flap is used to close the pharyngeal wall.

Endoscopic carbon dioxide laser resection is a unique method of conservative surgical management. It is performed endoscopically and is thus less invasive, and it is the only surgical intervention of the hypopharynx that heals by secondary intention. In general, only select, small T1 and T2 lesions are amenable to this technique. The benefits of this surgical approach are cited as avoidance of tracheostomy and reconstruction; voice preservation; preservation of suprahyoid musculature, which minimizes loss of swallowing function; and reduced duration of hospitalization.[12]

There are two surgical procedures for advanced resectable disease. Total laryngectomy with partial or total pharyngectomy is indicated for extensive T3 and T4 lesions. Depending on the size of the surgical defect, primary closure may be possible with partial pharyngectomy, but preparation for reconstruction is necessary. When total pharyngectomy is performed, reconstruction is always required. Associated with this procedure is a very high rate of pharyngocutaenous fistulae. Total pharyngolaryngoesophagectomy is indicated for T4 lesions with involvement of the cervical esophagus. This procedure involves a transhiatal pull-through esophagectomy in addition to complete bilateral neck dissection. With regard to reconstruction, a gastric pull-up procedure is mandated, which involves a triple surgical approach via the neck, thorax, and abdomen. There is tremendous surgical morbidity and mortality associated with this operation.[26] Up to 20% of the patients with hypopharyngeal cancer are inoperable at the time of diagnosis.[27] Some contraindications to surgical intervention are as follows: carotid artery involvement, prevertebral musculature involvement, cervical spine involvement, and massive mediastinal nodal enlargement.

The most common postsurgical functional concerns are deglutition difficulties and speech dysfunction. Major intraoperative complications involve surgical bleeding and cranial nerve damage (X, XI, XII).[12] Involvement of the carotid artery can lead to catastrophic hemorrhage. Unilateral involvement of the hypoglossal nerve may be inconsequential functionally, but bilateral ligation can result in feeding, swallowing, and speaking difficulties. Transection of the vagus nerve has dire consequences especially when bilateral, because it causes vocal cord paralysis, which can progress to complete airway obstruction. In addition, the accessory nerve may be involved, resulting in gross motor deficits of the trapezius and other musculature. Clearly, many intraoperative complications have chronic sequelae. In the acute postoperative period, pulmonary embolus, gastric ulceration, and infection are common complications. Other complications more specific to hypopharyngeal surgery are postpharyngectomy pharyngocutaneous fistula development and pharyngoesophageal fistula development, especially when esophagectomy with gastric pull-up is performed. Poor surgical anastomosis, repair, or reconstruction can result in mediastinitis. An increased risk for postoperative aspiration-associated partial laryngectomy exists.[28] Finally, late-onset surgical complications involve pharyngoesophageal stenosis and strictures.[12,29] This occurs most frequently in postjejunal free flap reconstruction of a total laryngopharyngectomy, and unfortunately there is a high rate of gastrostomy dependence among these patients.

Another issue is the necessity of postoperative reconstruction. For the majority of conservative approaches, primary closure is safe and thus indicated. Generally, 4 cm (28 to 32 Fr) or more of pharyngeal mucosa is requisite for primary closure to allow for an adequate lumen for swallowing and to minimize the risk of stricture formation.[28] However, more invasive and radical approaches create larger surgical defects and thus may require additional tissue to achieve adequate closure. Both pedicled myocutaneous flaps or microvascular reconstruction with free flaps are options, and there are specific indications with unique advantages and disadvantages for each.[5,12] Pectoralis major myocutaneous free flaps are used for smaller partial pharyngectomy defects.

Larger surgical defects are repaired with either jejunal free-flap or tubed fasciocutaneous (i.e., radial forearm, latissimus dorsi, deltopectoral, and anterolateral thigh) free-flap reconstruction. Of note, jejunal free flaps are associated with a high rate of pharyngoesophageal stricture and stenosis (**Figs. 13.4** and **13.5**). As previously mentioned, a gastric pull-up is performed for disease with esophageal extension requiring total laryngopharyngoesophagectomy.[12]

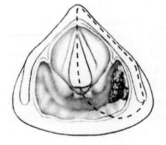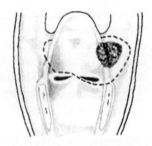

Figure 13.3 Resection of pyriform sinus neoplasm via supracricoid hemilaryngopharyngectomy—axial and coronal representation.

Adapted from: Papacharalampous GX, Kotsis GP, Vlastarakos PV, et al. Supracricoid hemilaryngopharynglctyomy for selected pyriform sinus carcinoma patients - a retrospective chart review. *World Journal of Surgical Oncology* 2009;7:65.

Radiotherapy

Therapeutic radiation is administered in three manners: definitive radiotherapy, postoperative/adjuvant radiotherapy,

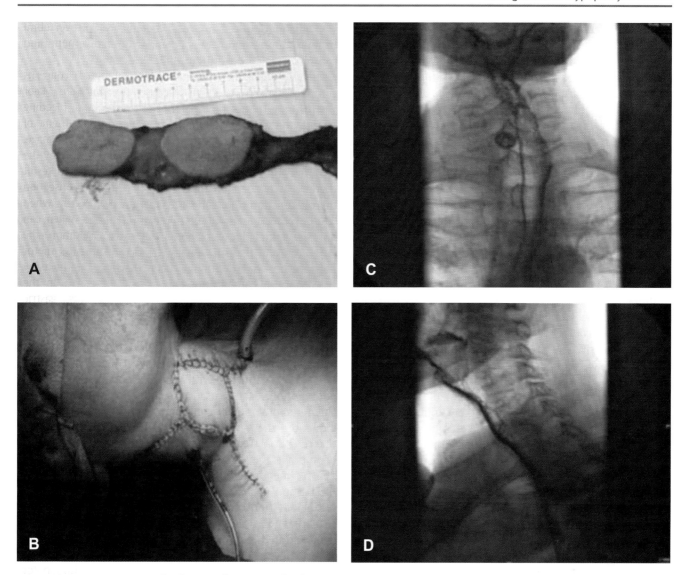

Figure 13.4   Reconstruction of a pharyngeal stenosis with a free radial forearm flap. (A) Flap design with monitor portion. (B) Status after flap insetting, monitor visible. (C and D) Barium swallow after surgery documenting resolution pharyngeal stenosis.

Adapted from: Simon C, Bulut V, Federspil PA, et al. *Radiation Oncology* 2011;6:109.

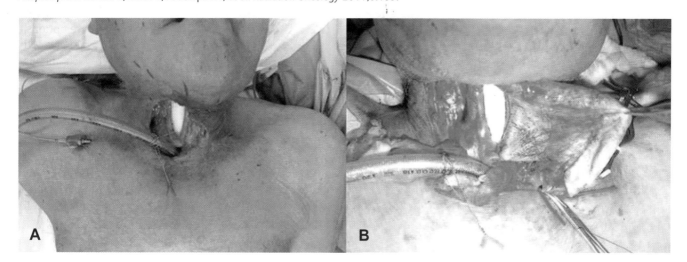

Figure 13.5   Anterior lateral thigh myocutaneous flap for hypopharyngeal reconstruction. (A) Preoperative view of the hypopharyngeal defect. (B) Intraoperative view of the inset flap.

Adapted from: Wehage I, Fansa H. Complex reconstructions in head and neck surgery: decision making. *Head and Neck Oncology* 2011;3:14.

and postoperative/adjuvant chemoradiation. As previously discussed, definitive radiotherapy is used as a primary single modality for "early" hypopharyngeal cancers of T1 and select T2 lesions. Recently, optimization of radiation dosing has become a topic of interest. Several studies have examined the conventional fractionation dose of 66 to 74 Gy at 2 Gy/fraction and compared it with altered fractionation regimens (**Fig. 13.6**). Hyperfractionation regimens use 81.6 Gy/7 wk with 1.2 Gy/fraction twice daily. Accelerated fractionation with concomitant boost administers 72 Gy/6 wk with 1.8 Gy/fraction and a 1.5-Gy boost as a second daily fraction for the final 12 treatment days.[19] Both hyperfractionated and accelerated fractionation radiotherapy regimens are superior to standard radiation dosing with regard to locoregional control and survival outcomes.[21–23] In addition to definitive radiotherapy, radiation can be used as an adjunctive therapy. In general, postoperative radiotherapy is administered within 6 weeks of surgery.

Radiotherapy is a therapeutic modality that is not devoid of toxicities, complications, and drawbacks. Radiation-induced mucositis is a well-characterized complication that generally results in dysphagia and odynophagia. Furthermore, the severity of mucositis has a dose-dependent relationship with radiation and is also more severe when chemotherapy and radiation are combined. Xerostomia, phlegm production, and dermatitis are other frequently reported acute manifestations. Another less-threatening complication is that of transient postradiotherapy taste alteration. However, the combination of change in taste sensation and painful mucosal ulceration can dramatically reduce appetite and nutritional intake; therefore, surveillance of patient nutritional status is important. In addition, analgesia should be provided to relieve the mucositis pain.

Radiation-induced mucosal edema is another acute complication of radiotherapy. Edema of the pharyngeal mucosa can also lead to deglutition difficulties. As was previously discussed in the patient evaluation section, anticipating these complications by placement of feeding tube or percutaneous gastrostomy tube should be considered. Radiation-induced hypothyroidism is an important late-onset toxicity of radiotherapy and this occurs with relative frequency. A 30 to 40% incidence of postradiation hypothyroidism has been reported in patients receiving external-beam radiation therapy. It is therefore prudent for a physician to assess thyroid function before and after therapy.[28,29] Other potential late-onset set manifestations of radiation therapy are cervical fibrosis, dental decay, osteoradionecrosis, cricopharyngeal strictures, and fistulas.[5] Finally, history of radiation to the head and neck has traditionally been a harbinger for increased risk of surgical complications.

Chemotherapy

With regard to the management of cancer of the hypopharynx, chemotherapy is never used as a single modality treatment with the exception of palliative intervention. It can be used as an induction before aggressive chemoradiotherapy or concurrently with radiation without induction. The rationale behind induction chemotherapy is that the initial treatment will reduce the local tumor burden to improve the chances of successful organ preservation. This regimen includes docetaxel, cisplatin, and 5-flurouracil (5-FU) and is also referred to as the TPF regimen. The recent addition of docetaxel to the standard regimen of cisplatin and 5-FU has been a minor revelation in that it has demonstrated improvement in progression-free survival,

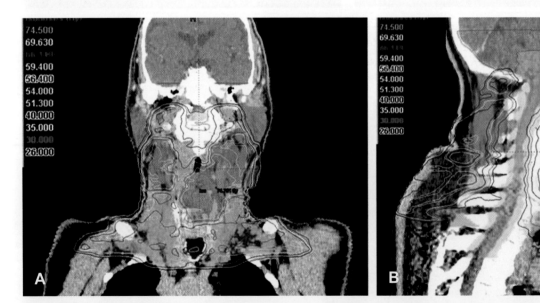

Figure 13.6 Intensity-modulated radiation therapy isodose plan for patients with T2N2c-staged hypopharyngeal cancer (A) Coronal view and (B) sagittal view.

Adapted from: Studer G, Huguenin PU, Davis JB, Kunz G, Lütolf UM, Glanzmann C. IMRT using simultaneously integrated boost (SIB) in head and neck cancer patients. *Radiation Oncology* 2006;1:7.

overall survival, and organ preservation.[30,31] For concurrent chemoradiotherapy and adjuvant chemotherapy, cisplatin is often used as the sole chemotherapeutic agent.[20]

Chemoradiotherapy

Several studies have demonstrated the survival advantages of combining chemotherapy with radiotherapy. A 2002 meta-analysis demonstrated that concurrent platinum-based chemoradiotherapy bestows significant survival benefit to patients with head and neck SCC.[32] Chemotherapy and radiotherapy both offer the potential benefit of organ preservation in comparison to a surgical approach. Specifically, with regard to hypopharynx management, if patients treated with chemoradiotherapy versus conventional surgical management were compared, larynx preservation was superior among the chemoradiotherapy cohort without compromising overall survival.[33] Furthermore, the concurrent administration of chemotherapy and radiation proved to have superior survival outcomes in comparison to regimens using the neoadjuvant/induction or adjuvant approach. However, all three combinations of chemotherapy and radiation yield modest survival benefits at the very least. Unfortunately, concomitant chemoradiotherapy was unable to prevent the occurrence of distant metastasis, which is a major cause of disease-related morbidity and mortality. It should also be noted that the toxicity of combined chemoradiotherapy is more severe than when either treatment modality is used alone.[21]

Follow-Up

Because of the high rate of treatment failure and high likelihood of recurrence, diligent surveillance of patients should be performed. Neck examination and fiberoptic laryngoscopy should be performed monthly during the year immediately after the initial treatment, every 2 months during the second posttreatment year, every 3 months during the third year, and every 6 months thereafter. There is also potential indication for PET scan imaging to monitor treatment response and recurrence. In addition, surveillance for second primary malignancy and metastases should be done once or twice annually with serial chest X-ray, LFTs, and TSH levels if patient underwent irradiation.

Future Directions in Management of Cancer of the Hypopharynx

Establishing a niche for biologic therapy is currently an intense area of investigation in the realm of clinical oncology. Biologic agents play a particularly important role in the management of head and neck SCCs because increased levels of epidermal growth factor receptor (EGFR) expression have been correlated with poorer prognosis, specifically with increased risk of relapse and decreased survival. Thus, inhibition of EGFR has become a molecular therapeutic target. Cetuximab, a monoclonal antibody against EGFR, has shown promise in the treatment of head and neck SCC. A 2006 randomized study compared radiotherapy alone with radiotherapy plus cetuximab in the treatment of stage III or IV locoregionally advanced SCC of the head and neck. It was found that treatment with concomitant high-dose radiotherapy plus cetuximab improves locoregional control and reduces mortality without increasing the common toxic effects associated with radiotherapy and did not negatively affect quality of life.[34–36] The next step in redefining treatment of cancer of the hypopharynx will be a comparison of cetuximab-based chemoradiotherapy and traditional chemoradiotherapy regimens (**Fig. 13.7**).

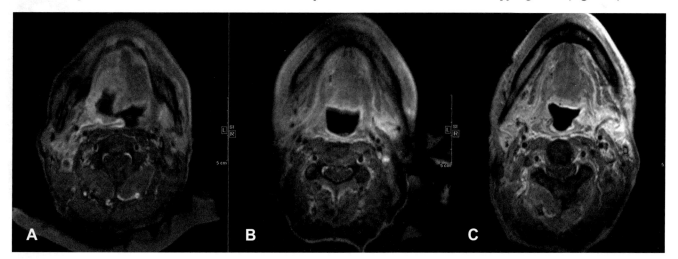

Figure 13.7 Patients with hypopharyngeal carcinoma treated in a phase II trial (REACH) of combined radiochemoimmunotherapy with weekly cetuximab, carboplatin/5-flurouracil, and intensity-modulated radiation therapy concomitant boost. (A) Pretreatment planning magnetic resonance imaging. (B) Complete remission 6 weeks after completion of therapy. (C) Continued response 4 months after completion of therapy.

Adapted from: Jensen AD, Krauss J, Potthoff K, et al. Radiochemoimmunotherapy with intensity-modulated concomitant boost: interum analysis of the REACH trial. *Radiation Oncology* 2012;7:57.

In addition, the advent of robotic surgery has offered new surgical options for the management of HNCs. Several prospective studies have identified robotic surgery as a safe and effective alternative with good preservation of swallowing function.[37–39] Finally, while great effort is concentrated on the development of new treatment modalities and improvement of patient survival measures, it is equally important to take quality-of-life issues into consideration. Quality of life, options for rehabilitation, and potential for permanent functional deficits should all be part of decision algorithm when deciding on patient management.

Conclusions

Hypopharyngeal cancer is associated with the poorest survival of all head and neck primary sites. Often, this disease remains silent until advanced stage. In fact, 80% are stage III or IV at presentation and 20% of the patients are inoperable at presentation. Thus, even at the time of diagnosis, treating patients with hypopharyngeal cancers is a daunting task. Furthermore, 50% of the patients develop recurrence within 1 year and locoregional recurrence is the most common cause of mortality within the first 2 years.[40]

References

1. Hoffman HT, Karnell LH, Funk GF, Robinson RA, Menck HR. The National Cancer Data Base report on cancer of the head and neck. Arch Otolaryngol Head Neck Surg 1998;124(9):951–962

2. Mendenhall WM, Riggs CE Jr, Cassisi NJ. Treatment of head and neck cancers. In: DeVita VT Jr, Hellman S, Rosenberg SA, eds. Cancer: Principles and Practice of Oncology. 7th ed. Philadelphia, PA: Lippincott Williams & Wilkins; 2005:662–732

3. Ward PH, Hanson DG. Reflux as an etiological factor of carcinoma of the laryngopharynx. Laryngoscope 1988;98(11):1195–1199

4. Curado MP, Hashibe M. Recent changes in the epidemiology of head and neck cancer. Curr Opin Oncol 2009;21(3):194–200

5. Quan H, Goldenberg D. Otolaryngology and Facial Plastic Surgery: Head & Neck Surgery: Hypopharyngeal Cancer. eMedicine Specialties; 2008, http://emedicine.medscape.com/article/1375268-overview

6. Garden AS. Organ preservation for carcinoma of the larynx and hypopharynx. Hematol Oncol Clin North Am 2001;15(2):243–260

7. Kantarjian HM, Wolff RA, Koller CA, eds. Head and Neck Cancer. The M.D. Anderson Manual of Medical Oncology. New York, NY: McGraw-Hill; 2006

8. Diaz EM Jr, Sturgis EM, Laramore GE, Sabichi AL, Lippman SM, Clayman G. Neoplasms of the head and neck. In: Kufe DW, Pollock RE, Weichselbaum RR, et al, eds. Holland-Frei Cancer Medicine. 6th ed. Hamilton, ON: BC Decker; 2003:647–698

9. Barnes L, Johnson JT. Pathologic and clinical considerations in the evaluation of major head and neck specimens resected for cancer, part I. Pathol Annu 1986;21(Pt 1):173–250

10. Pignon JP, Bourhis J, Domenge C, Designé L. Chemotherapy added to locoregional treatment for head and neck squamous-cell carcinoma: three meta-analyses of updated individual data. MACH-NC Collaborative Group. Meta-Analysis of Chemotherapy on Head and Neck Cancer. Lancet 2000;355(9208):949–955

11. Summary Staging Manual SEER – 2000. Definition of anatomic sites within the head and neck adapted from the Summary Staging Guide 1977 published by the SEER Program, and the AJCC Cancer Staging Manual Fifth Edition published by the American Joint Committee on Cancer Staging

12. Flint PW, Haughey BH, Lund VJ, et al. Neoplasms of the hypopharynx and cervical esophagus. In: Cummings CW, Haughey BH, Thomas JR, Harker LA, eds. Otolaryngology: Head and Neck Surgery. 4th ed. New York, NY: Mosby; 2005:245–278

13. Million RR, Mancuso AA. Pharyngeal walls, pyriform sinus, post-cricoid pharynx. In: Million R, Cassissi NJ, eds. Management of Head and Neck Cancer: A Multidisciplinary Approach. Philadelphia, PA: Lippincott; 1994:505–532

14. Hoffman HT, Karnell LH, Shah JP, et al. Hypopharyngeal cancer patient care evaluation. Laryngoscope 1997;107(8):1005–1017

15. Kotwall C, Sako K, Razack MS, Rao U, Bakamjian V, Shedd DP. Metastatic patterns in squamous cell cancer of the head and neck. Am J Surg 1987;154(4):439–442

16. Spector JG, Sessions DG, Haughey BH, et al. Delayed regional metastases, distant metastases, and second primary malignancies in squamous cell carcinomas of the larynx and hypopharynx. Laryngoscope 2001;111(6):1079–1087

17. Marur S, Forastiere AA. Head and neck cancer: changing epidemiology, diagnosis, and treatment. Mayo Clin Proc 2008;83(4):489–501

18. American Joint Committee on Cancer. AJCC Cancer Staging Manual. 7th ed. New York: Springer;2010

19. National Comprehensive Cancer Network. NCCN Clinical Practice Guidelines in Oncology™ Head and Neck Cancers Version 1. Fort Washington, PA: National Comprehensive Cancer Network; 2010

20. Cooper JS, Pajak TF, Forastiere AA, et al; Radiation Therapy Oncology Group 9501/Intergroup. Postoperative concurrent radiotherapy and chemotherapy for high-risk squamous-cell carcinoma of the head and neck. N Engl J Med 2004;350(19):1937–1944

21. Budach W, Hehr T, Budach V, Belka C, Dietz K. A meta-analysis of hyperfractionated and accelerated radiotherapy and combined chemotherapy and radiotherapy regimens in unresected locally advanced squamous cell carcinoma of the head and neck. BMC Cancer 2006;6:28

22. Fu KK, Pajak TF, Trotti A, et al. A Radiation Therapy Oncology Group (RTOG) phase III randomized study to compare hyperfractionation and two variants of accelerated fractionation to standard fractionation radiotherapy for head and neck squamous cell carcinomas: first report of RTOG 9003. Int J Radiat Oncol Biol Phys 2000;48(1):7–16

23. Bourhis J, Overgaard J, Audry H, et al; Meta-Analysis of Radiotherapy in Carcinomas of Head and neck (MARCH) Collaborative Group. Hyperfractionated or accelerated radiotherapy in head and neck cancer: a meta-analysis. Lancet 2006;368(9538):843–854

24. Lefebvre JL, Chevalier D, Luboinski B, Kirkpatrick A, Collette L, Sahmoud T; EORTC Head and Neck Cancer Cooperative Group. Larynx preservation in pyriform sinus cancer: preliminary results of a European Organization for Research and Treatment of Cancer phase III trial. J Natl Cancer Inst 1996;88(13):890–899

25. Gourin CG, Johnson JT. A contemporary review of indications for primary surgical care of patients with squamous cell carcinoma of the head and neck. Laryngoscope 2009;119(11):2124–2134

26. Wein Richard O, Chandra Rakesh K, Weber Randal S. Disorders of the head and neck. In: Brunicardi FC, Andersen DK, Billiar TR, et al, eds. Schwartz's Principles of Surgery. 9e. New York, NY: McGraw-Hill; 2011:961–994

27. Hall SF, Groome PA, Irish J, O'Sullivan B. The natural history of patients with squamous cell carcinoma of the hypopharynx. Laryngoscope 2008;118(8):1362–1371

28. Turner SL, Tiver KW, Boyages SC. Thyroid dysfunction following radiotherapy for head and neck cancer. Int J Radiat Oncol Biol Phys 1995;31(2):279–283

29. Constine LS. What else don't we know about the late effects of radiation in patients treated for head and neck cancer? Int J Radiat Oncol Biol Phys 1995;31(2):427–429

30. Hitt R, López-Pousa A, Martínez-Trufero J, et al. Phase III study comparing cisplatin plus fluorouracil to paclitaxel, cisplatin, and fluorouracil induction chemotherapy followed by chemoradiotherapy in locally advanced head and neck cancer. J Clin Oncol 2005;23(34):8636–8645

31. Vermorken JB, Remenar E, van Herpen C, et al; EORTC 24971/TAX 323 Study Group. Cisplatin, fluorouracil, and docetaxel in unresectable head and neck cancer. N Engl J Med 2007;357(17):1695–1704

32. Monnerat C, Faivre S, Temam S, Bourhis J, Raymond E. End points for new agents in induction chemotherapy for locally advanced head and neck cancers. Ann Oncol 2002;13(7):995–1006

33. Al-Sarraf M. Treatment of locally advanced head and neck cancer: historical and critical review. Cancer Contr 2002;9(5):387–399

34. Bonner JA, Harari PM, Giralt J, et al. Radiotherapy plus cetuximab for squamous-cell carcinoma of the head and neck. N Engl J Med 2006;354(6):567–578

35. Mell LK, Weichselbaum RR. More on cetuximab in head and neck cancer. N Engl J Med 2007;357(21):2201–2202, author reply 2202–2203

36. Mesía R, Rivera F, Kawecki A, et al. Quality of life of patients receiving platinum-based chemotherapy plus cetuximab first line for recurrent and/or metastatic squamous cell carcinoma of the head and neck. Ann Oncol 2010;21(10):1967–1973

37. Boudreaux BA, Rosenthal EL, Magnuson JS, et al. Robot-assisted surgery for upper aerodigestive tract neoplasms. Arch Otolaryngol Head Neck Surg 2009;135(4):397–401

38. Iseli TA, Kulbersh BD, Iseli CE, Carroll WR, Rosenthal EL, Magnuson JS. Functional outcomes after transoral robotic surgery for head and neck cancer. Otolaryngol Head Neck Surg 2009;141(2):166–171

39. Moore EJ, Olsen KD, Kasperbauer JL. Transoral robotic surgery for oropharyngeal squamous cell carcinoma: a prospective study of feasibility and functional outcomes. Laryngoscope 2009;119(11):2156–2164

40. Gourin CG, Johnson JT. A contemporary review of indications for primary surgical care of patients with squamous cell carcinoma of the head and neck. Laryngoscope 2009;119(11):2124–2134

14 Larynx and Laryngeal Neoplasms

Ryan Winters and Paul Friedlander

Core Messages

- Most true neoplasms in the adult larynx represent malignancy.

- Hoarseness persisting beyond 2 weeks is a "warning sign," particularly in patients with risk factors for laryngeal carcinoma, and warrants prompt referral for evaluation by an otolaryngologist.

- Smoking, especially when combined with alcohol consumption, is the most important risk factor for laryngeal cancer.

- Early-stage laryngeal cancer can be treated with single modality therapy, while late-stage laryngeal cancer fares best with combined modality therapy.

The larynx is a complex structure with multiple functions connecting the pharynx with the trachea and is divided into three sections for oncologic descriptive purposes: the supraglottis, glottis, and subglottis (**Fig. 14.1**). The supraglottis extends from the tip of the epiglottis superiorly to the true vocal cords (TVCs) inferiorly; this area encompasses both the laryngeal vestibule and the ventricle. The glottis comprises the TVC proper and the space between them—the rima glottidis. The subglottis extends from the undersurface of the TVCs superiorly to the inferior margin of the cricoid cartilage inferiorly. Laterally, the larynx extends to the lateral aspect of the thyroid and cricoid cartilages, and the posterior margin is defined by the posterior aspect of the arytenoid cartilages and interarytenoid space in the supraglottis, while the "party wall"—that is, the common wall shared by the posterior larynx/trachea and the cervical esophagus—defines the posterior aspect of the glottis and subglottis. The anterior boundaries of the larynx are the vallecula and preepiglottic space, the anterior surfaces of the thyroid cartilage, cricothyroid membrane, and cricoid cartilage, as well as the paraglottic space more laterally (**Fig. 14.2**).

While there are many different neoplasms that can arise in the larynx, in adults the vast majority are malignant. Of these, greater than 90% are squamous cell carcinoma (SCC) and greater than 75% of these arise initially in the TVCs.[1,2] SCC of the larynx is strongly associated with smoking tobacco; greater than 95% of laryngeal SCC is diagnosed in smokers or former smokers.[1] A synergistic effect between tobacco use and alcohol consumption has been described; thus, patients who are both smokers and heavy drinkers are among the highest risk for cancers of the upper aerodigestive tract. A recent discovery is that of the role of human papillomavirus (HPV) in certain subtypes of SCC in the head and neck. While HPV appears to be more actively involved in the pathogenesis of tumors of the pharynx, rather than the larynx, precise mechanisms and risk factors are an area of active ongoing research.

Many laryngeal neoplasms present at an advanced stage owing to a combination of vague early symptoms and patient denial. The most common presenting symptom of laryngeal cancer is hoarseness, though other common symptoms are globus sensation, hemoptysis, weight loss, odynophagia or sore throat, persistent cough, or earache.[2,3]

Neoplasms

There are many neoplasms that can arise in the adult larynx, and the majority of these are malignant. As mentioned above, the most common malignant neoplasm is SCC, though others are possible and will be discussed in further detail. Of the rarer benign neoplasms, papilloma deserves special mention. Benign neoplasms present in much the same way as malignancy; however, weight loss may not be present. A history of childhood recurrent respiratory papillomatosis (RRP) may portend adult benign papillomatosis, but these may arise de novo as well in the absence of a childhood history.

Benign

Papilloma

There are a multitude of subtypes of HPV, and the most common causative subtypes of RRP are HPV 6 and 11 compared with those associated with aerodigestive malignancy, where HPV 16 dominates.[4] Verrucous or cauliflower-like lesions are traditionally thought to occur at areas of squamociliary junctions, such as the TVCs, but can be extensive. RRP is classically described as a disease of childhood that may persist into adulthood, with a significant subset of patients clearing the recurrent infections by puberty. Those whose infections do not spontaneously

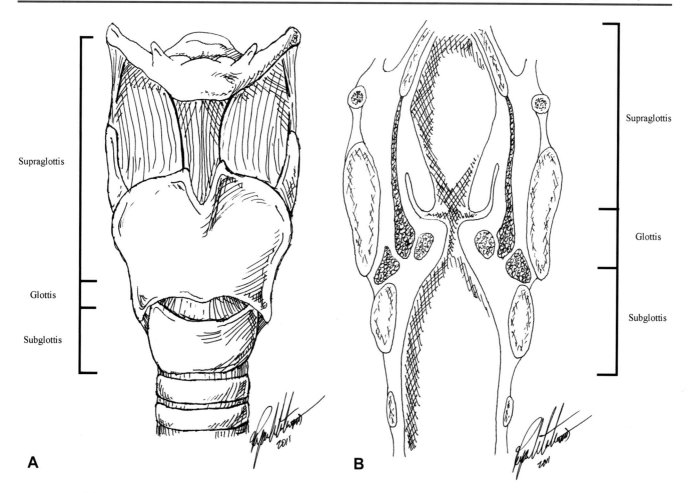

Supraglottis

Glottis

Subglottis

Supraglottis

Glottis

Subglottis

A   **B**

Figure 14.1   (A) Anterior and (B) coronal views of the larynx defining the supraglottis, glottis, and subglottis.

regress tend to have a heavier burden of disease, and these benign papillomas may spread throughout the aerodigestive tract to involve the oral and nasal cavities and bronchi, and may eventually undergo malignant degeneration. As the same HPV subtype responsible for RRP has also been described in genital papillomatosis, a vertical transmission model has been proposed. Indeed, half of all patients with RRP are born to mothers with active papillomatosis in the vaginal canal.[5] These lesions may arise de novo in adulthood as well, and in those who do tend to have milder disease, but with less risk of malignant transformation. Surgical debulking remains the mainstay of treatment, with adjunct therapy such as local injection of cidofovir, or other antivirals, representing an area of ongoing clinical research as to the long-term effects on recurrence and severity.

Malignant

SCC accounts for the great majority of laryngeal malignancies (> 90%), but there are other rare malignant tumors that can occur as well. While the bulk of the remainder of this chapter is devoted to the diagnosis and management of SCC, several of these rare, non-SCC tumors that deserve mention as well.

Minor Salivary Gland Tumors

Rests of minor salivary gland tumors exist throughout the upper aerodigestive tract. While the bulk of these lie in the oropharynx and hypopharynx, a small number of these exist in the larynx, particularly the supraglottis and subglottis. Ganly et al reviewed their experience of 33 years at Memorial Sloan-Kettering Cancer Center, a major international tertiary referral center, and identified 12 patients with such tumors[6]; of these, 10 had adenoid cystic carcinoma and 2 had myoepithelial carcinoma. Tumor site was 48% supraglottis and 52% subglottis, and most (10 patients) were treated with combined surgery and radiation therapy (XRT). Fifty-eight percent developed recurrent disease; of these, 50% locoregional and 50% distant recurrence were observed. The authors advocate aggressive surgical treatment, usually requiring total laryngectomy, based on the propensity for perineural and submucosal spread, as well as high recurrence rates.

Neuroendocrine Tumors

Neuroendocrine neoplasms in the larynx can be classified into two distinct groups: those of neural origin and those of epithelial origin. Laryngeal tumors of neural origin are paragangliomas, while those of epithelial origin are either carcinoid tumors or neuroendocrine carcinoma. Each of

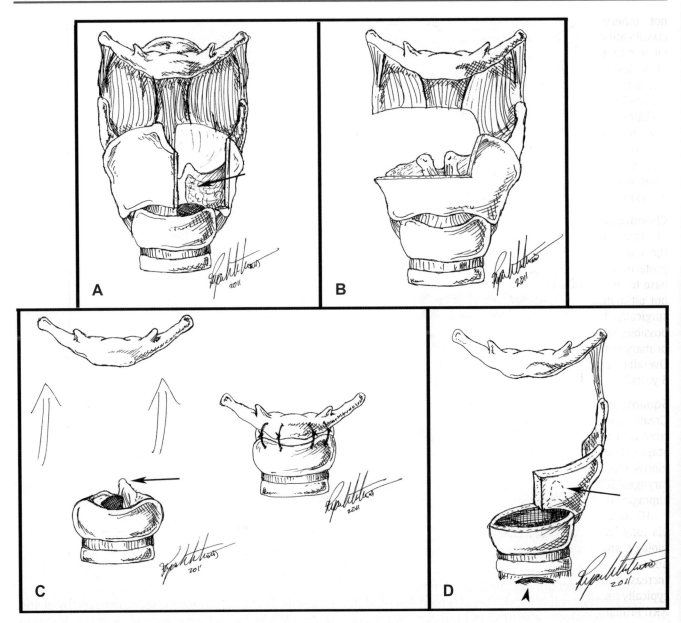

Figure 14.2   (A) Anterior view of the larynx after left vertical partial laryngectomy. Arrow denotes the cut surface where left true vocal cord (TVC) was removed, but ipsilateral arytenoid was spared. (B) Anterior view after supraglottic laryngectomy. Note preservation of both TVCs and arytenoids. (C) Anterior view of the larynx after supracricoid laryngectomy before (left) and after (right) cricohyoidopexy. Arrow denotes preservation of left arytenoid. (D) Anterior view of the larynx after near-total laryngectomy. Arrow denotes preserved left arytenoids (dotted line), and arrowhead denotes permanent tracheostomy necessary for respiration.

these tumor groups warrants a different management strategy. Paragangliomas display a female preponderance of nearly 3:1 and respond well to conservative surgical resection, with larynx preservation as appropriate. Carcinoid tumors, of which typical and atypical variants exist, are another treatment dilemma in themselves. Typical carcinoid tumor is exceedingly rare, but warrants only local resection as lymphatic spread has not been described. Likewise, chemotherapy and XRT have not been successful in reported cases. Atypical carcinoid tumor, the distinction being based on histologic criteria, has a high likelihood of locoregional lymphatic spread, and therefore elective neck dissection is

necessary. The mainstay of treatment remains surgical, as results with chemotherapeutic agents and XRT have been disappointing. Primary neuroendocrine carcinoma of the larynx is a rare, aggressive tumor, and the surgical results are not satisfactory. Surgery is reserved for salvage situations, and chemotherapy remains the modality of choice for treatment. Despite this, long-term survival is poor, with 16% survival at 5-year posttreatment reported.[7]

Adenocarcinoma

This group of carcinomas denotes those of glandular origin, but the most common subtype, "adenocarcinoma, not otherwise specified," prohibits further histologic classification. These tumors are exceedingly rare, comprising far less than 1% of all laryngeal malignancies.[8] So rare are these lesions that there are no agreed upon staging or treatment algorithms available. Primarily the realm of case reports in the literature, treatment often includes wide local excision, sparing as much of the larynx as possible, with adjuvant XRT after surgery. Survival of several years after such treatment has been reported. As with many non-SCC malignancies of the larynx, these lesions often present as submucosal masses, rather than the mucosal lesions often associated with SCC and its subtypes.

Chondrosarcoma

Chondrosarcoma is a mesenchymal tumor, very rare in the head and neck, and classically presents as a tumor of the posterior cricoid cartilage, though described from the skull base to the cervical spine. These tumors are slow growing but ultimately locally aggressive and are treated primarily surgically, with larynx preservation when oncologically possible. XRT can be used in a salvage or adjunct fashion, but primary surgical resection remains the treatment of choice. Overall disease-free survival has been reported to be 73% at 5 years.[9]

Squamous Cell Carcinoma

Greater than 90% of laryngeal malignancies are SCC, and from a treatment perspective, these are classified as early-stage (T1 and T2) and late-stage (T3 and T4) tumors. The glottis represents the most common primary subsite for laryngeal SCC, accounting for 75% of tumors, followed by the supraglottis (approximately 20%) and subglottis (≤ 5%).[2]

Historically, all laryngeal SCCs were treated surgically via total laryngectomy. As advances were made in tumor biology, anatomy, surgical technique, XRT, chemotherapy, and immunotherapy, efforts in laryngeal preservation increased. Currently, early-stage (T1 and T2) tumors are typically treated with single modality therapy, often primary XRT. Primary surgical resection may be an option for some patients in the form of partial laryngectomy, and this will be discussed in greater detail later.

Until the mid-1980, second-advanced laryngeal cancers were treated primarily with surgery (often total laryngectomy and adjuvant XRT). An interest in combined modality therapy (chemotherapy and XRT) began in mid-1980s. The landmark Veterans Affairs cooperative trial established combined chemotherapy and XRT as an acceptable alternative for patients with advanced laryngeal carcinoma who traditionally would require total laryngectomy.[10] Recent data from the National Cancer Database (NCDB) have challenged the shift of advanced laryngeal cancer treatment to nonsurgical therapy. Investigators demonstrated for late-stage glottic, early-stage supraglottic, and T3N0M0 supraglottic SCC 5-year survival rates of only 59.2% for patients treated with combined chemotherapy and XRT and 42.7% for patients treated with XRT alone, as compared with 65.2% for patients treated with surgery plus XRT and 63.3%

for those treated with surgery alone.[11] These, and other, data suggest that surgery may provide a survival advantage, particularly in late-stage SCC.

Whichever treatment modalities are chosen, it is imperative to treat not only the primary tumor but also the local and regional lymphatics as appropriate. Most of the larynx, with the exception of the glottis, is served by a rich lymphatic network with predictable drainage patterns. When describing these lymphatics, the neck is divided into five levels. The supraglottis drains primarily to levels II, III, and IV and may drain bilaterally. Thus in supraglottic SCC, both sides of the neck may harbor metastasis, either clinically/radiographically evident or occult. It is necessary to address these bilateral lymphatic beds in the treatment of supraglottic tumors, via either surgical neck dissection or XRT. The overall rate of occult metastasis is significant, being 16% in early-stage tumors and up to 62% in late-stage supraglottic SCC.[12]

Glottic SCC is somewhat unique. The glottis itself has a paucity of lymphatics; therefore, the rate of metastasis to the lymph nodes of the neck is significantly lower (< 10% of the patients with tumors confined to the glottis) than that observed in supra- or subglottic SCC. Tumors of the glottis may grow to be quite large and locally invasive (T3), but still may not metastasize to the lymphatics of the neck. Indeed, this subset of T3N0M0 glottic SCC, that is, large locally advanced tumors without regional or distant metastasis, was the only subset of patients that showed equal 5-year survival with either primary surgery plus XRT or primary chemotherapy plus XRT (65.6%) in the NCDB study.[11] Elective neck dissection or irradiation is not routinely recommended for early-stage glottic SCC. In late-stage glottic SCC, some authors recommend treatment of the ipsilateral neck, particularly levels II and III, even if the patient is clinically and radiographically N0.[13] It is important to note, however, that if a glottic SCC extends into the supraglottis or subglottis, the relevant lymphatics of these areas must be addressed as if the primary tumor were supraglottic or subglottic.

Subglottic SCC represents approximately 1% of all laryngeal tumors, and it often presents at an advanced stage with airway obstruction. These tumors have a much poorer prognosis than either glottic or supraglottic SCC, and they frequently present with metastatic disease in the neck. Garas and McGuirt reported a 25-year experience with subglottic SCC; 80% of the patients presented with either T3 or T4 disease, and the 5-year survival rate was 25%.[14] As in the supraglottis, lymphatic drainage can be bilateral, chiefly involving levels III and IV, but also frequently involving the central compartment of the neck, sometimes known as level VI, which is a space containing the Delphian lymph nodes extending from the cricoid cartilage superiorly to the sterna notch inferiorly and laterally bordered by the common carotid arteries. Further drainage along this lymphatic pathway allows metastatic disease entry into the pretracheal lymph nodes and the lymph nodes of the mediastinum.

Surgical Approaches

When considering surgical treatment of SCC of the larynx, total laryngectomy is the historical standard against which other surgical modalities are compared. It allows oncologically sound resection of the intact tumor plus a surrounding cuff of normal tissue at all margins. Removal of the entire larynx, however, carries with it real morbidity not only from the loss of natural voice but also from the loss of the sense of smell and much of the sense of taste, as well as a decrease in the ability to cough effectively. Such sequelae are the driving force behind the development of partial laryngectomy, also called organ-preservation surgery, where portions of the larynx are left intact, hoping for more natural function and improved quality of life. When considering organ-preservation surgery, it is important to determine whether the larynx is "competent" or not. A competent larynx is one that, despite the tumor, is able to perform the most basic of laryngeal functions of protecting the trachea and lower airways from oropharyngeal contents and subsequent aspiration, while allowing for adequate respiration.

Vocal cord function plays a large role in laryngeal competence. Vocal cords may become paralyzed or weakened by tumor involvement of the cord or the recurrent laryngeal nerves that control them. If the vocal cords cannot close completely because of paralysis or tumor, oropharyngeal contents and secretions may pass through them and into the trachea, potentiating aspiration pneumonia. If the vocal cords cannot open fully because of paralysis or bulky tumor burden, there will not be an adequate airway for the patient to breathe comfortably. In either of these situations, careful consideration should be given to total laryngectomy as the safest surgical treatment option. Organ-preservation surgery makes sense only if the preserved organ is going to be functional for the patient. It is also crucial to counsel any patient undergoing a partial laryngectomy that findings at surgery may require conversion to total laryngectomy, and they must be amenable to this possibility before entering the operating room.

Total Laryngectomy

First performed by Billroth in 1873, it was not until the mid-20th century that total laryngectomy was recognized as a safe, oncologically sound operation. Modern indications for total laryngectomy include late-stage tumors, specifically, T3 SCC, where supracricoid or supraglottic laryngectomy is not possible; T4 SCC, where supracricoid or near-total laryngectomy is not possible; and any tumor with invasion into the surrounding soft tissue of the neck, extensive involvement of the thyroid or cricoid cartilage, or extending beyond the posterior one-third of the tongue base. Also, it is indicated for patients with late-stage tumors in whom XRT alone or chemotherapy plus XRT are not possible for any reason.[15] To perform a total laryngectomy, the surgeon removes the hyoid bone, thyroid and cricoid cartilages, and upper tracheal rings. The opening of the trachea is diverted to the skin of the neck, creating a permanent stoma for respiration. The arytenoid cartilages and interarytenoid tissue are removed, and the party wall is dissected free. The resulting pharyngeal defect is sutured closed in a layered fashion, thus completely separating the oropharynx from the airway. With removal of the entire larynx, the ability to produce the native voice is lost; however, vocal rehabilitation is possible and can allow for speech. Handheld devices such as the electrolarynx, learning the technique of esophageal speech wherein air is swallowed and expelled via the esophagus, neopharynx, and mouth to create sound, or surgical insertion of a tracheoesophageal prosthesis to allow for speech with the tracheostoma occluded are all possible. Patients may also choose to use writing for communication.

Vertical Partial Laryngectomy

Indications for vertical partial laryngectomy include early-stage SCC (T1 and T2) with a mobile contralateral cord, no cartilaginous involvement by tumor, no involvement of the body of the arytenoid by tumor, and maximum subglottic extension of 5 mm. This procedure can be performed via traditional open approach, or endoscopically for smaller lesions in a procedure termed endoscopic cordectomy using an operating microscope. In an open procedure, the thyroid cartilage is exposed and the perichondrium overlying the affected side of the larynx is elevated and preserved for use in closure. Using an oscillating saw, a vertical cut is made in the cartilage at the midline if there is no anterior commissure involvement by the tumor to be resected or on the contralateral side of the thyroid cartilage to allow for a 5 to 7 mm margin of uninvolved tissue if anterior commissure involvement is present. The entire ipsilateral supraglottis, excepting the epiglottis, is removed, and the ipsilateral arytenoid may be spared if uninvolved. The involved TVC, and anterior commissure, if uninvolved, is taken. If there is anterior commissure involvement, up to one-third of the contralateral TVC may be resected and good outcomes still achieved. The ipsilateral cricothyroid membrane and even a small amount of upper ipsilateral cricoid cartilage may also be resected if warranted (**Fig. 14.2**). Reconstruction of the tissue defect can be achieved by using local strap muscles or the epiglottis, and it often ultimately heals into a scarred band resembling a rudimentary vocal fold, sometimes referred to as a "neo-cord."

For endoscopic cordectomy, an operating laryngoscope is placed into the mouth to expose the larynx. Using the operating microscope and microlaryngeal instruments or a laser, the affected TVC is excised under direct visualization, taking with it a 5-mm cuff of normal surrounding mucosa. The specimen is then freed from the underlying cartilage, taking perichondrium. Ultimate outcomes include normal swallowing function, though many patients require some rehabilitation under the auspices of a speech and language pathologist for swallowing techniques. Vocal rehabilitation typically proceeds well, with most patients satisfied with their voice, which does tend to have a "breathy" quality.

Supraglottic Laryngectomy

Indications for a supraglottic laryngectomy include tumors confined to the supraglottis, with no extension onto the TVCs and minimal medial pyriform sinus involvement above the TVCs. Indications also include supraglottic tumors that are T3 by way of preepiglottic space involvement only. Typically, both arytenoid cartilages are left in situ in supraglottic laryngectomy; however, select patients may tolerate resection of one arytenoid cartilage. All patients considered for this procedure must have good pulmonary reserve and cough reflex, as aspiration is frequent, and the ability to cough to clear secretions is paramount. Tissue removed in supraglottic laryngectomy includes the epiglottis, preepiglottic space, and upper portion of the thyroid cartilage down to the midpoint of the laryngeal ventricle, truly removing the entire supraglottis. The arytenoids and both TVCs are left intact (**Fig. 14.2**), allowing for normal voice postoperatively. The patient will need to be evaluated by a speech and language pathologist for safe swallowing techniques to minimize the risk of aspiration.

Supracricoid Laryngectomy

This is an extension of the supraglottic laryngectomy, removing all the same structures as by that procedure, as well as one arytenoid cartilage and possibly some of the upper ipsilateral cricoid cartilage. One arytenoid and vocal cord must be left unresected (**Fig. 14.2**). This procedure is nearly always performed with concomitant cricohyoidopexy, wherein the cricoid cartilage is tethered to and suspended from the hyoid bone, elevating it for further protection from aspiration during deglutition. Indications for supracricoid laryngectomy are the same as for supraglottic laryngectomy, but also include T3 SCC because of unilateral TVC fixation, or very minimal invasion of the thyroid cartilage. As with supraglottic laryngectomy, patients need good pulmonary function and reserve to tolerate this procedure well, and they will likely require prolonged postoperative rehabilitation for speech and swallowing. Ultimate outcomes that can be expected are normal swallowing function and recovery of laryngeal speech, though voice quality may be poor. These patients often require prolonged tracheostomy, but they can be decannulated as rehabilitation progresses.

Near-Total Laryngectomy

Indications for this procedure include T3 and T4 SCC not amenable to supraglottic or supracricoid laryngectomy but with one uninvolved arytenoid and laryngeal ventricle, unilateral transglottic SCC with TVC fixation, or patients who would otherwise be candidates for supraglottic or supracricoid laryngectomy but have poor pulmonary reserve. Important contraindications are subglottic extension below the cricoids or salvage situations after XRT failure. In near-total laryngectomy, the entire supraglottis is

removed bilaterally, together with the ipsilateral glottis and arytenoid cartilage, and resection can also include a portion of the ipsilateral upper cricoid cartilage. Patients are left with a single arytenoid and TVC and ultimately speak via a surgically created laryngoesophageal fistula. A permanent tracheostomy is left in place for respiration. Ultimately these patients can be expected to recover normal deglutition after rehabilitation in conjunction with a speech and language pathologist. In practice, this is a rarely performed procedure that is technically difficult and best reserved for those few practitioners with extensive experience in its use.

Radiation Therapy

XRT is a very important part of the treatment of head and neck cancers, including laryngeal SCC. There are a variety of methods to deliver ionizing radiation to tumors, but in the head and neck, external beam therapy predominates. In this technique, an externally located radiation source delivers a beam of radiation to a precise area of tissue, this being determined before treatment is begun based on clinical examination and radiographic imaging. XRT can be used as a solo treatment modality or can be combined with surgery or with chemotherapy, which will be discussed in further detail later in the chapter.

Radiation Therapy as Solo Treatment

When using XRT as a solo treatment of laryngeal SCC, it is necessary to define not only the precise areas to be irradiated that contain the primary tumor but also if the neck needs to be irradiated as well to control known or occult metastasis. As discussed previously, early-stage laryngeal SCC (T1 and T2) may be amenable to single modality treatment. Typically, the neck is included in the irradiated field if clinical evidence of metastasis is evident or if the risk of occult metastasis is felt to be 15% or greater. The total dose of radiation given is measured in Gray (Gy) and is based on the size of the tumor, as well as the tolerance of surrounding normal tissues to radiation exposure. Doses of 60 to 65 Gy are used for small, early-stage tumors of the larynx with control rates of greater than 90% reported, while 70 to 75 Gy are necessary for larger, T3 to T4 laryngeal SCC to achieve 90 to 100% local control rates.[16] These doses are typically given in daily sessions over a period of 6 to 7 weeks, and complications such as mucositis or dermatitis may necessitate breaks in therapy, though too long a hiatus from treatment leads to a decrease in efficacy and ultimately poorer tumor control.

Radiation Therapy Combined with Surgery

More advanced, late-stage tumors are best treated with combined modality therapy, such as XRT plus surgery or XRT plus chemotherapy (discussed later). Local surgical failures in laryngeal SCC are often the result of microscopic residual disease intentionally (to avoid morbidity or mortality) or inadvertently left behind after primary surgical resection.

XRT plays a role in eliminating such microscopic disease. Primary surgery with postoperative XRT facilitates the surgical resection and postoperative healing, as nonirradiated tissue heals far more effectively than does irradiated tissue. A larger total dose of radiation can be given postoperatively, and this dose can be adjusted based on the amount (if any) of obvious residual disease postresection. Disadvantages to this algorithm include the possibility of delay in commencing XRT if wound healing is slow or if surgical site infection occurs. Results of postoperative XRT are not as favorable if treatment is delayed 6 weeks or more postoperatively.[17,18]

Chemotherapy

Historically, chemotherapy was used for palliation in cases of unresectable or metastatic advanced laryngeal cancer. Currently, chemotherapy in laryngeal SCC is not used as a single-treatment modality when a cure of the disease is intended but is always combined with XRT. Indications for chemotherapy are locoregionally advanced, late-stage (T3 and T4) SCC. The most widely used chemotherapeutic agents are cisplatin and carboplatin, with cisplatin perhaps being slightly more efficacious but having a more severe side-effect profile as well. Schema for the use of chemotherapy broadly fall into three categories: (1) induction chemotherapy, wherein chemotherapy is given before definitive XRT or surgery, which is performed later; (2) concurrent chemotherapy plus XRT, wherein chemotherapy cycles are given during the patient's ongoing XRT; and (3) adjuvant chemotherapy, wherein surgical resection is first performed and concurrent chemotherapy plus XRT are begun postoperatively.

Induction Chemotherapy

In 1991, the U.S. Department of Veterans Affairs Study Group conducted a large, randomized controlled trial (RCT) of 332 patients to determine whether induction chemotherapy with definitive XRT was more effective than total laryngectomy with postoperative XRT for stages 3 and 4 laryngeal SCC. Overall, survival rates between the control and experimental arms of the surgery were comparable, and 64% of the patients in the experimental arm of the study retained their larynx at 2-year posttreatment, the remaining 36% required salvage laryngectomy for residual or recurrent SCC.[10] Factors associated with treatment failure were T4 disease and supraglottic primary site. Of note, the authors did mention in their study that chemotherapy plus XRT was not compared with XRT alone; therefore, some questions remained unanswered about the actual benefit of the chemotherapy. A similarly designed study sponsored by the European Organization for Research and Treatment of Cancer (EORTC) Cooperative Group, conducted in 1996, gave similar results. There was no difference in the overall 5-year survival between the two groups, and no direct comparison between chemotherapy plus XRT and XRT alone was made; the precise benefit of the induction chemotherapy remained

somewhat in question.[19] Of note, both these studies did suggest that the rate of distant metastasis may be slowed or decreased with the addition of chemotherapy, and further studies using other treatment schemes for chemotherapy were conducted.

Concurrent Chemotherapy

Based on the data described in the Veterans Affairs Laryngeal Study and the EORTC study, a prospective RCT was conducted in 2003 to compare XRT, induction chemotherapy plus XRT, and concurrent chemotherapy plus XRT in patients with stage 3 or 4 laryngeal SCC. The rate of larynx preservation was higher (84%) in patients receiving concurrent chemotherapy plus XRT than in either of the other two arms of the study.[20] There was no significant difference in overall 5-year survival between any of the treatment groups, though rates of locoregional recurrence were lower at 2 years in the concurrent chemotherapy plus XRT group, as well as a decrease in the rate of distant metastasis in this same group at 5-year posttreatment. Other authors have reported similar findings, improving disease-free survival, not to be confused with overall survival, by 15 to 20% using concurrent chemotherapy plus XRT.[21,22]

Adjuvant Chemotherapy

Indications for adjuvant chemotherapy plus XRT after primary surgical resection in laryngeal SCC include positive surgical margins, perineural or perivascular invasion, extracapsular extension in cervical lymph node metastasis, or cervical nodal disease in level IV or V of the neck. All these are associated with higher local and locoregional recurrence rates. Two prospective RCTs addressed the efficacy of adjuvant chemotherapy plus XRT in locally advanced head and neck SCC, the Radiation Therapy Oncology Group Trial 9501 and the EORTC Trial 22931 in 2004. Subsequent combined analysis of the two similar trials found advantages in both locoregional control and overall survival in patients receiving adjuvant therapy.[23] Adjuvant therapy is best used in patients with adverse clinical or histologic features and improves local control and disease-free survival, and it may improve overall survival as well.

Clinical Pearls

- Most true neoplasms of the adult larynx are malignant, and most of these are squamous cell carcinomas (SCCs).

- Including surgical resection in the treatment of laryngeal SCC may increase long-term (> 5 years) survival.

- Concurrent chemotherapy with radiation therapy (XRT) and adjuvant chemotherapy with XRT after surgical resection both improve overall survival.

- Multiple options for voice rehabilitation exist after total laryngectomy.

Pitfalls

- Delays in commencement of postoperative radiation therapy results in poorer outcomes.

- Patients with poor lung function are suboptimal candidates for partial laryngectomy.

- Partial laryngectomy should only be offered to patients with a competent larynx.

References

1. American Academy of Otolaryngology – Head & Neck Surgery Health. Fact Sheet: Laryngeal (Voice Box) Cancer. Available from: http://www.entnet.org/HealthInformation/laryngealCancer.cfm. Accessed October 1, 2012

2. Bailey BJ. Early glottic and supraglottic carcinoma: vertical partial laryngectomy and laryngoplasty. In: Bailey BJ, Johnson JT, Newlands SD, eds. Head and Neck Surgery—Otolaryngology. 4th ed. Philadelphia, PA: Lippincott, Williams & Wilkins; 2006:1441

3. Miziara ID, Cahali MB, Murakami MS, Figueiredo LA, Guimaraes JR. Cancer of the larynx: correlation of clinical characteristics, site of origin, stage, histology and diagnostic delay. Rev Laryngol Otol Rhinol (Bord) 1998;119(2):101–104

4. Goon PKC, Stanley MA, Ebmeyer J, et al. HPV & head and neck cancer: a descriptive update. Head Neck Oncol 2009;1:36

5. Wiatrak BJ, Wiatrak DW, Broker TR, Lewis L. Recurrent respiratory papillomatosis: a longitudinal study comparing severity associated with human papilloma viral types 6 and 11 and other risk factors in a large pediatric population. Laryngoscope 2004;114(11 Pt 2, Suppl 104):1–23

6. Ganly I, Patel SG, Coleman M, Ghossein R, Carlson D, Shah JP. Malignant minor salivary gland tumors of the larynx. Arch Otolaryngol Head Neck Surg 2006;132(7):767–770

7. Ferlito A, Barnes L, Rinaldo A, Gnepp DR, Milroy CM. A review of neuroendocrine neoplasms of the larynx: update on diagnosis and treatment. J Laryngol Otol 1998;112(9):827–834

8. Haberman PJ, Haberman RS II. Laryngeal adenocarcinoma, not otherwise specified, treated with carbon dioxide laser excision and postoperative radiotherapy. Ann Otol Rhinol Laryngol 1992;101(11):920–924

9. Hong P, Taylor SM, Trites JR, Bullock M, Nasser JG, Hart RD. Chondrosarcoma of the head and neck: report of 11 cases and literature review. J Otolaryngol Head Neck Surg 2009;38(2):279–285

10. Wolf GT; The Department of Veterans Affairs Laryngeal Cancer Study Group. Induction chemotherapy plus radiation compared with surgery plus radiation in patients with advanced laryngeal cancer. N Engl J Med 1991;324(24):1685–1690

11. Hoffman HT, Porter K, Karnell LH, et al. Laryngeal cancer in the United States: changes in demographics, patterns of care, and survival. Laryngoscope 2006;116(9 Pt 2, Suppl 111)1–13

12. Dünne AA, Davis RK, Dalchow CV, Sesterhenn AM, Werner JA. Early supraglottic cancer: how extensive must surgical resection be, if used alone? J Laryngol Otol 2006;120(9):764–769

13. Pennings RJ, Marres HA, den Heeten A, van den Hoogen FJ. Efficacy of diagnostic upper-node procedures during laryngectomy for glottic carcinoma. Am J Surg 2009;197(5):666–673

14. Garas J, McGuirt WF Sr. Squamous cell carcinoma of the subglottis. Am J Otolaryngol 2006;27(1):1–4

15. Smith RV, Fried MP. Advanced cancer of the larynx. In: Bailey BJ, Johnson JT, Newlands SD, eds. Head and Neck Surgery—Otolaryngology. 4th ed. Philadelphia, PA: Lippincott, Williams & Wilkins; 2006:1762

16. Shukovsky LJ. Dose, time, volume relationships in squamous cell carcinoma of the supraglottic larynx. Am J Roentgenol Radium Ther Nucl Med 1970;108(1):27–29

17. Vikram B, Strong EW, Shah JP, Spiro R. Failure at the primary site following multimodality treatment in advanced head and neck cancer. Head Neck Surg 1984;6(3):720–723

18. Hussey DH. Principles of radiation oncology. In: Bailey BJ, Johnson JT, Newlands SD, eds. Head and Neck Surgery—Otolaryngology. 4th ed. Philadelphia, PA: Lippincott, Williams & Wilkins; 2006:1727

19. Lefebvre JL, Chevalier D, Luboinski B, et al; EORTC Head and Neck Cancer Cooperative Group. Larynx preservation in pyriform sinus cancer: preliminary results of a European Organization for Research and Treatment of Cancer phase III trial. J Natl Cancer Inst 1996;88(13):890–899

20. Weber RS, Berkey BA, Forastiere AA, et al. Outcome of salvage total laryngectomy following organ preservation therapy: the Radiation Therapy Oncology Group trial 91-11. Arch Otolaryngol Head Neck Surg 2003;129(1):44–49

21. Olmi P, Crispino S, Fallai C, et al. Locoregionally advanced carcinoma of the oropharynx: conventional radiotherapy vs. accelerated hyperfractionated radiotherapy vs. concomitant radiotherapy and chemotherapy—a multicenter randomized trial. Int J Radiat Oncol Biol Phys 2003;55(1):78–92

22. Adelstein DJ, Li Y, Adams GL, et al. An intergroup phase III comparison of standard radiation therapy and two schedules of concurrent chemoradiotherapy in patients with unresectable squamous cell head and neck cancer. J Clin Oncol 2003;21(1):92–98

23. Bernier J, Cooper JS, Pajak TF, et al. Defining risk levels in locally advanced head and neck cancers: a comparative analysis of concurrent postoperative radiation plus chemotherapy trials of the EORTC (#22931) and RTOG (# 9501). Head Neck 2005;27(10):843–850

15 Ethmoid and Anterior Skull Base Neoplasms

Gilad Horowitz, Dan M. Fliss, and Ziv Gil

Core Messages

- Tumors of the nasal cavity and paranasal sinuses account for only 3% of all head and neck tumors, and ethmoid tumors are found in 20 to 30% of all paranasal malignancies.

- Primary ethmoid tumors invade via the route of least resistance, which includes the nasal cavity, paranasal sinuses, nasopharynx, lamina papyracea, and cribriform plate.

- The most common of malignant neoplasms in this group is squamous cell carcinoma, and the most common benign tumor is inverted papilloma.

- Signs and symptoms can often be misleading and initially interpreted as infectious and benign disease. A high degree of suspicion is necessary for any symptom suggestive of a growing tumor in the nasal cavity and sinuses.

- The physical examination should always include a fiberoptic endoscopic evaluation of the nose, sinuses, nasopharynx, and oropharynx. Special attention should also be paid to the presence of facial asymmetry, proptosis, serous otitis media, and cranial nerve palsies.

- Computed tomography (CT) and magnetic resonance imaging (MRI) are the modalities of choice for staging and follow-up of skull base tumors. The main advantage of CT scans is their superiority in delineating the architecture of the bones, and the main advantage of MRI is its supremacy in delineating among soft-tissue structures.

- Tissue diagnosis is crucial for the tailoring of treatment and should always be performed after a proper imaging work-up. Tissue is usually obtained by means of endoscopic biopsy under local anesthesia.

- Malignant tumors of the ethmoids and anterior skull base are almost always treated by surgery. Exceptions are lymphomas and small cell carcinomas, which are managed by chemoradiation.

- The classical resections of malignant tumors of the anterior skull base and ethmoids are performed via the open craniofacial approach. Recent developments in minimally invasive modalities have led to the popularization of endoscopic surgery for resection of both benign and malignant tumors.

- The overall 5-year survival of patients with malignant tumors of the anterior skull base is 50%. Their prognosis depends, above all else, on histology and margin status.

- The overall quality of life in the majority of patients after anterior skull base tumor extirpation can be classified as "good," with significant improvement taking place within 6 months after surgery.

Tumors involving the ethmoid sinus and anterior skull base represent a group of varying histologies with distinct clinical implications. The route of spread of tumors originating in the anterior skull base and ethmoid sinuses is determined by the complex anatomy of the craniofacial compartments. Over the last four decades, advancements in imaging modalities, development of minimally invasive techniques, and refinements in surgical and reconstructive methods have enabled an increasing number of patients with skull base neoplasms to undergo curative surgical resections. Benign tumors of the ethmoid complex are usually treated by endoscopic surgery, whereas malignant tumors with anterior skull base invasion are treated by craniofacial resection or endonasal surgery with adjuvant radiation therapy.

This chapter reviews the evaluation and management of the ethmoid complex and anterior skull base neoplasms. The surgical results and quality of life (QOL) of these patients are also discussed.

Epidemiology

Tumors of the nasal cavity and paranasal sinuses account for only 3% of all head and neck tumors, and ethmoid tumors are found in 20 to 30% of all paranasal malignancies. Malignant tumors involving the anterior skull base arise from the respiratory epithelium or glandular tissues of the paranasal mucosa.[1] An overwhelming majority of patients with ethmoid sinus malignancy have locally advanced tumors with skull base invasion. It is not uncommon for these patients to have undergone limited surgical manipulations, such as functional endoscopic sinus surgery and sumbucosal resection, before their referral to a skull base surgical team.[2]

Routes of Spread

Lesions of the ethmoid sinuses can be divided into primary and secondary tumors. Primary tumors originate in the ethmoid compartment, whereas secondary tumors invade the skull base from the nasal cavity; maxillary, frontal, and sphenoid sinuses; or the skin (**Fig. 15.1**). Rarely, these tumors originate in the globe, brain, meninges, or infratemporal fossa (**Fig. 15.2**). Neoplasms arising from the nasal cavity, nasopharynx, paranasal sinuses, and other structures that are in proximity to the anterior base of the skull can interrupt the continuity of the cranial valet, causing cerebrospinal fluid (CSF) leak and pneumocephalus (**Fig. 15.3**). Primary ethmoid tumors usually invade via the route of least resistance, which includes the sphenoid sinus and nasopharynx posteriorly and the nasal cavity and maxillary sinus inferiorly. Other routes of least resistance are the lamina papyracea (medial orbital wall) and cribriform plate. Primary ethmoid tumors can invade the dura or brain via direct extension through the fovea ethmoidalis (the roof of the ethmoids) and cribriform plate or involve the orbit via lateral extension through the lamina papyracea (**Fig. 15.4**).

Pathology

Tumors in this area can be of ectodermal, endodermal, or mesodermal origin (**Tables 15.1** and **15.2**).

Tumors Originating from the Sinonasal Epithelium

Tumors of the ethmoids and anterior skull base generally originate from the sinonasal mucosa (i.e., the schneiderian

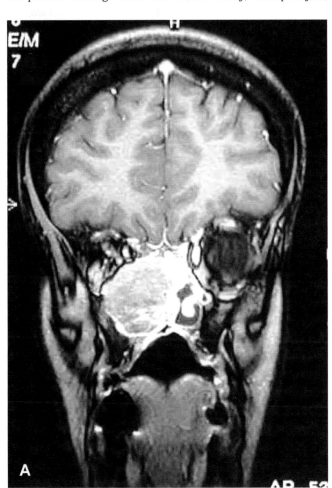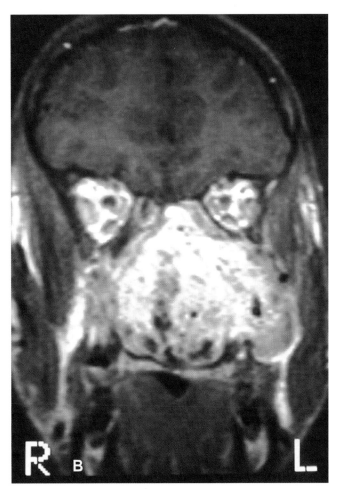

Figure 15.1 Primary and secondary tumors of the ethmoid sinuses. (A) Coronal magnetic resonance imaging (MRI) with gadolinium showing primary osteosarcoma of the ethmoid sinuses, with invasion into the nasal cavity. (B) MRI showing juvenile angiofibroma of the maxillary sinus, with secondary invasion into the ethmoid sinuses.

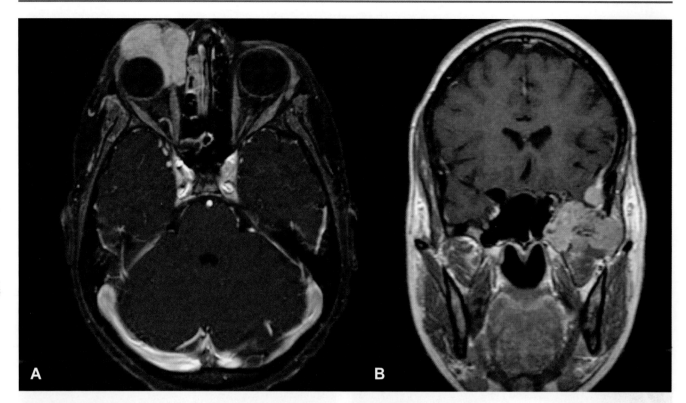

Figure 15.2 (A) Magnetic resonance imaging showing adenocarcinoma originating in the right orbit with invasion into the anterior skull base. (B) Infratemporal fossa involvement of rhabdomyosarcoma.

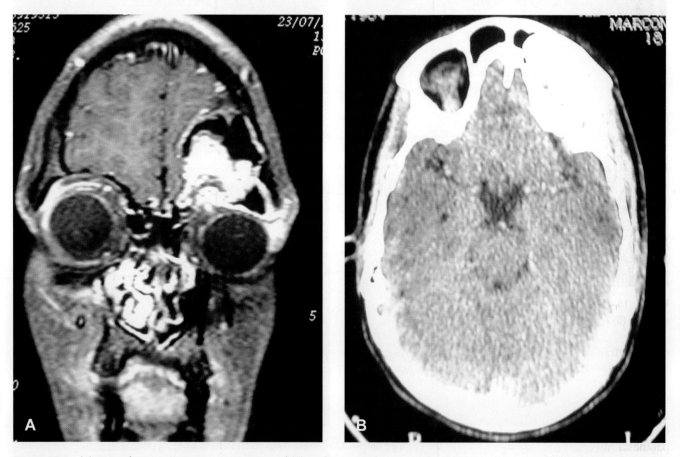

Figure 15.3 (A) Coronal magnetic resonance imaging and (B) axial computed tomography showing osteoma originating in the orbital roof, causing cerebrospinal fluid leak and pneumocephalus.

Table 15.1 Benign Pathologies of Ethmoid Sinus and Anterior Base of Skull

Papilloma
Pleomorphic adenoma
Dermoid
Fibroma
Chondroma
Osteoma
Neurofibroma
Vascular and lymphatic malformations
Nasal glioma
Schneiderian papilloma: inverted, papillary, cylindrical
Angiofibroma
Fibrous dysplasia
Ossifying fibroma
Giant cell tumor

Adapted from reference 8.

Table 15.2 Malignant Pathologies of Ethmoid Sinus and Anterior Base of Skull

Squamous cell carcinoma
Basaloid squamous
Adenosquamous
Adenoid cystic carcinoma
Mucoepidermoid carcinoma
Adenocarcinoma
Mucosal melanoma
Olfactory neuroblastoma (esthesioneuroblastoma)
Sinonasal undifferentiated carcinoma
Chordoma
Chondrosarcoma
Osteogenic sarcoma
Fibrosarcoma
Malignant fibrous histiocytoma
Hemangiopericytoma
Angiosarcoma
Rhabdomyosarcoma
Lymphoma
Plasmacytoma
Metastatic

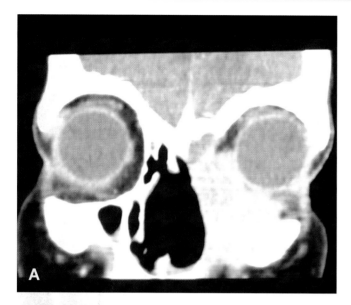

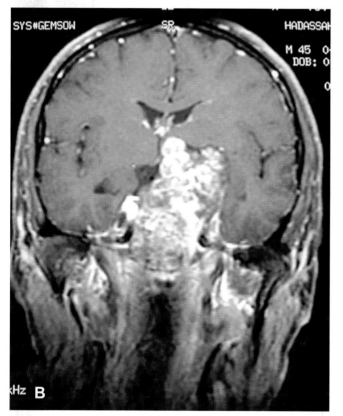

Figure 15.4 (A) Recurrent esthesioneuroblastoma with orbital invasion. (B) High-grade sarcoma with massive brain invasion.

epithelium). The most common of malignant neoplasms in this group is squamous cell carcinoma (SCC), and the most common benign tumor is inverted papilloma. Other carcinomas of the nasal mucosa include sinonasal undifferentiated carcinoma, adenocarcinoma, and mucosal melanoma. Salivary gland tumors are derived from the minor salivary glands of the paranasal mucosa and are usually of malignant origin. Adenoid cystic carcinoma and mucoepidermoid carcinoma are the most common of these tumors.

Bone and Fibrous Tumors

Another group of tumors are the ones that originate in the bony structures of the craniofacial skeleton. These bony lesions include benign conditions, such as fibrous dysplasia, osteoma, and ossifying fibroma, as well as malignant neoplasms, such as osteosarcoma (**Fig. 15.5**).

Vascular Tumors

Vascular tumors include angiofibroma, paraganglioma, arteriovenous malformation, and hemangioma, all of which are benign conditions (**Fig. 15.6**). Malignant vascular tumors are rare, and they include hemangiopericytoma, malignant paraganglioma, and angiosarcoma.

Tumors of Muscle and Nerve Origin

Tumors that are derived from muscle tissue are mainly malignant, and the most representative of this group is rhabdomyosarcoma. Common benign nerve cell tumors include schwannoma and neurofibroma, which usually arise in cranial nerves. The malignant tumors in this group are esthesioneuroblastoma and malignant peripheral nerve sheath tumor. Chordoma and chondrosarcoma are malignant soft-tissue tumors that usually arise from the clivus. Head and neck tumors are notorious for their ability to invade nerves. Adenoid cystic carcinomas, sinonasal SCC, and SCC of the skin are among the most common neurotrophic tumors in this group (**Fig. 15.7**). Tumors that infiltrate the base of the skull via nerve dissemination can eventually involve the dura and brain.[3]

Presenting Signs and Symptoms

Signs and symptoms can often be misleading and initially interpreted as infectious and benign disease. Because early detection is probably the most important factor in improving prognosis, a high degree of suspicion is necessary for any symptom suggestive of a growing tumor in the nasal cavity and sinuses. The most common signs and symptoms of malignant neoplasms are listed in **Table 15.3**. There may also be locoregional neck metastases in fewer than 10% of the patients with malignant tumors. The physical examination should always include a fiberoptic endoscopic evaluation of the nose, sinuses, nasopharynx, and oropharynx. Special attention should also be paid to the presence of facial asymmetry, proptosis, serous otitis media, cranial nerve palsies, and suspicious neck nodes (**Fig. 15.8**).

Radiological Evaluation

All patients with suspected craniofacial neoplasm should undergo a radiological evaluation. Imaging is critical for the evaluation of location, size, and extent of disease and for differential diagnosis. Imaging is also important for guiding a transnasal biopsy. Computed tomography (CT) and magnetic resonance imaging (MRI) are the modalities of choice for staging and follow-up of skull base tumors. The main advantage of CT scans is their superiority in delineating the architecture of the bones. Adding contrast enhancement to the study increases tumor definition from adjacent soft tissue. Bone destruction and soft-tissue invasion suggest an aggressive behavior pattern. Widening of the foraminas in the base of the skull can indicate perineural spread. The main advantage of MRI is its supremacy in delineating among soft-tissue structures, especially muscles, brain, and dura. Moreover, MRI best evaluates brain, cavernous sinus, carotid artery, perineural invasion (**Fig. 15.9**), and intraorbital invasion (**Fig. 15.10**). Dural thickening or enhancement may suggest dural involvement. Perhaps one of the most significant advantages of MRI is its ability to distinguish the tumor from retained secretions secondary to obstruction of sinus drainage. This is best demonstrated with a T2-MRI scan (**Fig. 15.11**). Positron emission tomography-CT is used for further assessment of the patient's metastatic status (**Fig. 15.12**). Its superiority in the delineation of regional and distant metastases has made MRI a highly valuable tool both in the preoperative evaluation and for follow-up because it can help distinguish between postoperative changes and tumor recurrence.

Tissue Diagnosis

Tissue diagnosis is crucial for the individual tailoring of treatment and should always be performed after a proper imaging work-up. Tissue is usually obtained by means of endoscopic biopsy under local anesthesia. An adequate specimen of the tissue should be obtained, with care being taken to avoid crushing it. If the lesion is suspected for being of a lymphoproliferative nature, the fresh tissue should be immersed in saline rather than fixed in formalin. Biopsy should be avoided if the nasal mass is suspected to be as an encephalocele, because the procedure can lead to CSF leak and meningitis. Similarly, biopsy is contraindicated for suspected vascular lesions, such as juvenile angiofibromas, hemangiopericytomas, and hemangiomas. The biopsy specimen should be examined by a pathologist who is an expert in the field of head and neck cancer (HNC).

Tailoring of Treatment

Malignant tumors of the ethmoids and anterior skull base are almost always treated by surgery. Exceptions are lymphomas and small cell carcinomas, which are managed by chemoradiation. Surgery is contraindicated in highly malignant neoplasms when the tumor infiltrates the internal carotid artery or cavernous sinus, and when there is evidence of high volume disease in the brain parenchyma (**Fig. 15.13**). The goals of surgery are complete tumor resection and preservation of function. The classical resections of malignant tumors of the anterior skull base and ethmoids are performed via transfacial or transcranial open approaches. Recent developments in minimally invasive modalities have led to the popularization of endoscopic surgery for resection of benign and malignant tumors of the anterior skull base and paranasal sinuses.[4]

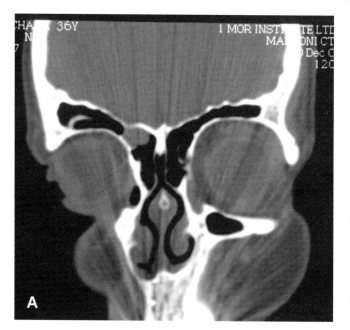

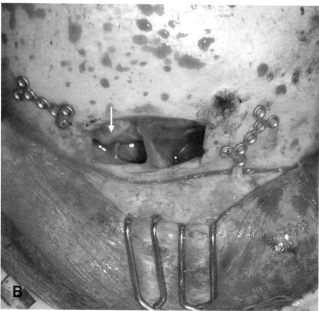

Figure 15.5   Osteoma of the right frontal bone. (A) Coronal computed tomography. (B) Intraoperative view. The arrow indicates the osteoma.

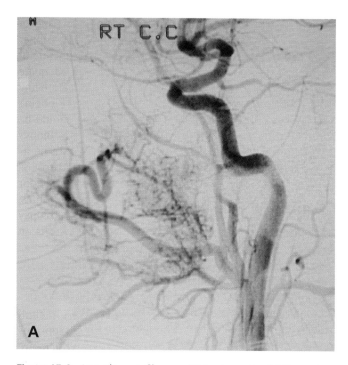

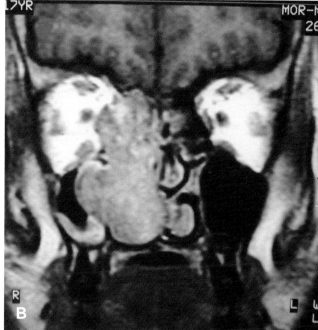

Figure 15.6   Juvenile angiofibroma. (A) Angiography. (B) Coronal magnetic resonance imaging.

Open Surgical Approaches

The surgical approach should include extirpation of the cribriform plate for all malignant tumors and for those benign tumors with involvement of the roof of the ethmoids. The classical transfacial-transethmoid approaches remain viable surgical techniques only for benign tumors that do not involve the anterior skull base.

Craniofacial Approach and Its Modifications

In cases of tumor extension superiorly or laterally to the paranasal sinuses, transfacial approaches alone cannot provide adequate exposure of the tumor, and so other supplementary techniques are needed to allow safe resection and reconstruction. The craniofacial approach is

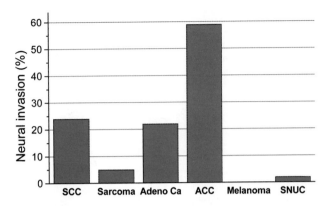

Figure 15.7 Incidence of perineural invasion according to pathology. ACC, adenoid cystic carcinoma; SCC, squamous cell carcinoma; SNUC, sinonasal undifferentiated carcinoma.

Adapted from reference 9.

the workhorse technique for resection of tumors involving the ethmoid sinuses and cribriform plate. It combines frontal craniotomy via a coronal flap and transfacial approach via a lateral rhinotomy incision. It is performed with suprastracture or infrastructure maxillectomy (**Fig. 15.14**). The surgery is performed by a multidisciplinary team that includes skull base surgeons from the disciplines of otolaryngology and neurosurgery. Using the craniofacial approach, which was first described by Katcham in the 1960s, both benign and malignant tumors can be extirpated in a single procedure that is performed simultaneously above and below the anterior skull base. The procedure involves minimal morbidity and a relatively low rate of severe complications. A complete resection of the tumor is achieved in more than 50% of the patients with malignant neoplasm. The subcranial approach, an alternative to resection of anterior skull base tumors, involves osteotomies of the anterior table of the frontal sinus, the medial orbital wall bilaterally, and the upper segment of the nasal bones. It allows simultaneous intradural and extradural tumor

Table 15.3 Signs and Symptoms Suggestive of Malignant Neoplasm

Epistaxis

Anosmia

Nasal obstruction

Headache

Facial pain

Changes in vision

Proptosis

Facial numbness

Facial asymmetry

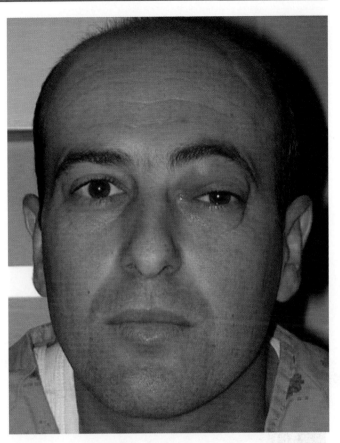

Figure 15.8 Preoperative picture of a patient with orbital invasion of squamous cell carcinoma originating in the ethmoid sinuses.

removal through a subfrontal access, thereby eliminating the need for facial incisions and minimizing the extent of frontal lobe manipulation (**Fig. 15.15**).[5]

Other Transfacial Approaches

Conventional transfacial approaches involve various skin incisions and osteotomies of the maxillary, frontal, and ethmoid bones (**Fig. 15.16**). The conventional exposure of the suprastructure of the maxilla requires a lateral rhinotomy incision, whereas a total maxillectomy is usually performed via the Weber-Fergusson incision. The Lynch incision can be used to approach the frontal sinus lateral to the supraorbital nerve, where endoscopic resection is not feasible. Lateral rhinotomy may be combined with a Lynch incision to gain exposure to the ethmoid sinuses, anterior skull base, and frontal sinus. A Dieffenbach incision combined with a lateral rhinotomy incision is used for tumors that extend to the infraorbital rim, lateral orbital wall, and zygoma. These approaches offer wide access to the ethmoid sinuses and allow an anterior and posterior ethmoidectomy via a facial incision. Thanks to the technical developments in minimally invasive techniques, these procedures are now usually performed by transnasal endoscopic surgery, eliminating the need for a facial incision and yielding

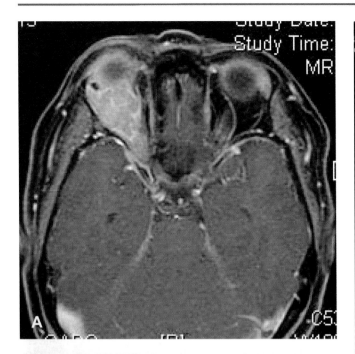

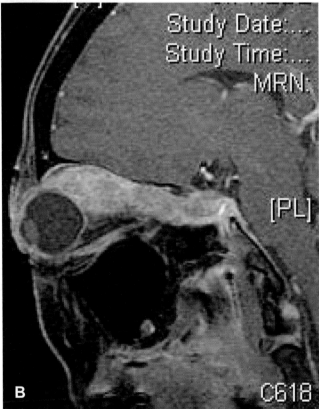

Figure 15.9   Neural invasion along the optic nerve of adenoid cystic carcinoma.

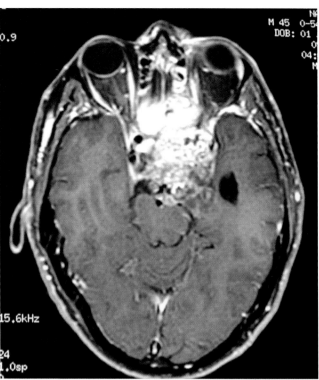

Figure 15.10   Cavernous sinus invasion by esthesioneuroblastoma.

Endoscopic Surgery

The endoscopic approach provides excellent access to the paranasal sinuses and skull base and, therefore, it has become a popular alternative to open procedures for the treatment of benign tumors and selected malignant neoplasms. Recent refinements in endoscopic techniques together with the development of specialized surgical instruments allow complete radical resection of complex anatomic structures through full endonasal or combined endoscopic and open approaches, without compromising any oncological principles (**Fig. 15.17**). This innovative surgical approach avoids facial incisions and open craniotomy and may subsequently reduce postoperative morbidity and the risk of complications after radiotherapy.

With the accumulation of greater experience, endoscopic approaches have also been applied to neoplasms of the anterior skull base. Recent data have suggested the technical feasibility, satisfactory survival, and low complication rates of endoscopic surgery for sinonasal neoplasms with skull base involvement. Important contraindications of endoscopic surgery include soft tissue, skin, and orbital involvement.

Reconstruction

When tumors arising in the anterior skull base and ethmoid sinuses invade both soft and hard tissues of the skull base, tumor resection may create extensive skull base defects and produce a free conduit between the paranasal sinuses and the intracranial space. After tumor extirpation, skull

excellent results. Several clear-cut indications for choosing transfacial approaches include involvement of the skin or underlying bone, tumors invading the lateral area of the frontal sinus, involvement of the anterior wall of the frontal sinus, intraorbital involvement, and nasal bone or piriform aperture invasion.

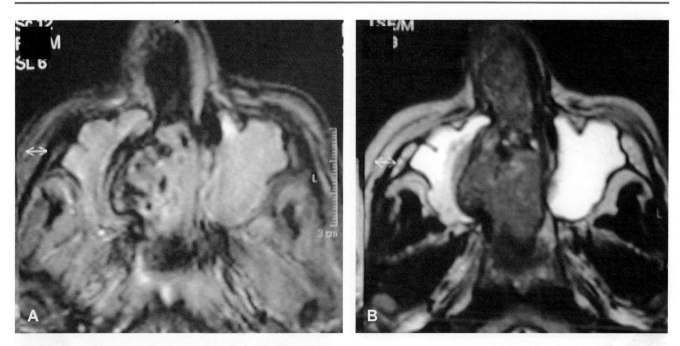

Figure 15.11 Squamous cell carcinoma of the ethmoid cavity. (A) T1-magnetic resonance imaging (MRI) without gadolinium. (B) T2-MRI showing secretion in the maxillary sinuses.

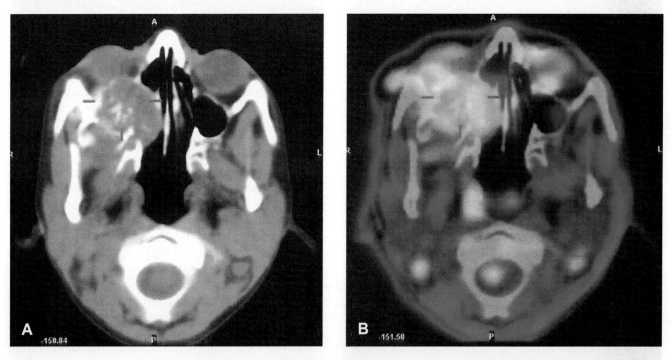

Figure 15.12 Positron emission tomography (PET)-computed tomography (CT) of a patient with osteosarcoma. (A) CT scan. (B) Fusion of PET and CT showing the tumor marked with a red cross.

base defects require precise and durable reconstruction[1] to form a fluid-tight dural seal,[2] provide a barrier between the contaminated sinonasal space and the sterile subdural compartment,[3] prevent airflow into the intracranial space,[4] maintain a functional sinonasal system,[6] and provide a good cosmetic outcome. A variety of approaches have been developed to accomplish these goals. Whatever the choice, failure to create adequate reconstruction harbors serious

complications; among them are CSF leak, meningitis, brain herniation, and tension pneumocephalus. Surgeons commonly use combinations of methods to accomplish satisfactory anterior skull base reconstruction. Thus, there is no single "gold standard" technique that is both simple and reliable for reducing the morbidity and mortality associated with anterior cranial base operations. Previous reports have provided evidence showing that the long-term viability of

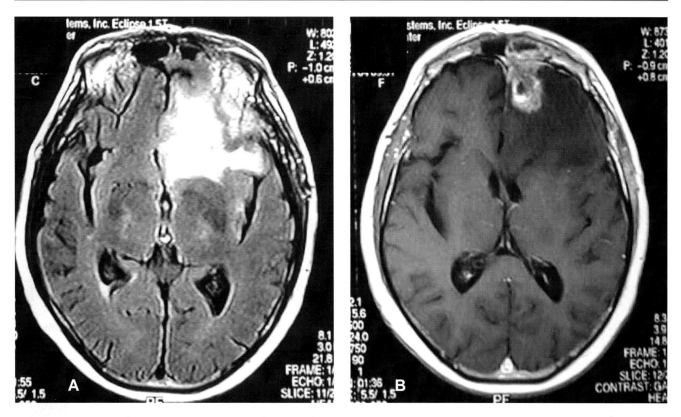

Figure 15.13   Massive brain invasion of patients with sinonasal undifferentiated carcinoma. (A) T1-magnetic resonance imaging (MRI) with gadolinium showing enhancement of the tumor. (B) T2-MRI showing severe brain edema.

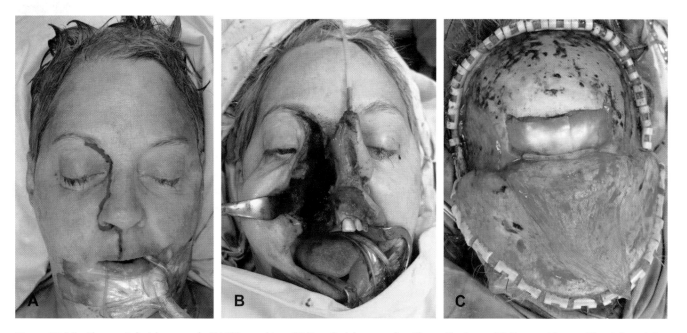

Figure 15.14   The craniofacial approach. (A) Skin marking. (B) Transfacial approach with maxillectomy. (C) Bicoronal flap and frontal craniotomy.

a graft is achievable without an overlying vascularized flap, such as a pericranial flap (**Fig. 15.18**), a temporoparietal flap, a temporalis muscle flap, and free flaps (**Fig. 15.19**). For endoscopic reconstruction, a vascularized nasoseptal flap offers a high-quality means of reconstruction for defects of the sella, planum sphenoidale, and cribriform plate (**Fig. 15.20**). A nonvascularized fascia lata flap provides a simple, inexpensive, and versatile means of skull base reconstruction after both endoscopic and open approaches. Histological findings indicate that fascia lata grafts survive by means of local proliferation of a newly formed vascular layer embedded within the fascial sheath (**Fig. 15.21**).

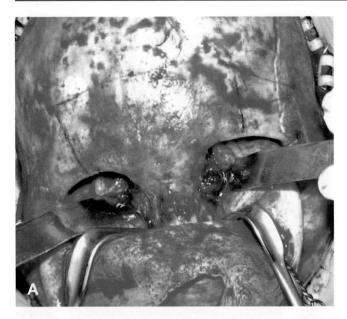 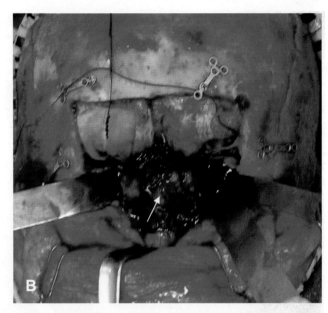

Figure 15.15 The subcranial approach. (A) Exposure of the frontal bone and orbits is performed via a coronal flap. (B) After craniotomy, which includes the frontal bone, nasal bones, and medial walls of the orbit, the tumor is exposed (arrow).

This feature provides long-term viability without the need for an overlying vascularized flap.

Complications

Postoperative anterior skull base tumor resection complications are encountered in approximately one-third of the patients.[2] The most frequent complications are listed in **Table 15.4**.[6] Despite the fact that the complication rate seems to be relatively high, the cases of serious complications, such as CSF leak, meningitis, intracranial hemorrhage, pneumocephalus, and neurological deficits, are less than 5% (**Fig. 15.22**). The postoperative mortality rate associated with anterior skull base tumor resection has remained around 3% for the past two decades. An increased risk of postoperative complications was noted in patients who had

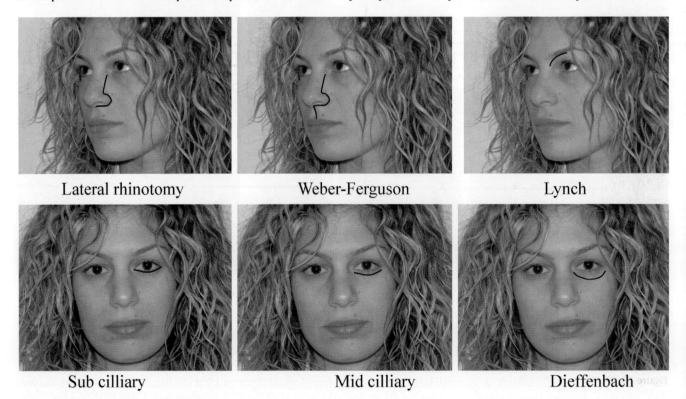

Lateral rhinotomy   Weber-Ferguson   Lynch

Sub cilliary   Mid cilliary   Dieffenbach

Figure 15.16 Transfacial approaches.

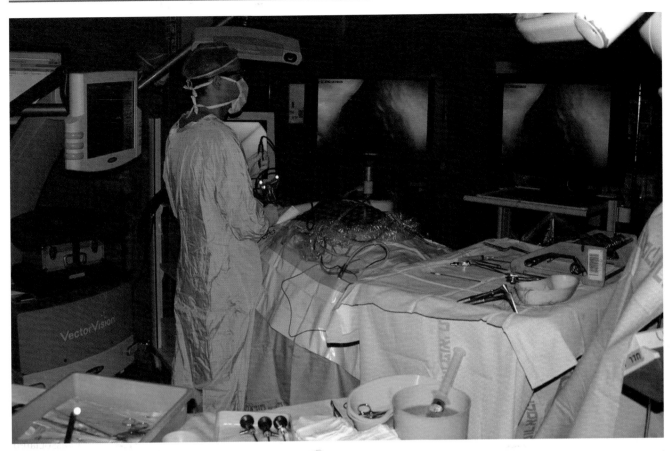

Figure 15.17   The neuroendoscopic surgical suite. Two three-dimensional screens are shown, as well as normal high-definition screen and intraoperative navigation system.

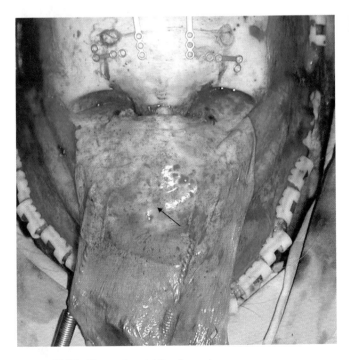

Figure 15.18   The pericranial flap (arrow).

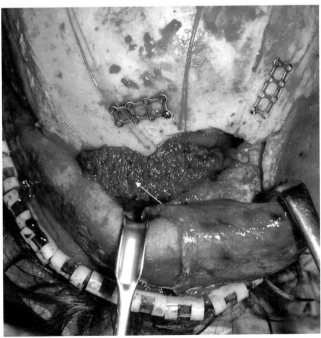

Figure 15.19   Reconstruction of the anterior skull base may be performed with a free flap, such as in this case, with a rectus abdominus flap.

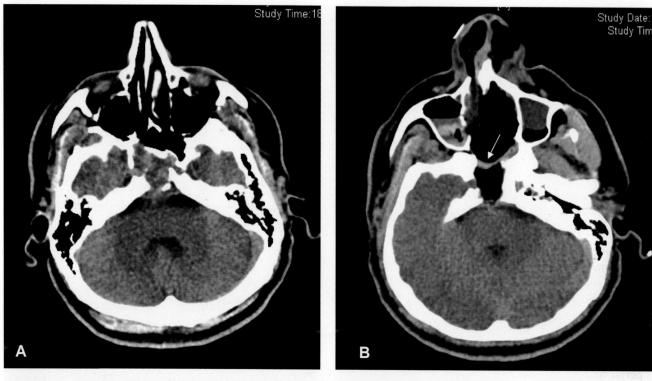

Figure 15.20 The nasal septal flap. (A) Preoperative computed tomography showing clival chordoma. (B) Postoperative image showing the nasal septal flap (arrow). The defect of the clivus was obliterated with fat and covered with the nasal septal flap.

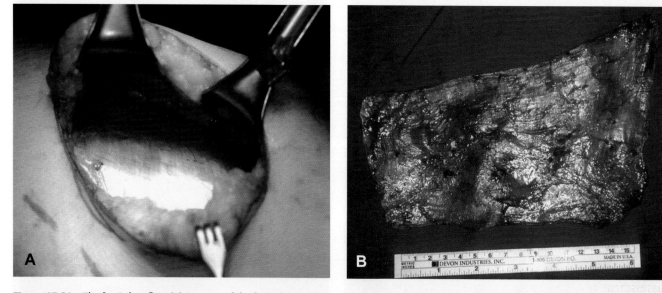

Figure 15.21 The fascia lata flap. (A) Exposure if the fascia lata is achieved with the lateral thigh skin incision. (B) Harvesting of the fascia lata flap.

been previously treated with external beam radiotherapy and in elderly patients.[2,6]

Adjuvant Therapy

The addition of postoperative radiotherapy is the accepted standard of care for patients with malignant tumors of the head and neck. Adjuvant radiotherapy is routinely used for esthesioneuroblastoma, SCC, adenoid cystic carcinoma,

and adenocarcinoma of the anterior skull base, with an improvement of up to 10% in 5-year overall survival. Adjuvant radiation therapy can also enable better local tumor control in patients with mucosal melanoma. The utility of chemoradiation as an adjuvant treatment modality after tumor removal is a subject that warrants further study. Neoadjuvant radiotherapy, with or without chemoradiation, has been associated with good results in patients with esthesioneuroblastoma, and further studies are required to

Table 15.4 Incidence of Postoperative Complications after Craniofacial Resection

Complications	N (%) 1973–1995	1996–2005	p
Intracranial[a]	12 (10.5)	16 (13)	NS
Wound[b]	32 (28)	9 (7.5)	< 0.0001
Systemic[c]	7 (6)	7 (5.8)	NS
Ocular[d]	5 (4.4)	4 (3.3)	NS
Mortality	5 (4.4)	4 (3.3)	NS
Total	60 (52)	40 (33)	0.002

[a]Intracranial: cerebrospinal fluid leak, meningitis, encephalitis, pneumocephalus, intracranial hematoma.
[b]Wound: infection, dehiscence, flap necrosis, fistula.
[c]Systemic: myocardial infarction, arrhythmia, systemic infections, pulmonary, urinary tract, metabolic.
[d]Ocular: diplopia, blindness, orbital cellulitis.

evaluate its use in other skull base cancers. One distinct group of patients who are primarily treated with chemoradiation includes children with soft-tissue sarcomas in whom surgery is performed only as salvage treatment.

Outcome

The overall 5-year survival rate of patients with malignant tumors of the anterior skull base is 50%.[2] Their prognosis depends, above all else, on histology and margin status (**Fig. 15.23**).[7] Other factors that have an effect on survival are orbital, dural, and brain invasion. Most patients with tumor recurrence will die of local disease that is followed by distant metastases.

Quality of Life

QOL is assessed in an effort to improve treatment modalities, to promote restoration of patients' daily functions, and to accelerate their return to a normal lifestyle. The estimation of the influence of surgical procedures on QOL can serve as a means by which the most appropriate surgical approach can be selected for a given patient. A detailed understanding of the different aspects of QOL helps surgeons improve assessment and management of patients, identify specific impediments as early as possible during follow-up, and implement specific medical interventions for patients with increased risk and poor outcome. Furthermore, early access of patients to detailed information about their disease can yield better adjustment to an imminent medical condition. The technical development of anterior skull base surgery has had a major positive impact on the long-term survival of patients with lesions involving the anterior base of the skull and adjacent paranasal sinuses. Nevertheless, this procedure may carry considerable risk as well as serious morbidity. Several studies have already used the anterior

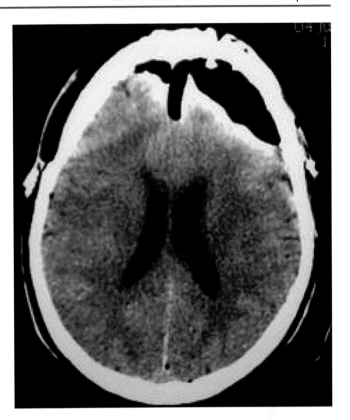

Figure 15.22 Postoperative computed tomography showing pneumocephalus with signs of brain compression.

skull base surgery QOL questionnaire, a disease-specific instrument recently developed at the Tel Aviv Medical Center, to investigate the effect of surgery on patients' QOL. The overall QOL in the majority of patients after anterior skull base tumor extirpation can be classified as "good," with significant improvement taking place within 6 months after surgery. Prospective studies revealed that the financial and emotional QOL domains had the worse impact on these patients. Old age, malignancy, comorbidity, radiotherapy,

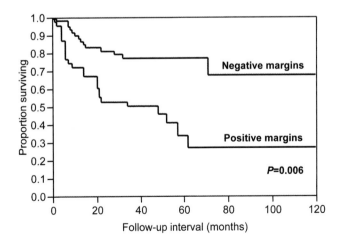

Figure 15.23 Survival curves showing the impact of margin status on survival.

Adapted from reference 10.

and extensive surgery were found to be negative prognostic factors for QOL measures. It was also shown that pain control regimens, antidepressants, and other psychological modalities, including group support, can improve QOL measures in these patients. A multidisciplinary team approach emerged as being the best intervention modality for enhancing the health-related and overall QOL of patients with skull base tumors.

Conclusions

Tumors arising in the ethmoid sinuses and anterior skull base are uncommon. Whereas most HNCs are more likely to be discovered by the patient or by the physician during a routine physical examination, sinonasal malignancies are not accessible to self-examination and are often diagnosed late, thus resulting in poor prognosis. There is a variety of tumors arising from the sinonasal epithelium, and due to the complicated differential diagnosis of these tumors, immunocytochemical staining is frequently required to establish the diagnosis. Except for lymphoma and soft-tissue sarcomas in children, surgery is considered the treatment of choice for most tumors. The high rate of local recurrence mandates that all lesions undergo wide surgical resection and adjuvant radiation therapy. Local failure is a significant cause of morbidity and mortality in these patients. The utility of other treatment modalities, such as chemoradiation or biological therapy, has not been established. Most patients with benign tumors are treated with endoscopic approaches, whereas the efficacy of endonasal surgery for the treatment of patients with malignant neoplasms awaits the results of further studies.

References

1. Batra PS, Luong A, Kanowitz SJ, et al. Outcomes of minimally invasive endoscopic resection of anterior skull base neoplasms. Laryngoscope 2010;120(1):9–16
2. Bentz BG, Bilsky MH, Shah JP, Kraus D. Anterior skull base surgery for malignant tumors: a multivariate analysis of 27 years of experience. Head Neck 2003;25(7):515–520
3. Cantù G, Riccio S, Bimbi G, et al. Craniofacial resection for malignant tumours involving the anterior skull base. Eur Arch Otorhinolaryngol 2006;263(7):647–652
4. Gil Z, Carlson DL, Gupta A, et al. Patterns and incidence of neural invasion in patients with cancers of the paranasal sinuses. Arch Otolaryngol Head Neck Surg 2009;135(2):173–179
5. Fliss Dm, Abergel A, Canel O, Margalit N, Gil Z. Combined subcranial approaches for excision of complex anterior skull base tumors. Arch Otolaryngol head Neck surg 2007;133:888–896
6. Gil Z, Patel SG, Bilsky M, Shah JP, Kraus DH. Complications after craniofacial resection for malignant tumors: are complication trends changing? Otolaryngol Head Neck Surg 2009;140(2):218–223
7. Patel SG, Singh B, Polluri A, et al. Craniofacial surgery for malignant skull base tumors: report of an international collaborative study. Cancer 2003;98(6):1179–1187
8. Hanna EY, Kupferman M, DeMonte F. Surgical management of tumors of the nasal cavity, paranasal sinuses, orbit, and anterior skull base. In: Hanna E, Demonte F, eds. comprehensive management of Skull Base Tumors. New York, NY: Informa Health Care USA, Inc; 2008
9. Gil Z, Carlson DL, Gupta A, et al. Patterns and incidence of neural invasion in patients with cancers of the paranasal sinuses. Arch Otolaryngol Head Neck Surg 2009;135(2):173–179
10. Gil Z, Patel SG, Singh B, et al; International Collaborative Study Group. Analysis of prognostic factors in 146 patients with anterior skull base sarcoma: an international collaborative study. Cancer 2007;110(5):1033–1041

16 Maxillary Sinus Neoplasms

J. Kenneth Byrd and Joshua Hornig

Core Messages

- Because of the anatomic boundaries of the maxillary sinuses, masses typically present with minimal vague symptoms until they are very locally advanced.

- There are more than 70 benign and malignant types of sinonasal tumors. The maxillary sinus is the most frequent site of malignancy within the paranasal sinuses.

- Inverted papilloma is the most common benign tumor, and squamous cell carcinoma is the most common malignant tumor.

- Surgical resection is the mainstay of treatment.

- Adjuvant radiation to the primary site and neck or chemoradiation may be indicated after resection, depending on the adverse pathologic features.

- Endoscopic and endoscopic-assisted resection of benign tumors has been proven to be as effective as open resection but may be of limited benefit for malignant tumors because of the advanced stage at presentation.

- Reconstruction versus obturation of the surgical defect should be decided on the basis of individual patient.

The paired maxillary sinuses are the largest of the paranasal sinuses and are the first to develop in utero. They resemble an inverted pyramid in shape and are bounded anteriorly by the anterior maxilla and skin, posteriorly by the pterygopalatine fossa, superiorly by the inferior orbital wall and infraorbital nerve, inferiorly by the maxillary alveolar process and tooth roots, and medially by the lateral nasal wall and contents of the nasal cavity. Tumors of the maxillary sinuses tend to present late in their course because of the lack of early symptoms and may present with ocular, nasal, or oral symptoms.

Patients tend to present with vague symptoms initially, including nasal obstruction, epistaxis, or nasal discharge. Expansion into adjacent structures, including the nasal cavity, orbit, or infratemporal or pterygopalatine fossas, may occur in benign or malignant processes. As the tumor enlarges, patients begin to complain of diplopia, facial pain, swelling of the hard palate, or loose teeth. Numbness of the cheek suggests infraorbital nerve involvement and is worrisome for malignancy. Signs of maxillary sinus tumors on physical examination include a medially expanded lateral nasal wall, hypoesthesia of the maxillary teeth or cheek, proptosis, extraocular muscle weakness, trismus, or lesions of the oral maxilla.

Neoplasms

There are more than 70 pathologic entities that have been described for the sinonasal cavity, more than half of which

are malignant.[1] **Table 16.1** lists some of the more common benign and malignant tumors that may involve the maxillary sinus.

Benign Neoplasms

Inverted papillomas (IPs) are the most common benign sinonasal tumors, occurring with a yearly incidence of 0.2 to 0.6 per 100,000. They are more common in males (3:1), and they typically present with unilateral nasal obstruction in the fifth and sixth decades of life. They most commonly originate from the lateral nasal wall, followed by the maxillary sinus, and are bilateral in approximately 5% of the cases. Unilateral nasal polyposis should raise the suspicion of IPs. They are associated with a 9% risk of concurrent or delayed malignancy and have a rate of recurrence as high as 71% if incompletely excised.[2] Histologically, they appear as proliferative respiratory epithelium with inversion into the stroma, with or without squamous metaplasia, and without invasion. Cylindrical cell papillomas are less common than IPs and typically arise from the lateral nasal wall but have been described in the maxillary sinus. Because of the potential for malignancy and a high-recurrence rate, traditional surgical approaches for IPs have been lateral rhinotomy or midface degloving, but an aggressive endoscopic technique has been shown in numerous studies to be equally efficacious with less morbidity.[2,3]

Table 16.1 Common Benign and Notable Malignant Primary Tumors of the Maxillary Sinuses

	Benign	Malignant
Epithelial	Inverted papilloma Cylindrical papilloma Exophytic papilloma	Squamous cell carcinoma Cylindrical cell carcinoma Sinonasal tract mucosal melanoma
Salivary	Adenoma	Adenocarcinoma Adenoid cystic carcinoma Mucoepidermoid carcinoma
Neuroendocrine	Neurofibroma	Esthesioneuroblastoma Small cell carcinoma Sinonasal undifferentiated carcinoma
Soft tissue	Fibroma leiomyoma	Rhabdomyosarcoma Osteosarcoma Chondrosarcoma Hemangiopericytoma
Hematopoietic		Lymphoma Plasmacytoma

Malignant Neoplasms

Malignant neoplasms of the paranasal sinuses are rare, with a yearly incidence of less than 1 per 100,000. The maxillary sinus is the most common site within the paranasal sinuses, followed by the ethmoid sinuses, sphenoid sinuses, and frontal sinuses. Risk factors for sinonasal malignancies include wood exposure, work in the leather or textile industry, and exposure to metals and chemicals including aluminum, nickel, and chromium. Heavy cigarette smoking has also been implicated, as have the Epstein-Barr virus and the human papillomavirus.[1]

Squamous cell carcinoma (SCC) is the most common subtype in adults, accounting for 40 to 50% of malignant sinonasal tumors, followed by adenocarcinomas (13 to 19%) and adenoid cystic carcinoma (ACC) (6 to 10%).[1] The American Joint Committee on Cancer (AJCC) staging system is used for these tumor types (**Table 16.2**). Treatment is most often surgery followed by adjuvant therapy (when indicated).[4] As in ACC, it is important to ensure that adjacent nerves are free of disease in SCC, as perineural spread is not uncommon and may lead to recurrence or spread to the central nervous system. Unlike other head and neck SCCs, the degree of involvement of cervical lymph nodes is not completely clear, and therefore treatment of the neck is controversial, and will be discussed later in this chapter.

The maxillary sinus is the most common site of sinonasal ACC. Histologic patterns of ACC include cribriform, tubular, and solid; the solid subtype has the worst prognosis. The

Table 16.2 AJCC Staging for Epithelial Malignancies of the Maxillary Sinus

T1	Limited to maxillary sinus without bony erosion/ destruction
T2	Bone erosion/destruction with extension into the middle meatus or hard palate
T3	Involvement of the posterior wall of the maxillary sinus, pterygopalatine fossa, ethmoid sinuses, medial or inferior orbital wall, or soft tissue
T4	Moderately advanced
T4a	Involvement of pterygoid plates, cribriform plate, infratemporal fossa, sphenoid or frontal sinuses, or skin
T4b	Very advanced Involvement of orbital apex, dura, brain, nasopharynx, or clivus, or any cranial nerve other than V2

Adapted from reference 40.

AJCC, Amnerican Joint Committe on Cancer.

5-year survival rates have been reported to range from approximately 60 to 70%.[5] Rates of perineural invasion (PNI) of 20 to 80% have been described for ACC,[6] which may be related to its high-recurrence rate despite aggressive surgical treatment and postoperative radiation.[5] Recurrence and distant metastases are common, the lung being the most common site. In a recent series of 105 patients from MD Anderson, most patients presented with advanced stage (T3/T4) disease and 98% of the patients were node negative. Thirty percent of the patients developed distant metastases, 40% of the patients had PNI, and 65% of the patients treated with postoperative radiation eventually developed recurrence. A significant survival advantage was found for patients treated with surgery and postoperative radiation over other treatments.[5]

Neuroendocrine tumors of the sinuses have been divided into four subtypes: esthesioneuroblastoma (ENB), sinonasal undifferentiated carcinoma (SNUC), neuroendocrine carcinoma, and small cell carcinoma (SmCC). Because of prognosis, these have been divided into ENB and non-ENB categories. ENB has the best prognosis by far, followed by SNUC and neuroendocrine carcinoma; SmCC has the worst prognosis.[7] Neuroendocrine tumors of the nasal cavity and paranasal sinuses typically involve the olfactory epithelium most frequently, but cases of maxillary ENB,[8] SmCC,[9] SNUC,[10] and neuroendocrine carcinoma have been reported.[11] The Kadish staging system is used for ENB (**Table 16.3**). Because of the patterns of failure, the treatment for ENB is usually limited to local therapy, including surgery and/or radiation, and multimodality therapy including chemotherapy for non-ENB neuroendocrine tumors due to their propensity for distant metastasis.[7] The optimal sequence for the management of SNUC is controversial; definitive radiation may increase the resectability of a tumor, but it carries a higher risk of radiation damage to surrounding structures.

Table 16.3 Kadish Staging for Olfactory Esthesioneuroblastoma

Stage A	Confined to nasal cavity
Stage B	Tumor extending into paranasal sinuses
Stage C	Orbital, skull base, or cranial extent, or distant metastases

Craniofacial resection, radiation, chemotherapy, and treatment of the neck should all be considered because of the propensity for cervical and distant metastases.

Nonepithelial soft tissue malignancies of the paranasal sinuses are rare and include many subtypes, many of which have only been published as case reports and series.[1] Rhabdomyosarcoma is the most common paranasal sinus malignancy in childhood and is classified as parameningeal when involving the sinuses. It is divided into four subtypes: (1) embryonal, which presents early in life; (2) alveolar, which presents in the second decade of life; (3) pleomorph and; (4) mixed.[1] The embryonal form has the best prognosis. Sinonasal rhabdomyosarcoma presents in adults as well, but much less frequently. Prognosis is worse than in children, with a 5-year survival rate of 30% for adults compared with approximately 70% for children, according to a study of 171 patients and literature review in Italy.[12] However, this may represent differences in histologic subtypes and treatment regimens. Multimodality therapy is required for the treatment of these aggressive tumors; chemoradiation is the treatment of choice for advanced tumors, with surgical intervention for residual disease. Early stage tumors may be resected initially if there is no skull base invasion; complete excision is possible, and cosmetic deformity is minimal.[13]

Sinonasal tract mucosal malignant melanoma (STMMM) may have an appearance similar to that of neuroendocrine and soft tissue tumors described above, but immunohistochemical stains are positive for S-100, melan A, tyrosinase, and HMB-45. It is a rare tumor that accounts for only up to 2% of all melanomas and 4% of head and neck melanomas; it typically presents in the sixth to seventh decades of life. Compared with other melanomas and mucosal melanomas, it has a poorer prognosis, with a 5-year survival rate of only 20 to 40% and a high propensity for distant metastasis (> 50%). Several staging systems have been proposed for STMMM, including the widely used system proposed by Ballantyne, which classifies localized melanomas (stage I), those with cervical lymphadenopathy (stage II), and those with distant metastases (stage III),[14] and the AJCC maxillary sinus staging system[4] (**Table 16.1**). A recent publication from the MD Anderson Cancer Center reported a 5-year survival rate of 27.3% for tumors specifically within the maxillary sinus. Treatment is typically multimodality, involving surgical resection, postoperative radiation, and sometimes chemotherapy. However, in the MD Anderson series, overall survival was not improved with radiation chemotherapy, or immunotherapy, although

locoregional recurrence was less in patients treated with > 54 Gy than in patients treated with 30 to 50 Gy.[15]

Benign and malignant tumors of odontogenic origin can also involve the maxillary sinus via extension from the maxillary alveolus. They may arise at any age and are classified into three categories by the World Health Organization according to the odontogenic tissue of origin.[16] Tumors may present with similar signs and symptoms to other maxillary sinus tumors, but may also present with dental symptoms including alveolar swelling or pain, loose teeth, or change in occlusion. Although benign odontogenic tumors and cysts grow slowly, malignant tumors may present more rapidly and with pain or paresthesias. Odontogenic tumors vary in radiographic appearance depending on their origin, but they are based on erupted or unerupted maxillary teeth. The most common odontogenic tumor is the odontoma, a well-differentiated tumor based on mesenchymal and epithelial tooth elements. It is treated with simple removal, has no malignant potential, and does not recur. Ameloblastoma is the second most common tumor of odontogenic origin, is epithelial in origin, and is aggressively invasive. It is more common in the mandible than in the maxilla. Treatment is excision along with a rim of normal tissue due to its high rate of recurrence.[16] Keratocysticodontogenic tumors, formerly known as odontogenickeratocysts, are aggressive, recurrent parakeratinized epithelial cysts that may occur sporadically or be associated with Gorlin syndrome. Aggressive surgical treatment may be required for cure.

Numerous metastatic tumors to the paranasal sinuses have been described, most frequently from the kidney, and the maxillary sinus is the most frequently affected sinus.[17] Endoscopic biopsy should confirm the diagnosis, and treatment should be directed at relieving symptoms. Hematopoietic malignancies, including lymphomas, may also arise within the sinonasal tract, including the maxillary sinus. The role of the surgeon is diagnostic, and treatment should entail expedient referral to a medical oncologist.

Prognosis

Tumors of the maxillary sinus commonly present with advanced stage because of minimal symptomatology until expansion beyond its boundaries. Ohngren noted in 1933 that tumors of the paranasal sinuses that arise superior to an imaginary line drawn from the medial canthus to the angle of the mandible had a worse prognosis than those arising inferior to the line. Poor prognostic factors in carcinomas of the maxillary sinus have been found to be advanced age, advanced T stage (T4), node positivity (associated with distant metastases), and male sex.[18,19] A study from Memorial Sloan-Kettering Cancer Center recently demonstrated that PNI is common in ACC, SCC, and SNUC (55, 60, and 30%, respectively). The study found that PNI is associated with positive margins, but its effect on survival is disputed.[6] Field cancerization seen in other head and neck primaries appears to be less significant in

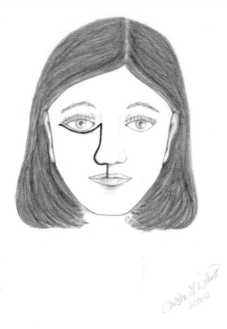

Figure 16.1 Depending on the amount of exposure necessary to resect the tumor, lateral rhinotomy (black), Weber-Ferguson (green), and lip split (red) may be necessary. (*Credit to artist for recreating:* Christina S.T. Wilhoit, Research Specialist, Department of Otolaryngology–Head and Neck Surgery, Medical University of South Carolina, Charleston, South Carolina, United States.)

sinonasal tumors. A review of 2475 patients treated for sinonasal head and neck SCC at Johns Hopkins University revealed 0.2% incidence of a second sinonasal primary cancer.[20] In addition, although its role has not been defined, investigators at the MD Anderson Cancer Center found that in stage III/IV SCCs of the paranasal sinuses, response to induction chemotherapy was predictive of better prognosis and improved treatment outcome in patients treated with definitive surgical treatment or concurrent chemoradiotherapy.[21] Local failure remains the most common cause of mortality in patients with maxillary sinus cancers; 5-year local control rates fall in the 55 to 60% range, and 5-year overall survival rate has been reported to be approximately 45% in a recent review of the literature.[22]

Surgical Approaches

Surgical resection of benign and malignant tumors remains the mainstay of treatment. External access, including midface degloving and lateral rhinotomy, are the traditional approaches used (**Figs. 16.1** and **16.2**). Total maxillectomy involves removal of the entire maxillary structure with or without orbital exenteration. Open en-bloc medial maxillectomy was described in 1977 by Sessions as a modification of the procedure to spare the eye, palate, and facial structure. With the development of sophisticated optics and endoscopic instruments, more and more surgeons are advocating endoscopic resection for removal of

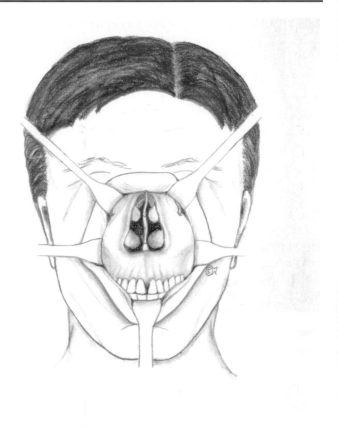

Figure 16.2 Midfacial degloving exposure. (*Credit to artist for recreating:* Christina S.T. Wilhoit, Research Specialist, Department of Otolaryngology–Head and Neck Surgery, Medical University of South Carolina, Charleston, South Carolina, United States.)

benign tumors, including IP.[3] Harvey et al divided the nasal cavity into five zones that may be accessed intranasally with different instruments and approaches, including maxillary antrostomy/medial maxillectomy (zone 2), medial buttress resection/nasolacrimal duct resection (zone 3), transseptal approach and anterior maxillary drilling (zone 4), and an open approach (zone 5).[23] The role of endoscopic resection has been controversial for malignant tumors of the paranasal sinuses and skull base, although multiple reports have demonstrated good outcomes with preservation of oncologic cure in the endoscopic group. However, the advanced presentation of most maxillary sinus tumors often necessitates palatal and soft tissue resection, although endoscopic tumor mapping and endoscopic-assisted resection may be of benefit. Endoscopic-assisted resection of less bulky sinonasal melanomas has been described with success in appropriately selected patients.[15]

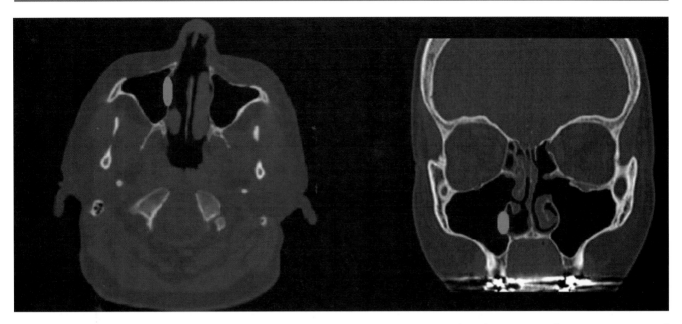

Figure 16.3 Axial and coronal depiction of a medially based tumor that does not extend into the palate or surrounding structures. Potential surgical approaches include endoscopic medial maxillectomy, midfacial degloving, or lateral rhinotomy.

Figs. 16.3 to **16.5** show examples of tumor locations and proposed surgical approaches.

Adjuvant Treatment and Treatment of the Neck

Treatment of the clinically negative neck is controversial.[24,25] Ipsilateral levels I and II are most commonly involved, and a wide range of incidences of initial and delayed nodal metastasis has been reported. For carcinomas of the maxillary sinus, a combination of surgery and radiotherapy has been shown to improve local control and survival compared with radiation alone.[18] Involvement of retropharyngeal nodes is possible with spread to the hard palate; attention should be paid to these nodes while imaging given potential patterns of spread, although definitive evidence is lacking. According to the National Comprehensive Cancer Network guidelines, postoperative radiation is recommended to the primary site

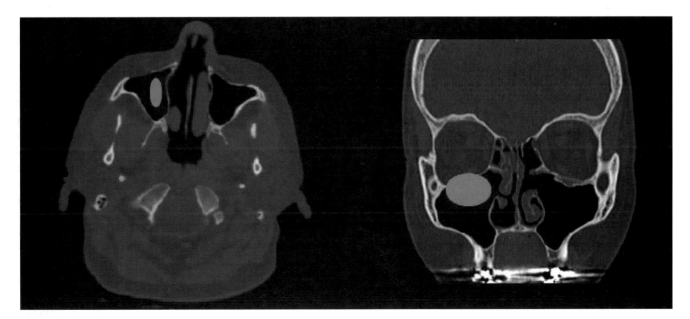

Figure 16.4 Axial and coronal depiction of a superiorly based tumor involving the orbital floor. Potential approaches include lateral rhinotomy or Weber-Ferguson, combined open and endoscopic, or combined midfacial degloving and lateral rhinotomy.

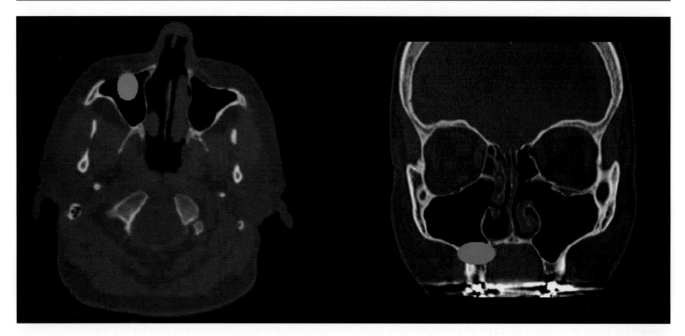

Figure 16.5 Axial and coronal depiction of an inferiorly based tumor involving the maxillary alveolar ridge and palate. Midfacial degloving or lateral rhinotomy with lip split may be considered.

in T1-2N0 with PNI and T3-4aN0 without adverse features, and to both the primary and the neck after resection and neck dissection in node-positive patients without adverse features. Postoperative chemoradiation to the primary site and the neck is recommended for patients with T3-4a tumors with adverse features regardless of nodal status. Patients with T4b tumors may be treated with definitive radiotherapy or chemoradiation or enrolled in a clinical trial.[4] Gamma knife radiosurgery and proton beam therapy have been reported as case reports in the literature for patients with locally advanced tumors.[26,27]

A large study of paranasal sinus tumors including 399 maxillary sinus tumors reported 8.3% node-positive disease at the time of treatment across all histologies. The rate was higher in SCC (10.3%) and SNUC (15.4%). The authors of that study now advocate elective neck irradiation or neck dissection T2N0 or greater tumors, based on a 5-year delayed neck failure rate of 18%; this rate of failure was even higher in SCC (26%).[19] The authors postulate that T2 tumors behave in the same way as oral cavity tumors because of their involvement of the hard palate, which has a richer lymphatic network than the nasal cavity and sinuses. A study of 97 patients treated with radiotherapy for maxillary sinus cancer by Le et al revealed a similar rate of delayed nodal metastasis for SCC (14%); however, no neck relapses were noted in T2 tumors.[18]

The role of neck dissection for sinonasal rhabdomyosarcoma is controversial, with some authors advocating follow-up only and others advocating for elective neck dissection (END) in the alveolar subtype when surgery is a treatment modality.[13] As in other head and neck melanomas and mucosal melanomas, END is not routinely performed. However, adjuvant radiation may help improve locoregional control.[15]

As in other cancers of the head and neck region, the role of induction chemotherapy has not been completely elucidated, but it may provide prognostic value and guide surgical versus nonsurgical treatment.[21] Ongoing research and clinical trials will likely provide valuable information in the near future.

Reconstruction

Several classification systems have been proposed for surgical defects involving the maxilla. At our institution, the defects are classified by a system similar to those proposed by Brown et al and Okay et al, which address the horizontal and vertical components of the defect.[28,29] The option to reconstruct the defect versus plan for obturation should be discussed thoroughly with the patient preoperatively, considering the patient's long-term prognosis and medical comorbidities that would preclude a complex, lengthy reconstructive procedure. The advantages of obturation include decreased perioperative risk, improved surveillance, and excellent speech and swallowing outcomes. However, patients may be dissatisfied with obturator cleaning and maintenance, appearance, discomfort, air escape around the obturator, and the need for adjustment. Most importantly, a skilled prosthodontist is needed to fashion and fit a functional prosthesis (**Figs. 16.6** to **16.8**).

Reconstructive options include local or regional pedicled flaps and free tissue transfer. Pedicled flaps include the rotational palatal flap, buccal flap, submental island flap, and temporalis flap. Free flap options include fasciocutaneous or myocutaneous flaps and osseocutaneous flaps, which provide more structural support and the possibility of

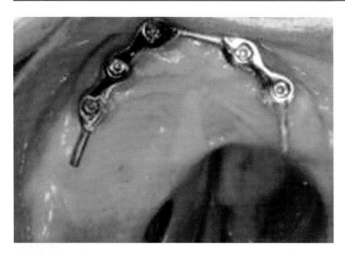

Figure 16.6 This patient has had a subtotal resection of her left secondary palate and soft palate. Permanent implants were placed by a skilled prosthodontist for definitive obturation.

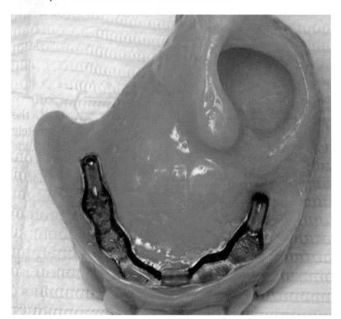

Figure 16.7 Definitive obturator for the patient shown in Fig. 16.6.

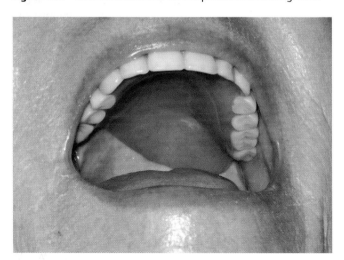

Figure 16.8 Definitive obturator in place.

dental implants (**Figs. 16.9** and **16.10**). Choosing the appropriate reconstructive material should take into account the composition of the defect in size and material, overall health of the patient, and the potential need for future dental rehabilitation. Preoperative consultation with a skilled maxillofacial prosthodontist and a microvascular reconstructive surgeon is advised.

Studies comparing obturation and free flap outcomes have been scarce in the literature. The largest study to our knowledge compared 10 obturated patients and 18 patients who underwent free tissue transfer. Satisfaction outcomes were similar, but there was a borderline trend for obturator patients to have more pain, report concern about their appearance and upper teeth, and report lower satisfaction.[30]

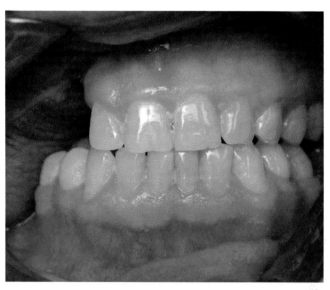

Figure 16.9 Free-flap reconstruction of a palatal and cheek defect.

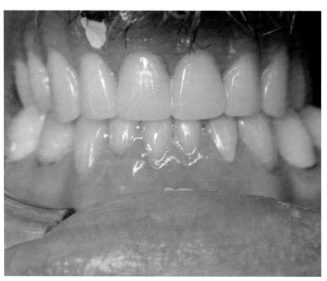

Figure 16.10 A patient with free-flap reconstruction of the hard palate; resection appliance in place.

Pearls and Pitfalls

- In cases that require total or partial maxillectomy, tracheostomy is not always necessary.

- If a lip-splitting incision is required, careful reapproximation of the vermilion border is paramount for the best postoperative cosmesis.

- Large maxillary defects do not heal by secondary intention; split-thickness skin grafting and bolstering or free-flap reconstruction is typically required for successful healing.

- Resection of the coronoid process of the mandible is required for successful obturation.

- Gauze packing and antibiotics should be maintained after skin grafting of the maxillary defects for 5 to 7 days.

- Free-flap reconstruction of the maxilla and palate requires a long pedicle length, and every effort should be made to preserve the maximal length of the facial artery and vein in preparation for the anastomosis.

- Involvement of the premaxilla is a determining factor in reconstruction; it portends a poor prognosis with obturation.

- Patients with orbital floor involvement are poor obturator candidates.

- Failure to evaluate for perineural invasion of the pterygopalatine fossa and V2, especially in adenoid cystic carcinoma, may lead to recurrence.

- Orbital exenteration should be avoided unless there is involvement of the orbital soft tissues.

References

1. Götte K, Hörmann K. Sinonasal malignancy: what's new? ORL J Otorhinolaryngol Relat Spec 2004;66(2):85–97

2. Krouse JH. Endoscopic treatment of inverted papilloma: safety and efficacy. Am J Otolaryngol 2001;22(2):87–99

3. Reh DD, Lane AP. The role of endoscopic sinus surgery in the management of sinonasal inverted papilloma. Curr Opin Otolaryngol Head Neck Surg 2009;17(1):6–10

4. National Comprehensive Cancer Network. Head and neck cancers: NCCN clinical practice guidelines in oncology. 2010. Available from: www.nccn.org. Accessed 9/2/2010

5. Lupinetti AD, Roberts DB, Williams MD, et al. Sinonasal adenoid cystic carcinoma: the M. D. Anderson Cancer Center experience. Cancer 2007;110(12):2726–2731

6. Gil Z, Carlson DL, Gupta A, et al. Patterns and incidence of neural invasion in patients with cancers of the paranasal sinuses. Arch Otolaryngol Head Neck Surg 2009;135(2):173–179

7. Rosenthal DI, Barker JL Jr, El-Naggar AK, et al. Sinonasal malignancies with neuroendocrine differentiation: patterns of failure according to histologic phenotype. Cancer 2004;101(11):2567–2573

8. Bitiutskiĭ PG, Kozhanov LG, Kats VA, Volchenko NN. [Esthesioneuroblastoma of the maxillary sinus]. Sov Med 1983;(7):91–92

9. Renner G. Small cell carcinoma of the head and neck: a review. Semin Oncol 2007;34(1):3–14

10. Sharara N, Muller S, Olson J, Grist WJ, Grossniklaus HE. Sinonasal undifferentiated carcinoma with orbital invasion: report of three cases. Ophthal Plast Reconstr Surg 2001;17(4):288–292

11. Yamamoto R, Hosokawa S, Yamatodani T, Morita S, Okamura J, Mineta H. [Eight cases of neuroendcrine carcinoma of the head and neck]. Nippon JibiinkokaGakkaiKaiho 2008;111(7):517–522

12. Ferrari A, Dileo P, Casanova M, et al. Rhabdomyosarcoma in adults: a retrospective analysis of 171 patients treated at a single institution. Cancer 2003;98(3):571–580

13. Gradoni P, Giordano D, Oretti G, Fantoni M, Ferri T. The role of surgery in children with head and neck rhabdomyosarcoma and Ewing's sarcoma. Surg Oncol 2010;19(4):e103–e109

14. Ballantyne AJ. Malignant melanoma of the skin of the head and neck: an analysis of 405 cases. Am J Surg 1970;120(4):425–431

15. Moreno MA, Roberts DB, Kupferman ME, et al. Mucosal melanoma of the nose and paranasal sinuses, a contemporary experience from the M. D. Anderson Cancer Center. Cancer 2010;116(9):2215–2223

16. Press SG. Odontogenic tumors of the maxillary sinus. Curr Opin Otolaryngol Head Neck Surg 2008;16(1):47–54

17. Prescher A, Brors D. [Metastases to the paranasal sinuses: case report and review of the literature]. Laryngorhinootologie 2001;80(10):583–594

18. Le QT, Fu KK, Kaplan M, Terris DJ, Fee WE, Goffinet DR. Treatment of maxillary sinus carcinoma: a comparison of the 1997 and 1977 American Joint Committee on Cancer staging systems. Cancer 1999;86(9):1700–1711

19. Cantù G, Bimbi G, Miceli R, et al. Lymph node metastases in malignant tumors of the paranasal sinuses: prognostic value and treatment. Arch Otolaryngol Head Neck Surg 2008;134(2):170–177

20. Wolpoe ME, Goldenberg D, Koch WM. Squamous cell carcinoma of the sinonasal cavity arising as a second primary in individuals with head and neck cancer. Laryngoscope 2006;116(5):696–699

21. Hanna EY, Cardenas AD, DeMonte F, et al. Induction chemotherapy for advanced squamous cell carcinoma of the paranasal sinuses. Arch Otolaryngol Head Neck Surg 2011;137(1):78–81

22. Khademi B, Moradi A, Hoseini S, Mohammadianpanah M. Malignant neoplasms of the sinonasal tract: report of 71 patients and literature review and analysis. Oral Maxillofac Surg 2009;13(4):191–199

23. Harvey RJ, Sheehan PO, Debnath NI, Schlosser RJ. Transseptal approach for extended endoscopic resections of the maxilla and infratemporal fossa. Am J Rhinol Allergy 2009;23(4):426–432

24. Dulguerov P, Jacobsen MS, Allal AS, Lehmann W, Calcaterra T. Nasal and paranasal sinus carcinoma: are we making progress? A series of 220 patients and a systematic review. Cancer 2001;92(12):3012–3029

25. Katz TS, Mendenhall WM, Morris CG, Amdur RJ, Hinerman RW, Villaret DB. Malignant tumors of the nasal cavity and paranasal sinuses. Head Neck 2002;24(9):821–829

26. Kawaguchi K, Yamada H, Horie A, Sato K. Radiosurgical treatment of maxillary squamous cell carcinoma. Int J Oral Maxillofac Surg 2009;38(11):1205–1207

27. Chera BS, Malyapa R, Louis D, et al. Proton therapy for maxillary sinus carcinoma. Am J Clin Oncol 2009;32(3):296–303

28. Brown JS, Rogers SN, McNally DN, Boyle M. A modified classification for the maxillectomy defect. Head Neck 2000;22(1):17–26

29. Okay DJ, Genden E, Buchbinder D, Urken M. Prosthodontic guidelines for surgical reconstruction of the maxilla: a classification system of defects. J Prosthet Dent 2001;86(4):352–363

30. Rogers SN, Lowe D, McNally D, Brown JS, Vaughan ED. Health-related quality of life after maxillectomy: a comparison between prosthetic obturation and free flap. J Oral Maxillofac Surg 2003;61(2):174–181

17 The Unknown Primary

Allen O. Mitchell and Brent R. Driskill

Core Messages

- Evaluation of the unknown primary mandates a methodical process.

- A thorough history and physical examination is beneficial in the identification of a primary lesion.

- The location of lymph node metastases can guide the identification of the primary tumor.

- Although the examination and biopsy in the clinic may be definitive, evaluation in the operating room is often necessary.

- Identification of the primary decreases patient morbidity via more focused radiation therapy portals.

- A positron emission tomography scan is complementary to history, physical examination, triple endoscopy with biopsy, and conventional imaging.

The views expressed in this chapter are those of the authors and do not necessarily reflect the official policy or position of the Department of Navy, the Department of Defense, or the U.S. government.

I am a military service member. This work was prepared as part of my official duties. Title 17 U.S.C. 106 provides that "Copyright protection under this title is not available for any work of the United States Government." Title 17 U.S.C. 101 defines a U.S. government work as a work prepared by a military service member or employee of the U.S. government as part of a person's official duties.

Carcinoma of unknown primary (CUP) is defined as the presence of histologically confirmed metastatic cancer in a patient without an identifiable primary tumor despite a standardized diagnostic approach that includes medical history, physical examination, appropriate laboratories, panendoscopy, and conventional imaging.

Metastasis to a regional lymph node is often the initial presentation of a primary head and neck carcinoma. Although the primary lesion may often be readily identified during a thorough head and neck examination, in 3 to 5% of the cases there is no apparent aerodigestive lesion.[1] Recent advances in imaging hold promise for improved detection; however, the work-up of the patient with CUP remains a challenge. Discovery of the primary tumor improves patient morbidity by decreasing the necessary volume of irradiated tissue. In a small percentage of patients, the primary will not be identified after a thorough evaluation including fiberoptic nasopharyngeal and laryngeal endoscopy, panendoscopy with biopsies, and appropriate imaging. Controversy surrounds the further evaluation and management of this patient population.

Background

The true incidence of CUP of the head and neck has not been definitively determined. American Cancer Society (ACS) data from 2010 lists the incidence of "Other & unspecified primary sites" as 30,680 for an incidence of 2% of all cancers. This number has been consistent with previous years. However, there is no specific data for cervical squamous cell CUP versus other anatomic locations. The estimated number of deaths is 44,030 for an overall cancer death rate of 7%. The larger number of deaths versus incidence may reflect lack of specificity in recording the underlying cause of death or an undercount in the case estimate.[2] The true rate of CUP could be estimated at around 2%, possibly lower because of other anatomic sites being included in the ACS numbers or higher because of undercounting of cases. One interesting question that could not be answered in our data review is whether the true incidence of CUP is decreasing in response to advances in imaging technology. This question will probably remain elusive because of the relative infrequency of head and neck squamous cell carcinoma (HNSCC) of unknown primary. In addition, a patient who is identified as having CUP may later develop a primary tumor, thereby removing himself or herself from the CUP population. A commonly quoted estimate of the incidence of CUP in multiple references is 2 to 9% of all head and neck cancers (HNCs). It includes numerous tumor types and locations. Squamous cell carcinoma is responsible for 90% of all cervical metastasis of unknown primary.[3]

The risk factors for CUP are the same as those for known primary squamous cell carcinoma of the head and neck: alcohol, tobacco exposure, and human papillomavirus (HPV).

Different theories attempt to explain the phenomenon of the unknown primary. One thought is that the primary exists and the work-up just failed to locate it; however, even long-term follow-up often fails to identify a primary tumor. Other theories are that the primary tumor regressed after early metastasis or that the tumor sloughed off into the digestive tract.

The most common presentation of CUP is a new, painless neck mass, increasing in size, present in a patient with a long history of tobacco and alcohol abuse. HPV-related carcinoma may present in patients without the tobacco and alcohol history. The absence of the most common presentation should not preclude a thorough evaluation.

Diagnosis

Localization of the primary tumor is paramount to reduction of patient morbidity and will allow for surgical resection and/or a higher radiation dosage to the site of the primary, thereby decreasing overall patient morbidity.

History

The first, and most critical, step in the evaluation of any patient with a new cervical mass is a thorough history and physical examination. The temporal development of the mass, location, and changes in size and color should be noted. The history should include etiologic factors: tobacco and alcohol history as well as standard HNC review of system questions (**Table 17.1**). Consideration should also be made for environmental exposures that put patients at risk for nasopharyngeal squamous cell carcinoma: wood dust and nickel exposure. Recent immigration from China or Hong Kong could indicate an increased risk of nasopharyngeal carcinoma. Medical and surgical history should be reviewed. Often, the HNC patient population has significant comorbidities that preclude aggressive therapy. Ensure you ask your patient about pertinent drug allergies.

Physical Examination

All skin areas of the head and neck should be inspected. Careful visualization and palpation of hair-bearing scalp

Table 17.1 Questions for History-Taking

History of head and neck carcinoma/skin cancer
Dysphagia/aspiration
Unintentional weight loss
Night sweats
Hoarseness
Odynophagia
Hemoptysis
New masses or ulcers
Stridor
Change in denture fit
Otalgia
Unexplained fevers

areas is required. Physical examination consists of direct inspection of all pharyngeal and laryngeal mucosal surfaces. Palpation of the tongue base and tonsils can reveal subtle masses not appreciated on visual examination and should be performed on every patient who can tolerate it. The neck should be palpated, and the level of the mass should be determined. A small subset of patients will have multiple neck metastases. Levels II and III are the most common neck levels of presentation. Direct examination with a mirror may allow visualization of the laryngeal anatomy; however, a patient with a severe gag-reflex will often allow only a limited view. Fiberoptic examination is the preferred method for evaluation in nearly all cases (**Fig. 17.1**). After proper topical anesthesia and vasoconstriction, this modality allows an excellent view that is well tolerated by most patients and is recordable for documentation, peer review, and later comparison.

Location of the Mass

The mass location can indicate a likely primary source. **Table 17.2** illustrates potential primary sites on the basis of the location of the cervical metastases. Special consideration should be given to occipital nodes for a scalp primary and supraclavicular nodes for a nonhead and neck primary.

Laboratory Studies

Screening laboratory studies of the patient with CUP should include complete blood cell count, liver-associated enzymes, and thyroid function tests, modified as appropriate for any comorbidities. The usefulness of routine screening laboratories has been questioned in the general population,[4] however; HNC patients have a higher prevalence of comorbidities and often undergo larger surgical procedures. This fact may justify the routine usage of screening laboratories in these patients.

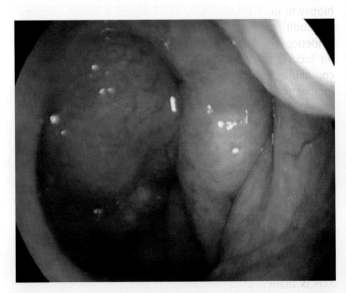

Figure 17.1 Examination of the nasopharynx may reveal the primary lesion, in this case a nasopharyngeal carcinoma.

Table 17.2 Lymph Node Metastases—Potential Primary Sites

Level	Possible Primary
Ia	Floor of mouth, oral tongue
Ib	Mandibular alveolus, floor of mouth, oral tongue, retromolar trigone, pharynx, oropharynx
II	Ib sites, plus supraglottis, piriform, glottis
III	Tongue, oropharynx, supraglottis, piriform, glottis
IV	Pharynx, oropharynx, piriform, supraglottis
V	Oropharynx
Occipital	Scalp
Supraclavicular node	Discuss possibility of nonhead and neck origin and likely sites: breast, lung, gastrointestinal tract associated with thoracic duct

Adapted from reference 16.

Some authors have recommended testing for Epstein-Barr virus antibody titers in the setting of nonkeratinizing or poorly differentiated carcinoma, when a nasopharyngeal primary might be suspected. As noted by Neel in 1985, positive viral capsid antigen IgA and early antigen tests may indicate the presence of World Health Organization type 2 and 3 nasopharyngeal carcinomas. Patients with type 1 carcinoma exhibit a lower incidence of these antigen responses.[5]

Tissue Diagnosis

After history and physical examination, fine-needle aspiration (FNA) will provide the best opportunity for the diagnosis of malignancy. Traditionally, incisional/excisional biopsy of neck masses has been discouraged because of the possibility of hindering cure. However, there is contradictory evidence in the literature about the effect of open biopsy on locoregional control and ultimate survival. The most compelling reason to first consider nonsurgical techniques for diagnosis is that there is a high probability that a diagnosis may be made without resorting to open biopsy.

FNA, either direct or under ultrasound guidance, can usually be performed in an office setting. Whenever possible, the aspirate should be assessed for adequacy during the procedure. In our institution, a cytopathology technician is called to the clinic room. **Fig. 17.2** illustrates a typical setup for this procedure. The patient's skin is prepped with alcohol or Betadine swabs and draped with a blue towel. Local anesthesia with lidocaine is infrequently required. A 22- to 25-gauge needle is connected to either suction tubing or a biopsy gun. Insertion into the tumor along the long axis is made. When the bevel of the needle is subdermal, suction is applied. Some surgeons prefer not to use suction. Gentle back-and-forth motion is made for several passes.

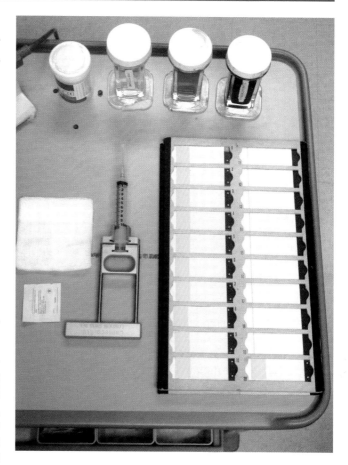

Figure 17.2 Setup for fine-needle aspiration.

Then, the needle is withdrawn off suction and passed to the cytopathologist for immediate staining and a preliminary read.

Cellular analysis of the aspirate or surgical specimen by the pathologist with light microscopy, special staining, immunohistochemistry, and even electron microscopy can aid in determining tissue origin. The ease of diagnosis of tissue type is related to the degree of differentiation in the tumor. For poorly differentiated tumors, more complex analysis is often necessary. Special staining for keratin, S-100, or mucin can aid in diagnosis. Electron microscopy can detect cellular features not seen with light microscopy. DNA amplification of Epstein-Barr virus has been used to detect occult nasopharyngeal carcinoma. **Figs. 17.3** and **17.4** illustrate the FNA appearance of moderately differentiated squamous cell carcinoma.

The great majority of tumors will be classified as squamous cell carcinoma, likely relating to the most common site of origin in Waldeyer ring. However, other sites of origin should be considered. The thyroid, parathyroid, cervical nerves, and larynx can produce neck masses. The possibility of distant metastasis to the neck should also be considered, especially with level 4 and 5 neck masses. Establishing the tissue diagnosis of squamous cell carcinoma in the first clinical visit can greatly aid in diagnostic and therapeutic planning. This knowledge may also help determine the need for dental

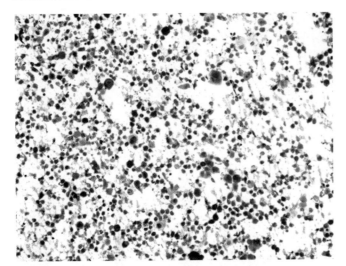

Figure 17.3 Light micrograph of fine-needle aspiration specimen. Magnification ×20.

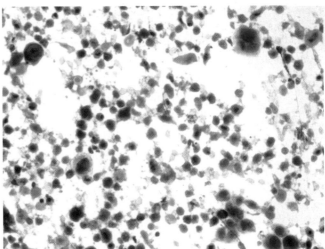

Figure 17.4 Light micrograph of fine-needle aspiration specimen. Magnification ×40.

extractions. Hematology/oncology and radiation oncology consults can also be made confidently. Once a diagnosis of carcinoma is made, insurance approval for positron emission tomography (PET) scanning can also be secured.

Imaging

Before the direct laryngoscopy with biopsy, imaging should be performed to allow for more directed biopsies. The common patient population at risk for CUP has significant risk factors for lung cancer. Screening for pulmonary metastasis, whether by chest radiograph, computed tomography (CT) scan, magnetic resonance imaging (MRI), or 2-[fluorine-18] fluoro-2-deoxy-d-glucose (FDG)-PET, is necessary. Discovery of a new lung mass could be the source of metastasis or a synchronous primary, either of which would significantly alter the patient's staging and treatment.

CT with contrast remains the best initial radiographic study. PET is usually not undertaken until a firm diagnosis of malignancy is made. Traditionally, plain chest radiography served to screen for metastases, but more recently, CT scanning of the chest with cuts thorough the liver has provided a more precise evaluation. The likelihood of benign incidental findings complicating the work-up must be considered. Sinus X-rays were also commonly performed in the past; however, CT scanning of the head and neck has largely replaced this practice. Some practitioners perform CT scanning of the chest in lieu of bronchoscopy. Contrast radiography of the esophagus has also been used in place of esophagoscopy.

More recently, PET scanning has become more popular, though its cost and low sensitivity for smaller lesions must be considered. PET scanning has been shown to be insensitive for lesions smaller than 0.5 to 1 cm. The sensitivity of PET is 31% for detecting a primary lesion and 20% in patients who have had negative previous imaging. MRI may also be considered, though its cost is higher versus that of CT, has increased acquisition time, and similar sensitivity.

Evaluation in the Operating Room

If examination in the clinic setting fails to identify a primary lesion, examination under anesthesia is indicated. Traditionally, this consists of direct laryngoscopy with nasopharyngoscopy, and rigid or flexible bronchoscopy and esophagoscopy. Direct laryngoscopy should include visualization of all subsites of the oral cavity, oropharynx, hypopharynx, supraglottis, and glottis. The tonsils and base of tongue should be palpated with the patient fully relaxed. Some providers prefer to use a high-definition (HD) Hopkins rod attached to an HD monitor to visualize the subsites. This provides a closer view, multiple provider review, recording, and discussion. The nasal cavity and nasopharynx should be suctioned and a Hopkins rod passed for visualization. Straight forceps can be passed in the opposite nostril for directed biopsy. Rigid or flexible bronchoscopy and esophagoscopy can be performed on the basis of provider preference. Often, direct laryngoscopy with biopsy of the tumor is performed, and then all other procedures are performed while the frozen section is analyzed. **Figs. 17.5** and **17.6** illustrate typical setup, instruments used, and examination technique.

If no abnormality on direct laryngoscopy is noted, random or directed biopsies should be performed. CUP biopsy forceps typically provide adequate tissue when sampling all directed biopsy sites with the exception of the tonsils. Directed biopsies of the base of tongue, nasopharynx, and piriform sinuses are recommended.[6] However, no data exist to support or refute this practice. The detection rate of random guided (directed) biopsies ranges from 5 to 16%.[7]

The tonsils are a large volume of tissue and a common source of occult malignancy.[8] A small biopsy of the tonsil has an unacceptable rate of a false-negative test result. If tonsils are present, tonsillectomy should be performed. The primary tumor detection rate for tonsillectomy ranged from 17 to 39% in a recent systematic literature review of 39 articles.[7] In this same review, 4 of 3291 patients had an occult tonsillar primary in the contralateral tonsil.[7] When tonsillectomy has

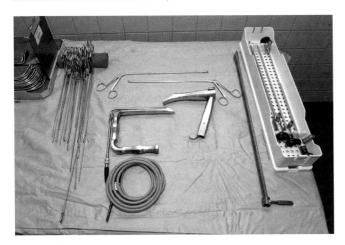

Figure 17.5 Basic instrumentation of panendoscopy includes laryngoscopes, esophagoscope, Hopkin rods, biopsy instruments, and suction.

been previously performed, biopsy of the tonsillar fossae is advised. When primary tumors are located, whether during initial work-up or in a delayed fashion, the greatest majority are located in either the tonsil or the tongue base.[7]

In patients with a high index of suspicion for metastatic squamous cell carcinoma, open biopsy may be considered with preparations for definitive treatment if the frozen biopsy is positive. A high degree of trust in the frozen section analysis is required with this strategy. A false positive on the frozen section would result in unnecessary surgical procedures and increased morbidity. In addition to the diagnostic evaluation, additional procedures to include dental extractions and percutaneous endoscopic gastrostomy are often performed.

Positron Emission Tomography

PET is a nuclear medicine study in which a radionuclide is injected into the bloodstream of a patient and absorbed by metabolically active tissue. The tracer used is FDG, an analogue of glucose, which is absorbed intracellularly in greater quantities by more metabolic cells, such as brain or malignant cells. The FDG is taken up by cells in the normal glucose pathway, but it becomes trapped because of the 2-deoxy addition. Within these metabolically active cells, the FDG undergoes decay and emits a positron, a positively charged particle that is the opposite of an electron. Within a short distance, the positron encounters an electron and their mutual annihilation produces two gamma rays traveling in opposite directions.

The detector in a PET scanner is a ring around the patient that can detect the oppositely moving photons at the same or close to the same instant. Roughly, the middle point in a straight line between these points represents the source and would be represented on the image produced as a point of uptake. The image is produced in a similar fashion to a CT scan; however, the number of data points is approximately 1000 times less, therefore producing a less precise image. Three-

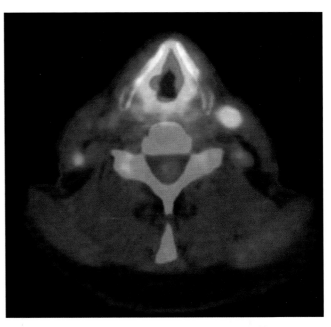

Figure 17.6 This positron emission tomography-computed tomography image fusion shows a hypermetabolic focus in the left neck.

dimensional images can be produced, and a fourth dimension, of uptake change over time, can be considered. **Fig. 17.6** illustrates typical PET-CT image of a metastatic lymph node.

Modern scanners have a cylinder of detectors, and can also include a CT scanner for PET-CT scanning. Typically, patients must fast for 4 to 6 hours before the study to increase the cellular uptake of FDG. The blood sugar level of a patient is tested to ensure that there is no hyperglycemia. An hour's wait between injection of the radiotracer and scanning is standard practice. Patients must be able to lay still for 30 minutes to an hour for the study. There is a radiation exposure with the procedure, somewhat higher than with a chest CT. The key advantage of PET scanning is that the study images physiologic activity. PET scanning uses the high metabolic activity of tumors compared with background tissues to advantageously visualize malignancy. This complements traditional anatomic studies. The images produced are far inferior in quality to conventional CT or MRI scans, but the completely different imaging strategy more than makes up for this. Current estimates are that a tumor volume of 1 cm is required for detection. The degree of uptake does not correlate with tumor histological grade; therefore, PET has largely been used to localize tumors. PET scanning detects an additional 10 to 20% of primary tumors that may have been missed on panendoscopy.[7] No level 1 data exist to support or refute PET scanning in patients with CUP; however, in the authors' opinion, PET is reasonably sensitive and cost-effective after an adequate work-up of CUP has failed to locate the primary.

A recent retrospective study[9] of 183 consecutive patients with head and neck CUP over a 10-year period compared the detection rate of preoperative imaging modalities, including CT, MRI, PET, and PET-CT. The overall imaging detection rate was 45.9%, increasing to 60.9% with directed biopsies. The individual modality detection rate was as follows: CT-neck, 14 of 46 (9.6%); MRI, 0 of 13 (0%); PET, 6 of 41 (14.6%); and PET-CT fusion, 23 of 52 (44.2%).

One additional reason to include FDG-PET or PET-CT fusion is the detection of other regional or distant metastasis.

Table 17.3 lists some studies evaluating PET in the evaluation of CUP of the head and neck. A broad range of sensitivity and false-positive rate was noted. The author recommendations also ranged from positive to no effect on primary detection rate. PET scanning, at this point, has a complementary role to conventional imaging in the detection of the primary tumor.

Recommended Evaluation

Table 17.4 lists a recommended approach for the evaluation of CUP based on our literature review.

Prognosis

Numerous studies have attempted to classify prognostic factors in CUP; however, no level 1 data exist. Counterintuitively, subsequent detection of the primary lesion has been noted to have a poor prognostic significance, with a 5-year survival rate of 20 to 30%.[10] In contrast, some large series have demonstrated that subsequent detection of the primary lesion does not change the survival rate.[11]

Nodal stage is one of the best-studied prognostic factors. Several studies have shown that a lower nodal stage, variously defined in the studies as N1 or N1-2a, conveys a significant survival advantage.[10–12] Extracapsular spread (ECS) is another important histological factor that adversely affects prognosis.[9,11,12] Davidson et al from Memorial Sloan-Kettering performed a multivariate analysis of neck control, including patient, tumor, and treatment variables that revealed that ECS was the only significant predictor of neck failure.[9]

Well-differentiated tumors had a higher rate of distant metastasis and a lower survival rate.[11] Locoregional recurrence, as expected, implies a poorer prognosis and is more common in higher nodal stage patients.[10,11]

Conflicting studies exist on the prognostic significance of the level of metastasis (I through V). Huang et al[10] demonstrated no difference, whereas some studies have shown worse prognosis with supraclavicular or level IV metastasis.

Conflicting data exist regarding the effect of gender, with some studies showing females to have a higher survival rate and others demonstrating no difference.

Management

One fundamental problem in the management of patients with head and neck CUP is how to balance the morbidity of treating all possible occult sites with irradiation versus the risk of careful observation. The 3-year survival rate ranges from 35 to 59% when patients with squamous or undifferentiated tumors are treated with radical radiation therapy, surgery, or both. The 5-year disease-specific survival rates were 85% in patients with a solitary node and 58% in patients with multiple nodes. No prospective double-blinded randomized clinical trial exists comparing these treatment strategies; therefore, all strategies presented are reasonable recommendations based on the limited data.

It is not uncommon, in a referral institution, to see patients with unsuspected carcinoma discovered on the final path from a routine lymph node excision. In these cases, neck irradiation is the prudent course of action.

Table 17.3 Example of Studies Evaluating PET for Carcinoma of Unknown Primary

Study	Journal	Year	Study Type	N	Sensitivity (%)	FP (%)	Pos/Neg	Comments
Jungehülsing et al[18]	Otolaryngol Head Neck Surg	2000	Prospective	27	26	0	+	
Greven et al[4]	Cancer	1999	Prospective	13	8	46	−	
Mukherji et al[19]	Radiology	1996	Prospective	18	82	62	+	
Waltonen et al[20]	Arch Otolaryngol Head Neck Surg	2009	Retrospective	41	14.6	2.4	−	Positive for PET-CT
Rusthoven et al[21]	Cancer	2004	Review	302	88.3	39.3		
Cianchetti et al[17]	Laryngoscope	2009	Restrospective	21	32.4	28.6	−	Did not have an effect on the detection rate

PET, positron emission tomography; FP, false positive; Pos, positive; Neg, negative; CT, computed tomography.

Table 17.4 Recommended Approach for the Evaluation of CUP

History

Physical examination with FFL, palpation of tongue base/tonsils

Laboratories: CBC, LFTs, EBV, p16, BMP

FNA

CT scan neck/chest (consider MRI)

If all negative, then PET or PET-CT

Panendoscopy with nasopharyngoscopy with biopsy

Tonsillectomy and directed biopsies (tonsillar fossa biopsy if previous tonsillectomy)

If all above negative, then excisional biopsy (possible neck dissection) with immunohistochemistry

CUP, carcinoma of unknown primary; FFL, flexible fiberoptic laryngoscopy; CBC, compelete blood cell count; LFTs, liver function tests; EBV, Epstein-Barr virus; BMP, basic metabolic panel; FNA, fine-needle aspiration; CT, computed tomography; MRI, magnetic resonance imaging; PET, positron emission tomography.

Neck management options include observation, neck dissection, neck irradiation, both neck dissection and neck irradiation, and/or extended (comprehensive) field irradiation to potential primary sites, often including the nasopharynx (**Table 17.5**).

The first decision point is nodal stage. The data available support multimodal therapy for later nodal stage, greater than N2a. Other information available after excisional biopsy would include the presence of additional nodes upstaging the patient, ECS, histological grade, and the presence or absence of soft tissue invasion. Furthermore, surgical treatment of the neck or neck irradiation could be determined on the basis of these factors.

For N1-N2a disease, excisional biopsy at the time of panendoscopy is reasonable and has been supported by the literature.[11,12] Some survival benefit has been shown with

Table 17.5 Management of the Neck

N1

- Excisional biopsy
- Additional nodes present intraoperatively—ipsilateral neck dissection
- ECS, multiple noses, or residual neck disease on histology—ipsilateral neck irradiation

N2a
- Selective neck dissection
- ECS or residual neck disease present—ipsilateral neck irradiation

N2b–N4
- Selective ipsilateral neck dissection followed by postoperative ipsilateral neck irradiation

Note: Patient discovered to have stage N1–N2a squamous cell carcinoma of the neck after diagnostic excisional biopsy—neck irradiation.

ECS, extracapsular spread.

this option.[11,12] This strategy provides tissue for analysis and determination of histological grade. Additional nodal disease noted at the time of excisional biopsy should prompt a selective neck dissection. These prognostic factors can help determine the need for neck dissection, neck irradiation, or both.

A more aggressive, but reasonable, route would be elective neck dissection at the time of panendoscopy for N1-N2a stage disease. The advantages over just excisional biopsy would be clinical staging of the neck. Spiro in his series at Memorial Sloan-Kettering found that the pathologic N stage was higher than the clinical stage 34% of the time. Early surgical treatment is potentially curative therapy. Morbidity from selective neck dissections by experienced providers is minimal. The patient should be counseled and accept the possibility of a purely diagnostic neck dissection. The information gained is useful to guide therapy.

The MD Anderson retrospective series by Wang et al[9] demonstrated no difference in survival rates for early stage neck disease; however, improvement was seen with surgical therapy for later stage (N2b or higher) neck disease. Colltier's series also demonstrated improved survival when the neck was treated surgically and adjuvant neck irradiation was given along with primary site irradiation.[12] Harper et al from Perth demonstrated no difference in neck control with radiotherapy (RT) alone versus RT with neck dissection for early stage disease; however, combined therapy had improved neck control in N2B and N3A disease.[6]

Davidson et al from Memorial Sloan-Kettering demonstrated a 74% survival rate with surgery and RT versus 15% for surgery alone and 11% for RT alone. Their strategy was combined modality therapy for later stage neck disease (N2-N3) or in N1 disease with or multiple nodes.[13]

Another article to support initial neck dissection was by Reddy and Marks from Loyola University who found a 5-year disease-free survival rate of 61% in patients who had a lymph node dissection before RT versus 37% for those who had an excisional biopsy.[14]

In review of the literature regarding surgical therapy for CUP, several conclusions can be drawn. N1-N2a disease does very well regardless of the modality of treatment. However, if neck dissection is performed, approximately one-third of the patients will be upstaged, and if the neck is treated with irradiation only, important prognostic information such as ECS and multiple nodes will be lost. N2b and greater neck disease has a much graver prognosis and clearly benefits from combined modality therapy.

The timing, preoperative versus postoperative, and the extent of radiation therapy are controversial. The advantages of postoperative radiation are determination of the extent of neck disease and potentially the source. Also, the extent of radiation portals is controversial. In addition to the ipsilateral neck, should the contralateral neck be included? The likely primary sites of the upper aerodigestive tract are included in most protocols, and the nasopharynx in some. Typically, the location of the node, high and posterior, and demographic factors are considered in irradiating the nasopharynx because of the morbidity associated with it.

Another question is whether to treat the necks bilaterally. The argument for treating both necks is that the primary carcinoma could be located in an area with bilateral drainage, and there is risk for metastasis to the contralateral neck. Reddy et al from Loyola University found that bilateral neck irradiation conferred 53% survival compared with 47% for the unilateral neck irradiation group.[14] The cost of the survival improvement was xerostomia in 100% of the bilateral neck irradiation group versus the unilateral group.

Improvement in management via neck irradiation may come with intensity-modulated radiotherapy (IMRT). IMRT is a form of three-dimensional conformal RT that more accurately maximizes radiation dose to the target tissue while minimizing the radiation dose to the surrounding tissue. The target tissue is still identified through CT imaging, and radiation is delivered via linear accelerators as in conventional RT; the unique feature of IMRT is its ability to conform the shape of the beam from any angle. Beam conformation is achieved through dynamic multileaf collimators that have 120 computer-controlled, moveable leaves to shape the beam to more accurately target tumor tissue. One recent small series by Madani out of Belgium compared IMRT with their historical control group for CUP HNSCC patients. The two groups had an equivalent overall survival; however, grade 3 dysphagia was reduced from 50 to 4.5%, and xerostomia was reduced from 53.4 to 11.8%.[15]

Conclusions

The evaluation and management of the patient with unknown primary carcinoma demands a systematic and methodical approach. Correct identification of the primary tumor is critical to ensure appropriate treatment. The most significant prognostic factors are extracapsular extension and multiple nodes. Early stage disease (N1-N2a) should be treated with excisional biopsy or selective neck dissection followed by neck irradiation based on the histologic factors of extracapsular extension or multiple nodes. N2b-N4 disease should be treated surgically followed by adjuvant neck and primary site irradiation. New advances in imaging may improve diagnostic evaluation.

Clinical Pearls

- Fine-needle aspiration (FNA) is the preferred method for the identification of malignancy in the neck mass.

- Evaluation of a needle aspiration specimen for adequacy at the time of FNA can improve diagnostic accuracy.

- Insufflation during nasopharyngoscopy can aid in visualizing the limits of the piriform sinuses and hypopharynx.

- In patients with carcinoma of unknown primary who have had an adequate evaluation and no identification of the primary tumor, positron emission tomography scanning may improve detection rates.

- Incisional or excisional biopsy for the diagnosis of a neck mass has not been definitively shown to worsen prognosis.

- Bilateral neck irradiation may increase survival slightly, but those patients will endure a higher rate of side effects.

- The nasopharynx may be spared radiation if physical examination and imaging do not reveal malignancy in that location and the patient has no high-risk factors for nasopharyngeal carcinoma.

References

1. Talmi YP, Wolf GT, Hazuka M, Krause CJ. Unknown primary of the head and neck. J Laryngol Otol 1996;110(4):353–356

2. American Cancer Society. Cancer facts and figures. 2010. Available from: http://www.cancer.org/docroot/STT/stt_0.asp. Accessed Nov 2011

3. Jereczek-Fossa BA, Jassem J, Orecchia R. Cervical lymph node metastases of squamous cell carcinoma from an unknown primary. Cancer Treat Rev 2004;30(2):153–164

4. Greven KM, Keyes JW Jr, Williams DW III, McGuirt WF, Joyce WT III. Occult primary tumors of the head and neck: lack of benefit from positron emission tomography imaging with 2-[F-18]fluoro-2-deoxy-D-glucose. Cancer 1999;86(1):114–118

5. DeSanto LW, Neel HB III. Squamous cell carcinoma: metastasis to the neck from an unknown or undiscovered primary. Otolaryngol Clin North Am 1985;18(3):505–513

6. Harper CS, Mendenhall WM, Parsons JT, Stringer SP, Cassisi NJ, Million RR. Cancer in neck nodes with unknown primary site: role of mucosal radiotherapy. Head Neck 1990;12(6):463–469

7. Rohman GT, Samant S. SP197—occult primary head and neck carcinoma: a systematic review. Otolaryngol Head Neck Surg 2009;141(Suppl 3):158–159

8. Randall DA, Johnstone PA, Foss RD, Martin PJ. Tonsillectomy in diagnosis of the unknown primary tumor of the head and neck. Otolaryngol Head Neck Surg 2000;122(1):52–55

9. Davidson BJ, Spiro RH, Patel S, Patel K, Shah JP. Cervical metastases of occult origin: the impact of combined modality therapy. Am J Surg 1994;168(5):395–399

10. Huang CC, Tseng FY, Yeh TH, et al. Prognostic factors of unknown primary head and neck squamous cell carcinoma. Otolaryngol Head Neck Surg 2008;139(3):429–435

11. Wang RC, Goepfert H, Barber AE, Wolf P. Unknown primary squamous cell carcinoma metastatic to the neck. Arch Otolaryngol Head Neck Surg 1990;116(12):1388–1393

12. Colletier PJ, Garden AS, Morrison WH, Goepfert H, Geara F, Ang KK. Postoperative radiation for squamous cell carcinoma metastatic to cervical lymph nodes from an unknown primary site: outcomes and patterns of failure. Head Neck 1998;20(8):674–681

13. Davidson BJ, Harter KW. Metastatic cancer to the neck from an unknown primary site. In: Harrison LB, Sessions RB, Hong WK, eds. Head and Neck Cancer: A Multidisciplinary Approach. 2nd ed. Philadelphia, PA: Lippincott Williams & Wilkins; 2004:245–265

14. Reddy SP, Marks JE. Metastatic carcinoma in the cervical lymph nodes from an unknown primary site: results of bilateral neck plus mucosal irradiation vs. ipsilateral neck irradiation. Int J Radiat Oncol Biol Phys 1997;37(4):797–802

15. Madani I, Vakaet L, Bonte K, Boterberg T, De Neve W. Intensity-modulated radiotherapy for cervical lymph node metastases from unknown primary cancer. Int J Radiat Oncol Biol Phys 2008;71(4):1158–1166

16. Byers RM, Wolf PF, Ballantyne AJ. Rationale for elective modified neck dissection. Head Neck Surg 1988;10(3):160–167

17. Cianchetti M, Mancuso AA, Amdur RJ, et al. Diagnostic evaluation of squamous cell carcinoma metastatic to cervical lymph nodes from an unknown head and neck primary site. Laryngoscope 2009;119(12):2348–2354

18. Jungehülsing M, Scheidhauer K, Damm M, et al. 2[F]-fluoro-2-deoxy-D-glucose positron emission tomography is a sensitive tool for the detection of occult primary cancer (carcinoma of unknown primary syndrome) with head and neck lymph node manifestation. Otolaryngol Head Neck Surg 2000;123(3):294–301

19. Mukherji SK, Drane WE, Mancuso AA, Parsons JT, Mendenhall WM, Stringer S. Occult primary tumors of the head and neck: detection with 2-[F-18] fluoro-2-deoxy-D-glucose SPECT. Radiology 1996;199(3):761–766

20. Waltonen JD, Ozer E, Hall NC, Schuller DE, Agrawal A. Metastatic carcinoma of the neck of unknown primary origin: evolution and efficacy of the modern workup. Arch Otolaryngol Head Neck Surg 2009;135(10):1024–1029

21. Rusthoven KE, Koshy M, Paulino AC. The role of fluorodeoxyglucose positron emission tomography in cervical lymph node metastases from an unknown primary tumor. Cancer 2004;101(11):2641–2649

18 Hypopharynx and Cervical Esophagus Cancer

S. Lewis Cooper and Anand Sharma

Core Messages

- Work-up should include direct laryngoscopy and biopsy for hypopharyngeal tumors and endoscopic ultrasound for tumors of the cervical esophagus.

- The primary management for locally advanced cancers of the cervical esophagus and hypopharynx is chemoradiotherapy with surgical salvage for those with persistent local disease after treatment.

- Cancers of the cervical esophagus and lower hypopharynx have a high incidence of nodal metastasis, and careful attention must be paid to management of the neck.

- Superficial cancers of the hypopharynx and cervical esophagus may be managed with endoscopic surgery or other larynx-preserving surgeries in centers with experience with these techniques.

Cancers of the hypopharynx and cervical esophagus are relatively uncommon, together accounting for less than 10% of cancers of the upper aerodigestive tract and less than 5% of cancers of the head and neck.[1-3] Cancers of the cervical esophagus account for only approximately 5% of all esophageal cancers. The incidence of cancers of the hypopharynx and cervical esophagus is currently 1:100,000 in North America and has been steadily decreasing, with a drop of more than 30% in each site between 1975 and 2001.[2] No significant improvements in survival have been seen in population-based registries in either carcinoma of the hypopharynx or cervical esophagus.[2,3]

Epidemiology

Squamous cell carcinoma (SCC) is the predominant histology, comprising more than 95% of cancers of the hypopharynx and 85% of cancers of the cervical esophagus. Adenocarcinoma is the second most common histology in the cervical esophagus, comprising 9% of the cases. Other less common histologies include lymphoma, adenoid cystic carcinoma, and small cell carcinoma.[2]

The most common age range at presentation for cancers of the hypopharynx and cervical esophagus is 50 to 80 years. Men are two to three times more likely to be diagnosed than women. Smoking and alcohol are the two largest risk factors for the development of SCC of the hypopharynx and cervical esophagus. Cigarette smoking increases the risk, with an odds ratio (OR) of 3 to 5, and this risk is modified by the age at which started smoking, total number of years smoked, number of packs smoked in a day,

and current smoking status.[4,5] The risk of SCC of the head and neck and esophagus remains elevated up to at least 10 years after smoking cessation. Cigar and pipe smoking also increases the risk of cancers of the upper aerodigestive tract but not to the same degree as cigarette smoking. Those who abuse alcohol also have an increased risk of cancers of the upper aerodigestive tract, and this effect is multiplicative in those who smoke as well, with an increased OR of up to 35. There is also evidence that the use of alcohol in individuals with polymorphisms in alcohol dehydrogenase and aldehyde dehydrogenase increases the risk for cancers of the upper aerodigestive tract.[6]

Infection with the human papillomavirus (HPV) has been implicated in the pathogenesis of cancers of the upper aerodigestive tract, and HPV16 is the predominant genotype. The oropharynx is the site with the highest incidence of HPV-related SCC, with up to 50% of the cases in North America associated with HPV. HPV association is not as common in other cancers of the aerodigestive tract, with one review revealing an incidence of 13.8% in cancers of the larynx and hypopharynx in North America with higher incidence in other parts of the world.[7] A meta-analysis of patients with head and neck cancer demonstrated an improved prognosis in HPV-related oropharyngeal cancer but not HPV-related cancers of the oral cavity, larynx, and hypopharynx.[8]

Anatomy

The hypopharynx and cervical esophagus are adjacent structures in the head and neck. The hypopharynx begins inferior to the oropharynx, and the superior border is

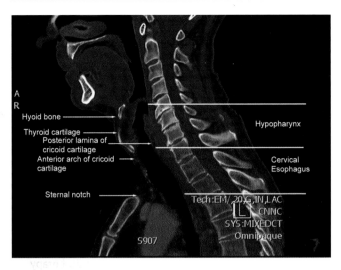

Figure 18.1 Sagittal computed tomography of the neck revealing the anatomic boundaries of the hypopharynx and cervical esophagus.

the vallecula. This begins at a plane at the superior border of the hyoid bone. The inferior border of the hypopharynx is the cervical esophagus, which begins at a plane at the inferior border of the cricoid cartilage. The inferior border of the cervical esophagus is at the thoracic inlet, which begins at a plane at the sternal notch (**Fig. 18.1** and **Table 18.1**). The length of the cervical esophagus can vary on the basis of age, gender, and body habitus, but measurements on endoscopy are generally 15 to 20 cm from the incisors.

The hypopharynx consists of three subsites: the postcricoid region, pyriform sinuses, and lateral and posterior hypopharyngeal walls. The postcricoid region is posterior to the arytenoid and cricoid cartilages and forms the anterior border of the hypopharynx, connecting the two pyriform sinuses. The right and left pyriform sinuses begin at the pharyngoepiglottic fold and extend down to the cervical esophagus and are bound laterally by the lateral hypopharyngeal wall.

Lymphatic Drainage

Both the hypopharynx and the cervical esophagus have a rich lymphatic drainage that is commonly bilateral. The upper hypopharynx drains through an anterior collecting

system with lymphatics from the supraglottic larynx that exit the thyrohyoid membrane to drain to levels II and III. The posterior collecting system drains the inferior hypopharynx and exits the superior constrictor muscle to drain to lateral retropharyngeal, paratracheal, and internal jugular chain lymph nodes. Locally advanced SCCs of the hypopharynx can also involve levels IV and V. Contralateral lymph-node metastases are common as bilateral lymphatic drainage occurs along superficial lymphatics of the posterior pharyngeal wall.[9]

The lymphatic drainage of the esophagus is concentrated in the submucosal layer, but lymphatic channels also exist in the lamina propria. Lymphatics penetrate the muscularis propria to drain to regional lymph nodes. Even superficial tumors have access to this rich lymphatic drainage system and have a propensity for lymph-node metastasis.[10] SCC of the cervical esophagus can result in metastases to cervical, upper mediastinal as well as recurrent nerve lymph nodes.[11] The number of lymph nodes involved, and not the location, is related to prognosis, and this is reflected in the current edition of the American Joint Committee on Cancer (AJCC) staging manual.

Patient Evaluation and Staging

Cancers of the hypopharynx and cervical esophagus often present with advanced disease. The most common presenting symptom is dysphagia. Dysphagia can present with "sticking" of certain solid foods such as meats and can progress to complete dysphagia to solid foods and then liquids. Weight loss can occur because of dysphagia, dietary changes, and tumor anorexia. Patients can also have hoarseness due to recurrent laryngeal nerve involvement or involvement of the cricoarytenoid joint or the cricoarytenoid muscle. Unilateral or bilateral otalgia can also be present in cancer of the hypopharynx due to referred pain from cranial nerves IX and X. Other symptoms can include hemoptysis, cough, and anemia. Complete obstruction of the cervical esophagus can result in an inability to clear secretions, and erosion into the trachea can result in tracheoesophageal fistula.

Work-up of cancers of the hypopharynx and cervical esophagus should start with a thorough physical examination. Lesions in the superior hypopharynx may be seen with mirror examination or fiberoptic laryngoscopy (**Fig. 18.2**).

Table 18.1 Anatomic Boundaries of the Hypopharynx and Cervical Esophagus

	Hypopharynx	**Cervical Esophagus**
Superior border	Vallecula	Plane at inferior border of the cricoid cartilage
Inferior border	Plane at inferior border of the cricoid cartilage	Plane at sternal notch
Anterior border	Arytenoid and cricoid cartilage	Trachea
Posterior border	Prevertebral cervical fascia	Prevertebral cervical fascia
Lateral border	Carotid sheath	Carotid sheath

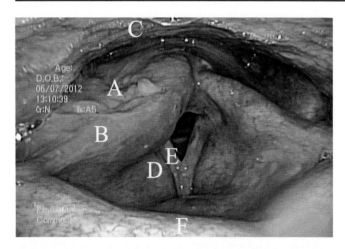

Figure 18.2 A right pyriform sinus tumor. Structures as follows: (A) right pyriform sinus tumor, (B) right aryepiglottic fold, (C) posterior pharyngeal wall, (D) right false cord, (E) right true cord, and (F) epiglottis.

However, lesions in the lower hypopharynx and cervical esophagus may not be seen with either mirror examination or laryngoscopy and requires rigid endoscopy. Palpation of the neck can reveal the presence of suspicious cervical nodes. Diagnosis should be made by biopsy performed during endoscopy. Fine-needle aspiration for cytology may be performed on suspicious cervical lymph nodes with a sensitivity of 89.5% and a specificity of 96.5 to 98.5%.[12]

Imaging studies play an important role in the work-up of SCC of the hypopharynx and cervical esophagus as physical examination, laryngoscopy, and endoscopy often cannot determine the extent of local invasion or regional and distant dissemination to accurately stage the patient (**Tables 18.2** and **18.3**). Computed tomography (CT) imaging can identify the invasion of adjacent structures and cortical bone as well as retropharyngeal, paratracheal, and upper mediastinal lymph-node metastases (**Fig. 18.3**). A study found that CT imaging upstaged the primary tumor (T) or regional lymph node (N) stage in 90% of hypopharynx cancers, with two-thirds of these upstaged in the T stage and one-third upstaged in the N stage.[13] In head and neck cancers, CT imaging increases the sensitivity for detecting cervical node metastases compared with physical examination from 74 to 83%, with the specificity increasing from 81 to 83%.[14] The sensitivity of CT imaging for regional nodal metastasis is lower for esophageal carcinoma at 50%, with a specificity of 83%.[15]

Positron emission tomography (PET) has improved sensitivity compared with CT in detecting regional nodal metastasis as well as distant metastasis. One study showed an increase in sensitivity from 82 to 90% for detecting nodal metastasis in SCC of the head and neck with PET compared with CT imaging.[16] In esophageal cancer, PET increased the sensitivity in detecting regional nodal metastasis from 50 to 57%. While providing modest increases in sensitivity for detecting regional nodal metastasis, in esophageal carcinoma PET improves the sensitivity in detecting distant

metastasis from 52% to 71%, with the specificity increasing from 91% to 93%.[15] Integrated PET-CT can improve the accuracy of PET alone by providing anatomic correlation to areas of increased ^{18}F-flouro-2-deoxy-D-glucose uptake and decreasing the number of equivocal lesions.[17] In detecting distant metastases, PET-CT has a sensitivity of 97.5%, a specificity of 92.6%, a positive predictive value of 62.9%, and a negative predictive value of 99.7%.[18] While PET-CT is very good at ruling out distant metastasis, positive findings should be interpreted with caution and confirmed histologically when possible.

To properly assess T and N stages in SCC of the cervical esophagus, endoscopic ultrasound (EUS) should be performed. EUS can visualize the different layers of the esophageal wall and determine the depth of invasion into these layers to assess the T stage (**Fig. 18.4**). Superficial esophageal carcinomas can be further subclassified into M 1-3 on the basis of the depth of mucosal invasion and SM 1-3 on the basis of the depth of submucosal invasion (**Table 18.4**). The accuracy of EUS for T stage depends on operator experience, depth of the tumor invasion, or the presence of a malignant stricture but is generally between 80 and 90%.[19] The sensitivity and specificity for detecting regional nodal metastasis with EUS are 80 and 70%, respectively.[15]

Treatment

The management of SCC of the cervical esophagus and hypopharynx is complex and should be managed in a multidisciplinary setting including otolaryngology, thoracic surgery, medical oncology, radiation oncology, diagnostic radiology, pathology, gastroenterology, dentistry, speech and language pathology, and nutrition. The optimal management of SCC of the cervical esophagus is controversial, and there is considerable regional variation in treatment. Most patients with carcinoma of the hypopharynx or cervical esophagus present with locally advanced disease, and some institutions prefer surgical resection with either adjuvant or neoadjuvant chemotherapy or chemoradiotherapy, and other institutions prefer definitive chemoradiotherapy with surgical salvage for local failure. In the case of early stage disease, less invasive options may be available.

Endoscopy—Cervical Esophagus

Superficial SCC of the cervical esophagus was traditionally managed surgically with esophagectomy. However, endoscopic treatments are now being used for carefully selected superficial lesions. Tumor invasion into the submucosa is associated with a 38% risk of lymph-node metastasis, and endoscopic management alone should be avoided in these patients because of the increased risk of recurrence.[20] Patients with M3 tumors that exhibit lymphovascular invasion also have an increased risk of lymph-node involvement (up to 18%) and may require

Table 18.2   American Joint Committe on Cancer Staging for Hypopharynx

Primary tumor (T)	
• T1	Tumor limited to one subsite of the hypopharynx and/or 2 cm or less in greatest dimension
• T2	Tumor invades more than one subsite of the hypopharynx or an adjacent site, or measures more than 2 cm, but not more than 4 cm in greatest dimension without fixation of the hemilarynx
• T3	Tumor more than 4 cm in greatest dimension or with fixation of hemilarynx or extension into the esophagus
• T4a	Moderately advanced local disease. Tumor invades thyroid/cricoid cartilage, hyoid bone, thyroid gland, or central compartment soft tissue[a]
• T4b	Very advanced local disease. Tumor invades prevertebral fascia, encases carotid artery, or involves mediastinal structures
Regional lymph nodes (N)	
• Nx	Regional lymph nodes cannot be assessed
• N0	No regional lymph-node metastasis
• N1	Metastasis in a single ipsilateral lymph node, 3 cm or less in greatest dimension
• N2	Metastasis in a single ipsilateral lymph node, more than 3 cm but not more than 6 cm in greatest dimension, or in multiple ipsilateral lymph nodes, not more than 6 cm in greatest dimension, or in bilateral or contralateral lymph nodes, not more than 6 cm in greatest dimension
• N2a	Metastasis in a single ipsilateral lymph node, more than 3 cm but not more than 6 cm in greatest dimension
• N2b	Metastasis in multiple ipsilateral lymph nodes, not more than 6 cm in greatest dimension
• N2c	Metastasis in bilateral or contralateral lymph nodes, not more than 6 cm in greatest dimension
• N3	Metastasis in a lymph node, more than 6 cm in greatest dimension[b]
Distant metastasis (M)	
• M0	No distant metastasis
• M1	Distant metastasis

Source: Edge SB, Byrd DR, Compton CC, Fritz AG, Greene FL, Trotti A. *AJCC Cancer Staging Manual*. 7th ed. New York: Springer; 2010.
[a]Central compartment soft tissue includes prelaryngeal strap muscles and subcutaneous fat.
[b]Metastasis at level VII is considered regional lymph-node metastasis.

further therapy.[21] Endoscopic mucosal resection (EMR) has been in use for more than 20 years and can yield equivalent local control and survival and reduced morbidity compared with esophagectomy in esophageal carcinoma confined to the mucosa.[20] EMR should not be used in patients with cirrhosis and esophageal varices and should be used with caution in patients with multifocal disease. Lesions greater than 2 cm often require piecemeal resection and are more likely to experience local recurrence after EMR.

Endoscopic mucosal dissection (EMD) has been in use for more than 10 years and allows for en-bloc resection of larger lesions. A meta-analysis revealed that EMD produced higher rates of en-bloc resection and complete resection and lower rates of local recurrence compared with EMR. However, EMD was associated with longer procedure times as well as increased rates of bleeding and perforation.[22] There is limited experience with endoscopic therapies such as EMR plus photodynamic therapy, argon plasma coagulation,

Table 18.3 American Joint Committe on Cancer Staging for Esophagus

Primary tumor (T)[a]

- Tx   Primary tumor cannot be assessed
- T0   No evidence of primary tumor
- Tis   High-grade dysplasia[b]
- T1   Tumor invades lamina propria, muscularis mucosae, or submucosa
- T1a   Tumor invades lamina propria or muscularis mucosae
- T1b   Tumor invades submucosa
- T2   Tumor invades muscularis propria
- T3   Tumor invades adventitia
- T4   Tumor invades adjacent structures
- T4a   Resectable tumor invading pleura, pericardium, or diaphragm
- T4b   Unresectable tumor invading other adjacent structures, such as aorta, vertebral body, and trachea

Regional lymph nodes (N)[c]

- Nx   Regional lymph nodes cannot be assessed
- N0   No regional lymph-node metastasis
- N1   Metastasis in one to two regional lymph nodes
- N2   Metastasis in three to six regional lymph nodes
- N3   Metastasis in seven or more regional lymph nodes

Distant metastasis (M)

- M0   No distant metastasis
- M1   Distant metastasis

Source: Edge SB, Byrd DR, Compton CC, Fritz AG, Greene FL, Trotti A. *AJCC Cancer Staging Manual*. 7th ed. New York: Springer; 2010.

[a]At least maximal dimension of the tumor must be recorded, and multiple tumors require the T(m) suffix.

[b]High-grade dysplasia includes all noninvasive neoplastic epithelia, formerly called carcinoma in situ, a diagnosis that is no longer used for columnar mucosae anywhere in the gastrointestinal tract.

[c]Number must be recorded for total number of regional nodes sampled and total number of reported nodes with metastasis.

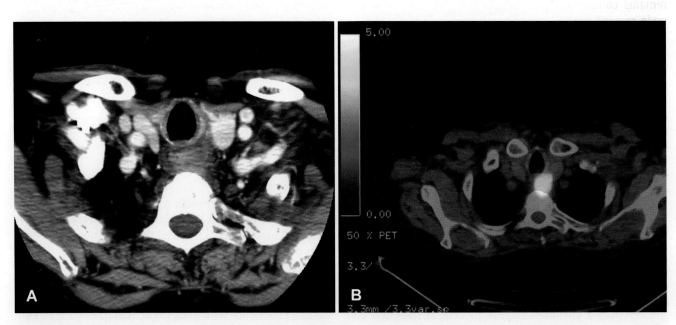

Figure 18.3 Cervical esophagus primary seen on axial (A) contrasted computed tomography (CT) of the neck and (B) positron emission tomography (PET)-CT.

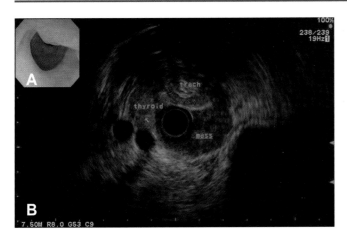

Figure 18.4 Cervical esophagus primary as seen (A) on endoscopy and (B) with endoscopic ultrasound.

radiofrequency ablation, and laser ablation, and the use of these techniques in superficial esophageal carcinoma remains investigational.

Surgery—Cervical Esophagus

Surgical resection for carcinoma of the cervical esophagus involves either cervical or total esophagectomy. Esophagectomy (cervical or total) and reconstruction are complex operative procedures that require specialized postoperative care, and best results are obtained by high-volume surgeons (> 6 per year) and high-volume hospitals (> 19 per year).[23] If there is extension into the hypopharynx and involvement of the larynx, then a laryngopharyngectomy may be required as well. The thyroid may also be involved and a hemithyroidectomy or complete thyroidectomy may be required.[24] The extent of lymph-node dissection remains controversial. In the cervical esophagus, lymph-node regions at the highest risk of metastasis include the lower cervical nodes and upper mediastinal lymph nodes. Lymph-node regions containing clinically positive nodes should be dissected. Some authors recommend routine dissection of clinically uninvolved cervical lymph nodes and upper mediastinal lymph nodes in carcinoma of the cervical esophagus because of the high risk of lymph-node metastasis.[25,26] The therapeutic benefit and prognostic information obtained from a more extensive lymph-node

dissection must be weighed against the extended operative times and increased surgical morbidity with increased risk of vessel injury, fistula, and postoperative hypocalcemia. Results of recent reported series of surgery for SCC of the esophagus are listed in **Table 18.5.**

Several reconstructive options are available after resection of carcinoma of the cervical esophagus, and the method chosen depends on the extent of resection, patient characteristics, and surgeon preference. The two most common methods of reconstruction are the gastric pull-up and free jejunal graft. The gastric pull-up is used if a total esophagectomy is performed and is advantageous in that microvascular reconstruction is not required. If a cervical esophagectomy is performed, then a jejunal graft may be used. Advantages of the jejunal graft include ease of harvesting, close approximation of lumen size to the esophagus, and peristalsis; however, microvascular reconstruction is required, and some authors have reported a higher rate of complications compared with gastric pull-up.[24,27] Other reconstructive options include ileocolon graft or myocutaneous free tissue transfer.

Cervical esophagectomy or total esophagectomy with or without laryngopharyngectomy has an operative mortality rate of 4 to 9.8% in modern series.[27–31] These results compare favorably to older series that reported operative mortality rates of 11 to 24%.[24] Rates of anastomotic leak from jejunal graft or gastric pull-up range from 4 to 26.6%.[27–32] One series that used neoadjuvant chemoradiotherapy reported an anastomotic leak rate of 29.4% for reoperation.[29] The surgical series vary significantly in the details of how complications are reported, and standardization of reporting is needed to compare results from different institutions. The operative complication rates reported vary from 9.3 to 74.3%.[27,30,31,33] Operative mortality has improved in large, modern series, but these results are applicable to only those institutions that have a relatively large volume of cervical esophageal cancers and experience in these surgical techniques and aggressive postoperative management.

Surgery—Hypopharynx

Locally advanced SCC of the hypopharynx often requires laryngopharyngectomy. However, some larynx-preserving strategies are possible in early stage SCC limited to the

Table 18.4 Staging of Superficial Esophageal Cancers

AJCC Stage	Superficial Stage	Mucosal Layer
Tis	M1	Epithelial layer
T1a	M2	Lamina propria
	M3	Muscularis mucosa
T1b	SM1	First one-third of the submucosa
	SM2	Middle one-third of the submucosa
	SM3	Last one-third of the submucosa

AJCC, American Joint Committee on Cancer.

Table 18.5 Results of Surgery for Cervical Esophagus

Author	Number of Patients	Surgery	Reconstruction	Neoadjuvant/Adjuvant Therapy	Toxicity	Local Control	Survival
Tong et al[28]	62	PLE (59.6% R0, 40.4% R1/2)	Gastric pull-up (preferred) or ileocolon transfer	RT: 50% CTRT: 11%	Anastamotic leak: 10% Hospital mortality: 7.1%	Not reported	2-y OS: 37.6% Median survival for R0: 22.4 mo Median survival for R1/R2: 9.8 mo
Chou et al[40]	15	PLE	Gastric pull-up	CTRT for T3, N1, or M1a	Not reported	Not reported	Mean DSS: 36.2 mo
Kadota et al[32]	32	Cervical esophagectomy	Jejunal transfer	RT: 6.2% CT: 9.4%	Anastamotic leak: 12.5%	5-year LRFS: 75%	5-y DFS: 41%
Ott et al[29]	109	Cervical esophagectomy with 15% laryngectomy 4% partial laryngectomy	Jejunal transfer	Neoadjuvant CTRT: 86%	Hospital mortality: 2.8% Reoperation: 29.4% Anastamotic leak: 26.6%	R0 resection: 72.5% LRFS: 70% if R0 resection	5-y OS: 47%
Daiko et al[30]	74	Cervical esophagectomy: 75% Total esophagectomy: 25% (68% of all patients also received laryngopharyngectomy)	Jejunal transfer: 68% Gastric pull-up: 25% Colon transfer: 1.4%	None	Operative morbidity: 34% Hospital mortality: 4% Anastamotic leak: 4%	Local control: 51.4%	3-y OS: 42% 5-y OS: 33%
Wang et al[31]	41	PLE	Gastric pull-up: 95.1% Colon transfer: 4.9%	Neoadjuvant RT: 14.6% Adjuvant RT: 51.2%	Hospital mortality: 9.8% Anastamotic leak: 22%	Local control: 87.8% LR control: 73.2%	5-y OS: 31.5%
Shirakawa et al[33]	54 (23 HP and 31 CE)	PLE: 89% Cervical esopgagectomy: 11%	Jejunal transfer	Not reported	Operative morbidity: 9.3%	Not reported	5-y OS: 46.7%
Triboulet et al[27]	209 (131 HP and 78 CE)	PLE	Gastric pull-up: 60.8% Jejunal transfer: 36.8% Colon transfer: 2.4%	Neoadjuvant CTRT: 10.5% Neoadjuvant CT: 7.2% Neoadjuvant RT: 2.4% Adjuvant RT: 73%	Hospital mortality: 4.8% Postoperative morbidity: 38.3% Anastamotic leak: 22.5%	Local control: 78% LR control: 55%	5-y OS: 24% 5-y OS: 14% for CE

PLE, pharyngolaryngoesophagectomy; RT, radiotherapy; CTRT, chemoradiotherapy; OS, overall survival; y, year; mo, month; DSS, disease-specific survival; CT, chemotherapy; LRFS, locoregional recurrence-free survival; DFS, disease-free survival; LR, locoregional; HP, hypopharynx; CE, cervical esophagus.

hypopharynx. For tumors isolated to the lateral wall of the pyriform sinus and without involvement of the apex, a partial lateral pharyngectomy may be performed with acceptable local control.[34] The supraglottic hemipharyngolaryngectomy can also be used for some early tumors of the posterior pharyngeal wall and pyriform sinus and involves removal of the ipsilateral laryngeal vestibule and supraglottic pyriform sinus.[35] Some larger tumors in carefully selected patients with carcinoma of the pyriform sinus may be amenable to a supracricoid hemilaryngopharyngectomy (SCHLP), but poor local control was seen if the apex of the pyriform sinus was involved. The SCHLP involves removal of the supraglottis, thyroid cartilage, as well as false and true cords. The cricoid cartilage, hyoid bone, and an arytenoid are spared, resulting in low rates of permanent gastrostomy (0.7%) and completion laryngectomy (1.5%).[36] Transoral laser microsurgery in the hands of an experienced surgeon can also yield excellent local control in select cases.[37] The use of EMR for carcinoma of the hypopharynx with early invasion has been reported in one small series and is an area for future study, but the use of EMR in this setting remains investigational.[38] Careful consideration should be given to the management of the neck in any organ-preserving strategy as even early stage SCC of the hypopharynx has a high incidence of nodal metastasis. Neck dissection or adjuvant radiotherapy should be performed in the majority of cases. Some institutions have decided to closely follow patients with T1 tumors while others treat the neck in all cases.[35,37] Patients with poor lung function may not be optimal candidates for partial laryngopharyngectomy.

Neoadjuvant Therapy

Disappointing survival rates after esophagectomy alone with high rates of locoregional and distant recurrence led investigators to pursue strategies to improve the survival rates. There have been numerous randomized trials investigating neoadjuvant chemotherapy or chemoradiotherapy for esophageal cancer. One meta-analysis found a significant survival benefit to neoadjuvant chemoradiotherapy (13% absolute difference at 2 years), but the benefit of neoadjuvant chemotherapy was not significant in SCC.[39] Unfortunately, many of these randomized trials excluded carcinoma of the cervical esophagus. The few randomized trials that did allow carcinoma of the cervical esophagus included only a few patients with tumors of this location, making it difficult to apply these results to the cervical esophagus. One large retrospective study included 94 patients who underwent neoadjuvant chemoradiotherapy followed by cervical esophagectomy with free jejunal graft. The complete response rate to chemoradiotherapy was 26.6%, with a larynx-preservation rate of 85.3% and a 5-year survival rate of 47%. The reoperation rate was 29.4%, with 74.3% of all patients having a minor or major complication.[29] These are encouraging results with respect to survival, but this approach requires care in a large center with expertise in microvascular surgery and management of postoperative complications from this approach. Combined modality approaches with neoadjuvant chemoradiotherapy should be investigated further and might likely result in improved survival compared with surgery alone in the cervical esophagus.

Adjuvant Therapy

There is limited evidence for adjuvant chemoradiotherapy in SCC of the esophagus. Many retrospective surgical series of cervical esophageal cancer use adjuvant chemotherapy, radiotherapy, or both.[27,28,31,32,40] The role of adjuvant radiotherapy and chemoradiotherapy in SCC of the hypopharynx is well established. Adjuvant radiotherapy improves local control and disease-specific survival in SCC of the head and neck and should be given in cases of pT3/T4 tumors, nodal extracapsular extension, close or positive margins, pN2/N3 disease, perineural invasion, or lymphovascular invasion.[41] The risk of local recurrence increases with the addition of each additional risk factor. The dose for adjuvant radiotherapy that was found to be the minimum effective dose in one trial was 57.6 Gy. If there was extracapsular extension, then higher rates of local failure were seen below 63 Gy.[41] We recommend 60 Gy in 30 fractions to the primary tumor bed unless there is extracapsular extension or positive margins. We recommend 66 Gy in 33 fractions to the nodal regions exhibiting extracapsular extension or to areas of microscopic positive margins, and 70 Gy in 35 fractions in cases of gross residual disease. Undissected at-risk nodal regions that are clinically negative should receive 50 to 56 Gy. In SCC of the cervical esophagus, we would use the same risk factors listed above to determine whether adjuvant radiotherapy is indicated provided neoadjuvant radiotherapy was not used.

Even with postoperative radiotherapy, 5-year survival rates for locally advanced head and neck cancer remained approximately 40%. Two large randomized trials (RTOG 95–01 and EORTC 22931) investigated adjuvant radiotherapy alone compared with radiotherapy with concurrent cisplatin (100 mg/m^2 on days 1, 22, and 43). RTOG 95–01 included patients with positive margins, extracapsular extension, or two or more positive lymph nodes and gave 60 to 66 Gy in 30 to 33 fractions. EORTC 22931 included patients with positive margins, extracapsular extension, perineural invasion, lymphovascular invasion, stage III or IV disease, or level IV or V lymph nodes with oropharyngeal and oral cavity primaries and gave 66 Gy in 33 fractions. Both trials saw significant improvements in disease-free survival and local control in the chemoradiotherapy arm while EORTC 22931 also produced an improvement in overall survival. A combined analysis of the two trials revealed that the overall survival benefit was significant in patients with positive margins and extracapsular extension, and these patients should receive concurrent cisplatin if possible.[42] Other patients with multiple risk factors may benefit from adjuvant chemoradiotherapy, and this decision should be made on a case-by-case basis. Clinical trials investigating additional agents in addition to cisplatin and adjuvant radiotherapy are being performed, but results are not available at this time.

As the majority of SCCs of the head and neck overexpress the epidermal growth factor receptor (EGFR), agents that target this receptor are the focus of many of these trials.

Radiotherapy and Chemoradiotherapy

Because of disappointing results of surgery alone or surgery combined with neoadjuvant or adjuvant radiotherapy (5-year survival rate of 4 to 27%) for SCC of the cervical esophagus, an organ-preserving approach using radiotherapy or chemoradiotherapy has been investigated. Results with radiotherapy alone resulted in a 5-year survival rate of 15 to 32%.[24] Because equivalent survival rates could be obtained with radiotherapy without the operative morbidity and mortality, definitive radiotherapy became the treatment of choice for SCC of the cervical esophagus. Two randomized trials have been performed investigating radiotherapy alone compared with chemoradiotherapy in SCC of the esophagus (RTOG 85–01 and ECOG EST-1282) and found an overall survival benefit to chemoradiotherapy, but neither of these trials included cervical esophagus primaries.[43,44] In locally advanced (stages III and IV) SCC of the head and neck, multiple trials have investigated the addition of chemotherapy to radiation therapy. A meta-analysis revealed a benefit of 6.5 to 8% in overall survival at 5 years for concurrent chemotherapy, and the benefit was greatest in patients receiving platinum-based chemotherapy. The benefit of chemotherapy decreased with increasing age and was no longer significant in patients older than 71 years.[45] None of these trials included cervical esophagus primaries, but these results have been extrapolated to SCC of the cervical esophagus in an attempt to improve local control and survival. Current guidelines recommend chemoradiotherapy as the treatment of choice for SCC of the cervical esophagus. Modern series of chemoradiation for SCC of the cervical esophagus are listed in **Table 18.6**.

In the hypopharynx, attempts were made to pursue organ conservation and a randomized clinical trial (EORTC 24891) also revealed that an organ-preserving approach could be used in SCC of the hypopharynx with chemotherapy and radiotherapy with equivalent survival rates.[46] Patients who had a complete response to induction chemotherapy received 70 Gy, and nonresponders received surgery with adjuvant radiotherapy. A subsequent randomized trial revealed that concurrent chemoradiotherapy (70 Gy/35 fractions with cisplatin 100 mg/m² on days 1, 22, and 43) produced higher rates of laryngeal preservation and improved local control compared with induction chemotherapy followed by radiotherapy.[47] In the larynx, there is some indication that T4 tumors may have improved survival with laryngectomy, and hypopharyngeal tumors with significant invasion of the laryngeal cartilage should be offered laryngopharyngectomy if chemoradiotherapy will not produce a functional larynx.[48] Radiotherapy alone can produce excellent local control for stage I and II tumors. One single institution series saw an ultimate local control rate of 96 and 84% for T1 and T2 tumors, respectively. The local control rate with a functional larynx was 83%, and patients with a tumor volume of more than 6.5 cm³ had worse local control.[49]

Dose and Volumes

The optimal dose and fractionation for SCC of the cervical esophagus remains controversial. A large-dose escalation trial (Intergroup 0123) comparing 50.4 Gy to 64.8 Gy with concurrent fluorouracil (5-FU) and cisplatin in esophageal cancer did not produce an improvement in local control or overall survival and had higher treatment-related mortality (9% compared with 2%). However, of 11 treatment-related deaths in the high-dose arm, 7 deaths occurred in patients who had received less than 50.4 Gy.[50] Patients with SCC of the cervical esophagus were allowed on this trial but represented a minority of patients. In light of these results, the standard dose for esophageal cancer remains 50 to 50.4 Gy. However, many institutions feel that these results do not apply to SCC of the cervical esophagus and that it should be treated to higher doses as an SCC of the head and neck. Many of the modern series give 60 to 70 Gy with concurrent chemotherapy with treatment mortality ranging from 0 to 6%.[28,51–56] We give 60 to 70 Gy to the primary tumor and involved lymph nodes and 56.1 Gy concurrently to the at-risk nodal regions. For SCC confined to the cervical esophagus, we treat the paratracheal nodes down to the carina as well as the low cervical nodes (levels III and IV) if the neck is clinically uninvolved (**Fig. 18.5**). If there is extension into the hypopharynx, then the levels treated may be modified depending on the extent of hypopharynx involved.

In SCC of the head and neck, many different dose and fractionation schedules have been used. Results from several randomized trials have consistently shown that hyperfractionation regimens and accelerated fractionation produce significantly improved local control and survival in the setting of radiotherapy alone and this was shown in a meta-analysis.[45] Although accelerated or hyperfractionated regimens have been tested with concurrent chemotherapy because of increased acute and late toxicity and because of the demands placed on the patient and facility, altered fractionation regimens have not been widely used in the United States.[57,58] We give 70 Gy in 35 fractions in almost all cases of SCC of the hypopharynx. We give 56.1 Gy concurrently to the clinically uninvolved, at-risk nodal regions (levels II to V and retropharyngeal).

Results

Unfortunately, the overall survival in SCC of the cervical esophagus treated with chemoradiotherapy remains poor, with 5-year survival rates ranging from 18.6 to 55%. In the one series reporting a 5-year overall survival rate of 55%, 80% of the patients had tumors staged T1-T3N0. The most common acute toxicities are mucositis/esophagitis with grade 3 to 4 events occurring in approximately 15% of the patients.[28,52–56] Grade 3 to 4 leukopenia can occur in up to a quarter of patients. Esophageal stricture can also occur in 5 to 10% of the patients. One series saw that patients receiving chemoradiotherapy had worse posttreatment dysphagia scores than patients

Table 18.6 Results of Chemoradiotherapy for Cervical Esophagus

Author	Number of Patients	Radiation Therapy	Chemotherapy	Toxicity	Local Control	Survival
Tong et al[28]	21	60–68 Gy/30–34 fx	Cisplatin 100 mg/m² on days 1 and 22 and 5-FU continuous infusion days 1–5 and 22–26	Grade 5 toxicity: 4.8% Grade 3 mucositis: 9.5% Grade 3 esophageal stricture: 4.8% Vocal cord paralysis requiring tracheotomy: 9.5%	CR: 29%	Median survival: 24.9 mo 2-y OS: 46.9%
Chou et al[40]	14	60–70 Gy at 1.8–2 Gy/fx	Cisplatin (60 mg/m²) on day 1 and 5-FU (600 mg/m²) and leucovorin (20 mg/m²) on days 1–5 × 2–3 cycles	Not reported	Not reported	Mean DSS: 34.4 mo
Huang et al[51]	71 (50 curative intent)	1997–2000: 54 Gy/20 fx 2001–2005: 70 Gy/35 fx	1997–2000: 5-FU (1000 mg/m²) on days 1–4 + mitomycin C (10 mg/m²) OR cisplatin (75 mg/m²) on day 1 2001–2005: cisplatin (100 mg/m²) on days 1, 22, and 43	Severe posttreatment dysphasia: 45%	CR: 91% 1997–2000: 2-y LRFS: 48% 2001–2005: 2-y LRFS 46%	5-y OS: 28% 1997–2000: 2-y OS: 52% 2001–2005: 2-y OS: 43%
Uno et al[47]	21 (6 of these neoadjuvant)	60–74 Gy at 2 Gy/fx 40 Gy/20 fx (neoadjuvant)	1. Cisplatin (15 mg/m²) on days 1–5 and 5-FU (500 mg/d for 5 d per week) 2. Cisplatin 5 mg and 5-FU 250 mg daily 3. Two patients no chemotherapy	Grade 5 toxicity: 1 Grade 3 toxicities: 8	CR: 58% if CTRT CR: 75% if T1–3 CR: 22% if T4 LRF: 47%	2-y OS: 41% 5-y OS: 27%
Wang et al[53]	35	24.5–64.8 Gy (median 50.4 Gy/28 fx)	Induction: Various regimens including 5-FU, cisplatin, paclitaxel, or carboplatin Concurrent: 57% 5-FU, 34% cisplatin and 5-FU, 3% carboplatin and 5-FU, 3% irinotecan and 5-FU, 3% carboplatin	Not reported	CR: 62.9% CR: 79.2% if ≥ 50 Gy CR: 27.3% if < 50 Gy 5-y LRFS: 47.7%	5-y OS: 18.6% 5-y DSS: 27.6% 5-y DSS: 44% if ≥ 50 Gy
Yamada et al[54]	27	44–73.7 Gy (mean 66 Gy)	85% received cisplatin (50–80 mg/m²) on days 1, 22, and 43 and 5-FU (500–750 mg/m²) on days 2–5, 23–26, and 44–47	Grade 3 mucositis: 15% Grade 3 leukopenia: 26%	CR: 48% Local control: 52% Local control: 70% if ≥ 60 Gy	5-y OS: 37.9% 5-y DFS: 13%
Burmeister et al[55]	34	50.4 Gy/20 fx–65 Gy/33 fx	1. 5-FU (800 mg/m² daily) days 2–5 and 23–26 2. 5-FU as above and cisplatin (80 mg/m²) on days 1 and 22 3. 5-FU as above and cisplatin (20 mg/m²) days 1–5, 22–26	Grade 4 esophagitis: 15% Grade 5 toxicity: 6%	CR: 91% Local control: 88% Local recurrence: 1	5-y OS: 55%
Stuschke et al[56]	17	60 Gy/30 fx–65 Gy/30 fx	Induction: Cisplatin, 5-FU, and etoposide OR cisplatin and 5-FU Concurrent: Cisplatin (75 mg/m²) on days 2 and 8 and etoposide (80–100 mg/m²) on days 4–6	Grade 4 toxicity: 12% Grade 3 esophagitis: 12%	CR: 47% Local control: 33%	3-y OS: 24%

fx, fraction; 5-FU, fluorouracil; CR, complete response; mo, month; y, year; OS, overall survival; DSS, disease-specific survival; LRFS, locoregional recurrence-free survival; CTRT, chemoradiotherapy; LRF, locoregional failure; DFS, disease-free survival.

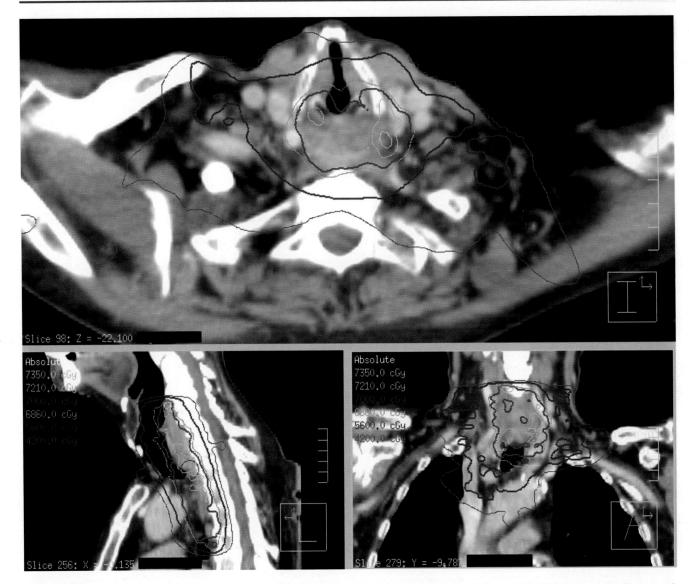

Figure 18.5 Radiotherapy plan for patient receiving 70 Gy in 35 fractions to cervical esophageal primary and 56.1 Gy concurrently to at-risk nodal regions.

who underwent surgical resection, although survival was not different. Because of the significant operative morbidity and overall poor survival, chemoradiotherapy remains the treatment of choice for SCC of the cervical esophagus. Isolated local failures may be salvaged surgically.

Palliation

In patients presenting with metastatic SCC of the cervical esophagus or hypopharynx, chemotherapy is the primary treatment modality. The performance status and comorbidities of the patient as well as the clinical course should be taken into account when deciding to initiate therapy and selecting the regimen. There are no biomarkers in this setting to aid in the selection of a specific regimen, and there is no one chemotherapy regimen that

has clearly shown superiority. Commonly used regimens that are active in SCC of the head and neck include cisplatin, cisplatin and 5-FU, cisplatin and paclitaxel, cisplatin and cetuximab, or cisplatin with 5-FU and cetuximab.[59] Carboplatin is often substituted for cisplatin in those with poor renal function. Cetuximab alone also may be used in the second-line treatment of metastatic SCC of the head and neck. Other agents such as vinorelbine, pemetrexed, mTOR inhibitors, and EGFR tyrosine kinase inhibitors continue to be investigated to treat metastatic SCC of the head and neck.

In the setting of metastatic SCC of the hypopharynx and cervical esophagus, the site of local disease can cause significant morbidity. In the case of airway compromise, a tracheostomy may need to be performed. Palliative approaches for dysphagia include chemotherapy, external beam radiotherapy, stent

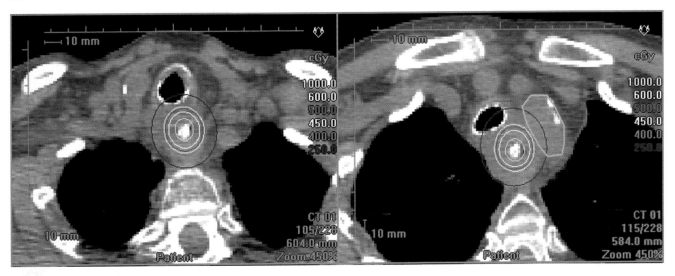

Figure 18.6 Radiotherapy plan for patient who received 10 Gy in two fractions high-dose rate brachytherapy for palliation of a locally advanced cervical esophagus primary. He was unable to swallow his secretions before treatment, and he was able to swallow most of his secretions 1 month after radiotherapy.

placement, and intraluminal brachytherapy. One randomized trial compared brachytherapy to stent placement for patients with dysphagia from esophageal cancer. Tumor growth within 3 cm of the upper esophageal sphincter was an exclusion criterion. Patients who received stent placement had more immediate improvement in dysphagia, but patients who received brachytherapy had better long-term relief and improved quality of life.[60] For tumors involving the lower cervical esophagus, brachytherapy should be considered to relieve dysphagia (**Fig. 18.6**). There are many patient and institutional factors in selecting the appropriate therapy for palliation of local symptoms from hypopharyngeal and cervical esophageal primaries, and multidisciplinary evaluation is essential.

Conclusions

SCCs of the cervical esophagus and hypopharynx are uncommon tumors that have been declining in incidence in the United States because of the declining rates of smoking. Unfortunately, most of these cancers present with locally advanced disease, and the prognosis has not significantly improved. Superficial lesions may be managed endoscopically or with larynx-preserving surgery in centers with experience in these techniques, but careful attention must be paid to the neck because of the high rate of nodal metastasis. Definitive chemoradiotherapy is the treatment of choice for locally advanced disease. However, if the larynx is involved to the point that it will not remain functional after chemoradiotherapy, then laryngopharyngectomy should be offered followed by adjuvant radiotherapy or chemoradiotherapy. Cancers of the hypopharynx and cervical esophagus require multidisciplinary management in centers with experience treating these sites.

Clinical Pearls

- Tracheoesophageal fistula should be ruled out by bronchoscopy in advanced (T3/4) cases of cervical esophageal cancer.

- Laryngopharyngectomy should be offered for cancers of the hypopharynx with significant laryngeal invasion that will result in a nonfunctioning larynx after chemoradiotherapy.

- Cancers of the cervical esophagus and lower hypopharynx can metastasize to paratracheal lymph nodes, and these should be included in radiation treatment planning.

- Retropharyngeal nodal coverage should be added if part of hypopharyngeal mucosa is involved in primary cervical esophageal cancer.

- Patients treated with radiation therapy should be carefully followed for hypothyroidism.

- Cancers of the hypopharynx and cervical esophagus are uncommon and often present with locally advanced disease.

- Because of their complexity and rarity, cancers of the cervical esophagus and hypopharynx require careful multidisciplinary management at centers with experience with these sites.

- Chemoradiotherapy is the preferred management for locally advanced cancers of the cervical esophagus and hypopharynx.

References

1. Popescu CR, Bertesteanu SVG, Mirea D, Grigore R, Lonescu D, Popescu B. The epidemiology of hypopharynx and cervical esophagus cancer. J Med Life 2010;3(4):396–401
2. Davies L, Welch HG. Epidemiology of head and neck cancer in the United States. Otolaryngol Head Neck Surg 2006;135(3):451–457
3. Gupta S, Kong W, Peng Y, Miao Q, Mackillop WJ. Temporal trends in the incidence and survival of cancers of the upper aerodigestive tract in Ontario and the United States. Int J Cancer 2009;125(9):2159–2165
4. Blot WJ, McLaughlin JK, Winn DM, et al. Smoking and drinking in relation to oral and pharyngeal cancer. Cancer Res 1988;48(11):3282–3287
5. Pandeya N, Williams G, Green AC, Webb PM, Whiteman DC; Australian Cancer Study. Alcohol consumption and the risks of adenocarcinoma and squamous cell carcinoma of the esophagus. Gastroenterology 2009;136(4):1215–1224, e1–e2
6. Druesne-Pecollo N, Tehard B, Mallet Y, et al. Alcohol and genetic polymorphisms: effect on risk of alcohol-related cancer. Lancet Oncol 2009;10(2):173–180
7. Kreimer AR, Clifford GM, Boyle P, Franceschi S. Human papillomavirus types in head and neck squamous cell carcinomas worldwide: a systematic review. Cancer Epidemiol Biomarkers Prev 2005;14(2):467–475
8. Ragin CC, Taioli E. Survival of squamous cell carcinoma of the head and neck in relation to human papillomavirus infection: review and meta-analysis. Int J Cancer 2007;121(8):1813–1820
9. Mukherji SK, Armao D, Joshi VM. Cervical nodal metastases in squamous cell carcinoma of the head and neck: what to expect. Head Neck 2001;23(11):995–1005
10. Edge SB, Byrd DR, Compton CC, Fritz AG, Greene FL, Trotti A. AJCC Cancer Staging Manual. 7th ed. New York: Springer; 2010
11. Tachimori Y, Nagai Y, Kanamori N, Hokamura N, Igaki H. Pattern of lymph node metastases of esophageal squamous cell carcinoma based on the anatomical lymphatic drainage system. Dis Esophagus 2011;24(1):33–38
12. Tandon S, Shahab R, Benton JI, Ghosh SK, Sheard J, Jones TM. Fine-needle aspiration cytology in a regional head and neck cancer center: comparison with a systematic review and meta-analysis. Head Neck 2008;30(9):1246–1252
13. Prehn RB, Pasic TR, Harari PM, Brown WD, Ford CN. Influence of computed tomography on pretherapeutic tumor staging in head and neck cancer patients. Otolaryngol Head Neck Surg 1998;119(6):628–633
14. Merritt RM, Williams MF, James TH, Porubsky ES. Detection of cervical metastasis: a meta-analysis comparing computed tomography with physical examination. Arch Otolaryngol Head Neck Surg 1997;123(2):149–152
15. van Vliet EPM, Heijenbrok-Kal MH, Hunink MGM, Kuipers EJ, Siersema PD. Staging investigations for oesophageal cancer: a meta-analysis. Br J Cancer 2008;98(3):547–557
16. Adams S, Baum RP, Stuckensen T, Bitter K, Hör G. Prospective comparison of 18F-FDG PET with conventional imaging modalities (CT, MRI, US) in lymph node staging of head and neck cancer. Eur J Nucl Med 1998;25(9):1255–1260
17. Schöder H, Yeung HWD, Gonen M, Kraus D, Larson SM. Head and neck cancer: clinical usefulness and accuracy of PET/CT image fusion. Radiology 2004;231(1):65–72
18. Kim SY, Roh JL, Yeo NK, et al. Combined 18F-fluorodeoxyglucose-positron emission tomography and computed tomography as a primary screening method for detecting second primary cancers and distant metastases in patients with head and neck cancer. Ann Oncol 2007;18(10):1698–1703
19. Rösch T. Endosonographic staging of esophageal cancer: a review of literature results. Gastrointest Endosc Clin North Am 1995;5(3):537–547
20. Fujita H, Sueyoshi S, Yamana H, et al. Optimum treatment strategy for superficial esophageal cancer: endoscopic mucosal resection versus radical esophagectomy. World J Surg 2001;25(4):424–431
21. Eguchi T, Nakanishi Y, Shimoda T, et al. Histopathological criteria for additional treatment after endoscopic mucosal resection for esophageal cancer: analysis of 464 surgically resected cases. Mod Pathol 2006;19(3):475–480
22. Cao Y, Liao C, Tan A, Gao Y, Mo Z, Gao F. Meta-analysis of endoscopic submucosal dissection versus endoscopic mucosal resection for tumors of the gastrointestinal tract. Endoscopy 2009;41(9):751–757
23. Ng T, Vezeridis MP. Advances in the surgical treatment of esophageal cancer. J Surg Oncol 2010;101(8):725–729
24. Mendenhall WM, Sombeck MD, Parsons JT, Kasper ME, Stringer SP, Vogel SB. Management of cervical esophageal carcinoma. Semin Radiat Oncol 1994;4(3):179–191
25. de Bree R, Leemans CR, Silver CE, et al. Paratracheal lymph node dissection in cancer of the larynx, hypopharynx, and cervical esophagus: the need for guidelines. Head Neck 2011;33(6):912–916
26. Stiles BM, Mirza F, Port JL, et al. Predictors of cervical and recurrent laryngeal lymph node metastases from esophageal cancer. Ann Thorac Surg 2010;90(6):1805–1811, discussion 1811
27. Triboulet JP, Mariette C, Chevalier D, Amrouni H. Surgical management of carcinoma of the hypopharynx and cervical esophagus: analysis of 209 cases. Arch Surg 2001;136(10):1164–1170
28. Tong DKH, Law S, Kwong DLW, Wei WI, Ng RWM, Wong KH. Current management of cervical esophageal cancer. World J Surg 2011;35(3):600–607
29. Ott K, Lordick F, Molls M, Bartels H, Biemer E, Siewert JR. Limited resection and free jejunal graft interposition for squamous cell carcinoma of the cervical oesophagus. Br J Surg 2009;96(3):258–266
30. Daiko H, Hayashi R, Saikawa M, et al. Surgical management of carcinoma of the cervical esophagus. J Surg Oncol 2007;96(2):166–172
31. Wang HW, Chu PY, Kuo KT, et al. A reappraisal of surgical management for squamous cell carcinoma in the pharyngoesophageal junction. J Surg Oncol 2006;93(6):468–476
32. Kadota H, Sakuraba M, Kimata Y, Hayashi R, Ebihara S, Kato H. Larynx-preserving esophagectomy and jejunal transfer for cervical esophageal carcinoma. Laryngoscope 2009;119(7):1274–1280
33. Shirakawa Y, Naomoto Y, Noma K, et al. Free jejunal graft for hypopharyngeal and esophageal reconstruction. Langenbecks Arch Surg 2004;389(5):387–390
34. Holsinger FC, Motamed M, Garcia D, Brasnu D, Ménard M, Laccourreye O. Resection of selected invasive squamous cell carcinoma of the pyriform sinus by means of the lateral pharyngotomy approach: the partial lateral pharyngectomy. Head Neck 2006;28(8):705–711
35. Makeieff M, Mercante G, Jouzdani E, Garrel R, Crampette L, Guerrier B. Supraglottic hemipharyngolaryngectomy for the treatment of T1 and T2 carcinomas of laryngeal margin and piriform sinus. Head Neck 2004;26(8):701–705
36. Laccourreye O, Ishoo E, de Mones E, Garcia D, Kania R, Hans S. Supracricoid hemilaryngopharyngectomy in patients with invasive squamous cell carcinoma of the pyriform sinus, part I: technique, complications, and long-term functional outcome. Ann Otol Rhinol Laryngol 2005;114(1 Pt 1):25–34

37. Martin A, Jäckel MC, Christiansen H, Mahmoodzada M, Kron M, Steiner W. Organ preserving transoral laser microsurgery for cancer of the hypopharynx. Laryngoscope 2008;118(3): 398–402

38. Shimizu Y, Yoshida T, Kato M, et al. Long-term outcome after endoscopic resection in patients with hypopharyngeal carcinoma invading the subepithelium: a case series. Endoscopy 2009;41(4): 374–376

39. Gebski V, Burmeister B, Smithers BM, Foo K, Zalcberg J, Simes J; Australasian Gastro-Intestinal Trials Group. Survival benefits from neoadjuvant chemoradiotherapy or chemotherapy in oesophageal carcinoma: a meta-analysis. Lancet Oncol 2007;8(3): 226–234

40. Chou SH, Li HP, Lee JY, Huang MF, Lee CH, Lee KW. Radical resection or chemoradiotherapy for cervical esophageal cancer? World J Surg 2010;34(8):1832–1839

41. Peters LJ, Goepfert H, Ang KK, et al. Evaluation of the dose for postoperative radiation therapy of head and neck cancer: first report of a prospective randomized trial. Int J Radiat Oncol Biol Phys 1993;26(1):3–11

42. Bernier J, Cooper JS, Pajak TF, et al. Defining risk levels in locally advanced head and neck cancers: a comparative analysis of concurrent postoperative radiation plus chemotherapy trials of the EORTC (#22931) and RTOG (# 9501). Head Neck 2005;27(10):843–850

43. Cooper JS, Guo MD, Herskovic A, et al; Radiation Therapy Oncology Group. Chemoradiotherapy of locally advanced esophageal cancer: long-term follow-up of a prospective randomized trial (RTOG 85-01). JAMA 1999;281(17):1623–1627

44. Smith TJ, Ryan LM, Douglass HO Jr, et al. Combined chemoradiotherapy vs. radiotherapy alone for early stage squamous cell carcinoma of the esophagus: a study of the Eastern Cooperative Oncology Group. Int J Radiat Oncol Biol Phys 1998;42(2):269–276

45. Pignon JP, Maitre A, Bourhis J. Meta-analysis of chemotherapy in head and neck cancer (MACH-NC): an update. Int J Radiat Biol Phys 2007;69:S112–S114

46. Lefebvre JL, Chevalier D, Luboinski B, Kirkpatrick A, Collette L, Sahmoud T; EORTC Head and Neck Cancer Cooperative Group. Larynx preservation in pyriform sinus cancer: preliminary results of a European Organization for Research and Treatment of Cancer phase III trial. J Natl Cancer Inst 1996;88(13):890–899

47. Prades JM, Lallemant B, Garrel R, et al. Randomized phase III trial comparing induction chemotherapy followed by radiotherapy to concomitant chemoradiotherapy for laryngeal preservation in T3M0 pyriform sinus carcinoma. Acta Otolaryngol 2010;130(1): 150–155

48. Chen AY, Halpern M. Factors predictive of survival in advanced laryngeal cancer. Arch Otolaryngol Head Neck Surg 2007;133(12):1270–1276

49. Rabbani A, Amdur RJ, Mancuso AA, et al. Definitive radiotherapy for T1-T2 squamous cell carcinoma of pyriform sinus. Int J Radiat Oncol Biol Phys 2008;72(2):351–355

50. Minsky BD, Pajak TF, Ginsberg RJ, et al. INT 0123 (Radiation Therapy Oncology Group 94-05) phase III trial of combined-modality therapy for esophageal cancer: high-dose versus standard-dose radiation therapy. J Clin Oncol 2002;20(5):1167–1174

51. Huang SH, Lockwood G, Brierley J, et al. Effect of concurrent high-dose cisplatin chemotherapy and conformal radiotherapy on cervical esophageal cancer survival. Int J Radiat Oncol Biol Phys 2008;71(3):735–740

52. Uno T, Isobe K, Kawakami H, et al. Concurrent chemoradiation for patients with squamous cell carcinoma of the cervical esophagus. Dis Esophagus 2007;20(1):12–18

53. Wang S, Liao Z, Chen Y, et al. Esophageal cancer located at the neck and upper thorax treated with concurrent chemoradiation: a single-institution experience. J Thorac Oncol 2006;1(3):252–259

54. Yamada K, Murakami M, Okamoto Y, et al. Treatment results of radiotherapy for carcinoma of the cervical esophagus. Acta Oncol 2006;45(8):1120–1125

55. Burmeister BH, Dickie G, Smithers BM, Hodge R, Morton K. Thirty-four patients with carcinoma of the cervical esophagus treated with chemoradiation therapy. Arch Otolaryngol Head Neck Surg 2000;126(2):205–208

56. Stuschke M, Stahl M, Wilke H, et al. Induction chemotherapy followed by concurrent chemotherapy and high-dose radiotherapy for locally advanced squamous cell carcinoma of the cervical oesophagus. Oncology 1999;57(2):99–105

57. Garden AS, Harris J, Trotti A, et al. Long-term results of concomitant boost radiation plus concurrent cisplatin for advanced head and neck carcinomas: a phase II trial of the Radiation Therapy Oncology Group (RTOG 99-14). Int J Radiat Oncol Biol Phys 2008;71(5):1351–1355

58. Brizel DM, Albers ME, Fisher SR, et al. Hyperfractionated irradiation with or without concurrent chemotherapy for locally advanced head and neck cancer. N Engl J Med 1998;338(25):1798–1804

59. Fury MG, Pfister DG. Current recommendations for systemic therapy of recurrent and/or metastatic head and neck squamous cell cancer. J Natl Compr Canc Netw 2011;9(6):681–689

60. Homs MYV, Steyerberg EW, Eijkenboom WMH, et al. Single-dose brachytherapy versus metal stent placement for the palliation of dysphagia from oesophageal cancer: multicentre randomised trial. Lancet 2004;364(9444):1497–1504

19 Tracheal Cancer: Aerodigestive Neoplasms of the Head and Neck

Nadia G. Mohyuddin and Jose P. Zevallos

Core Messages

- Primary tracheal tumors are rare and more than 90% of them are malignant. Patients often have nonspecific symptoms and this results in a delay of diagnosis.

- The two most common malignancies include squamous cell carcinoma and adenoid cystic carcinoma, the latter of which carries a slightly better overall survival.

- Secondary tracheal malignancies are more common and arise from direct invasion from the surrounding mediastinal and upper aerodigestive tract malignancies such as thyroid and esophageal cancers.

- Treatment of these malignancies requires a multidisciplinary team approach with surgical resection being the primary modality; however, alternative interventions include endotracheal/endobronchial stenting, radiation therapy, and chemotherapy.

- The best prognosis for long-term survival is in patients who receive complete surgical resection and have adenoid cystic carcinoma histology.

- Patients require close follow-up for several years with repeated bronchoscopies and radiographic imaging.

Primary tracheal malignancies are very rare, with an incidence of 0.1 per 100,000. More than 90% of primary tracheal tumors are malignant, of which the majority are present at an advanced stage. These tumors cause significant diagnostic and management challenges to the head and neck surgeon. Patients often present with nonspecific signs and symptoms, making the early diagnosis difficult. These tumors often require multimodality therapy including complex surgical resection and reconstruction, resulting in a long recovery period.

Optimal treatment of tracheal malignancies requires a multidisciplinary team including head and neck surgeons, thoracic surgeons, anesthesiologists, pathologists, radiation and medical oncologists, medical intensivists, pulmonologists, speech and language pathologists, as well as a well-trained nursing and support staff. Although several centers have reviewed their extensive experience with the management of primary tracheal malignancies, the rarity of these tumors has precluded the establishment of large clinical trials and defined treatment protocols. The purpose of this chapter is to review the diagnosis and management of tracheal malignancies. Emphasis will be placed on differential diagnosis, the importance of multimodality therapy, and surgical resection and reconstruction for these rare and interesting tumors. In addition, some of the current controversies and dilemmas are discussed.

Tracheal Anatomy

The average adult trachea is approximately 12 cm in length and 1.5 to 2.5 cm in width, and it is a hollow conduit connecting the larynx to the carina. It is divided in the proximal one-third cervical trachea and distal two-third thoracic trachea. Extension or flexion of the neck can either increase or decrease the amount of trachea above the sternal notch, respectively. There are 18 to 22 c-shaped incomplete cartilaginous rings, with each ring being approximately 4 mm in width and separated from one another by annular (intercartilaginous) ligaments. The trachealis muscle spans the length of the trachea, providing anterior and lateral support. This muscle is made of both longitudinal and transverse layers of smooth muscle. In addition, there is a posterior membranous portion of the trachea that separates the airway from the esophagus.[1,2]

The carina is approximately 38 cm from the incisors and is the bifurcation point of the trachea into the right and left main stem bronchi. It is held in position by the aortic arch. The right mainstem bronchus is more vertical, and this then divides into three upper, two middle, and five lower divisions. The left mainstem bronchus is further divided into two upper, two lingular, and four lower divisions.[1]

The mucosa of the tracheal lumen is made of ciliated pseudostratified columnar respiratory epithelium that overlies areolar and lymphoid tissue with elastic fibers, blood vessels, nerves, and mucous glands. In smokers, the cilia are destroyed and squamous metaplasias of the epithelium can result.[1]

The blood supply to the trachea is segmental and travels from lateral to medial. The primary arterial inflow is from the inferior thyroid artery off the thyrocervical trunk. This supplies the upper trachea and esophagus through three branches with distal anastomotic connections from the superior thyroid artery off the external carotid artery. The lower trachea and carina are supplied by the bronchial artery off the descending thoracic aorta. In addition, transverse intercartilaginous arteries extend into the tracheal wall and branch into the submucosa. This segmental blood supply can be easily violated and may lead to tracheal necrosis if extensive dissection along a significant length of the trachea is undertaken.[1,3]

Lymphatic drainage of the trachea is to the paratracheal, pretracheal, and subcarinal lymph nodes, with the primary echelon of nodes being closest to the tumor itself. It is rare for "skipped" nodal metastasis to occur.[1]

Surrounding the trachea are vital structures including the esophagus, thyroid gland, parathyroid glands, recurrent laryngeal nerves, great vessels, aorta, skeletal muscles, and other soft-tissue structures. These structures can often be the source of secondary tumors or can be directly invaded by primary tumors of the trachea.[1]

Diagnosis

Clinical Presentation

A high index of suspicion is required to diagnose primary tracheal malignancies as they often present with nonspecific signs and symptoms. In a series of 74 patients with primary tracheal malignancies treated at MD Anderson Cancer Center (MDACC), the most common presenting symptoms were most frequently dyspnea (55.4%), hemoptysis (48.6%), cough (41.9%), and hoarseness (35.1%).[4] Other presenting symptoms included dysphagia (28.4%), weight loss (30%), stridor (18.9%), sore throat (13.5%), history of asthma (6.8%), and wheezing (4.1%). Similarly, in a series of 270 patients with primary squamous cell carcinoma (SCC) and adenoid cystic carcinoma (ACC) of the trachea treated at Massachusetts General Hospital (MGH), the most common presenting symptoms were dyspnea and cough.[5] This group also noted that patients with SCC tended to present with hemoptysis. Unfortunately, in many cases, these symptoms were wrongfully attributed to adult-onset asthma or chronic obstructive pulmonary disease, thereby delaying diagnosis.[4,5] Furthermore, patients may not experience significant symptoms until 50 to 70% of the luminal diameter of the trachea is narrowed (**Fig. 19.1A**). In addition, exertional dyspnea and dyspnea at rest may not develop until the trachea has narrowed to less than 8 and 5 mm, respectively.[6,7]

Pulmonary function tests can detect obstruction in the upper airway and identify flow-volume loops that have characteristic flattening of both inspiratory and expiratory phases, providing further evidence of a fixed upper-airway obstruction.[2]

Imaging

Imaging studies are critical in the diagnosis and work-up of primary tracheal malignancies. These studies play a key role in depicting these tumors and assessing tumor extent within the tracheal lumen, airway wall, and surrounding structures before treatment planning.[8] Unfortunately, plain chest radiographs are often unremarkable in the setting of tracheal malignancies, although airway compression, tracheal narrowing, and postobstructive findings may be noted.

Thin-section contrast-enhanced computed tomography (CT) of the chest is the diagnostic imaging modality of choice for the evaluation of tracheal tumors. Furthermore, the development of multidetector CT scans has resulted in excellent axial source images and aided multiplanar three-dimensional (3D) reconstructed images. These high-resolution images allow the clinician to better delineate complex airway anatomy and tumor morphology.[9–11] A CT is usually performed at full inspiration but can be performed at the end of or during expiration to study the dynamics of the airway and the affect of a tumor on the distal airways and lung parenchyma.[8]

Although individual tumor histologies may show subtle differences, CT findings associated with tracheal neoplasms include a polypoid intraluminal mass of soft-tissue density with irregular, smooth, or lobulated contours (**Fig. 19.1B**). Eccentric narrowing of the airway or circumferential wall thickening of the trachea creating localized stenosis can also be evaluated by using CT, as well as tumor extension through the tracheal wall and into the surrounding structures in the neck and mediastinum (**Figs. 19.1B** and **19.2A, B**).[8] CT with intravenous contrast is also the study of choice for the evaluation of suspected nodal metastases.

Several authors have studied the benefit of positron emission tomography (PET) in the evaluation of tracheal tumors.[12,13] Specifically, PET and fused PET/CT images are useful in differentiating malignant from benign tumors of the trachea. Park et al found that SCC often demonstrates high standardized uptake values (SUVs) while ACC and other salivary gland malignancies show variable uptake depending on the grade of differentiation.[12] Benign neoplasms of the trachea will typically demonstrate decreased SUV. PET and PET/CT may also be helpful in diagnosing patients with suspected secondary malignancies or distant metastases, as well as in the evaluation of residual or recurrent disease after treatment. Current literature suggests using PET imaging no sooner than 8 weeks postradiation because of the increased risk of false-positive results if performed earlier.[14]

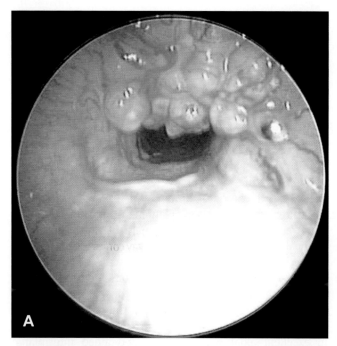

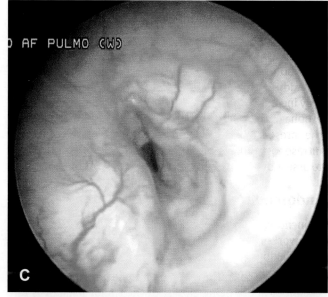

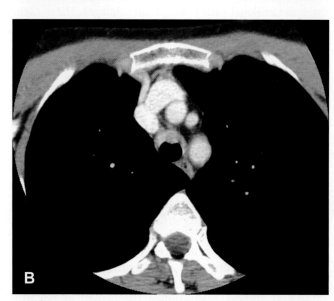

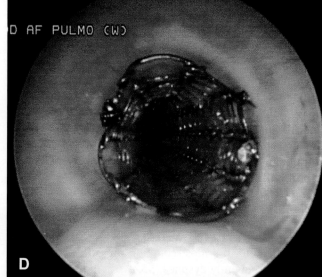

Figure 19.1 A 41-year-old female with progressive respiratory distress initially misdiagnosed as asthma was noted to have a primary tracheal lesion causing > 70% obstruction of the tracheal lumen. Biopsy revealed adenoid cystic carcinoma. Endoscopic (A) and radiographic (B) images of the airway show a lesion arising from the anterior mid-trachea. She refused conventional therapy and chose serial debridements followed by radiation therapy. She developed tracheal stenosis (C) and required endotracheal stent placement of her distal trachea (D) immediately proximal to the carina (E). She was initially diagnosed in 2003 and is currently alive with metastatic disease.

Image courtesy: These images are provided by Donald Donovan, MD, Bobby R. Alford Department of Otolaryngology/Head and Neck Surgery, Baylor College of Medicine Houston, Texas, United States.

The routine use of magnetic resonance imaging (MRI) has no significant advantage over present-day CT images except in the face of ACC. For these tumors, MRI offers superior evaluation of the surrounding soft tissue and extent of tumor involvement.[2]

Additional work-up for patients with tracheal tumors may include direct laryngoscopy and esophagoscopy, barium esophagram to evaluate the patency of the esophagus or the presence of a tracheoesophageal fistula, endoscopic ultrasonography, and fluoroscopy of the trachea and larynx to assess dynamic motion of these structures.[15]

Endoscopy

Bronchoscopy is an essential component in the diagnosis and work-up of patients with tracheal malignancies. While both flexible and rigid bronchoscopies allow for excellent visualization of the trachea and bronchi, rigid bronchoscopy is often preferred in the setting of airway compromise. Rigid bronchoscopy can be both diagnostic and therapeutic and allows for biopsy of tracheal lesions, dilation of a compromised airway, and ventilation.[16] Several scopes of different diameters and lengths should be available when planning endoscopy and airway intervention in a patient with suspected tracheal cancer.

Another novel imaging modality is virtual bronchoscopy (VB).[17,18] This technique is noninvasive and uses CT scan images along with commercial software to examine 2D and 3D anatomic details. Images from multiple directions are created with extreme precision to adequately view intraluminal and extraluminal pathology. It has also proven to be useful in determining airway patency distal to the lesion, evaluating the length of airway stenosis, as well as helping to establish the feasibility of endobronchial procedures including dilations, stent placements, and laser ablation. The main limitation of VB is in its inability to adequately evaluate the mucosal surface of the respiratory tract. More specifically, mucosal irregularity, color, or friability cannot be assessed; thus, using VB for routine surveillance is not warranted. There is promising research that suggests that new aerosolized contrast agents or spectroscopic techniques can potentially differentiate between benign and malignant mucosal tissues within the respiratory tract, thus enhancing the sensitivity and specificity of VB to diagnose preinvasive cancers.[18]

Tracheal Neoplasms

Close to 90% of primary tracheal neoplasms in adults are malignant. However, most malignant neoplasms of the trachea are secondarily due to direct extension from laryngeal, thyroid, esophageal, bronchogenic, or other metastatic tumors.[19,20] In children, nearly 70% of tracheal neoplasms are benign.[21] **Table 19.1** outlines a variety of primary neoplasms, both benign and malignant, of the adult tracheobronchial tree.

Benign Tracheal Neoplasms

Although this chapter focuses on malignant tracheal lesions, it is noteworthy to know that approximately 10% of adult primary tracheal tumors are benign.[19] The most common benign tumor is squamous papilloma caused by the human papillomavirus.

Table 19.1 Classification of Primary Tracheobronchial Tumors

Mesenchymal	Epithelial	Salivary
Benign • Fibroma • Benign fibrous histiocytoma • Hemangioma • Paraganglioma • Glomus tumor • Leiomyoma • Chondroma • Schwannoma	Benign • Papilloma	Benign • Pleomorphic adenoma • Mucous gland adenoma • Myoepithelioma • Oncocytoma
Malignant • Chondrosarcoma • Rhabdomyosarcoma • Hemangiopericytoma • Hodgkin lymphoma • Non-Hodgkin lymphoma • Malignant fibrous histiocytoma	Malignant • Squamous cell carcinoma • Adenocarcinoma • Large cell undifferentiated carcinoma • Neuroendocrine tumors • Typical and atypical carcinoid • Large cell neuroendocrine • Small cell carcinoma	Malignant • Adenoid cystic carcinoma • Mucoepidermoid carcinoma • Carcinoma ex pleomorphic adenoma
Other • Granular cell tumor • Hamartoma • Fibromatosis		

Other benign lesions include pleomorphic adenoma, granular cell tumor, and benign cartilaginous tumors.

Malignant Tracheal Neoplasms

Squamous Cell Carcinoma

SCC makes up the majority of primary tracheal malignancies, accounting for 36 to 59% of primary tracheal malignancies in most large series.[2,4,5,19,22] Primary tracheal SCC is associated with smoking, has a male predominance, occurs in the sixth and seventh decades of life, and has a propensity for regional nodal metastasis.[2] Macroscopically, SCC appears as a large mass within the central airways with either exophytic or ulcerative component. It can be multifocal in approximately 10% of the patients, but majority of SCCs will occur in the distal trachea.[8] Regional extent into the esophagus or mainstem bronchus is frequent.

Primary tracheal SCC is associated with worse outcomes compared with other tracheal malignancies, with overall 5-year survival rate ranging from 7.3 to 39%.[5] It is well established that surgical resection is the mainstay of the treatment for SCC and resectabilty affords patients' improved disease-specific and overall survival. A landmark study by Gaissert et al demonstrated that mean survival time was 38 months for resected tracheal SCC and 8.8 months for unresectable tumors undergoing chemotherapy and radiation.[5] This study also demonstrates that locoregional recurrence is the main determinant of disease-specific survival in patients with tracheal squamous cell cancer.[5]

A study by Honings et al from MGH demonstrated specific pathologic features of primary tracheal SCC that may serve as prognostic predictors of survival.[23] On the basis of a histologic review of 59 resected tracheal SCC specimens, they identified completeness of resection, involvement of the thyroid gland, and lymphatic invasion as predictors of survival.[23] Although patients with well-differentiated tumors had a better overall survival than those with moderately or poorly differentiated tumors, this difference did not achieve statistical significance. This study emphasizes the importance of clear surgical margins and suggests that the invasion of the thyroid gland may preclude a surgical cure.[23]

Adenoid Cystic Carcinoma

ACC represents the second most common primary tracheal malignancy. In a large observational study by Urdaneta et al, ACC accounted for 16.3% of tumors.[24] In other series, ACC represents up to 40% of all tracheal malignancies.[2,4,5,19,22] It has been shown to occur equally in males and females and presents most commonly in the fifth decade of life.[25]

ACC is an aggressive malignancy of salivary gland origin that is characterized by local invasion and perineural spread. Almost half of tracheal ACCs are found in the proximal trachea, with the most common presenting symptoms being dyspnea, cough, and hoarseness. Because of the later findings, patients are often referred to an otolaryngologist first.[25] These tumors tend to be locally recurrent, particularly with inadequate surgical margins (**Fig. 19.1**). Nodal and

paratracheal metastases develop late in the course, with distant metastases occurring in the lungs, liver, or bones. Unlike SCC of the trachea, smoking is not associated with the development of ACC. Also, in contrast to SCC, the prognosis for resected ACC is much better with 5- and 10-year survival rates of 52 and 29%.[5] Although surgery is the mainstay of the treatment for this malignancy, other modalities have been investigated and are discussed in the "Management of Tracheal Malignancies" section.

The remaining 30% of primary tracheal neoplasms are a heterogeneous group of epithelial, salivary, and mesenchymal tumors.[19,20]

Pediatric Tracheal Malignancies

In contrast to adult patients, the vast majority of pediatric tracheal tumors are benign.[21] Primary tracheal cancers arising in children are extremely rare, with only 14 cases reported in the literature.[21] There is often a significant delay in diagnosis, as the early symptoms are wrongfully attributed to asthma or upper airway infection. Romão et al published their experience with two cases of tracheal cancer in children and performed a literature review.[26] Mucoepidermoid carcinoma accounted for the majority of these cancers, and when complete surgical resection was feasible, the prognosis was generally good. The average age at presentation among the cases reviewed in this study was 7 years, and the delay from the onset of symptoms to diagnosis ranged from 2 weeks to 2 years.[26]

Secondary Tracheal Malignancies

Secondary malignancies of the trachea arise as a result of either direct invasion or metastasis and are more common than primary tumors.[19,20] A wide variety of metastatic tumors have been described in the trachea, most commonly from thyroid malignancies; however, SCC from other sites in the head and neck, esophageal carcinoma, melanoma, sarcoma, tumor of breast, and colorectal tumor are also known to invade the trachea.

Thyroid cancer is the most commonly invasive tumor of the trachea. Aerodigestive tract invasion has been reported in approximately 7 to 16% of all cases of thyroid carcinoma.[27] Although anaplastic thyroid cancer is often associated with tracheal invasion, a study of patients with thyroid cancer with tracheal invasion by Gaissert et al demonstrated that 76% of tumors were well-differentiated carcinomas.[27] Sites of invasion include all portions of the endolarynx, trachea, esophagus, strap muscles, and recurrent laryngeal nerve.[28] While the prognosis of well-differentiated thyroid cancer is excellent, laryngeal or tracheal invasion is an independent predictor of death.[27,29] McConahey et al found that laryngotracheal invasion was the direct cause of death in 36% of the patients with locally advanced thyroid cancer.[30]

Controversy exists regarding the extent of resection required to treat thyroid cancer with tracheal invasion. Several authors recommend radical complete resection irrespective of the degree of invasion to be the most oncologically sound procedure.[31,32] However, many authors have demonstrated no difference in survival for patients with locally invasive well-differentiated thyroid carcinoma treated by radical resection of aerodigestive tract structures and those treated by near-complete conservative surgery.[28] Czaja and McCaffrey found no difference in survival for patients undergoing shave excision versus radical resection if gross tumor did not remain.[29] Although there is debate regarding the extent of resection, there is generally agreement on the need for radical resection when tracheal mucosa has been invaded.

Staging

An official staging system for primary tracheal malignancies has not been universally adopted to date by the American Joint Committee on Cancer. However, a TNM (tumor, node, metastasis) staging system (**Table 19.2**) developed by Bhattacharyya is widely accepted and validated.[33] He proposed a TNM system for primary tracheal malignancies, in which T1 and T2 tumors are limited to the trachea and differentiated by size of less than or greater than 2 cm. T3 tumors have spread outside the trachea without invasion of adjacent structures, while T4 tumors have invaded adjacent structures or organs. Unlike other sites in the head and neck, regional nodal disease is defined as the absence (N0) or presence (N1) of metastatic lymph nodes. Overall stage is defined as follows: stage I, T1N0; stage II, T2N0; stage III, T3N0; stage IV, T4N0 or any N1 disease.[33]

Management of Tracheal Malignancies

Surgery

Surgery for primary tracheal cancer may involve acute surgical management for tracheal obstruction as well as definitive surgical resection. According to Grillo, therapeutic goals of the initial emergent management of tumor-related obstruction are as follows: (1) to facilitate safe anesthesia

Table 19.2 Primary Tumor and Nodal Staging for Tracheal Carcinoma

Staging	Definition
T stage	
• T1	Confined to trachea < 2 cm
• T2	Confined to trachea > 2 cm
• T3	Spread to outside the trachea but not to adjacent organs or structures
• T4	Spread to adjacent organs or structures
• Tx	Unknown or cannot be assessed
N stage	
• N0	No evidence of regional nodal disease
• N1	Positive regional nodal disease
• Nx	Unknown or cannot be assessed

Note: No universally agreed upon staging system exists; however, this description by Bhattacharyya is most commonly used.
Adapted from reference 33.

for resection; (2) to permit delay of resection for study, to clear obstructive pneumonia, to wean from high doses of steroids, and to stabilize medical conditions; and (3) to allow palliative irradiation, external or brachytherapy.[34] If obstruction is due to extrinsic compression by a tumor, an internal stent or Y-tube stent can provide temporary relief (**Fig. 19.2**).[35,36] Blockage by a tumor must be removed rather than dilated.[34]

Surgical resection is the primary treatment modality in most cases of primary tracheal malignancies and is the only modality that has consistently demonstrated the potential for cure and long-term survival.[2,5,11] In addition, it is the primary treatment modality for benign tumors of the trachea. In a large study by Gaissert et al, it was demonstrated that those patients undergoing surgery had better overall survival than those treated by other modalities.[5] They also reported that disease-free survival was longer in patients who had complete resection than in those whose resection was incomplete ($p < 0.05$), in those with negative airway margins than in those who had positive airway margins ($p < 0.05$), and in patients with adenoid cystic histology compared with patients with squamous histology ($p < 0.001$).[2,5]

It is important to note that resection requires multidisciplinary collaboration between head and neck surgeons, thoracic surgeons, and skilled anesthesiologists because of the inherent danger associated with airway manipulation. Acute and long-term operative complications should also be considered.

Contraindications for surgery include greater than 50% involvement of the adult trachea or 30% involvement of the juvenile trachea, extension to vital surrounding structures, extensive nodal involvement, metastatic disease, or a mediastinum that has received radiation dose of more than 60 Gy or has been operated on.[2] In addition, patients should have a proper medical evaluation preoperatively, as these procedures are high-risk and preexisting medical conditions can preclude the operation.

Anesthesia

When performed surgery on the airway including the larynx, trachea, and bronchi, it is crucial to have an anesthesiologist who is skilled in managing these complex cases. It is not infrequent to have patients in respiratory distress, and urgently establishing a secure airway is of utmost importance, which must be done in a timely manner. Use of inhalation agents, slow induction of anesthesia, and maintaining spontaneous ventilation with the initial avoidance of muscle relaxants maybe necessary in several of these cases.[37] The use of jet ventilation has been well established in various airway surgeries, and as such, it has a critical role in procedures performed on patients with endoluminal disease.[38,39] A catheter is placed beyond the lesion to provide ventilation to the distal airways. However, care must be taken to allow egress of gas and to prevent breath stacking, which can lead to barotrauma.[37] Another option is cardiopulmonary bypass for extensive intrathoracic tracheal and vascular surgery.

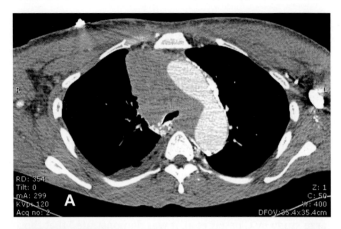

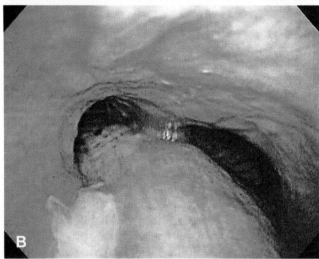

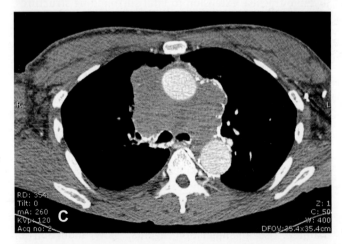

Figure 19.2 A 74-year-old male with extensive mediastinal large cell neuroendocrine tumor causing significant extrinsic distal tracheal (A), carinal (B), and bilateral (C) main stem bronchi compression.

Surgical Procedures

A detailed discussion of all the surgical techniques is beyond the scope of this chapter; however, an excellent description of various procedures can be found in the classic text by Grillo.[40]

Surgical evaluation with rigid bronchoscopy can be both diagnostic and therapeutic. This technique allows ventilation while simultaneously allowing the surgeon to perform a complete endoscopic evaluation as well as biopsies, debridements, dilations, and stent placements.

The maximum amount of trachea that can be safely resected for an end-to-end primary anastomosis is one-half of the adult trachea and one-third of the juvenile trachea.[41,42] An important consideration with tracheal resection is to dissect only the lymphatics immediately surrounding the resected segment of trachea, as any extensive proximal or distal paratracheal dissection could jeopardize the vasculature and result in tracheal necrosis.[1,3] Ideally, the patient's neck should be flexed to facilitate the anastomosis and prevent excessive tension on the suture line; resorbable vicryl sutures should be used to decrease the risk for suture line granulation tissue development; and the endotracheal tube cuff should be distal to the anastomosis to prevent future stenosis. Postoperatively, a guardian chin stitch or "Grillo" stitch is placed from the patient's submental crease to the presternal skin to prevent hyperextension and potential anastomosis rupture (**Fig. 19.3**).

There are several lengthening procedures that can be performed to assist with complete mobilization of the trachea.[43-45] Supralaryngeal release procedures include suprahyoid (release all muscles attached to the superior hyoid exposing the preepiglottic space), infrahyoid (sectioning of the strap muscles above the thyroid cartilage), or complete (removal of the hyoid bone) laryngeal release. This allows an additional 5 cm of length. Infralaryngeal release consists of various thoracic procedures including mobilization of the right hilum, division of the pulmonary ligament, intrapericardial dissection of the pulmonary vessels, and division of the left main bronchus from the carina and reimplantation into the right bronchial system in and end-to-side anastomosis. These techniques allow an additional 6 cm of length. Another infralaryngeal release that gains an additional 2 cm of length is the incision of the annular ligaments between the tracheal rings. Care must be taken to avoid circumferential incisions, as this can lead to vascular injury and tracheal necrosis.[43-45]

A cervical collar incision is used for exposure of the upper cervical and mediastinal trachea, while a median sternotomy exposes the remaining mediastinal trachea.[46] Distal tracheal or carinal resection may require a right posterolateral thoracotomy. Carinal resections are higher risk and require single lung ventilation throughout the procedure. There is also an increased morbidity and mortality associated with this procedure.[47]

Additional procedures for the distal airway include bronchial sleeve resection and sleeve lobectomy. The former involves removal of a circumferential portion of the bronchus while sparing the lung parenchyma. The latter, however, consists of removal of both the bronchus and the associated pulmonary lobe.

Another procedure that can be performed in rare instances is the cervicomediastinal exenteration with mediastinal tracheostomy.[48,49] This carries a high risk for morbidity

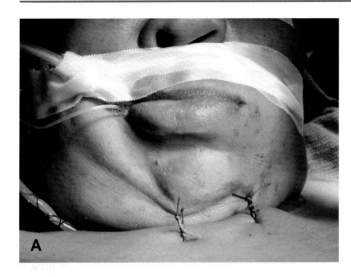

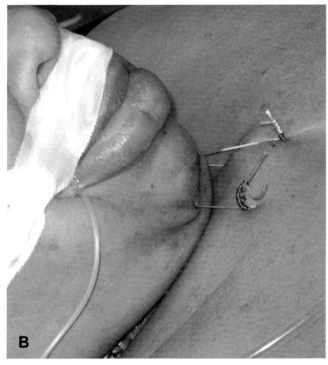

Figure 19.3 A guardian chin stitch or "Grillo" stitch is placed from the patient's submental crease to the anterior sternal skin to prevent hyperextension of the neck and potential anastomotic rupture after primary tracheal resection with end-to-end anastomosis. (A) Frontal view; (B) lateral view.

and mortality and is very rarely performed. It involves removal of the medial heads of the clavicles, manubrium, costal cartilages 1 and 2, larynx, pharynx, esophagus, and majority of trachea. Esophageal reconstruction is warranted, with either a free tissue transfer or a gastric pull-up. The innominate artery may need to be divided; thus, intraoperative electroencephalogram and preoperative vascular studies are necessary. A mediastinal tracheostoma is created in the center of the chest. This heroic procedure, when performed on carefully selected patients, can result in acceptable palliation.[48,49]

Postoperatively, it is critical to avoid mechanical ventilation once surgery is completed; keep the patient's neck in a flexed position, control secretions, use prophylactic antibiotics and antireflux medications, and administer steroids and racemic epinephrine as needed. If a patient requires reintubation, it is best for the operating surgeon to place the tube under direct visualization through either flexible or rigid bronchoscopy. In addition, the tube should be of a small diameter and the cuff should be inflated either distal to or proximal from the suture line. Positive pressure ventilation should also be avoided, as this can force air through the suture line and cause anastomotic disruption.

Stenting

Endotracheal and endobronchial stents are an alternative for patients who are surgically unresectable or medically inoperable (**Fig. 19.1D, E**). When performed on the properly selected patient, reliable and durable palliation can be achieved in 80 to 90% of the cases with the use of either silicone or expandable stents.[35] There are several different types, shapes, and materials of available stents on the market; however, before using such devices, it is important to understand the goals of stenting. An ideal stent is (1) easy to insert, (2) able to be adjusted or removed without the risk of migration, (3) capable of maintaining airway patency, (4) firm enough to resist compressive forces yet compliant enough to prevent airway erosion, (5) conformable to airway contours, (6) biocompatible and rarely results in infection or granulation tissue development, and (7) noninterfering with normal mobilization of secretions and mucociliary clearance.[36]

Complications

Airway resection is a major undertaking and when performed at centers that are experienced in these technically challenging cases, the morbidity and mortality is low. Nonetheless, complications include infection, bleeding, vocal cord dysfunction, laryngeal/tracheal edema, suture line granulation tissue, aspiration, malacia, stenosis, tracheoesophageal fistula, anastomotic leak or rupture, tracheal necrosis, complete suture line dehiscence, and death.

In a study of 32 patients undergoing tracheal or carinal resection for primary malignancies, Liu et al reported major postoperative complications in 31% of the patients, including pulmonary empyema, dysphonia due to recurrent laryngeal injury, and acute postoperative respiratory failure requiring mechanical ventilation.[11] No operative deaths were reported; however, 3 patients (9.4%) died in the early postoperative period owing to acute respiratory distress syndrome, myocardial infarction, and bleeding gastric ulcer, respectively. In addition, three patients developed anastomotic stenosis requiring bronchoscopy and dilatation.[11]

Adjuvant Therapies

Radiation Therapy

Radiation therapy in the treatment of tracheal cancer has traditionally been reserved for patients with positive margins and extra tracheal invasion, nodal involvement, and unresectable disease. Several small series have examined the role of radiation therapy in the postoperative setting, as definitive treatment for clinically localized disease, and in cases of inoperable cancers.[4,5,50,51] Although standardized treatment protocols for the use of radiation therapy have not been established, radiation therapy should be considered postoperatively when pathologic features of aggressive disease (lymphatic or perineural invasion and close or positive surgical margins) are present. In recent years, intensity-modulated radiation therapy (IMRT) has become the gold standard. IMRT is administered such that the maximum dosage of radiation is delivered to the tumor while minimizing exposure to the surrounding normal tissue, thus limiting morbidity to potentially vital structures. In addition, the use of PET/CT-directed IMRT therapy has shown favorable results.[52]

A study by Webb et al from MDACC demonstrated improved disease-specific and overall survival in patients with tracheal carcinoma who received postoperative radiation, although this trend was not statistically significant.[4] They suggested that adjuvant postoperative radiotherapy be given to most patients with SCC of the trachea, even with negative margins. Furthermore, they advocated postoperative radiotherapy for patients with tracheal ACC given the propensity for perineural spread and local recurrence.[4]

Neutron therapy has also been investigated for locally advanced ACC of the trachea.[53] Citing promising results in the treatment of ACC in other head and neck sites, Bittner et al at the University of Washington examined the role of neutron therapy in 20 patients with locally advanced unresectable primary ACC.[53] They found that a 5-year locoregional control rate was 54.1% and the overall 5-year survival rate was 89.4%.[53]

Chemotherapy

The role of chemotherapy in the management of primary tracheal cancers is unclear. In a series from MDACC chemotherapy was used in 12 of 45 patients, and the most commonly used agents were etoposide, adriamycin, doxorubicin, cisplatin, and cyclophosphamide. In the majority of cases, chemotherapy was used in combination with local therapy. Although they acknowledge the lack of data on the use of chemotherapy for primary tracheal cancers, the MD Anderson group suggests its role for palliation of distant metastatic disease and for radiosensitization.[4]

Follow-Up and Management

Primary tracheal SCC is associated with worse outcomes compared with other tracheal malignancies, with the overall 5- and 10-year survival rate for resectable disease being 39 and 18%, respectively.[5] A landmark study by Gaissert et al at MGH demonstrated that mean survival time was 38 months for resected tracheal SCC and 8.8 months for unresectable

tumors undergoing chemotherapy and radiation.[5] Patients with primary ACC tracheal malignancies have a better 5- and 10-year survival rate for resectable disease of 52 and 29%, while unresectable disease resulted in 33 and 10% survival rate, respectively.[5]

In a study of 92 patients with primary tracheal malignancies, Bhattacharyya demonstrated the validity of the TNM staging system in predicting survival.[33] Five-year unadjusted survival rates for stages I to IV tumors were 53, 70, 75, and 15%, respectively. Furthermore, this study demonstrated that a majority of patients with primary tracheal malignancies present with advanced disease (51% stage IV) and that SCC has a significantly worse 5-year survival than ACC (34 and 78%, respectively).[33]

Routine surveillance postoperatively includes serial bronchoscopies, CT scans and/or PET/CT images, and close clinical follow-up. The natural progression of ACC is less rapid compared with SCC. In addition, ACC can have much later recurrences and/or distant metastasis; therefore, these patients should be followed for a longer period of time (i.e., greater than 10 years) and periodically evaluated for bony and pulmonary metastasis.

Conclusions

Tracheal malignancies are rare tumors with nonspecific signs and symptoms and often presenting at advanced stages. The diagnosis and work-up require sophisticated imaging studies and endoscopic evaluation of the airway. The majority of primary malignancies of the trachea are SCC and ACC, while secondary metastases and direct invasion from thyroid cancer are also possible. The treatment of choice for most patients with tracheal cancer is complete resection, often followed by adjuvant radiation therapy. Chemotherapy can be considered in combination with radiation therapy in patients with unresectable disease or with distant metastases. Patients will require close postoperative follow-up with repeated bronchoscopy and radiographic imaging. Long-term survival is best seen in those patients with resectable disease and ACC histology.

References

1. Grillo HA. Anatomy of the trachea. In Grillo HC, ed. Surgery of the Trachea and Bronchi. Hamilton, London: BC Decker; 2004:39–60
2. Macchiarini P. Primary tracheal tumours. Lancet Oncol 2006;7(1):83–91
3. Salassa JR, Pearson BW, Payne WS. Gross and microscopical blood supply of the trachea. Ann Thorac Surg 1977;24(2):100–107
4. Webb BD, Walsh GL, Roberts DB, Sturgis EM. Primary tracheal malignant neoplasms: the University of Texas MD Anderson Cancer Center experience. J Am Coll Surg 2006;202(2):237–246
5. Gaissert HA, Grillo HC, Shadmehr MB, et al. Long-term survival after resection of primary adenoid cystic and squamous cell carcinoma of the trachea and carina. Ann Thorac Surg 2004;78(6):1889–1896, discussion 1896–1897

6. Hollingsworth HM. Wheezing and stridor. Clin Chest Med 1987;8(2):231–240

7. Geffin B, Grillo HC, Cooper JD, Pontoppidan H. Stenosis following tracheostomy for respiratory care. JAMA 1971;216(12):1984–1988

8. Ferretti GR, Bithigoffer C, Righini CA, Arbib F, Lantuejoul S, Jankowski A. Imaging of tumors of the trachea and central bronchi. Radiol Clin North Am 2009;47(2):227–241

9. Lee KS, Yoon JH, Kim TK, Kim JS, Chung MP, Kwon OJ. Evaluation of tracheobronchial disease with helical CT with multiplanar and three-dimensional reconstruction: correlation with bronchoscopy. Radiographics 1997;17(3):555–567, discussion 568–570

10. LoCicero J III, Costello P, Campos CT, et al. Spiral CT with multiplanar and three-dimensional reconstructions accurately predicts tracheobronchial pathology. Ann Thorac Surg 1996;62(3):811–817

11. Liu XY, Liu FY, Wang Z, Chen G. Management and surgical resection for tumors of the trachea and carina: experience with 32 patients. World J Surg 2009;33(12):2593–2598

12. Park CM, Goo JM, Lee HJ, Kim MA, Lee CH, Kang MJ. Tumors in the tracheobronchial tree: CT and FDG PET features. Radiographics 2009;29(1):55–71

13. Kwak SH, Lee KS, Chung MJ, Jeong YJ, Kim GY, Kwon OJ. Adenoid cystic carcinoma of the airways: helical CT and histopathologic correlation. AJR Am J Roentgenol 2004;183(2):277–281

14. Agarwal V, Branstetter BF IV, Johnson JT. Indications for PET/CT in the head and neck. Otolaryngol Clin North Am 2008;41(1):23–49, v

15. Shepard JO, Weber AL. Imaging the larynx and trachea In: Grillo HC, ed. Surgery of the Trachea and Bronchi. Hamilton, London BC Decker; 2004: 103–160

16. Ferson PF, Eibling DE. Tracheoscopy and bronchoscopy. In Myers EN, ed. Operative Otolaryngology Head and Neck Surgery. New York: Saunders Elsevier; 2008:565–575

17. Bauer TL, Steiner KV. Virtual bronchoscopy: clinical applications and limitations. Surg Oncol Clin N Am 2007;16(2):323–328

18. Finkelstein SE, Summers RM, Nguyen DM, Schrump DS. Virtual bronchoscopy for evaluation of airway disease. Thorac Surg Clin 2004;14(1):79–86

19. Beheshti J, Mark EJ, Graeme-Cook F. Epithelial tumor of the trachea. In: Grillo HC, ed. Surgery of the Trachea and Bronchi. Hamilton, London: BC Decker; 2004:73–85

20. Beheshti J, Mark EJ. Mesenchymal tumor of the trachea. In: Grillo HC, ed. Surgery of the Trachea and Bronchi. Hamilton, London: BC Decker; 2004:86–97

21. Desai DP, Holinger LD, Gonzalez-Crussi F. Tracheal neoplasms in children. Ann Otol Rhinol Laryngol 1998;107(9 Pt 1):790–796

22. Grillo HC, Mathisen DJ. Primary tracheal tumors: treatment and results. Ann Thorac Surg 1990;49(1):69–77

23. Honings J, Gaissert HA, Ruangchira-Urai R, et al. Pathologic characteristics of resected squamous cell carcinoma of the trachea: prognostic factors based on an analysis of 59 cases. Virchows Arch 2009;455(5):423–429

24. Urdaneta AI, Yu JB, Wilson LD. Population based cancer registry analysis of primary tracheal carcinoma. Am J Clin Oncol 2011;34(1):32–37

25. Azar T, Abdul-Karim FW, Tucker HM. Adenoid cystic carcinoma of the trachea. Laryngoscope 1998;108(9):1297–1300

26. Romão RL, de Barros F, Maksoud Filho JG, et al. Malignant tumor of the trachea in children: diagnostic pitfalls and surgical management. J Pediatr Surg 2009;44(11):e1–e4

27. Gaissert HA, Honings J, Grillo HC, et al. Segmental laryngotracheal and tracheal resection for invasive thyroid carcinoma. Ann Thorac Surg 2007;83(6):1952–1959

28. McCaffrey JC. Aerodigestive tract invasion by well-differentiated thyroid carcinoma: diagnosis, management, prognosis, and biology. Laryngoscope 2006;116(1):1–11

29. Czaja JM, McCaffrey TV. The surgical management of laryngotracheal invasion by well-differentiated papillary thyroid carcinoma. Arch Otolaryngol Head Neck Surg 1997;123(5):484–490

30. McConahey WM, Hay ID, Woolner LB, van Heerden JA, Taylor WF. Papillary thyroid cancer treated at the Mayo Clinic, 1946 through 1970: initial manifestations, pathologic findings, therapy, and outcome. Mayo Clin Proc 1986;61(12):978–996

31. Nishida T, Nakao K, Hamaji M. Differentiated thyroid carcinoma with airway invasion: indication for tracheal resection based on the extent of cancer invasion. J Thorac Cardiovasc Surg 1997;114(1):84–92

32. Yang CC, Lee CH, Wang LS, Huang BS, Hsu WH, Huang MH. Resectional treatment for thyroid cancer with tracheal invasion: a long-term follow-up study. Arch Surg 2000;135(6):704–707

33. Bhattacharyya N. Contemporary staging and prognosis for primary tracheal malignancies: a population-based analysis. Otolaryngol Head Neck Surg 2004;131(5):639–642

34. Grillo H. Urgent treatment of tracheal obstruction. In: Grillo HC, ed. Surgery of the Trachea and Bronchi. Hamilton, London: BC Decker; 2004:471–478

35. Wood DE. Management of malignant tracheobronchial obstruction. Surg Clin North Am 2002;82(3):621–642

36. Wood DJ. Tracheal and bronchial stenting. In Grillo HC, ed. Surgery of the Trachea and Bronchi. Hamilton, London: BC Decker; 2004:763–790

37. Alfille P. Anesthesia for tracheal surgery. In: Grillo HC, ed. Surgery of the Trachea and Bronchi. Hamilton, London: BC Decker; 2004: 453–470

38. Cay DL. Venturi for tracheal reconstruction. Anaesth Intensive Care 1978;6(2):171

39. Giunta F, Chiaranda M, Manani G, Giron GP. Clinical uses of high frequency jet ventilation in anaesthesia. Br J Anaesth 1989; 63(7 Suppl 1):102S–106S

40. Grillo H. Surgery of the Trachea and Bronchi. Hamilton, London: BC Decker; 2004

41. Mulliken JB, Grillo HC. The limits of tracheal resection with primary anastomosis: further anatomical studies in man. J Thorac Cardiovasc Surg 1968;55(3):418–421

42. Wright CD, Graham BB, Grillo HC, Wain JC, Mathisen DJ. Pediatric tracheal surgery. Ann Thorac Surg 2002;74(2):308–313, discussion 314

43. Dedo HH, Fishman NH. Laryngeal release and sleeve resection for tracheal stenosis. Ann Otol Rhinol Laryngol 1969;78(2):285–296

44. Montgomery WW. The surgical management of supraglottic and subglottic stenosis. Ann Otol Rhinol Laryngol 1968;77(3):534–546

45. Grillo HC. Tracheal reconstruction: anterior approach and extended resection. In Grillo HC, ed. Surgery of the Trachea and Bronchi. Hamilton, London: BC Decker; 2004:517–548

46. Pearson FG, Cardoso P, Keshavjee S. In: Pearson FG, Cooper JD, Deslauriers J, Ginsberg RJ, Hiebert C, Patterson GA, Urschel HC, eds. Thoracic Surgery. New York: Churchill Livingstone; 1995: 285–298

47. Mathisen DJ, Grillo HC. Carinal resection for bronchogenic carcinoma. J Thorac Cardiovasc Surg 1991;102(1):16–22, discussion 22–23

48. Madsen JC, Mathisen DJ, Grillo HC. Cervical exenteration. Semin Thorac Cardiovasc Surg 1992;4(4):292–299

49. Grillo HC. Cervicomediastinal exenteration and mediastinal tracheostomy. In: Grillo HC, ed. Surgery of the Trachea and Bronchi. Hamilton, London: BC Decker; 2004:681–692

50. Schraube P, Latz D, Wannenmacher M. Treatment of primary squamous cell carcinoma of the trachea: the role of radiation therapy. Radiother Oncol 1994;33(3):254–258

51. Jeremic B, Shibamoto Y, Acimovic L, Milisavljevic S. Radiotherapy for primary squamous cell carcinoma of the trachea. Radiother Oncol 1996;41(2):135–138

52. Haresh KP, Prabhakar R, Rath GK, Sharma DN, Julka PK, Subramani V. Adenoid cystic carcinoma of the trachea treated with PET-CT based intensity modulated radiotherapy. J Thorac Oncol 2008;3(7):793–795

53. Bittner N, Koh WJ, Laramore GE, Patel S, Mulligan MS, Douglas JG. Treatment of locally advanced adenoid cystic carcinoma of the trachea with neutron radiotherapy. Int J Radiat Oncol Biol Phys 2008;72(2):410–414

20 Parapharyngeal Space Tumors

Anupam Mishra, Raghav C. Dwivedi, and Rehan A. Kazi

Core Messages

- Parapharyngeal space is a deep-seated fascial space associated with adjoining fascial spaces and the infratemporal fossa having a complex anatomy.

- Parapharyngeal space lesions are diagnosed late with imaging and fine-needle aspiration cytology.

- Angiography is important to characterize the vascularity of the lesion and for assessment of the cerebral circulation where the internal carotid artery is at risk of being damaged during surgery.

- Most parapharyngeal space tumors are benign and can be surgically resected completely with excellent results. The use of transparotid with or without transcervical approach is sufficient in most of the cases.

- Primary malignancy of parapharyngeal space carries a relatively satisfactory outcome, while prognosis of a metastatic disease is dismal.

- Owing to anatomic complexity and high morbidity associated with surgical clearance especially of an extensive/invasive disease, a balance needs to be maintained between the advantage of surgery and the postoperative deterioration of the quality of life.

The parapharyngeal space (PPSp), previously known as lateral pharyngeal space, pharyngomaxillary space, pterygopharyngeal space, pterygomandibular space, or pharyngomasticatory space, is important by virtue of its location, although the tumors of the space are relatively uncommon (0.5% of all head and neck tumors). It is the most complex facial space of the suprahyoid segment of the neck in terms of anatomy. Traditionally, its sister accompaniment, the infratemporal fossa, has been dealt as a separate entity particularly by the anatomists, but pathologically they are often the seat of a single disease. Hence, they can be conceptualized as a single space, both being merely extension of one another. However, it is important to understand a few of the applied anatomic concerns with a surgeon's perspective. As per the traditional view, the medial pterygoid muscle separates these two compartments anteriorly while a free communication exists in the posterior half. The anatomic aspects are depicted in **Table 20.1**. The overall anatomic relationship can be resolved by defining the PPSp more accurately as per the radiologists, particularly with regard to the tumor spread. However, summarizing the surgical boundary (**Fig. 20.1A, B**), the PPSp is bounded medially by the pharyngobasilar fascia and the superior constrictor muscle while laterally by the ramus of the mandible. The prevertebral muscles form the posterior boundary. The styloid process with its attached muscles/fascia along with tensor palati fascial layer arbitrarily divides the PPSp into anterolateral prestyloid and posteromedial poststyloid compartments. Although the classical nomenclature of prestyloid and poststyloid PPSps still exists, current opinion to designate the poststyloid compartment as the carotid space and the prestyloid compartment as the true PPSp is being accepted. The prestyloid compartment ends at the level of the hyoid bone, while the poststyloid compartment continues inferiorly in the neck. The main structures in the prestyloid compartment consist of pterygoid and tensor palati muscles, fat, and the deep lobe of the parotid gland (enclosed in the deep parotid fascia). It is important to note that the masticator space containing the mandibular branch of the trigeminal nerve (V3) is not included in the PPSp but forms its immediate relation. It is formed by the splitting of the deep cervical fascia enclosing the muscles of mastication from the inferior margin of the mandible up to the skull base where it lodges the foramen ovale, a potential channel for tumor spread. Hence, its medial boundary, the medial pterygoid interpterygoid fascia, separates it from the prestyloid compartment of the PPSp. The poststyloid compartment consists of the carotid sheath with the carotid artery, the jugular vein, and the vagus nerve in addition to cranial nerves IX, XI, and XII, the sympathetic chain, and the internal maxillary artery.

The fascial subdivisions of the PPSp and the relationship with the adjoining fascial spaces are very important to decide the direction of the spread of the tumor. There are in general four fascial spaces in close relation with the

Table 20.1 Anatomy of the Infratemporal Fossa and the Prestyloid Parapharyngeal Space

	Intratemporal Fossa	Prestyloid Parapharyngeal Space
Shape boundaries	Inverted pyramid Roof: • Infratemporal surface of greater wing of sphenoid + squamous temporal bone Floor: (arbitrary) • Upper surface of medial pterygoid muscle and its attachment to the medial aspect of the lower part of the ascending ramus of the mandible Medial wall: • Lateral pterygoid plate (anteriorly) • Tensor palati and superior constrictor muscles (posteriorly) Lateral wall: • Inner aspect of zygomatic arch, masseter and temporalis muscle, ascending ramus of the mandible, uppermost part of the deep lobe of the parotid and styloid apparatus Anterior wall: • Posterolateral wall of the maxilla	Triangular Roof: • Angle between superior constrictor muscle and insertion of medial pterygoid muscle into the lateral pterygoid plate with minimal area of temporal bone medial to the foramen ovale and the spinosum Floor: • Descends into the neck medial to the carotid sheath Medial wall: • Lateral wall of the pharynx Lateral wall: • Under surface of medial pterygoid muscle (superiorly) • Deep lobe of the parotid and the styloid (posteriorly) Posteriorly: • Carotid sheath separates it from prevertebral muscles
Communication with	• Pterygopalatine fossa through pterygomaxillary fissure • Oral cavity through a gap between the anterior edge of the ascending ramus of the mandible and the posterolateral wall of the maxilla • Orbit through inferior orbital fissure	• Retropharyngeal space posteriorly
Contents	• Medial and lateral pterygoids and temporalis muscles • Maxillary artery with five branches (inferior alveolar, middle meningeal, accessory meningeal, deep auricular, and anterior tympanic) • Pterygoid venous plexus • V3	• Loose fibro/fatty tissue and salivary glandular tissue • Lower part of the PPSp is traversed by the superior laryngeal nerve and the pharyngeal branch of the vagus nerve • No muscle or lymph nodes are present in the PPSp

PPSp, parapharyngeal space.

PPSp. These are the pharyngeal mucosal space, masticator space, parotid space, and carotid space. **Fig. 20.2** depicts the topographical relation with respect to the PPSp. The pharyngeal mucosal space is somewhat anteromedial to the PPSp, while the masticator space is anterolateral. The parotid space is more lateral to the PPSp than posterolateral while the carotid space is posteromedial. Accordingly, the direction of extension of lesions in the adjoining spaces tends to displace the PPSp in a characteristic pattern. The medial wall of the PPSp is the most pliable of all walls followed by the retromandibular segment of the lateral wall. This results in an oropharyngeal bulge (**Fig. 20.3A**) and fullness of retromandibular sulcus (**Fig. 20.3B**), respectively, by any expanding lesion.

Pathology

It is worth mentioning that the primary tumors of the infratemporal fossa with PPSp extension are quite uncommon and mainly include the extracranial meningioma, fibrosarcoma, chondrosarcoma, lymphoma, angioma, and histiocytosis X.[1-3] On the other hand, the primary tumor of the PPSp is more frequent and is mostly the pleomorphic adenoma arising from detached islands of salivary gland tissue.[4,5] The lesion secondarily involving the PPSp is usually an extension from surrounding fascial spaces or sometimes metastasis from a distant primary. **Table 20.2** enumerates the various pathologies that can be encountered in adjoining fascial spaces.

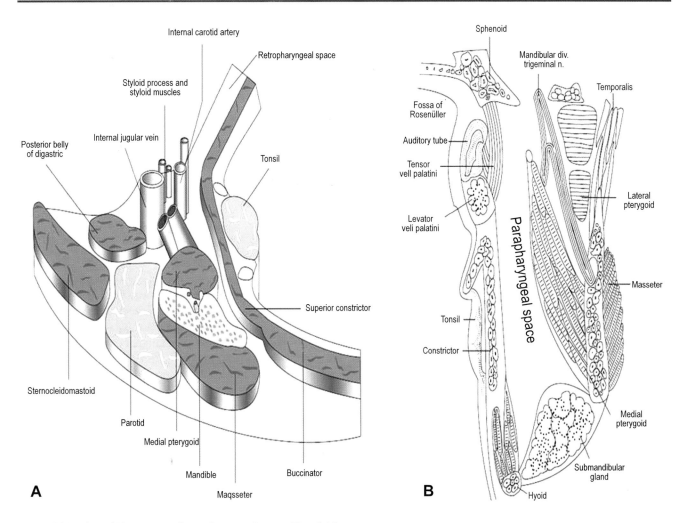

Figure 20.1   (A and B) Anatomy of parapharyngeal space. Div., division; n, nerve.

A review of several large series has revealed that salivary gland tumors (parotid origin), neurogenic tumors, paragangliomas, and lymphoma comprise approximately 80% of PPSp masses while the rest 20% includes other pathologic entities. Johnson et al[6] in an analysis of 213 cases from four series found that neurogenous tumors are likely to be encountered more than expected and in accordance schwannomas were seen in 20% of all PPSp tumors. Similarly, Carrau et al[7] in their series reported that neurogenic tumors comprised 57% of all PPSp cases. However, malignant tumors in different series were seen in 20,[7] 27,[8] 31,[9] and up to 52% of all PPSp cases.[10] **Table 20.3** enumerates the types of pathologies as reported from National Cancer Institute Egypt.[10] The more common pathologies need further discussion.

The commonest tumefaction to involve the PPSp is a salivary gland tumor in the prestyloid compartment. It mostly originates from the deep lobe of the parotid gland but can also arise from the isolated salivary glandular tissue in the PPSp itself. In the former case, the parapharyngeal fat is displaced medially while the latter situation is characterized by the presence of a fat plane between the tumor and the deep lobe of the parotid gland. Almost always, the histology

reveals a benign pleomorphic adenoma but the occurrence of uncommon pathologies such as oncocytoma, Warthin tumor, or even malignant salivary tumors is well known. Pleomorphic adenoma is a very slow growing tumor and when within the PPSp displaces the parotid gland laterally, the medial pterygoid muscle superolaterally, and the faucial region of the lateral wall of the oropharynx medially. The route of extension from the deep lobe of the parotid gland to the PPSp is through the stylomandibular tunnel, which is formed by the posterior border of the ascending ramus of the mandible, the styloid process, and the stylomandibular ligament. This narrow tunnel gives a constriction in the gross appearance of tumor, resulting in a dumb-bell configuration.[11] Such a dumb-bell tumor can be delivered only when the stylomandibular ligament is incised during surgery, thereby releasing the constriction and "widening" the tunnel. Rarely does the pleomorphic adenoma grow large enough to cause bone erosion even if it extends in the infratemporal fossa up to the skull base. On the other hand, malignant salivary gland tumors are likely to grow rapidly and infiltrate the surrounding structures including the pterygoid and masseter muscles (masticator space),

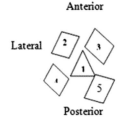

1. Parapharyngeal space
2. Masticator space
3. Pharyngeal mucosal space
4. Parotid space
5. Carotid space

Figure 20.2 Relationship of parapharyngeal space with adjoining fascial spaces.

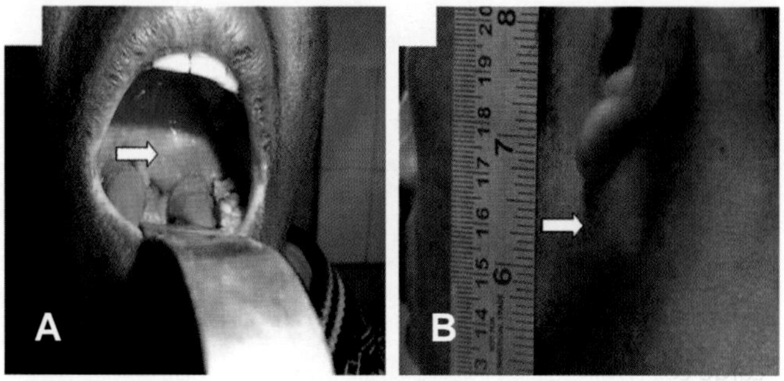

Figure 20.3 (A) Oropharyngeal bulge. (B) Fullness of retromandibular sulcus.

infratemporal fossa, skull base and eustachian tube, and facial nerve and auriculotemporal nerves (laterally in the parotid space).

The neurovascular bundle is mainly located in the poststyloid compartment or the carotid space. Hence, the classical neurogenous lumps originate in this space. Overall, the nerves involved by the latter include the vagus nerve, the hypoglossal nerve, and the sympathetic chain. The common neurogenous tumors extending into the PPSp region include schwannoma and neurofibroma while ganglioneuroma and neuroblastoma are rarely encountered. The schwannoma is the commonest neurogenous tumor of the head and neck region. It originates from schwann cells and hence grows along the course of the nerve, taking a somewhat longitudinal spindle shape. Because they are situated along the nerve sheath with no infiltration in

the nerve itself (unless a malignant counterpart of the schwannoma infiltrates the nerve), the tumor does not affect the structural or functional integrity of the nerve itself and hence can be surgically dissected away from that particular nerve of origin. Uncommonly, the nerve may theoretically be affected by compression if the tumor is large. Importantly, the histological features of malignancy (polymorphism and increased mitotic figures) often do not correlate with clinical malignancy[12–14] and is better decided by the physical examination along with imaging characteristics.

Neurofibroma, on the other hand, originates from the nerve fiber itself including the perineurium and hence situated within the nerve substance involving and splaying the nerve fibrils as it spreads between them.[15] Hence, it becomes impossible to surgically excise the tumor without sacrificing the involved nerve segment. This tumor may be

Table 20.2 Differential Diagnoses of Pathology in Adjoining Fascial Spaces

Pharyngeal Mucosal Space	Parotid Space	Carotid Space	Masticator Space
Squamous cell cancer	Congenital	Inflammatory	Congenital
Minor salivary gland tumor	• Hemangioma	• Abscess	• Hemangioma
Lymphoma	• Third branchial cleft cyst	Vascular	• Lymphangioma
Sarcoma	Inflammatory	• Carotid aneurysm	Inflammatory
	• Parotid abscess	• Carotid artery thrombosis	• Dental infection (abscess/
	• Lymphoepitheliod cyst	• Internal jugular vein	cellulitis)
	• Lymphadenitis	thrombosis	• Myositis
	Neoplastic	Neoplastic	Neoplastic
	• Pleomorphic adenorma	• Paraganglioma	• Osteoma
	• Warthin tumor	• Schwannoma	• Myoma
	• Lipoma	• Neurofibroma	• Osteosarcoma
	• Adenocarcinoma	• Meningioma (via jugular	• Rhabdomyosarcoma
	• Adenoid cystic carcinoma	foramen)	• Schwannoma
	• Mucoepidermoid	• Nodal metastasis	• NHL
	carcinoma		• Nodal metastasis
	• Squamous cell carcinoma		
	• Acnic cell carcinoma		
	• Lymphoma (NHL)		
	• Nodal metastasis from face		
	and scalp		

NHL, non-Hodgkin lymphoma.

Table 20.3 Frequency of Parapharyngeal Space Tumors

Pathology	% (N = 25)
Pleomorphic adenoma	16
Mucoepidermoid carcinoma	16
Paraganglioma	12
Neurofibroma	12
Large cell lymphoma	12
Undifferentiated carcinoma parotid	8
Fibrosarcoma	8
Branchial cyst	4
Malignant branchial cyst	4
Chondrosarcoma	4
Benign schwannoma	4

Adapted from reference 10.

associated with multiple subcutaneous nodules and café au lait spots characteristic of von Recklinghausen disease, which is known to be an autosomal-dominant disorder. It is important to note that malignant transformation is relatively uncommon in sporadic neurofibroma, and when it is associated with von Recklinghausen disease, the risk increases to 5 to 15%.[16] In reference to neurofibroma of the vagus nerve as a part of von Recklinghausen disease presenting as a PPSp tumor, it is important to examine optic and vestibulocochlear cranial nerves as these are more commonly involved than the vagus itself.

Paragangliomas are derived from paraganglionic cells that migrate in close association with autonomic ganglion cell and are seen predominantly in adrenal medulla where they are chromaffin positive producing catecholamines. Those in relation with the PPSp are glomus vagale (inferior vagal ganglion) and glomus jugulare (superior vagal ganglion). The paraganglionic cells are sensitive to changes in pH, and blood gas partial pressure of carbon dioxide more than oxygen. Paragangliomas arising from carotid bodies were known as carotid body tumor or incorrectly as chemodectoma. Not all paragangliomas are catecholamine secreting like adrenal medulla, and this applies more to those presenting as PPSp tumefaction. In gross appearance, the paragangliomas are reddish brown in color, richly vascular, and encapsulated. Histologically, a "Zellballen" pattern of epithelial cell clusters amid fibrovascular stroma is characteristic. They may be sporadic or familial but with female preponderance.

The sporadic variety is usually the vagal paraganglioma from superior and inferior ganglion, arising from the skull base around the jugular foramina and subsequently extending to the PPSp. Accordingly, a large glomus jugulare may be difficult to differentiate from a large glomus vagale.[17]

Owing to its extreme vascularity and complicated location posing difficulty in surgical excision, it is regarded as a cumbersome disease that needs a complete evaluation.[18] Also, vagal paragangliomas are relatively more common catecholomine secretors than is a carotid body tumor. Hence, it is reasonable to draw an index of suspicion for such a possibility during patient evaluation. A history of palpitations, liable hypertension along with tachycardia, and episodes of facial flushing suggest a secreting tumor. In such cases, a serum catecholamine assay and 24-hour urinary vanillylmandelic acid (VMA) estimation clinches the diagnosis. However, the metaiodobenzylguanidine scan may be helpful in borderline cases. A malignant counterpart of paraganglioma is diagnosed on the basis of locally aggressive behavior, as histological differentiation is unreliable and regional metastasis unknown.

The familial variety is inherited in an autosomal-dominant fashion[19-21] and carries more than four times the risk of harboring multiple lesions as compared with the sporadic variety.[21-23] The simultaneous occurrence of phaeochromocytoma is of great clinical significance,[22] and an attempt should be made to search for the latter in the familial variety when clinical features suggest a catecholamine-secreting tumor. A rare association with other endocrine tumors such as parathyroid adenoma and carcinoma thyroid has also been documented. The association with pheochromocytoma may suggest an association with multiple endocrine neoplasia syndrome especially MEN-2B. Hence, a thorough search for other endocrine neoplasias can be rewarding while dealing with the familial variety of paraganglioma.

Apart from the above-mentioned "common" tumors, other nonspecific tumors originating or extending in the PPSp are well known. For example, sarcomas can arise from various mesothelial benign tumors,[24] such as liposarcoma, synovial sarcoma,[25,26] leomyosarcoma,[27] and the more common malignant neurofibroma, especially associated with generalized neurofibromatosis. In general, fibrosarcomas are the most common sarcomas involving the PPSp. Among tumors of vascular origin, hemangiopericytoma[28] and intravascular papillary endothelial hyperplasia or Masson disease[29] have been reported. Among tumors of the adjoining infratemporal fossa, angiofibroma and extracranial meningioma can extend in the PPSp. The extension of an angiofibroma into the infratemporal fossa through the pterygomaxillary fissure is well known and as it enlarges it may extend in the PPSp downward. PPSp is the second most common site for the occurrence of extracranial meningioma after orbit.[30] That presenting in the PPSp originates from the dural sheath surrounding the trunk of the mandibular-trigeminal nerve and exits from the foramen ovale as it presents lower down in the PPSp. Very rarely, intracranial meningiomas may enlarge and extend through a single or multiple foramen of the skull base into the infratemporal fossa; hence, the PPSp displaces the structures in a complex manner. It is extremely uncommon to encounter a mandibular osseous or an amelogenous tumor arising from the ramus of the mandible to bulge into the PPSp.

Lymphatic metastasis commonly occurs in poststyloid PPSp from primary at the nasopharynx, the paranasal sinus (particularly the maxilla), the oropharynx (particularly the base of the tongue), and the parotid salivary gland. As about a third of the patients with undifferentiated nasopharyngeal cancer who develop distant metastasis[31] carry a grave prognosis, an effort should be made to properly image the PPSp at regular intervals to detect an occult metastasis. Similarly, an occult metastasis from a maxillary cancer has been suggested to be a contributory factor to the overall poor prognosis. Even papillary thyroid cancer,[32] medullary thyroid cancer,[33] and cancer of breast[33] have been reported to metastasize in the PPSp. Apart from metastasis along lymphatic channels, perineural spread (especially mandibular nerve) can be occasionally seen with adenoid cystic carcinoma or adenocarcinoma.

Infections involving the PPSp are seen as a part of the cellulites involving adjacent fascial spaces, most notably the masticator space with most commonly an odontogenic source.

Patient Work-Up

Clinical Features

The characteristic picture of a true PPSp tumefaction is the medial displacement of the lateral oropharyngeal wall including the tonsil (**Fig. 20.3A**). This is seen most often with the tumors of the deep lobe of the parotid gland, and a diameter of at least 3 cm is suggested for such a mass to be apparent intraorally.[34,35] Large tumors of the superficial lobe of the parotid gland may also present intraorally (dumb-bell tumors)[11] but more commonly present as neck swelling behind the angle of the mandible, often raising the ear lobule (**Fig. 20.3B**). The common symptoms related to intraoral expansion are foreign body sensation, subjective dysphasia, alteration of voice, and even obstructive sleep apnea,[34,36] Pharyngeal mucosal space tumors involving the PPSp laterally present predominantly with oropharyngeal symptoms and that too early in the course of disease.

The symptoms arising from an adjoining pathology of masticator space are characterized by trismus and swelling in neck/face. The trismus usually results from the involvement of pterygoid muscles by inflammation (infection), adjacent compression by benign tumor, or by malignant infiltration. Carotid space tumors usually present as a neck swelling, particularly the carotid body paraganglioma and nerve sheath tumor. These tumors may compress the adjoining nerves to present with cranial nerve palsies of different combinations. Similarly, the extension of such tumors superiorly toward the skull base may involve the jugular foramen, leading to jugular foramen syndromes involving cranial nerves (IX through XII) with or without the sympathetic chain (Vernet: IX, X, and XI; Schmidt: X and XI; Hughlings Jackson: X, XI,

and XII; Collet-Sicard: IX, X, XI, and XII; Villaret: IX, X, XI, and XII, Horner syndrome). Unlike the developed world, it is very common in underprivileged countries to find extensive/advanced malignancy with a varied combination(s) of symptoms. In addition, superior-based tumors of the carotid space may compress the cartilaginous part of the eustachian tube, causing middle ear problems (conductive deafness).

The occurrence of pain is common and is usually the result of nerve compression/invasion or a consequence of expansion of fascial spaces in the case of abscess/cellulites/inflammation, causing irritation. Other characteristic features of infection including fever and toxemia may be well evident. The associated pain may even lead to odynophagia at times while hoarseness of voice as a result of vagus involvement may be the initial presenting complain as well. Glossopharyngeal neuralgia with syncope is a theoretical possibility in parapharyngeal malignancy,[37] and this rare symptom complex has been reported in 30 cases of head and neck cancer till date. **Table 20.4** summarizes an institutional experience[10] of presenting features of PPSp tumors. The general examination should specially focus on the presence of palpitation, tachycardia, hypertension (catecholamine secreting), and presence of pulsatile lesion (carotid aneurysm) or arterial bruit (carotid body paraganglioma).

Investigations

The main investigating modalities consist of fine-needle aspiration cytology (FNAC), computed tomography (CT)/magnetic resonance imaging (MRI), and occasionally angiography. Currently, ultrasonography has become an indispensable tool at many centers and incisional biopsy is rarely required.

Fine-Needle Aspiration Cytology

In general, FNAC is the mainstay of immediate tissue diagnosis in the case of neck swellings. The same stands true for a PPSp tumefaction that presents as either a neck swelling or an oropharyngeal mass. In our tertiary care center in India, a few of the cases referred as a parapharyngeal tumor have

Table 20.4 Clinical Presentation of Parapharyngeal Space Tumors

Symptoms/Signs	% (*N* = 25)
Neck swelling	72
Parotid swelling	28
Otalgia	24
Facial palsy	16
Oral swelling	8
Dysphagia	8
Dysarthria	4
Horner syndrome	4

Adapted from reference 10.

revealed only chronic abscess on needle aspiration. Also, a theoretical possibility of aneurysm needs to be considered when the aspirate is frank blood. Our archival records indicate a single mortality with a PPSp aneurysm that was drained intraorally as a peritonsillar/parapharyngeal abscess. Such confusions of a tumor for an abscess or vice versa may be encountered more in the developing world owing to a higher prevalence of infection. A large tumor presenting in the PPSp does not create any difficulty in FNAC while a small tumor with minimal oropharyngeal presentation may be difficult to approach. Under such situation, we primarily carry out ultrasound-guided FNAC or even a CT-guided approach in case it fails. The majority of our patients are diagnosed on the basis of FNAC alone, but there are some limitations as well. Indian authors have reported an accuracy rate of 88% with FNAC,[38] which has been shown to improve with the addition of CT to the tune of 92%.[39] To reduce the diagnostic dilemma resulting from sampling errors or false-negative results, the histopathologists at our institute themselves collect (and examine) the aspirate from the patients. The pathologist may repeat such aspiration in the same sitting if a sufficient cytological material for an affective diagnosis cannot be obtained in the first instance. Apart from patient-related factors, an "inconclusive" tap is often seen with carotid body tumor where the desired cytological material is grossly diluted by the presence of blood and a dry tap is often encountered in recurrence after radiation therapy. Such situations are subject to be investigated by other means such as angiography and imaging. Immunocytochemistry is a valuable adjunct in some cases, but it is unfortunately not available at the majority of centers.

Imaging

Although a debate exists whether CT or MRI should be used as the primary modality, in reality both are equally good in assessing the PPSp.[40,41] While MRI provides a better tumor differentiation and better visualization of PPSp fat,[4] CT scan better delineates bony erosions that are critical with respect to the adjoining infratemporal fossa/skull base involvement. MRI also shows a better relationship of the mass to surrounding structures, particularly to the major blood vessels. At our institution in India, the cost factor prohibits the use of MRI as a primary modality of imaging and hence we use CT scanning for this purpose instead. Only if required we advise MRI; otherwise, our experience with CT scan is very satisfying. Image-guided FNAC is possible only with CT scan. However, a few studies have revealed a better anatomic localization with MRI—95 vs. 84% with CT scan.[42] In general, low-attenuation areas denote necrosis while high-attenuation areas reflect hemorrhage. The lack of visualization of a fat plane may indicate a tumor originating in the deep lobe of the parotid gland or a large tumor that is either compressing this plane or, rarely, invading it. MRI is superior to CT in such differentiation, and high-resolution images are often essential. We opt for MRI (a) to know the tissue details in the case of diagnostic dilemmas such as

accompanying vascularity that needs to be anticipated before surgery. The ability of MRI to visualize the tumor in three planes can be useful (a) in assessing carotid encasement, (b) in case of questionable recurrence where previous irradiation has been used, and (c) to assess the extensive tumor involvement of the infratemporal fossa and skull base. With the advances in imaging techniques, spiral CT consecutive volume data sets are useful for a 3-dimentional (3-D) assessment of a PPSp tumor.[43] In addition, the value of a positron emission tomography scan cannot be overemphasized in the case of questionable recurrence in the PPSp. The imaging characteristics of PPSp pathologies are depicted in **Table 20.5**.

As a radiological approach of diagnosis, the PPSp is considered as being located centrally surrounded by four fascial spaces and an understanding of interrelationships allows a logical approach to differentiate lesions arising in different spaces (**Fig. 20.2**). Unlike infiltrative malignancies (particularly squamous cell carcinoma) that tend to spread across fascial boundaries (**Fig. 20.4**), other tumors tend to be localized by fascial compartments. The displacement pattern of fat in the PPSp suggests the site of origin of the primary lesion, and the differential diagnoses can be shortlisted on the basis of the contents of that particular fascial space (**Table 20.2**). Tumors of pharyngeal mucosal space originate from the wall of the space and hence no clear delineation exists between it and the tumor. Benign and less aggressive tumors are likely to displace PPSp fat posterolaterally while infiltrating lesions diffusely replace it.

The tumor of the masticator space tends to displace the fat posteromedially. Because inflammatory pathology is most common, a CT scan should be regarded as the primary modality of imaging because abscess, dental infection, and osteomyelitis are better visualized on CT than on MRI. However, MRI is better suited to rule out perineural spread along the mandibular division of the trigeminal nerve. The direct evidence suggesting perineural spread can be nerve enlargement or enhancement as such or indirectly by the enlargement of the foramen ovale or denervation atrophy of muscles of mastication. Rhabdomyosarcoma should always be suspected if a child presents with a solid tumor in the masticator space. A parotid space tumor is likely to displace PPSp fat medially (**Fig. 20.5**), and the most common lesion is the parotid salivary gland neoplasm that has been discussed before.

The suprahyoid part of the carotid space is in direct relation with the PPSp, and a relative anatomic relationship amid its contents is helpful in deciding the precise anatomic origin of the lesion. The vagus nerve lies posterolateral to the carotid artery while the sympathetic trunk is posteromedial. Accordingly, the tumor arising from the vagus nerve would displace the carotid artery anteromedially while an uncommon tumor from the sympathetic chain would displace the artery anterolaterally. In general, tumors of the suprahyoid carotid space displace the PPSp fat and the internal carotid artery anteriorly and the internal jugular vein

Table 20.5 Imaging Characteristics of Parapharyngeal Space Lesions

Pathology	CT	T1W1-MRI	T2W1-MRI	Remarks
Squamous cell cancer	Minimal enhancement muscle attenuation, infiltrative masses	Intermediate signal intensity		
Lymphoma	Homogenous, diffusely infiltrative, low attenuation, minimal enhancement	Low to intermediate signal intensity	Slightly higher signal intensity	Less infiltrative and little bone erosion than sarcomas
Pleomorphic adenoma	Sharp margin, low (cyst/neurosis) or high (hemorrhage) attenuation	Low to intermediate signal intensity High signal (T1) in hemorrhage >1 d	High signal intensity	Displaces ICA posteriorly Calcification may be seen
Warthin tumor	Smooth margin, homogenous, occasionally cystic, multiple lesion ± bilateral involvement	Low signal intensity	High signal intensity	Cystic component has different intensity than solid
Adenoid cystic carcinoma	• Well-delineated parotid gland lesions • Malignant infiltrative margin of minor salivary gland lesions	Contrast MRI for postoperative recurrences and identify nerve enhancement to rule out perineural spread		
Mucoepidermoid	• Smooth, delineated margin, cystic areas with low attenuation (low grade) • Infilterative margins, homogenous with few cystic areas (high grade)	Low to intermediate signal intensity on both T1 and T2		
Acinic cell	Nonspecific benign-looking appearance, simulating pleomorphic adenoma on CT and MRI			
Paraganglioma	• Intense enhancement with contrast • Smooth contoured	Intense enhancement with characteristic salt and pepper appearance or vascular flow voids on T2W1		Angiography strictly indicated
Schwannoma	Solitary, well-delineated mass, enhancement with contrast	Isointense to muscle	Hyperintense	Displaces ICA anteriorly Calcification may be seen
Neurofibroma	• Regressive remodeling of skull base bone may occur • Multiple, delineated mass ± cystic • Low almost fully attenuated, may simulate a lipoma	Low to intermediate signal intensity	High signal intensity	Association with multiple neurofibromatosis may be seen
Meningioma	Bone erosion and remodeling with hyperostotic thickening of surrounding bone and skull base	Signal intensity similar to that of brain		
Osteosarcoma	Bone matrix and scattered calcification in diffuse infiltrative and destructive lesion Homogenous, diffusely infiltrative, low attenuation, surrounding bone erosion	Low to intermediate signal intensity	Slightly higher signal intensity on T2W1	CT characteristics are diagnostic More infiltrative and more bone erosion than lymphoma

	CT	T1WI	T2WI	
Metastatic node	Low attenuation, central necrosis with nodular irregularly thick walls	Low to intermediate signal intensity on T1W1, fat suppression contrast images	High signal intensity on T2W1	Primary tumor can be seen
Benign				
• Hemangioma	Lobular, enhancing, extending to overlying skin	Low to intermediate nonhomogenous signal intensity on T1W2	High signal intensity	Sites of high signal intensity on both T1W1 and T2W1 reflect prior hemorrhage and slow flow. Flow voids can be seen
• Hemangiopericytoma	Less distinct margin, bone erosion, marked contrast enhancement	Low to intermediate signal intensity	High signal intensity	Follow-up CT/MRI to detect recurrences
• Lymphangioma	Multicystic (cystic hygroma), increased attenuation of infection or hemorrhage	Low signal intensity on T1W2	High signal intensity	Rare in adults
• Branchial cyst	Uniform smooth wall, homogenous low attenuation	• Low or intermediate signal intensity • Cyst wall undefined	• High signal intensity in defined • Ill-defined cyst wall	Signal intensity vary with protein content
• Abscess	Thick enhancing, irregular rim about a central area of necrosis			• Multiple enlarged lymph nodes • May be associated with peritonsillar abscess • Peritonsillar abscess may be seen • Odontagenic abscess may be seen
• Cellulites	Poorly defined infilteration of PPSp fat and soft tissue planes in and around the PPSp			
• Myosits	Enlargement of muscle having ragged and fluffy border with infiltration and obliteration of PPSp fat			
• Vascular thrombosis	Tubular configuration of vessel with simulation of cystic mass	High signal intensity of slow-flowing or clotted blood on gradient echo		
• Vascular aneurysm	Peripheral rim calcification	Peripheral signal voids reflect calcifications		Angiography indicated
• Lipoma	May mimic lymphangioma	High signal intensity	Intermediate signal intensity	

CT, computed tomography; T1WI, T1- weighted image; T2WI, T2-weighted image; MRI, magnetic resonance imaging; ICA, internal carotid artery; PPSp, parapharyngeal space.

laterally. The two most common tumors of the carotid space are paraganglioma and nerve-sheath tumors. Also, it is not uncommon to mistake a dominant jugular vein or tortuous carotid artery for a pathology otherwise. Angiography under such circumstances resolves the issue. The common types of paragangliomas seen in the carotid space are carotid body tumor in the infrahyoid neck, and glomus vagale and glomus jugulare in the suprahyoid neck opposing the PPSp. Carotid body tumor tends to splay the carotid fork in the infrahyoid neck, whereas glomus vagale displaces the internal carotid artery anteriorly. Also, a feeding vessel from the ascending pharyngeal artery may be demonstrable in the latter while the former derives its blood supply from vasa vasorum. The characteristic feature of paraganglioma that differentiates it from nerve-sheath tumor is the presence of serpigenous flow voids, which, in turn, are apparent in MRI only if the tumor is at least 2 cm in size. Also, being more vascular, the paraganglioma enhances much more than a nerve-sheath tumor in a contrast-enhanced CT scan. MRI appearance of smooth margins of the paraganglioma can be used to differentiate it from vascular metastasis.[4]

Angiography

Carotid angiography is indicated especially preoperatively if the clinical and radiological findings suggest a vascular tumor. It is also helpful to diagnose anatomic variations such as dominant jugular vein or tortuous carotid artery. Apart from differentiating carotid body tumor from glomus vagale, it is useful in delineating glomus jugulare tumor in the jugular bulb that expands the jugular foramina. Despite advancements in angiography techniques, the carotid angiography still remains unparallel in identifying the feeding vessels.[44] Although it carries a risk of cerebrovascular episode, the chance of such an accident is remote. The recent development using a combination of digital subtraction technique and MRI further enhances the accuracy rate of diagnosis. Ideally, the measurement of cerebral blood flow preoperatively using the xenon CT-scan techniques is recommended.[44]

Ultrasonography

Ultrasonography has a special value in the evaluation of neck masses. It has an important role in diagnosing carotid artery aneurysm/thrombosis as well as the pattern of flowing blood in great vessels. The cystic and lymphangiomatous masses in the parotid area can be further evaluated. At out institution, we regularly use ultrasonography to exclude abscess/cellulitis in fascial spaces of the neck. We carry out ultrasound-guided FNAC at our institution routinely for clinically inaccessible tumors. The limitation of ultrasound with deeply located lesions is the complex bony framework around the tumor that often necessitates the use of a CT-guided FNAC. However, the use of ultrasonography has replaced the need of imaging in many clinical situations. A preliminary use of a transvaginal probe for transoral ultrasonography has been tried, and the results have been encouraging. The main advantage of the ultrasound

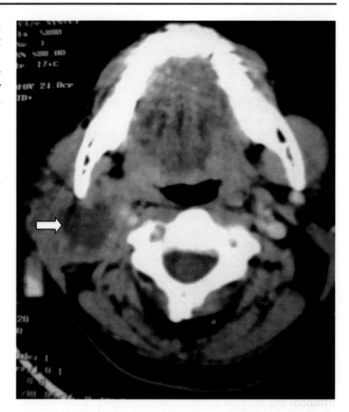

Figure 20.4 Computed tomography scan showing infiltrative lesion diffusely replacing the parapharyngeal space with no trace of normal fat interface.

technique lies in its safety, reduced cost, portability, and excellent patient compliance.

Incisional Biopsy

In situations in which tumors involving the PPSp, infratemporal fossa, and skull base are amenable to tissue diagnosis by FNAC, an incisional biopsy is indicated for the characterization of the lesion. Such incisional biopsy should never be performed intraorally for the fear of implantation seedlings. Hence, an external route is to be preferred. This requires a full patient preparation for operation under general anesthetic.

Other Investigations

Apart from the above-mentioned investigations focusing on tissue diagnosis and tumor localization for surgical feasibility, special investigations are needed to exclude specific pathologies. For example, urine VMA estimation and blood analysis is indicated to exclude a catecholamine-secreting tumor, and systemic investigations are needed for lymphoma and septicemia. In addition, relevant investigations to search for the distant spread of malignancy or to detect a distant primary is mandatory in many situations.

Surgical Approaches

The PPSp is anatomically a very complicated site, and its complete clearance is likely to result in extreme morbidity.

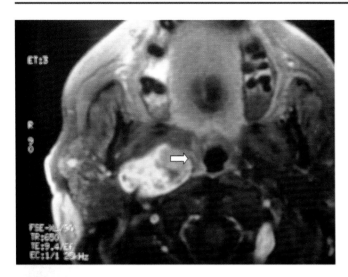

Figure 20.5 Magnetic resonance imaging axial cut showing a parotid space tumor displacing the parapharyngeal space medially.

Hence, a decision is to be made whether the disease clearance would increase survival at the cost of quality of life (QOL) or visa versa. The occurrence of too many rare histological entities prohibits the adoption of a universal protocol applicable to PPSp tumors in general. Hence, the rule of thumb to be followed while deciding to operate is whether (a) the tumor (benign/malignant) can be completely ressected and (b) the functional deficits are not too many to compromise QOL. The classical surgical approaches (transparotid, transcervical, and transmandibular) for PPSp tumors have been described with special emphasis on the parotid salivary gland tumors, paragangliomas, and nerve-sheath tumors. However, considering the proximity of the infratemporal fossa, a simultaneous clearance along with the PPSp sometimes necessitates infratemporal fossa approaches. In addition, many other techniques have been described by different authors to be adopted in specific situations and dealing with other pathologic entities as well.

Transparotid Approach

This is suited for small deep-lobe tumors of the parotid salivary gland. Through a modified Blair incision, the parotid gland is exposed, facial nerve is identified, and superficial parotidectomy performed as a prerequisite before dealing with a deep-lobe tumor. Very small deep-lobe tumors lateral to the stylomandibular tunnel are unlikely to displace the PPSp. They are best delivered from in between the two main branches of the facial nerve by retracting them apart after superficial parotidectomy. For small tumors medial to the stylomandibular tunnel, the stylomandibular ligament needs to be divided to release the bottleneck constriction across a dumb-bell tumor and facilitate its delivery. In such situations, anterior retraction of the angle of the mandible increases the exposure for easy delivery. For a relatively larger deep-lobe tumor not producing a significant oropharyngeal

bulge and where additional space is needed for delivery, it may be necessary to resort to a lateral mandibulotomy.[45–47] For a large deep-lobe tumor presenting with significant oropharyngeal bulge, other approaches are preferred as discussed later.

Transcervical Approach

This is predominantly indicated for poststyloid compartment lesions[7,47] especially when a vascular control of great vessels is needed or for resection of a medium-sized tumor of the lower PPSp involving both pre- and poststyloid compartments and extending in the neck. A routine transcervical exposure of the PPSp is obtained via the cervical part of the Blair incision. The incision is given at least two fingerbreadths below the lower border of the mandible and can be extended either anteriorly or backward as needed. While raising the skin flaps, care needs to be taken to avoid injury to the lower two peripheral branches of the facial nerve, specially the marginal mandibular. Occasionally, the submandibular gland may be excised to expose the digastric tendon and to obtain a better access for R0 tumor free margins resection.[47,48] The mass is palpated and the tissues over it, especially the styloglossus muscle and the stylohyoid ligament, are incised to expose the PPSp. A blunt finger dissection may be undertaken to enucleate the tumor and if needed the mandible may be dislocated anteriorly to obtain additional space. Alternatively, an angle mandibulotomy may be necessary. Although sometimes a poor local vascular control is obtained resulting in incomplete resection, a tie ligature (control) over the great vessels may facilitate a better intraoperative hemostasis.

Lateral Transmandibular Approach

The addition of mandibulotomy as a part of other approaches facilitates a better access for large deep-lobe parotid tumors located in the lower part of the infratemporal fossa and impinging over the PPSp (predominantly the prestyloid compartment). This is particularly suited when the tumor is adjacent to the oropharynx and producing an oropharyngeal bulge or when a malignancy is suspected.[45,46] During lateral mandibulotomy, care should be taken to divide the mandible above the lingula to preserve the mandibular nerve. This can be combined with a control over great vessels transcervically.

Transcervical-Transparotid Approach

This is suited for large tumors of the deep lobe of the parotid gland that neither extend superiorly to the skull base nor encase the petrous part of the internal carotid artery.[49] Stell et al advocate a vertical preauricular incision that extends beneath the mandible.[50] The parotid flap and a subplatysmal neck flaps are elevated. After identifying the facial nerve, its inferior branches are displaced superiorly to reach the deep lobe of the parotid gland. Subsequently, the tumor along with PPSp extensions is removed en bloc.[51,52] The advantage of this approach lies in control of carotid artery, jugular vein, and lower cranial nerves. This can be combined with osteotomy of the mandible if needed.

Traditional PPSp surgery mainly uses transcervical-transparotid approaches. Few authors have described the resection of PPSp tumors by using the transcervical approach alone in 90 to 100% of the cases.[13,48] Hughes et al published a series of 172 cases using the transcervical-transparotid approaches in 94% of resections, while using mandibular osteotomy in only 2% of resections.[53] Khafif et al reported 47 patients with tumors of the PPSp (12 malignant and 35 benign) and treated surgically during a 10-year period.[54] The transcervical (40%) and the transcervical-transparotid approaches (46%) were the most commonly performed surgical procedures followed by the orbitozygomatic-middle fossa approach (12%) and the transmandibular approach (2%). Sergi et al, on the other hand, advised the transparotid approach when the lesion was located higher and laterally and a combined transparotid and transmandibular approach when the tumor is lower and more medially located.[55]

Midline Transmandibular Oropharyngeal Approach

This approach is uncommonly used only for a very large benign or malignant tumor of the PPSp presenting as a predominant oropharyngeal bulge. It also provides a satisfactory exposure of the infratemporal fossa. A midline lower lip-splitting incision is given that surrounds the protuberance of the chin up to the mentum in the midline. Thereafter, the incision proceeds inferiorly and laterally parallel to and two fingerbreadths below the lower border of the mandible, preferably in the skin crease (just above the level of the hyoid), up to the anterior border of the sternomastoid muscle. A submandibular gland excision is performed to expose the digastric tendon and the lingual nerve. The visualization of the latter makes it easy to be saved while giving intraoral incision in the floor of the mouth. The digastric and omohyoid muscles are detached from the hyoid and retracted upward. The mandible is then split in the midline with a stepladder incision (for subsequent stability) only after making necessary drill holes for the subsequent plating or wiring. The mucous membrane of the floor of the mouth is then incised laterally and posteriorly medial to the horizontal ramus of the mandible and deepened to include the myelohyoid muscle. The horizontal ramus is swung laterally, and the course of the lingual nerve is identified. The incision of the mucous membrane is extended posteriorly onto the anterior pillar of the tonsil up to the soft palate. The latter part of the incision is deepened to include superior constrictor muscle of the pharynx, and the mandible is maximally retracted laterally to allow satisfactory visualization of the PPSp. The carotid sheath contents can be exposed once the incision extends to the maxillary tuberosity. The medial pterygoid

muscle may partially obstruct the access and that may be divided further to enable an easy delivery of the tumor. The respective muscles and mucous membrane are resutured while mandibulotomy edges are fixed with wires (or plate). Skin is closed over a suction drain.

Reconstructive Considerations

Mostly a primary closure of the surgical defect is routinely used over a suction drain. A reconstructive procedure can be performed when sacrifice of the facial nerve is required. In such situations, an interposition nerve graft should be used (the greater auricular nerve) during the same sitting. At times, a temporalis muscle sling can be rotated downward, passed subdermally, and sutured to the oral commissure to achieve better symmetry of the mouth. High-risk patients with a low life expectancy are unlikely to be benefited by the reconstruction of the facial nerve. If skin needs resection together with the tumor, a primary closure is performed if possible or else in selected cases, rotational flaps are required. Larger defects may need regional flaps (pectoralis major myocutaneous flap, temporalis muscle flap) or free flaps (a radial forearm fasciocutaneous flap, anterolateral thigh, or a scapular flap). Large mucosal oroparapharyngeal defects can be reconstructed with a radial-forearm fasciocutaneous flap. Combined skin and mucosal defects can be reconstructed with free flaps folded over themselves ("sandwiched"). Our institutional experience suggests that surgery of PPSp tumors may be performed in most patients via the transcervical or transcervical-transparotid approach with no need for any major reconstructive procedures.

Surgical Approaches to the Infratemporal Fossa

The involvement of the most superior segment of great vessels including the skull-base foramina is to be dealt extremely cautiously when surgery is contemplated. The occurrence of malignancy at this particular situation predicts a very high morbidity, and surgery should better be avoided unless a rare chance of complete cure is anticipated. Typically, Fisch type C approach is suited for extension within infratemporal and pterygopalatine fossae and provides good control over the internal carotid artery while risking the hearing and facial nerve functions. Fisch type D approach offers a limited preauricular access but preserves hearing as such. **Table 20.6** summarizes the indications of various infratemporal fossa approaches that may be undertaken in different situations. The surgical steps of various infratemporal approaches can be sought out elsewhere from surgical atlases. **Table 20.7** elaborates the advantages and disadvantages encountered with various approaches of the infratemporal fossa.

Approaches in Specific Situations

- For medial and anterior skull-base lesions, a lateral approach with significant morbidity has been practiced. Biller et al described a combination of a segmental Le-fort I osteotomy along with a transmandibular approach for a better functional outcome and a comparable oncological safety.[56]

- The combination of orbital frontal ethmoidal osteotomies with an extended frontal approach has been described[57,58] for a very large schwannoma that would alternatively be dealt transfacially by swinging the maxilla laterally.

- Anupam et al[59] described a combined internal and external approach to deal with a benign fibro-osseous tumor of mandibular ramus presenting in the infratemporal fossa and the PPSp, creating a bulge in the lateral wall of the oropharynx. This approach advocates an intraoral curved incision along the anterior tonsillar pillar exploring the mass attached at its base on bone, while simultaneously giving a transverse preauricular incision externally. The latter facilitates the elevation of the tumor from the underlying bone of the medial aspect of the ramus of the mandible by using a periosteal elevator and the subsequent division of the adherent part by an osteotome. This approach provides easy access and adequate visualization. It facilitates bimanual palpation, and hemostasis can be achieved more easily. The authors claim a better radical excision and reduced chances of iatrogenic mandibular fracture. Although the transoral approach has been discouraged, Goodwin and Chandler have considered this approach to give direct access to the PPSp. It is very useful when combined with other techniques, as it allows the deepest part of the tumor to be exposed, facilitating the removal of larger tumors.[41]

- A novel transorbital approach to the infratemporal fossa was described by Mishra et al in 2010.[60] The authors suggest this conservative surgical approach for selected infratemporal fossa involvement or inferolateral orbital tumor extending to the infratemporal fossa (**Fig. 20.6**). Excellent cosmetic and functional results outweigh the advantages of this technique over the classical open procedures (**Table 20.7**). The authors claim that the approach is suited for benign and early malignant tumor that presents as a small infratemporal fossa mass creating a diagnostic dilemma and would have been dealt with a lateral-approach incisional biopsy otherwise. Under such situations, a minimal access transorbital infratemporal fossa endoscopy and biopsy can be obtained (**Fig. 20.7**). For anterior-based infratemporal fossa tumors involving the PPSp and otherwise inaccessible for FNAC, biopsy can be approached through the transorbital route.

Surgical Results and Complications

Surgical results may be compromised because of a complex anatomy of the region and incomplete clearance, while complications may ensue because of extensive surgical manipulation for a lesion with a poor access otherwise. Hence, an effective preoperative counseling regarding the expected sequelae of surgical resection needs to be undertaken. This is an essential part of patient work-up.

An accurate assessment of the preoperative site and size of tumor is now possible with scanning techniques whereas angiography delineates the vascularity. Such an assessment allows for a less extensive procedure to be adequate in the majority of PPSp lesions. The biggest surgical challenge is to preserve the internal carotid artery in case of a massive glomus tumor or when invaded by a malignant process at immediate skull base. The former situation demands arterial grafting if the artery cannot be saved, whereas the latter situation indicates incurability, condemning a radical surgery. Tumor embolization is mostly required in infratemporal fossa approaches but uncommonly otherwise. We have used simple gelfoam for embolization intraoperatively, and the results have been quite encouraging without any long-term consequences. Only rarely is balloon occlusion needed for massive tumor encasing or invading the internal carotid artery. Above all, the most important but less required preoperative concern is to obtain a sufficient α and β sympathetic blockage with propranolol in the case of catecholamine-secreting tumors. The majority of surgical morbidity related to PPSp clearance is seen while dealing with paragangliomas.[6] Such a procedure runs a relatively high risk of precipitating cerebrovascular accident and cranial nerve palsies. The morbidities associated with various surgical approaches are summarized in **Table 20.7**.

Shahinian et al reported that patients undergoing an infratemporal fossa approach on average received 1.1 L of blood during surgery.[49] This was mainly due to blood loss from the rich pterygoid venous plexus. Preoperative information of the likelihood of blood transfusions and autotransfusions to the patient is to be encouraged.

Khafif et al in a series of 47 patients reported no surgery-associated mortalities.[54] The most common postoperative complication was facial nerve palsy (five patients), specially the marginal mandibular nerve with spontaneous resolution in all cases. Vocal cord paralysis due to vagal transection occurred in 11 of 14 patients with neurogenic tumors of the vagus nerve. One patient with a sympathetic chain schwannoma had Horner syndrome, and another patient had V2 deficit after the resection of a schwannoma of the trigeminal nerve. Other complications to occur singly in this series included pulmonary embolism, necrosis of a skin graft over a pectoralis major myocutaneous flap, a decubitus wound, and Frey syndrome.

To overcome the surgical morbidity associated with extensive dissection, a recent modality of the robotic surgery for the skull base holds potential as a minimally invasive approach. The animal model and preliminary patient data have documented the transoral robotic surgery to provide an excellent 3-D visualization and instrumentation. This has allowed successful PPSp and infratemporal fossa surgical

Table 20.6 Approaches to Infratemporal Fossa (Indications)

Approaches	Indications
Postauricular/temporal	Temporal bone lesions extending to the ITF
• Fisch type B	Pathology of petrous apex and clivus along the posterior part of the ITF
• Fisch type C	Pathology of anterior ITF, sella, and nasopharynx
Preauricular/subtemporal	Tumors originating at the anterior aspect of the temporal bone or the greater wing of the sphenoid and that extend to the ITF
• Fisch type D1	Anterior ITF tumor
• Fisch type D2	Lateral orbital wall lesions and high pterygopalatine fossa tumors
Transmaxillary/transfacial	• Sinonasal tumors that require maxillectomy and that invade the ITF, the masticator space, or the pterygomaxillary fossa • Tumors of the nasopharynx involving the maxilla and extending to the ITF
Endoscopic—Transnasal transantral transpterygopalatine fossa approach	• Benign tumors of nose, PNS, nasopharynx, extending in the ITF • Benign tumors of the ITF, e.g., trigeminal neurilemmoma • Skull base meningioma involving the ITF • Residual nasopharyngeal carcinoma after chemoradiation but not involving the ICA • Palliative debulking of cancers of sinuses, nose, and nasopharynx, e.g., adenoid cystic carcinoma
Transorbital approach to the ITF	Inferolateral-based orbital tumors with mild to moderate extension to the ITF and without invasion of pterygoid musculature

Adapted from reference 60.

ITF, infratemporal fossa; PNS, paranasal sinus; ICA, internal carotid artery.

resections from cadaver models to the first known human patient application.[61] However, continued development and investigation is needed in prospective human clinical trials before final conclusions can be drawn

Nonsurgical Management of Parapharyngeal Tumors

The use of radiation and chemotherapy depends on the type of PPSp tumor. The surgical clearance of the PPSp as a part of extended maxillectomy to take care of occult metastases to improve curability is associated with a very high morbidity.[62] Because the report does not support such a clearance, radiotherapy is best suited under such situations. The literature supports the use of radiation therapy of the PPSp mostly in cases of nasopharyngeal cancer extending into the same.[63–66] Teo et al claim a better locoregional control with a booster dose of radiation to the PPSp while treating nasopharyngeal cancer even without gross extension.[67] The metastasis may also be seen in oropharyngeal malignancies apart from nasopharyngeal and maxillary cancers. Under such situations in which complete R0 resection is not possible and the anticipated surgical morbidity outweighs the benefit, radiotherapy is definitely indicated. Similarly, the surgically difficult or unresectable paraganglioma, specially in elderly,

is better treated primarily with radiation, which has shown a growth reduction in carotid body tumors. The occurrence of metastasis from a distant primary may not need surgery and hence radiation therapy with or without chemotherapy may suffice. In general, any extensive malignancy of the head and neck involving the PPSp will need radiation therapy

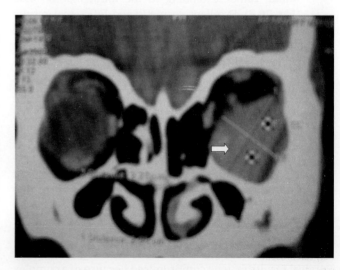

Figure 20.6 Computed tomography scan showing inferolateral orbital tumor extending to the infratemporal fossa.

Table 20.7 Approaches to the Infratemporal Fossa (Advantages and Disadvantages)

Approaches	Advantages	Disadvantages
Postauricular/temporal • Fisch type B • Fisch type C	Wide open radical excision	Total conductive deafness Sensorimotor loss (V3) Trismus VII palsy Bleeding from pterygoid plexus CSF leak Cosmetic disfiguration (zygomatic osteotomy)
Preauricular/subtemporal • Fisch type D1 • Fisch type D2	No conductive HI No VII palsy Petrous ICA not exposed Temporal craniotomy not needed.	Cosmetic disfiguration (orbitozygomatic osteotomy) Scarring, ankylosis of TMJ, and trismus Mandibular coronoidectomy may lead to malocclusion Anterior dislocation of mandibular condyle Potential for V3 nerve injury Troublesome bleeding from pterygoid plexus
Transmaxillary/transfacial	No conductive HI No VII palsy Petrous ICA not exposed Temporal craniotomy not needed Mandibular coronoidectomy not needed	Cosmetic disfiguration may need prosthetic reconstruction Injury/scarring of muscle results in trismus Bleeding (pterygoid plexus) Potential injury to frontal branch of the facial nerve Sensory motor loss from V2 and possibly V3 nerves
Endoscopic— Transnasal transantral transpterygopalatine fossa approach	Minimal morbidity as a result of minimal soft tissue manipulation as compared with open conventional approaches (no trismus, no VII injury, no V3 injury, minimal scarring, no cosmetic disfiguration, remote chances of CSF leak) Reduced patient cost of treatment Reduced postoperative hospitalization Best suited for benign ITF tumors Can be used to obtain biopsy	Expensive setup Two surgeons-four hand technique requiring expertise training Limited field of surgery not suited for radical excision of malignant tumors Potential damage to V2
Transorbital approach to ITF	Minimal morbidity (comparable to endoscopic approach) No morbidity with traction on eyeball Excellent cosmetic outcome No disfiguring osteotomies Minimal scarring No chances of trismus, VII injury, V3/V2 injury, CSF leak Can be used for benign and early malignant tumor Easy hemostasis Biopsy can be obtained	Not suited for extensive invasion of the ITF by malignant tumor Potential anesthesia of upper teeth (postsup alveolar nerve) and face (infraorbital nerve)

Adapted from reference 60.

CSF, cerebrospinal fluid; HI, hearing impairment; ICA, internal carotid artery; TMJ, temporomandibular joint; postsup, posterosuperior; ITF, infratemporal fossa.

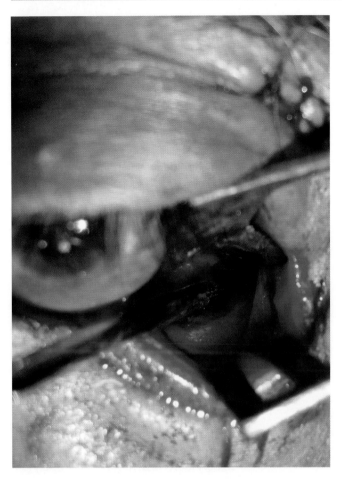

Figure 20.7 Minimal access transorbital infratemporal fossa approach (endoscopy).

even after a satisfactory resection. Because there are no studies evaluating the indications for radiation therapy after the resection of malignant tumors of the PPSp, we support the recommendations as described by Carrau et al.[68] Accordingly, the postoperative radiotherapy should be considered for patients with high-grade malignancies or when wide surgical margins cannot be achieved. More commonly, the recurrence of deep-lobe parotid pleomorphic adenoma has been seen to be very disseminated/extensive and complete surgical excision in that case is not possible. Radiation seems to be the only palliation is such cases sometimes. Controversy exists whether intraoperative tumor spillage as a result of intraoperative rupture or incomplete excision of pleomorphic adenoma of the parotid gland needs radiation therapy to prevent recurrence. The advocates of this policy[69] are opposed to the risk of inducing subsequent malignancy at a later date.[70] On the other hand, low-grade malignancies such as the desmoid tumor is less likely to recur with radiation therapy. Chemotherapy is primarily indicated in lymphoma where radiation may be added. Similarly, the combination of chemotherapy and radiation therapy is primarily indicated in sarcomatous involvement of the PPSp with excellent results obtained in rhabdomyosarcoma. In general, the aggressive tumors

may be subjected to chemoradiation rather than radiation alone for a better locoregional control. Teo et al have suggested doxorubicin for glandular malignancy and cisplatin and 5-florouracil for squamous cell cancer.[67] The recent advancements in radiotherapeutic techniques such as intensity-modulated radiation therapy (IMRT), proton therapy, and stereotactic (robotic) radiosurgery hold definite promise in future for controlling PPSp tumors.

Owing to the rarity of PPSp tumors, the customized protocol to deal with neck metastasis has not been standardized. It is beyond the scope of this chapter to elaborate the protocols for the management of metastatic neck disease that is standard for head and neck cancer elsewhere.

The adverse effects of radiation therapy are the same as elsewhere, but a theoretical possibility of temporal lobe necrosis has been suggested. However, practically the frequent occurrence of xerostomia adversely affects QOL. This probably results from the irradiation of parotid salivary glands because of anatomic proximity. Upcoming techniques such as IMRT and stereotactic radiosurgery are likely to spare the salivary gland and hence reduce xerostomia.

Prognosis

The cure in general depends on the nature and stage of the disease along with the quality of surgical clearance and adherence to postoperative chemoradiation. Excellent results have been reported for benign tumors, especially the salivary gland neoplasms, which have undergone proper preoperative work-up before a well-planned surgery. As far as malignant tumors are concerned, Hughes et al reported a recurrent disease in 27 of their 35 patients after a mean follow-up of 2.5 years (disease-free survival, 23%).[53] Katsantonis et al, however, reported a 3.5-year survival rate of 50% in a group of 18 patients with parotid tumors invading the PPSp after radical resections.[71] Bozza et al have lately reported a follow-up of 10 years for 12 patients (8 benign, 4 malignant).[72] All the benign pathologies were disease free at the end of follow-up while only one case of malignancy recurred. The recurrence was seen with adenocarcinoma (T3N1) only, and none of the others were more than T2N1 stage (squamous and papillary variety). Here, the improved disease-free survival reflected the nature and stage of pathology. The adenoid cystic variety constitutes a main part of recurrences seen at our institution. The metastatic disease performs much poorer as compared with primary malignancy in the PPSp. We have witnessed two dermal recurrences (with survival <3years from the time of diagnosis) in the past 10 years probably through perineural spread despite satisfactory resection of adenoid cystic carcinoma of the deep lobe of the parotid gland. The epidermoid variety of nasopharyngeal cancer is always incurable as it presents in an advanced stage (T4) while the spread of oropharyngeal and maxillary cancer also renders the patient inoperable. The overall survival and QOL may improve with radiation therapy, but the prognosis in terms of disease-free survival and recurrence is dismal in such cases. Chen et al reported a recurrence rate of 36% in patients with nasopharyngeal carcinoma extending to the PPSp.[63] The paucity of literature does not allow any conclusive predictions to be made about the behavior of malignant paraganglioma with respect to recurrence and survival. Hence, in the absence of a large series for follow-up studies, different cure rates have been reported with several smaller studies. Certain generalizations for improving prognosis and QOL can be made:

- A thorough preoperative work-up to facilitate better planning for an appropriate radical surgery is the most important aspect.
- Similarly for inoperable tumors, proper pretherapy counseling is an integral component of patient work-up.
- The progressive behavior of an inoperable malignant tumor can at least be controlled by chemoradiation.
- The treatment-induced toxicity may add to the morbidity and hence a balance needs to be maintained regarding the benefits and adverse effects influencing the QOL.

Conclusions

PPSp is anatomically a complex fascial space that harbors a multitude of pathologies either in itself or more commonly as extension from surrounding spaces. Early diagnosis is often difficult, and the diagnostic challenges are resolved by the triad of investigations, namely, FNAC, CT/ MRI/ ultrasound, and angiography. Assessment of cerebral blood flow is necessary when the internal carotid artery needs to be excised intraoperatively. The more common lesions are the salivary gland tumors, paraganglioma, and neurogenic tumors. The benign lesions usually show an excellent prognosis while malignant tumors are most of the times inoperable. Hence, the PPSp is a challenge for surgeons owing to the associated vital structures and the resultant high postoperative morbidity. The adjoining infratemporal fossa and skull base further add to the problem, specially in cases of extensive disease. The classical surgical approaches for PPSp tumors include transparotid, transcervical (or combined transcervical-transparotid), lateral mandibulotomy, and anterior-mandibulotomy-oropharyngeal approaches. Extensions in the infratemporal fossa can be dealt with Fisch approaches. The onset of transorbital infratemporal endoscopy is still in infancy but holds promise to replace more radical procedures meant to overcome diagnostic dilemma. Radiation therapy and chemotherapy play the most important role in dealing with malignant tumors, specially the inoperable ones. The morbidity associated with radical surgery is high, but the introduction of robotic surgery holds promise as the least invasive technique limiting the mutilation. Similarly, with the onset of IMRT, stereotactic radiosurgery, and proton therapy, the side effects of radiation are likely to be reduced. With an incidence of only 0.5% among all head and neck tumors, there is a paucity of literature to standardize the treatment and prognostic criteria. Considerable amount of work needs to be done for this yet "untouched" field.

References

1. Arena S, Hilal EY. Neurilemmomas of the infratemporal space: report of a case and review of the literature. Arch Otolaryngol 1976;102(3):180–184
2. Conley JJ. Tumours of the infratemporal fossa. Arch Otolaryngol 1964;79:498–504
3. Shaheen OH. Swellings of the infratemporal fossa. J Laryngol Otol 1982;96(9):817–836
4. Som PM, Biller HF, Lawson W. Tumors of the parapharyngeal space: preoperative evaluation, diagnosis and surgical approaches. Ann Otol Rhinol Laryngol 1981;90(80):3–15
5. Work WP, Gates GA. Tumors of the parotid gland and parapharyngeal space. Otolaryngol Clin North Am 1969;2:497–514
6. Johnson AT, Maran AG. Extracranial tumors of infratemporal fossa. J Laryngol Otol 1982;96(11):1017-1026
7. Carrau RL, Myers EN, Johnson JT. Management of tumors arising in the parapharyngeal space. Laryngoscope 1990;100(6): 583–589
8. Wasserman PG, Savargaonkar P. Paragangliomas: classification, pathology, and differential diagnosis. Otolaryngol Clin North Am 2001;34(5):845–862, v–vi
9. Batsakis JG, Sneige N. Parapharyngeal and retropharyngeal space diseases. Ann Otol Rhinol Laryngol 1989;98(4 Pt 1):320–321
10. Attia A, El-Shafiey M, El-Shazly S, Shouman T, Zaky I. Management of parapharyngeal space tumors at the National Cancer Institute, Egypt. J Egypt Natl Canc Inst 2004;16(1):34–42
11. Patey DH, Thackray AC. The pathological anatomy and treatment of parotid tumors with retropharyngeal extension (dumb-bell tumours): with a report of 4 personal cases. Br J Surg 1957;44:352–358
12. Fournier J, St Pierre S, Morrissette Y. Neurilemmoma of the parapharyngeal space: report of three cases and review of the literature. J Otolaryngol 1979;8(5):439–442
13. Hamza A, Fagan JJ, Weissman JL, Myers EN. Neurilemomas of the parapharyngeal space. Arch Otolaryngol Head Neck Surg 1997;123(6):622–626
14. Leu YS, Chang KC. Extracranial head and neck schwannomas: a review of 8 years experience. Acta Otolaryngol 2002;122(4): 435–437
15. Tandon DA, Bahadur S, Misra NK, Deka RC, Kapila K. Parapharyngeal neurofibromas. J Laryngol Otol 1992;106(3):243–246
16. Heard G. Malignant disease in von Recklinghausen's neurofibromatosis. Proc R Soc Med 1963;56:502–503
17. Black FO, Myers EN, Parnes SM. Surgical management of vagal chemodectomas. Laryngoscope 1977;87(8):1259–1269
18. Eriksen C, Girdhar-Gopal H, Lowry LD. Vagal paragangliomas: a report of nine cases. Am J Otolaryngol 1991;12(5):278–287
19. Batasakis J. Paragangliomas of the head and neck. In: Batsakis J, ed. Tumors of the Head and Neck: Clinical and Pathological Considerations. 2nd ed. Baltimore: Williams & Wilkins; 1979:369–380
20. Parkin JL. Familial multiple glomus tumors and pheochromocytomas. Ann Otol Rhinol Laryngol 1981;90(1 Pt 1):60–63
21. van Baars FM, Cremers CW, van den Broek P, Veldman JE. Familiar non-chromaffinic paragangliomas (glomus tumors): clinical and genetic aspects (abridged). Acta Otolaryngol 1981;91(5–6): 589–593

22. Irons GB, Weiland LH, Brown WL. Paragangliomas of the neck: clinical and pathologic analysis of 116 cases. Surg Clin North Am 1977;57(3):575–583

23. Spector GJ, Ciralsky R, Maisel RH, Ogura JH. IV. Multiple glomus tumors in the head and neck. Laryngoscope 1975;85(6): 1066–1075

24. Okabe Y, Shibutani K, Nishimura T, Furukawa M. Chondrosarcoma of the parapharyngeal space. J Laryngol Otol 1991;105(6):484–486

25. Bukachevsky RP, Pincus RL, Shechtman FG, Sarti E, Chodosh P. Synovial sarcoma of the head and neck. Head Neck 1992;14(1): 44–48

26. Hanada T, Iwashita M, Matsuzaki T, Hanamure Y, Fukuda K, Furuta S. Synovial sarcoma in the parapharyngeal space: case report and review of the literature. Auris Nasus Larynx 1999;26(1):91–94

27. Freije JE, Gluckman JL, Biddinger PW, Wiot G. Muscle tumors in the parapharyngeal space. Head Neck 1992;14(1):49–54

28. Llorente JL, Suárez C, Ablanedo P, Carreño M, Alvarez JC, Rodrigo JP. Hemangiopericytoma of the parapharyngeal space. Otolaryngol Head Neck Surg 1999;120(4):531–533

29. Pantanowitz L, Muc R, Spanger M, Sonnendecker H, McIntosh WA. Intravascular papillary endothelial hyperplasia (Masson's tumor) manifesting as a lateral neck mass. Ear Nose Throat J 2000;79(10):806–812, 809–810, 812 passim

30. Ducic Y, Ward G. Meningioma of the parapharyngeal space: case report. J Oral Maxillofac Surg 2000;58(8):905–908

31. Chiesa F, De Paoli F. Distant metastases from nasopharyngeal cancer. ORL J Otorhinolaryngol Relat Spec 2001;63(4):214–216

32. Sirotnak JJ, Loree TR, Penetrante R. Papillary carcinoma of the thyroid metastatic to the parapharyngeal space. Ear Nose Throat J 1997;76(5):342–344

33. Raut V, Sinnathuray AR, McClean G, Brooker D. Metastatic breast carcinoma in the parapharyngeal space. J Laryngol Otol 2001;115(9):750–752

34. Hamberger CA, Hamberger CB, Wersäll J, Wågermark J. Malignant catecholamine-producing tumour of the carotid body. Acta Pathol Microbiol Scand 1967;69(4):489–492

35. Whyte AM, Hourihan MD. The diagnosis of tumours involving the parapharyngeal space by computed tomography. Br J Radiol 1989;62(738):526–531

36. Moraitis D, Papakostas K, Karkanevatos A, Coast GJ, Jackson SR. Pleomorphic adenoma causing acute airway obstruction. J Laryngol Otol 2000;114(8):634–636

37. Ribeiro RT, Souza NA, Carvalho DdeS. Glossopharyngeal neuralgia with syncope as a sign of neck cancer recurrence. Arq Neuropsiquiatr 2007;65(4B):1233–1236

38. Mondal A, Raychoudhuri BK. Peroral fine needle aspiration cytology of parapharyngeal lesions. Acta Cytol 1993;3(107):1025-1028

39. Sack MJ, Weber RS, Weinstein GS, Chalian AA, Nisenbaum HL, Yousem DM. Image-guided fine-needle aspiration of the head and neck: five years' experience. Arch Otolaryngol Head Neck Surg 1998;124(10):1155–1161

40. Chong VF, Fan YF. Radiology of the parapharyngeal space. Australas Radiol 1998;42(3):278–283

41. Goodwin WJ Jr, Chandler JR. Transoral excision of lateral parapharyngeal space tumors presenting intraorally. Laryngoscope 1988;98(3):266–269

42. Miller FR, Wanamaker JR, Lavertu P, Wood BG. Magnetic resonance imaging and the management of parapharyngeal space tumors. Head Neck 1996;18(1):67–77

43. Sievers KW, Greess H, Baum U, Dobritz M, Lenz M. Paranasal sinuses and nasopharynx CT and MRI. Eur J Radiol 2000;33(3):185–202

44. de Vries EJ, Sekhar LN, Janecka IP, Schramm VL Jr, Horton JA, Eibling DE. Elective resection of the internal carotid artery without reconstruction. Laryngoscope 1988;98(9):960–966

45. Baker DC, Conley J. Treatment of massive deep lobe parotid tumors. Am J Surg 1979;138(4):572–575

46. Bozzetti A, Biglioli F, Gianni AB, Brusati R. Mandibulotomy for access to benign deep lobe parotid tumors with parapharyngeal extension: report of four cases. J Oral Maxillofac Surg 1998;56(2): 272–276

47. Olsen KD. Tumors and surgery of the parapharyngeal space. Laryngoscope 1994;104(5 Pt 2) (Suppl 63):1–28

48. Malone JP, Agrawal A, Schuller DE. Safety and efficacy of transcervical resection of parapharyngeal space neoplasms. Ann Otol Rhinol Laryngol 2001;110(12):1093–1098

49. Shahinian H, Dornier C, Fisch U. Parapharyngeal space tumors: the infratemporal fossa approach. Skull Base Surg 1995;5(2):73–81

50. Stell PM, Mansfield AO, Stoney PJ. Surgical approaches to tumors of the parapharyngeal space. Am J Otolaryngol 1985;6(2):92–97

51. Allison RS, Van der Waal I, Snow GB. Parapharyngeal tumours: a review of 23 cases. Clin Otolaryngol Allied Sci 1989;14(3): 199–203

52. Warrington G, Emery PJ, Gregory MM, Harrison DF. Pleomorphic salivary gland adenomas of the parapharyngeal space: review of nine cases. J Laryngol Otol 1981;95(2):205–218

53. Hughes KV III, Olsen KD, McCaffrey TV. Parapharyngeal space neoplasms. Head Neck 1995;17(2):124–130

54. Khafif A, Segev Y, Kaplan DM, Gil Z, Fliss DM. Surgical management of parapharyngeal space tumors: a 10-year review. Otolaryngol Head Neck Surg 2005;132(3):401–406

55. Sergi B, Limongelli A, Scarano E, Fetoni AR, Paludetti G. Giant deep lobe parotid gland pleomorphic adenoma involving the parapharyngeal space: report of three cases and review of the diagnostic and therapeutic approaches. Acta Otorhinolaryngol Ital 2008;28(5):261–265

56. Biller HF, Shugar JMA, Krespi YP. A new technique for wide-field exposure of the base of the skull. Arch Otolaryngol 1981;107(11):698–702

57. Schwartz TH, Bruce JN. Extended frontal approach with bilateral orbitofrontoethmoidal osteotomies for removal of a giant extracranial schwannoma in the nasopharynx, sphenoid sinus, and parapharyngeal space. Surg Neurol 2001;55(5):270–274

58. Shahinian HK, Suh RH, Jarrahy R. Combined infratemporal fossa and transfacial approach to excising massive tumors. Ear Nose Throat J 1999;78(5):350, 353–356

59. Anupam M, Shukla GK, Mishra SC, Bhatia N, Srivastava AN, Mishra N. Unusual solitary osteochondroma of the mandibular ramus. J Laryngol Otol 2002;116(1):65–66

60. Mishra A. Transorbital approach to infratemporal fossa: novel technique. J Laryngol Otol 2011;125(6):638–642

61. O'Malley BW Jr, Weinstein GS. Robotic skull base surgery: preclinical investigations to human clinical application. Arch Otolaryngol Head Neck Surg 2007;133(12):1215–1219

62. Umeda M, Minamikawa T, Yokoo S, Komori T. Metastasis of maxillary carcinoma to the parapharyngeal space: rationale and technique for concomitant en bloc parapharyngeal dissection. J Oral Maxillofac Surg 2002;60(4):408–413, discussion 413–414

63. Chen HJ, Leung SW, Su CY. Linear accelerator based radiosurgery as a salvage treatment for skull base and intracranial invasion of recurrent nasopharyngeal carcinomas. Am J Clin Oncol 2001;24(3):255–258

64. Hunt MA, Zelefsky MJ, Wolden S, et al. Treatment planning and delivery of intensity-modulated radiation therapy for primary

nasopharynx cancer. Int J Radiat Oncol Biol Phys 2001;49(3): 623–632

65. Lee AW, Sze WM, Yau TK, Yeung RM, Chappell R, Fowler JF. Retrospective analysis on treating nasopharyngeal carcinoma with accelerated fractionation (6 fractions per week) in comparison with conventional fractionation (5 fractions per week): report on 3-year tumor control and normal tissue toxicity. Radiother Oncol 2001;58(2):121–130

66. Levendag PC, Schmitz PI, Jansen PP, et al. Fractionated high-dose-rate brachytherapy in primary carcinoma of the nasopharynx. J Clin Oncol 1998;16(6):2213–2220

67. Teo PM, Chan AT, Lee WY, Leung TW, Johnson PJ. Enhancement of local control in locally advanced node-positive nasopharyngeal carcinoma by adjunctive chemotherapy. Int J Radiat Oncol Biol Phys 1999;43(2):261–271

68. Carrau RL, Johnson JT, Myers EN. Management of tumors of the parapharyngeal space. Oncology (Williston Park) 1997;11(5):633–640, discussion 640, 642

69. Rafla S. Mucous and Salivary Gland Tumours. Springfield, IL: Charles C. Thomas; 1970:104

70. Watkin G, Hobsley M. Should radiotherapy be used routinely in the management of benign parotid tumous. Br J Surg 1986;73:(8): 601-603

71. Katsantonis GP, Friedman WH, Rosenblum BN. The surgical management of advanced malignancies of the parotid gland. Otolaryngol Head Neck Surg 1989;101(6):633–640

72. Bozza F, Vigili MG, Ruscito P, Marzetti A, Marzetti F. Surgical management of parapharyngeal space tumours: results of 10-year follow-up. Acta Otorhinolaryngol Ital 2009;29(1):10–15

C. Salivary Neoplasms

21 Benign Salivary Gland Tumors

Hassan Arshad, Matthew O. Old, and Theodoros N. Teknos

Core Messages

- Benign neoplasms make up the majority of salivary gland pathology.

- The most common benign tumors of the salivary gland are pleomorphic adenomas and Warthin tumors.

- History and physical examination are often sufficient to determine if a lesion is benign or malignant but fine-needle aspiration is recommended.

- Complete surgical excisioin, not enucleation, is the preferred treatment for benign salivary neoplasms.

Benign salivary gland tumors make up the majority of salivary neoplasms. The most common of these are pleomorphic adenomas and Warthin tumors. In the pediatric population, the most common benign salivary tumor is a hemangioma. In addition to those mentioned, there exist several other types that will be covered here. This chapter will discuss the anatomy of salivary glands, the classification of the benign salivary neoplasms, and their management.

Anatomy

The major salivary glands are primarily composed of acini and their ducts. The acinar-ductal subunit comprises five kinds of cells: myoepithelial, acinar, intercalated ductal, striated ductal, and excretory ductal (remembered by the acronym MAISE). The acinar cells can be serous, mucinous, or mixed (seromucinous). These cells are surrounded by myoepithelial cells that are contractile in nature. Myoepithelial cells are also located around intercalated ducts. The acinus drains into the intercalated duct and then into the striated duct, which modifies the content of the primary secretion. Finally, the saliva moves to the excretory duct and then to the upper aerodigestive tract.

The largest of the paired major salivary glands is the parotid, located preauricularly. It is predominantly serous. The facial nerve exits the stylomastoid foramen and enters the gland, branching at the pes anserinus and then to the five major branches. The nerve arbitrarily divides the parotid into a superficial and deep lobe. Tumors involving the deep lobe may extend into the parapharyngeal space and will be covered in detail later in the chapter. The final excretory duct of the parotid is known as Stenson duct and empties into the buccal mucosa close to the maxillary second molars. Accessory parotid tissue, which is subject to the same

pathology as primary parotid tissue, can be located anterior to the parotid near Stenson duct.

The second largest of the three paired major salivary glands is the submandibular gland and is located in the submandibular triangle. It is considered mixed, but serous acini compose the majority of the gland. Superficial to the gland lies the facial vein, while the facial artery courses through the gland. Three nerves lie in close proximity to the gland: the marginal mandibular branch of the facial nerve, the lingual nerve, and the hypoglossal nerve. The main excretory duct of the gland is known as Wharton duct and drains into the floor of the mouth at the lingual frenulum.

The smallest of the major salivary glands are the paired sublingual glands, located anteriorly in the floor of the mouth. Mucinous acini predominate in these glands. The drainage goes directly in the floor of mouth via the ducts of Rivinus or may join the submandibular (Wharton) duct as the duct of Bartholin.

Classification of Benign Salivary Tumors

As of writing this chapter, the most recent classification of salivary gland tumors comes from the World Health Organization in 2005. The benign neoplasms included are listed in **Table 21.1**.

Pleomorphic Adenoma

Pleomorphic adenomas make up the majority of benign tumors in major and minor salivary glands, with most found in the parotid. They also account for 45 to 70% of all salivary tumors and up to 85% of benign tumors.[1,2] Grossly, pleomorphic adenomas can have a rubbery texture and a grayish yellow or tan appearance. Histologically, three

Table 21.1 World Health Organization Histological Classification of Benign Salivary Tumors

Pleomorphic adenoma

Warthin tumor (papillary cystadenoma lymphomatosum)

Basal cell adenoma

Myoepithelioma

Oncocytoma

Canalicular adenoma

Sebaceous adenoma

Lymphadenoma

Ductal papillomas

Cystadenoma

Hemangioma

types have been described: cellular, myxoid, and classic depending on the balance of epithelial/myoepithelial cells and the stromal component.[3] The epithelial cells are ductal while the myoepithelial cells can vary from spindle shaped to oval. Often there is a chondroid stroma or cartilaginous differentiation (**Fig. 21.1**). True to its name, pleomorphic adenomas have a wide variety of histopathologic appearances and can occasionally confuse the diagnosis with squamous cell carcinoma or mucoepidermoid carcinoma, depending on the epithelial differentiation. Up to 40% show "pseudopod" extensions into the normal parotid tissue and are likely responsible for recurrence after incomplete extirpation.[4] Malignant transformation is possible for these tumors and increases over time, with up to 10% becoming malignant over the lifetime of the patient.

Treatment involves complete tumor excision with a margin rather than enucleation. In the parotid gland, this usually entails a superficial parotidectomy with facial nerve preservation and complete gland removal for other major or minor salivary glands.

Warthin Tumor

Also known as papillary cystadenoma lymphomatosum, this tumor is the second most common benign salivary tumor. The vast majority occur in the parotid with only rare extraparotid occurrences. The "classic" patient is a 50- to 60-year-old, tobacco-smoking man. Although there is a male predominance, the percentage of men and women involved has become closer over the years. There is a strong predilection for tobacco smokers, and it typically affects patients in their 50s to 80s.[1,5] Up to 12.3% can present bilaterally.[6] Grossly, they are well circumscribed and cystic, often filled with a brownish or mucus-like fluid. Pathologic examination shows cystic structures with papillary projections lined with two layers of oncocytic cells, in a lymphoid stroma (**Fig. 21.2**). The latter feature can make it appear like a lymphoma on fine-needle aspiration (FNA) biopsy.

Malignant transformation is rare for these tumors, but the recommended treatment is complete surgical excision. Commonly, Warthin tumors involve the parotid tail so that superficial parotidectomy is sufficient for cure.

Basal Cell Adenoma

Basal cell adenomas were previously referred to as monomorphic adenomas, though this older classification probably also included canalicular adenomas as well. These rare tumors are three times more likely to be present in the parotid with the rest in minor salivary glands. They make up 1 to 3% of benign salivary gland neoplasms and the mean age at presentation is in the 50s. Pathologically, tumors are basaloid in appearance and can be solid, trabecular, membranous, or tubular (**Fig. 21.3**).[7,8] Treatment involves complete excision.

Oncocytomas

Oncocytes are cells that contain a deeply eosinophilic cytoplasm (because of an abundance of mitochondria) with

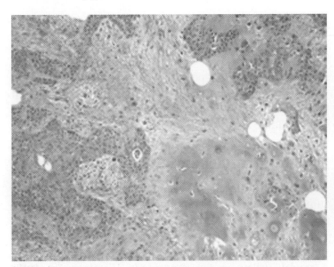

Figure 21.1 Pleomorphic adenoma (hematoxylin and eosin). Note the chondroid differentiation in the center right.

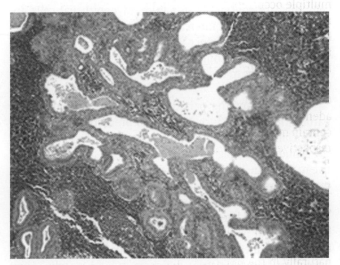

Figure 21.2 Warthin tumor (hematoxylin and eosin). Cystic spaces are lined with oncocytic epithelium with two layers of nuclei.

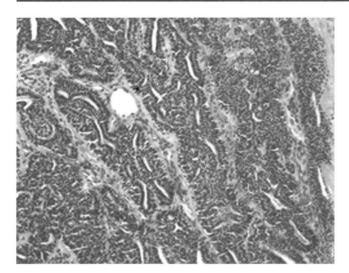

Figure 21.3 Basal cell adenoma (hematoxylin and eosin). Mixed tubular-trabecular type.

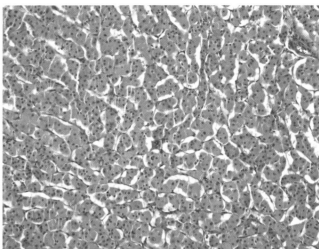

Figure 21.4 Oncocytoma (hematoxylin and eosin). Sheet of oncocytic cells with abundant eosinophilic cytoplasm.

round nuclei and a low nuclear to cytoplasmic ratio (**Fig. 21.4**). The most common oncocytic lesion in the head and neck is a Warthin tumor, but the term "oncocytoma" is reserved for a tumor consisting of "oncocytes arranged in solid sheets, collapsed trabeculae, or an organoid pattern."[9] The majority are found in the parotid gland, with the rest located in the oral cavity or sinonasal cavity.[10] Sinonasal oncocytomas may be locally aggressive without being malignant.

Canalicular Adenoma

Before 20 years ago, canalicular adenomas were classified together with basal cell adenomas as the monomorphic adenomas. Further histologic analysis has shown these two to be distinct tumors. These tumors almost exclusively occur in the minor salivary glands, usually arising in the upper lip. Rare cases of occurrences in the buccal mucosa, palatal mucosa, and parotid have been described. Very rarely, multiple occurrences can be found in the same patient. The mean age at presentation is between the 60s and 70s.[7,11,12] Pathology shows a well-encapsulated mass, with cuboidal to columnar cells arranged in a duct-like pattern, in a loose but vascular stroma (**Fig. 21.5**). Separation between some of the cells gives a "beads-on-a-string" characteristic.[13] Canalicular adenomas can be differentiated from basal call adenomas and pleomorphic adenomas in that they do not contain myoepithelial elements or chondroid differentiation, respectively. Treatment involves complete surgical excision.

Sebaceous Adenoma

Sebaceous adenomas are extremely rare, benign neoplasms that have been reported in the parotid gland, submandibular glands, and intraorally. Because sebaceous glands occur naturally in the oral cavity in a minority of the population, the origin of intraoral sebaceous adenomas is unclear. The mean age at presentation has been reported to be in the 60s.

Histologically, they show sebaceous cell nests in an acinar-like pattern, sometimes with squamous differentiation or oncocytic metaplasia.[14,15] Surgical excision is curative.

Myoepithelioma

These benign tumors are composed almost, if not completely, of myoepithelial cells. Myoepitheliomas may represent one extreme end of the spectrum of pleomorphic adenomas. Four subtypes have been described: plasmacytoid, spindle cell, reticular, and clear-cell type. These subtypes do not seem to indicate any prognostic significance (**Fig. 21.6**).[16,17] Most are found in the parotid gland or minor salivary gland and can be present in any age group.[18] The main differential diagnosis to consider is pleomorphic adenoma; however, treatment is the same with complete excision being satisfactory.

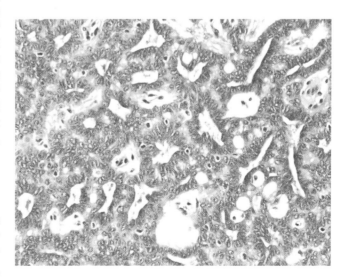

Figure 21.5 Canalicular adenoma (hematoxylin and eosin). Cuboidal to columnar cells arranged in a duct-like pattern, in a loose stroma.

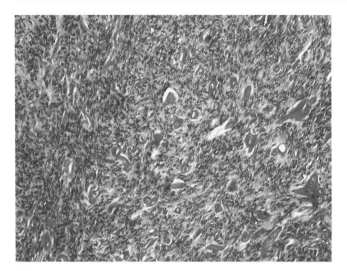

Figure 21.6 Myoepithelioma (hematoxylin and eosin), spindle-cell variant.

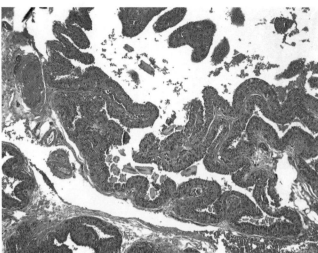

Figure 21.7 Intraductal papilloma (hematoxylin and eosin), also known as papillary cystadenoma. Papillary fronds are seen lined with cuboidal to columnar cells.

Lymphadenoma

Lymphadenomas can be subtyped into sebaceous and nonsebaceous varieties, depending on the presence of sebaceous differentiation. They show epithelial nests in a diffuse lymphoid background. Almost all are found in the parotid gland with only one case had been reported in the lip.[19] These tumors appear to arise in nodal tissue within glands. The differential diagnosis includes mucoepidermoid carcinoma. Foreign body type inflammatory reaction to sebum may help to differentiate the sebaceous adenoma from mucoepidermoid carcinoma.[20]

Ductal Papillomas

These tumors are divided into three types: intraductal papilloma, sialadenoma papilliferum, and inverted ductal papilloma. The vast majority are found in minor salivary glands, and those located intraorally represent 4.5% of benign salivary tumors.[7] They usually present in the sixth and seventh decades. Intraductal papilloma has also been called papillary cystadenoma. Sialadenoma papilliferum is a slow-growing exophytic lesion that is sometimes misdiagnosed as squamous papilloma. Inverted ductal papilloma is the rarest of the three types and is distinguished from intraductal form by its epithelial component proliferating within the duct itself (**Fig. 21.7**).[21]

Cystadenoma

Cystadenomas are related to intraductal papillomas and have been lumped together in literature. However, the term "papillary cystadenoma" should be used if the lesion is multicystic, rather than intraductal papilloma which is unicystic.[22] In addition, up to one-half of the cystadenomas are found in the parotid. Low-grade mucoepidermoid

carcinoma can appear similar to cystadenomas and must be distinguished.

Hemangioma

The most common benign parotid tumor of childhood is the hemangioma. These are true epithelial neoplasms and should be distinguished from vascular malformations (**Fig. 21.8**). Like other hemangiomas, those in the parotid typically present in the first few weeks after birth. This is followed by a rapid proliferative phase and then involution that is usually complete by the age of 5 years. Treatment may involve observation, surgery, high-dose systemic corticosteroids, or laser therapy.[23,24] Recurrence can be a problem after surgery. Surgery is not usually undertaken in the proliferative phase unless there is excessive bleeding or hemodynamic compromise. It is not uncommon to have a residual soft tissue deformity after involution, and at this stage, surgery can be offered to correct it. With the emergence of β-blockers as a viable and successful option to treat pediatric hemangiomas, the future of managing these tumors may change.[25]

Management

History and Physical Examination

Typically, benign tumors of the salivary glands are slow growing and painless. Questions during history taking should include those regarding onset, duration, rapidity of growth, pain, facial weakness, history of cutaneous neoplasm, and tobacco use. During physical examination, a thorough head and neck examination should be done including palpation of the parotid gland and neck (especially bimanual palpation of the submandibular region, if indicated) and testing of cranial nerves with regard to facial nerve function and cutaneous

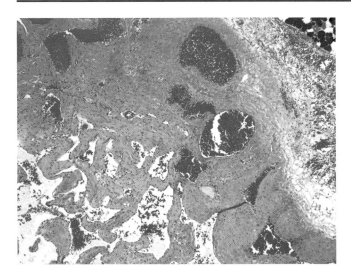

Figure 21.8 Hemangioma (hematoxylin and eosin). Closely spaced and immature capillaries are present.

sensation. Evaluation should be done of symptoms, such as rapid growth, pain, and/or facial nerve impairment, while not pathognomonic, should alert the clinician to the possibility of malignancy.

Imaging

At our institution, patients are typically referred after having undergone a computed tomography (CT) scan. This is usually adequate unless a malignancy is suspected. In that case, magnetic resonance imaging (MRI) may be added to look for perineural spread. Any of the three main imaging modalities (CT, MRI, and ultrasound) can be used in the work-up, and characteristic findings will be discussed for each.

Typically, benign tumors of the salivary glands will be circumscribed without evidence of invasion into surrounding tissues or perineural enhancement. On MRI, pleomorphic adenomas have a characteristic appearance with low to intermediate T1 signal and a hyperintense T2 signal. Postcontrast images with fat saturation on T1 sequences can further delineate the tumor.[26] Postcontrast images can show patchy enhancement, distinguishing it from Warthin tumors. The classic "dumbbell" shape can be seen for tumors involving the deep lobe. This shape results from compression by the stylomandibular ligament in the stylomandibular tunnel, creating the "bar" of the dumbbell. On CT, the tumor will appear well defined and spherical or lobulated. It will be hyperdense to the surrounding salivary tissue. Ultrasound shows a well-defined, hypoechoic mass. Larger tumors can be cystic with areas of hemorrhage.[27]

Warthin tumors are also low intensity on T1-weighted MRI images and hyperintense on T2 sequences. They show variable postcontrast enhancement, depending on how cystic the tumor is, but typically do not enhance well. On CT they are hypodense to the surrounding tissue. On ultrasonography they appear hypoechoic with multiseptated cysts.[19]

Benign tumors may appear hypermetabolic on positron emission tomography scans. In the case of a hypermetabolic parotid lesion, FNA should be done to guide treatment. If a Warthin tumor is suspected but FNA is inconclusive, a technetium scan can be done, as these tumors will accumulate technetium.[28]

Fine-Needle Aspiration

FNA is recommended for tumors of salivary origin. Though the argument can be made that the excision of these tumors is both diagnostic and therapeutic, FNA can help guide therapy especially if the patient has a contraindication to surgery or malignancy is suspected. Sensitivity and specificity of FNA for neoplasms of salivary origin have been reported as high as 92 and 100%, respectively.[29,30] In the case of nondiagnostic specimens, repeat FNA has been shown to be useful.[21] It is very helpful to have a cytopathologist present to determine adequacy of the sample. Ultrasound-guided FNA has shown to be superior in some reports.[31] False-negative cases can be seen for any case and should be kept in mind for Warthin tumors.

Surgery

Surgical management for benign tumors of the parotid gland usually involves superficial parotidectomy with facial nerve preservation. If the tumor involves the deep lobe, a total parotidectomy may be needed. The facial nerve should not be sacrificed even if the tumor is lying on the nerve. A particular conundrum happens when a diagnosis is not made before surgery and a frozen section during surgery shows a possible malignant tumor. If the patient's facial nerve was intact before surgery but appears to be involved by the tumor, the nerve should not be sacrificed until the permanent sections provide a conclusive diagnosis.

When performing a superficial parotidectomy, a cuff of normal tissue is included, especially in the case of a pleomorphic adenoma. Enucleation is strongly discouraged and can lead to incomplete excision and recurrence. For parapharyngeal space tumors, usually a cervical approach without mandibulotomy will suffice. This is covered in more detail in the following section. Benign tumors involving the submandibular or sublingual glands require complete excision of the involved gland. This is also true for minor salivary gland tumors.

During parotidectomy, it is recommended to use facial nerve monitoring for revision cases. The routine use of monitoring for primary cases is controversial but is becoming more common. Facial nerve monitoring may improve immediate postoperative paresis, but may not decrease the incidence of long-term dysfunction.[32–34] One must remember that facial nerve monitoring is not a substitute for a thorough understanding of the surgical anatomy. In addition, repeated and unnecessary stimulation of the nerve with the stimulator probe can lead to temporary postoperative nerve paresis or paralysis.

Parapharyngeal Space Tumors

Occasionally, benign tumors will extend or originate in the deep lobe with extension into the parapharyngeal space. Benign salivary tumors can also originate in the parapharyngeal space. In these cases, a transcervical approach without a mandibulotomy is usually sufficient.[35] Several maneuvers can increase access without dividing the mandible. Nasotracheal intubation can provide extra room for forward protrusion of the mandible. In addition, division of the diagastric and stylohyoid muscles and transection of the stylomandibular ligament and/or the styloid process can further increase exposure. The majority of these tumors can be resected by using these techniques. If a mandibulotomy is required, it can be done through a symphyseal or mandibular body osteotomy. For tumors completely confined to the parapharyngeal space, transoral robotic resection via the daVinci robot (Intuitive Surgical, Sunnyvale, California, United States) is a newer tool.[36] For this technique to be successful, there must be adequate oral exposure and the tumor must not be intimately involved with the great vessels of the neck.

Recurrent Pleomorphic Adenoma

Recurrent pleomorphic adenoma of the parotid gland can be a challenging problem. Surgical risk factors for recurrence include enucleation at time of initial surgery and tumor capsule rupture. As stated before, enucleation is not sufficient for tumor removal because of the pseudopod-like extensions of the neoplasm. Other risk factors may include younger age at time of excision, female gender, and genetic factors such as *MUC*1 expression. Time to recurrence can be from 1 to 20 years postoperatively, with most happening between 5 and 15 years. In addition, recurrences are typically multifocal.[37–40]

Treatment for recurrences involves total parotidectomy.[3] The risk of postoperative facial nerve injury increases with re-excision; therefore, nerve monitoring is recommended.[41] Postoperative radiotherapy has been shown to improve local control.[42] The incidence of malignant transformation in recurrences has been reported as high as 16%.[43]

References

1. de Oliveira FA, Duarte EC, Taveira CT, et al. Salivary gland tumor: a review of 599 cases in a Brazilian population. Head Neck Pathol 2009;3(4):271–275

2. Spiro RH. Salivary neoplasms: overview of a 35-year experience with 2,807 patients. Head Neck Surg 1986;8(3):177–184

3. Stennert E, Wittekindt C, Klussmann JP, Arnold G, Guntinas-Lichius O. Recurrent pleomorphic adenoma of the parotid gland: a prospective histopathological and immunohistochemical study. Laryngoscope 2004;114(1):158–163

4. Zbären P, Stauffer E. Pleomorphic adenoma of the parotid gland: histopathologic analysis of the capsular characteristics of 218 tumors. Head Neck 2007;29(8):751–757

5. Kotwall CA. Smoking as an etiologic factor in the development of Warthin's tumor of the parotid gland. Am J Surg 1992;164(6): 646–647

6. Teymoortash A, Krasnewicz Y, Werner JA. Clinical features of cystadenolymphoma (Warthin's tumor) of the parotid gland: a retrospective comparative study of 96 cases. Oral Oncol 2006;42(6):569–573

7. Buchner A, Merrell PW, Carpenter WM. Relative frequency of intra-oral minor salivary gland tumors: a study of 380 cases from northern California and comparison to reports from other parts of the world. J Oral Pathol Med 2007;36(4):207–214

8. Kawata R, Yoshimura K, Lee K, Araki M, Takenaka H, Tsuji M. Basal cell adenoma of the parotid gland: a clinicopathological study of nine cases—basal cell adenoma versus pleomorphic adenoma and Warthin's tumor. Eur Arch Otorhinolaryngol 2010;267(5): 779–783

9. Wakely PE Jr. Oncocytic and oncocyte-like lesions of the head and neck. Ann Diagn Pathol 2008;12(3):222–230

10. Kanazawa H, Furuya T, Murano A, Yamaki M. Oncocytoma of an intraoral minor salivary gland: report of a case and review of literature. J Oral Maxillofac Surg 2000;58(8):894–897

11. Philpott CM, Kendall C, Murty GE. Canalicular adenoma of the parotid gland. J Laryngol Otol 2005;119(1):59–60

12. Yih WY, Kratochvil FJ, Stewart JC. Intraoral minor salivary gland neoplasms: review of 213 cases. J Oral Maxillofac Surg 2005;63(6):805–810

13. Penner CR, Thompson L. Canalicular adenoma. Ear Nose Throat J 2005;84(3):132

14. Izutsu T, Kumamoto H, Kimizuka S, Ooya K. Sebaceous adenoma in the retromolar region: report of a case with a review of the English literature. Int J Oral Maxillofac Surg 2003;32(4):423–426

15. Zare-Mahmoodabadi R, Salehinejad J, Saghafi S, Ghazi N, Mahmoudi P, Harraji A. Sebaceous adenoma of the submandibular gland: a case report. J Oral Sci 2009;51(4):641–644

16. Dardick I. Myoepithelioma: definitions and diagnostic criteria. Ultrastruct Pathol 1995;19(5):335–345

17. Dardick I, Cavell S, Boivin M, et al. Salivary gland myoepithelioma variants. Histological, ultrastructural, and immunocytological features. Virchows Arch A Pathol Anat Histopathol 1989;416(1): 25–42

18. Alós L, Cardesa A, Bombí JA, Mallofré C, Cuchi A, Traserra J. Myoepithelial tumors of salivary glands: a clinicopathologic, immunohistochemical, ultrastructural, and flow-cytometric study. Semin Diagn Pathol 1996;13(2):138–147

19. Maruyama S, Cheng J, Inoue T, Takagi R, Saku T. Sebaceous lymphadenoma of the lip: report of a case of minor salivary gland origin. J Oral Pathol Med 2002;31(4):242–243

20. Rawlinson NJ, Almarzooqi S, Nicol K. Sebaceous lymphadenoma of the parotid gland in a 13-year-old girl: a case report. Head Neck Pathol 2010;4(2):144–147

21. Brennan PA, Davies B, Poller D, et al. Fine needle aspiration cytology (FNAC) of salivary gland tumours: repeat aspiration provides further information in cases with an unclear initial cytological diagnosis. Br J Oral Maxillofac Surg 2010;48(1):26–29

22. Brannon RB, Sciubba JJ, Giulani M. Ductal papillomas of salivary gland origin: a report of 19 cases and a review of the literature. Oral Surg Oral Med Oral Pathol Oral Radiol Endod 2001;92(1):68–77

23. Reinisch JF, Kim RY, Harshbarger RJ, Meara JG. Surgical management of parotid hemangioma. Plast Reconstr Surg 2004;113(7): 1940–1948

24. Sinno H, Thibaudeau S, Coughlin R, Chitte S, Williams B. Management of infantile parotid gland hemangiomas: a 40-year experience. Plast Reconstr Surg 2010;125(1):265–273

25. Buckmiller LM. Propranolol treatment for infantile hemangiomas. Curr Opin Otolaryngol Head Neck Surg 2009;17(6):458–459

26. Shah GV. MR imaging of salivary glands. Magn Reson Imaging Clin N Am 2002;10(4):631–662

27. Lee YY, Wong KT, King AD, Ahuja AT. Imaging of salivary gland tumours. Eur J Radiol 2008;66(3):419–436

28. Ozawa N, Okamura T, Koyama K, et al. Retrospective review: usefulness of a number of imaging modalities including CT, MRI, technetium-99m pertechnetate scintigraphy, gallium-67 scintigraphy and F-18-FDG PET in the differentiation of benign from malignant parotid masses. Radiat Med 2006;24(1):41–49

29. Elagoz S, Gulluoglu M, Yilmazbayhan D, Ozer H, Arslan I. The value of fine-needle aspiration cytology in salivary gland lesions, 1994–2004. ORL J Otorhinolaryngol Relat Spec 2007;69(1):51–56

30. Stewart CJ, MacKenzie K, McGarry GW, Mowat A. Fine-needle aspiration cytology of salivary gland: a review of 341 cases. Diagn Cytopathol 2000;22(3):139–146

31. Wu M. A comparative study of 200 head and neck FNAs performed by a cytopathologist with versus without ultrasound guidance: evidence for improved diagnostic value with ultrasound guidance. Diagn Cytopathol 2011;39(10):743–751

32. Grosheva M, Klussmann JP, Grimminger C, et al. Electromyographic facial nerve monitoring during parotidectomy for benign lesions does not improve the outcome of postoperative facial nerve function: a prospective two-center trial. Laryngoscope 2009;119(12):2299–2305

33. Meier JD, Wenig BL, Manders EC, Nenonene EK. Continuous intraoperative facial nerve monitoring in predicting postoperative injury during parotidectomy. Laryngoscope 2006;116(9):1569–1572

34. Terrell JE, Kileny PR, Yian C, et al. Clinical outcome of continuous facial nerve monitoring during primary parotidectomy. Arch Otolaryngol Head Neck Surg 1997;123(10):1081–1087

35. Zhi K, Ren W, Zhou H, Wen Y, Zhang Y. Management of parapharyngeal-space tumors. J Oral Maxillofac Surg 2009;67(6):1239–1244

36. O'Malley BW Jr, Quon H, Leonhardt FD, Chalian AA, Weinstein GS. Transoral robotic surgery for parapharyngeal space tumors. ORL J Otorhinolaryngol Relat Spec 2010;72(6):332–336

37. Hamada T, Matsukita S, Goto M, et al. Mucin expression in pleomorphic adenoma of salivary gland: a potential role for MUC1 as a marker to predict recurrence. J Clin Pathol 2004;57(8):813–821

38. Moonis G, Patel P, Koshkareva Y, Newman J, Loevner LA. Imaging characteristics of recurrent pleomorphic adenoma of the parotid gland. AJNR Am J Neuroradiol 2007;28(8):1532–1536

39. Redaelli de Zinis LO, Piccioni M, Antonelli AR, Nicolai P. Management and prognostic factors of recurrent pleomorphic adenoma of the parotid gland: personal experience and review of the literature. Eur Arch Otorhinolaryngol 2008;265(4):447–452

40. Wittekindt C, Streubel K, Arnold G, Stennert E, Guntinas-Lichius O. Recurrent pleomorphic adenoma of the parotid gland: analysis of 108 consecutive patients. Head Neck 2007;29(9):822–828

41. Glas AS, Vermey A, Hollema H, et al. Surgical treatment of recurrent pleomorphic adenoma of the parotid gland: a clinical analysis of 52 patients. Head Neck 2001;23(4):311–316

42. Chen AM, Garcia J, Bucci MK, Quivey JM, Eisele DW. Recurrent pleomorphic adenoma of the parotid gland: long-term outcome of patients treated with radiation therapy. Int J Radiat Oncol Biol Phys 2006;66(4):1031–1035

43. Makeieff M, Pelliccia P, Letois F, et al. Recurrent pleomorphic adenoma: results of surgical treatment. Ann Surg Oncol 2010;17(12):3308–3313

22 Salivary Gland Tumors

Barry T. Malin, Brendan P. O'Connell, and M. Boyd Gillespie

Core Messages

- The majority of salivary gland tumors present as asymptomatic masses with indolent progression. Timely, comprehensive evaluation and treatment of all salivary masses is critical, because of the complications associated with progression of benign lesions and the risk of malignancy.

- Ultrasound is the preferred imaging modality for presumed benign lesions of submandibular, sublingual, and superficial parotid tumors. Magnetic resonance imaging is warranted if any features suggestive of malignancy are present.

- Fine-needle aspiration is safe, rapid, inexpensive, and adequately sensitive, and is thus the optimal method for preoperative tissue sampling of salivary neoplasms.

- Surgical resection in eligible candidates is required for most benign and all malignant salivary neoplasms. In the setting of malignancy additional treatment, such as neck dissection or adjuvant radiation therapy, is variable and determination is based primarily on tumor stage and grade.

- Surgical approaches to excision of benign tumors of the superficial parotid gland vary with regards to planned extent or resection and facial nerve dissection, and the choice of techniques for excision of these masses remains controversial.

Salivary gland neoplasms arise within a common group of glands in the head and neck region: the parotid, submandibular, sublingual, and minor salivary glands. Most salivary gland tumors present as an asymptomatic, slowly enlarging mass in the region of a major salivary gland. Salivary gland cancers are relatively rare, accounting for only 20% of salivary tumors and 5% of all head and neck malignancies.[1] Up to 75% of salivary gland tumors are benign and the majority are asymptomatic. Both the asymptomatic quality and indolent growth rate of most salivary gland tumors may lead to an undue delay in diagnosis and provision of appropriate care. Comprehensive evaluation of salivary gland tumors is critical, as inappropriate treatment greatly increases the risk for persistent and recurrent disease. Moreover, failure to accurately diagnose and adequately treat malignant salivary disease can have grave consequences.

Imaging of Salivary Gland Tumors

Ultrasound (US), X-ray, computed tomography (CT), and magnetic resonance imaging (MRI) may be used in the detection and assessment of salivary gland tumors. Preoperative imaging may not be necessary in all cases of parotid masses, as surgical extirpation is the standard treatment modality. Imaging studies are mandated, however, in cases of suspected malignancy, and may be helpful in preoperative planning and patient counseling.

There are several advantages to imaging salivary gland tumors before treatment. Imaging helps confirm that the mass originates from the salivary gland and is not because of adjacent pathology (e.g., lipoma, adnexal mass, lymph node). Pretreatment scans assist operative planning by defining the relationship between the mass and nearby vital structures such as cranial nerves and blood vessels. Although no imaging modality can accurately depict the relationship of a parotid tumor mass to the facial nerve, the plane demarcated by the lateral border of the retromandibular vein can serve as a reasonable proxy for the level of the facial nerve. Assessment of the depth of the tumor relative to this plane can assist the surgeon in predicting the necessity of deep lobe extirpation.[2] Further, imaging can detect possible signs of malignancy not readily appreciable by physical examination, such as ill-defined tumor borders, invasion of surrounding structures (e.g., ear canal, muscle, bone), enhancement or thickening of the facial and trigeminal nerves, the presence of multifocal disease, and local nodal metastases.

US is the preferred imaging modality for suspected benign submandibular, sublingual, and superficial parotid tumors. Advantages of US include the fact that it can facilitate fine-needle aspiration (FNA) and it does not require administration of radiation. US is relatively inexpensive and can help characterize the following tumor characteristics: size and border regularity, the pattern of vascularity, multifocality, and adjacent lymphadenopathy. Disadvantages include the fact that US sensitivity and specificity are somewhat operator-dependent and that the ability to depict the deep aspects of the parotid gland and the parapharyngeal space is limited because of acoustic absorption, dispersion, and obscurement by the mandible.[3] Moreover, interpretation of US images of the salivary glands is more challenging than corresponding MRI or CT images for those without extensive experience.[4] US imaging is also unsuitable for assessing perineural spread, extraglandular invasion of bone or soft tissue, and oropharyngeal or retropharyngeal nodal metastases.[5]

If a malignant process is suspected, MRI with gadolinium is preferred because of its superior salivary tissue resolution, ability to assess marrow spaces, and capacity for revealing cranial nerve enhancement or thickening.[6] CT may be of value if MRI is unavailable or may serve as a useful adjunct to MRI if the tumor is fixed to the temporal bone or mandible, as it is superior in detecting bony involvement.

Fluorodeoxyglucose positron emission tomography is rarely indicated in the primary evaluation of salivary gland tumors because of the expense, lack of supporting evidence regarding its diagnostic value, and its high rate of false positives for malignancy in the setting of benign salivary tumors such as pleomorphic adenoma (PA) and Warthin tumor.[7] No imaging technique can reliably differentiate between benign and malignant salivary tumors; therefore, radiographic findings alone should not be used as a justification to defer adequate treatment of a salivary mass.

Fine-Needle Aspiration Biopsy of Salivary Gland Tumors

FNA biopsy is the preferred method for preoperative tissue sampling of salivary gland neoplasms. FNA is simple, rapid, and relatively inexpensive with little morbidity and low risk of malignant seeding. As surgical excision remains the standard treatment strategy for most salivary gland tumors, FNA may not substantially alter therapy. Therefore, performance of FNA is not mandated in all cases. Potential benefits to FNA include more accurate patient counseling regarding the likelihood of malignancy and operative risk. Surgical approaches may differ based on the expectation of malignancy. Moreover, even if benign pathology is confirmed on FNA, discrimination between the most common types of benign neoplasms may influence surgical techniques.[8] The overall sensitivity of FNA for detection of salivary gland neoplasia is 89.4% and its accuracy for discriminating between benign and malignant salivary tumors is 79.1%.[9] Diagnostic accuracy is enhanced with the use of US guidance.[10]

The diversity of tumor types can make cytopathologic diagnosis and subtyping based on FNA difficult. Diagnosis is further complicated by the potential for sampling error and the histologic similarities of tumor types with very different behaviors (so-called *look-alike* tumors). The common overlap in the cytopathologic morphologies also complicates malignancy determination; however, an experienced head and neck cytopathologist is often able to determine whether a salivary mass is likely benign or malignant based on cellular density, morphology, uniformity, and the presence

of mitotic figures with an overall accuracy of 80%.[11] Whereas a negative FNA finding does not eliminate the possibility of cancer and should not be used as the sole reason not to treat, a biopsy positive for malignancy greatly increases the true likelihood of cancer. With this information, the surgeon can plan an appropriate surgical approach and counsel the patient concerning the potential need for neck dissection, facial nerve resection, and reconstructive options.

The false-negative rate in US-guided FNA of major salivary gland tumors is 4.2%.[12] Although approximately 25% of initial FNA specimens are nondiagnostic, repeat FNA specimens may commonly lead to an ultimate cytopathologic diagnosis; sensitivity (85%) and specificity (93%) rates in detecting salivary gland malignancy on repeat FNA are comparable to those of initial specimens.[13] Overall, more than 90% of preoperative FNA specimens are interpreted as PA.[14] In a review of 879 FNA biopsies of major salivary gland tumors, Christensen et al found that FNA yielded accurate preoperative identification of tumor subtype in 97% of benign lesions and 71% of malignant lesions.[15]

Benign Salivary Gland Neoplasms

Roughly 75% of all salivary gland tumors are benign. Benign salivary gland neoplasms typically present as slow-growing, painless masses in the region of a salivary gland. Imaging is not mandated in suspected benign salivary gland neoplasms; however, it can assist with tumor characterization and preoperative planning, as the definitive treatment remains surgical excision. The histopathology of benign salivary gland tumors is extremely diverse, with the most common tumor being PA. Recently, the World Health Organization divided benign epithelial tumors into 10 subtypes.[16] A summary of these subtypes and their respective key features is provided in **Table 22.1**. Soft tissue tumors, such as hemangiomas, and hematolymphoid tumors, such as Hodgkin lymphomas, diffuse large B-cell lymphomas, and extranodal marginal zone B-cell lymphomas can, also be classified as benign salivary gland tumors.

Surgical Management of Benign Neoplasms

Although surgical excision is the mainstay of treatment for benign salivary gland neoplasms, the appropriate choice of surgical technique, particularly regarding the extent of parotid gland dissection, remains controversial. Debate over this issue has been shaped by multiple—sometimes competing—imperatives, including concerns regarding tumor recurrence, facial nerve preservation, and cosmetic considerations. In the first half of the 20th century, the preferred approach to surgical treatment of parotid neoplasms involved simple enucleation alone. Mid-century, a shift in the standard approach toward more extensive facial nerve dissection and comprehensive gland excision occurred. This change in prevailing surgical opinion was driven by multiple factors, including increased

Table 22.1 Benign Epithelial Salivary Tumors

Salivary Tumor	Gender Predilection	Most Commonly Affected Gland	Histologic Features	Other Features
PA	Female	Parotid	Luminal differentiation with varying mixture of epithelial, myoepithelial, and stromal components, surrounded by a false capsule	> 70% of all parotid masses High propensity for recurrence with inadequate resection or tumor spillage Risk of malignant generation to Ca-ex PA
Warthin tumor	Male	Parotid	Bilayered oncocytic epithelial cells arranged as papillary projections lining cystic spaces and a prominent lymphoid stroma	Bilateral in 10% of cases 1–12% rate of recurrence Selectively incorporates Tc99m pertechnetate on radionucleotide imaging
Basal cell adenoma	None	Parotid	Isomorphic basaloid cells and interlaced trabeculae with a well-defined basement membrane	Subdivided into solid, trabecular, tubular, and membranous growth patterns Most tumors display a combination of growth patterns
Oncocytoma	None	Parotid	Large epithelial cells with deeply eosinophilic, finely granular cystoplasm secondary to innumerable mitochondria	Selectively incorporates Tc99m pertechnetate on radionucleotide imaging Other salivary gland tumors have the potential to undergo oncocytic metaplasia and mimic oncocytomas
Cystadenoma	None	Minor salivary glands in the lip	The papillary subtype is most common and demonstrates intraluminal papillary projections lined by cuboidal to columnar cells	Mucus and papillary subtypes, with the latter being the most common Unicystic or multicystic growth
Canalicular adenoma	Female	Minor salivary glands in the lip	Columnar epithelial cells that form cords of single or double cell layers and a loose, highly vascular stroma	Multifocal in nature
Myoepithelioma	None	Major salivary glands	Spindle, plasmacytoid, epithelioid, and clear cells exhibiting myoepithelial differentiation	Malignant transformation is rare but has been reported
Ductal papilloma	None	Minor salivary glands	Papillary growth of the ductal epithelium	Can be subdivided into sialadenoma papilliferum, inverted papilloma, and intraductal papilloma
Lymphadenoma	Male	Major salivary glands	Epithelial component with sebaceous differentiation and prominent, reactive lymphoid proliferation	Malignant transformation is rare but has been reported to occur in the epithelial component
Sebaceous adenoma	Male	Parotid	Cells demonstrating sebaceous differentiation without atypia are arranged in nests forming acinar and duct-like structures with intervening fibrous stroma	Grossly solid or cystic

PA, pleomorphic adenoma; Ca-ex PA, carcinoma ex pleomorphic adenoma; Tc99m, technetium-99m.

recognition of the high rates of PA recurrence following enucleation. This shift in opinion was further supported by the findings of Patey and Thackray, who described the prevalence of microscopic PA extracapsular extension in a landmark histopathologic study in 1957.[17] The preferred approach to extirpation thus shifted toward superficial parotidectomy or en bloc excision of essentially all parotid tissue lateral to the plane of the facial nerve as the minimal acceptable degree of resection.

In recent years, there has been a resurgence of interest in subtotal parotid excision techniques. Several distinct techniques have been described: *enucleation, extracapsular dissection, limited parotidectomy, subtotal parotidectomy, partial-superficial parotidectomy, superficial parotidectomy*, and *total parotidectomy*. The partial-superficial parotidectomy approach, as described by Iizuka and Ishikawa, entails segmental resection in which facial nerve dissection is limited to the main trunk and the distal segmental branch proximate to the tumor.[18] The extracapsular dissection method, which uses dissection within the loose areolar plane surrounding the fibrotic PA pseudocapsule without directed facial nerve identification or dissection, was first comprehensively described by Gleave and has subsequently been elaborated upon by multiple authors.[19] Minimally invasive endoscopic techniques using facelift-type incisions have also recently been reported.[20] Although enucleation may be appropriate for some types of benign lesions, it is inadequate for resection of PA because of the unacceptably high rate of recurrence. However, the appropriate planned extent of excision for salivary benign neoplasms, and PAs of the parotid gland in particular, remains a matter of debate.

Some contemporary authors maintain that superficial parotidectomy constitutes the only suitable technique, reporting that complete ablation of the lateral lobe decreases the risk of tumor recurrence and facial nerve injury.[21] The body of literature in favor of more limited approaches in selected cases has grown, however, with extracapsular dissection emerging as the favored alternative. Riad et al have noted that even when resection is attempted with a superficial parotidectomy or a specified width of surrounding tissue cuff, close approximation of the tumor to the facial nerve occurs in many cases. Thus, the actual margin that can be obtained in the setting of facial nerve preservation is limited and often entails only a thin plane of tissue between the tumor capsule and the underlying facial nerve. In their recent review of 182 cases of parotid resections for PAs, resection margin had no apparent impact on recurrence rates; the only factor predictive of recurrence was intraoperatively recognized gross tumor spillage or pathologically confirmed surgical tumor puncture.[22] Witt compared results of partial superficial parotidectomy for PA using either 1- or 2-cm margins and reported no difference in outcomes or complication rates, while noting the fact that the effective margin of resection in a nerve-sparing approach is dictated not by the surgeon's planned width of

normal tissue cuff, but rather by the distance between the capsular plane and the most proximal facial nerve branch. Their group stressed that close abutment of the capsule to a facial nerve branch is a nearly ubiquitous finding in PA excisions.[23] In a review of 100 consecutive cases of superficial parotidectomy for PA, Donovan and Conley found that a significant margin of parotid tissue between the PA capsule and the facial nerve could not be achieved in more than 60% of cases. They argue that the achievement of "en bloc resection of parotid tumors" using superficial parotidectomy is an "illusion" in the majority of cases.[24] In a series of 162 parotid resections, Hancock highlighted the potential advantage of extracapsular dissection in decreasing the risk of gustatory sweating or Frey syndrome because of postoperative sympathetic–parasympathetic cross-innervation, with a reported rate of 25% prevalence following superficial parotidectomy as compared with 0% after extracapsular dissection.[25] Smith and Komisar reported no instances of capsular rupture, temporary or permanent paresis, or development of Frey syndrome in a series of 27 patients undergoing extracapsular dissection of parotid neoplasms.[26] McGurk et al reported significantly decreased rates of complications including transient facial nerve palsy, Frey syndrome, and neuroma when extracapsular dissection methods were employed for "simple" parotid masses; they advocated that the decision to employ an extracapsular dissection or superficial parotidectomy should be made intraoperatively following elevation of the skin flap based on the following characteristics: apparent tumor size, fixation, palpable nodal involvement, or palpable deep lobe extension.[27] **Table 22.2** provides an overview of the different surgical techniques employed for excision of parotid masses.

Benign Epithelial Tumors—Types

Pleomorphic Adenoma

PAs represent the most common benign neoplasm of the salivary glands. Overall, PAs account for more than 50% of all salivary neoplasms and more than 70% of parotid masses.[28] Although the role of risk factors in the development of salivary PAs has yet to be elucidated, PAs do exhibit a female predominance and bimodal age distribution.[29] The morphology of PAs is complex and highly variable, making accurate cytologic or histopathologic diagnosis occasionally difficult. Also known as *benign mixed tumors* because of their diverse morphology, PAs feature luminal differentiation and the presence of epithelial, myoepithelial, and stromal components in varying proportions. The morphologic plasticity demonstrated by PAs stems largely from the proliferative differentiation of salivary myoepithelial cells.[30] An additional histologic feature of PAs is envelopment by a false capsule, which develops as the result of a fibrotic reaction by the surrounding salivary parenchyma.[31] While PAs often appear to be grossly encapsulated, histologically

Table 22.2 Surgical Techniques for Excision of Parotid Masses

Surgical Technique	Plane of Dissection	Extent of Dissection	Approach to Facial Nerve	Comments
Enucleation	Intracapsular	Intracapsular contents	No CN VII identification	Not appropriate for most salivary masses High risk of recurrence
Extracapsular dissection	Extracapsular	Salivary gland tumor only	No attempt at CN VII identification Dissection and identification of CN VII branches only if they directly abut extracapsular plane	Technically more difficult May yield lower rate of complications in resection of benign lesions (controversial) Not appropriate for malignant neoplasms
Partial superficial parotidectomy	Intraglandular	Salivary gland tumor plus 1 or 2 cm margin Includes cuff of normal tissue	Segmental approach to CN VII identification and dissection Deliberate identification and complete dissection of CN VII elements associated with major segmental branch underlying superficial tumor mass	Specified margins may not be technically achievable Effective margin dependent on distance between capsular plane and nearest CN VII branch
Superficial parotidectomy	Intra/extraglandular	Superficial lobe (ideally includes all parotid tissue lateral to the plane of the facial nerve)	Directed identification and superficial dissection of all CN VII branches	Requires extensive nerve dissection High rate of postoperative Frey syndrome
Total parotidectomy	Intra/extraglandular	Entire parotid gland	Identification of all CN VII segments with dissection performed across lateral plane of facial nerve	Required for most malignant lesions Higher risk of permanent CN VII injury

CN, cranial nerve.

they feature areas of capsular disruption and small excrescences, often referred to as *pseudopodia*, the presence of which is related to the propensity for PAs to recur following surgical excision.[32] The cytopathologic hallmark of PA is a mixture of bland epithelial cells and chondromyxoid stroma with spindle features, but the relative predominance of epithelial versus mesenchymal matrix varies widely; the overall diagnostic accuracy of FNA for benign PA is 90%.[33]

Imaging characteristics of PAs have been summarized by Kakimoto et al. On MRI, PAs tend to feature well-defined margins, lobulated borders, inhomogeneity, and intermediate-high signal intensity with high enhancement. Lobulation of borders was a consistent feature of parotid PAs, but was typically not observed in PAs arising from submandibular or minor salivary glands. Although the PA capsule was consistently visualized using MRI, it is detectable on CT imaging in less than 5% of cases.[34] Although no imaging modality can reliably discriminate malignant from benign salivary gland tumors, certain imaging findings are suggestive of a malignant aggressiveness including low T1- and T2-signal intensities and muscular invasion.[35,36] Grayscale or color Doppler US modalities can help distinguish PAs from Warthin tumors preoperatively based on the degree of lobulation, cystic quality, and echogenicity, with Warthin tumors typically featuring anechoic cystic components and PAs having characteristic lobulations and an absence of anechoic cystic elements.[37] The presence of a lobulated contour, which is not observed on radiologic study of other types of benign salivary gland tumors, is the most specific feature of PA on ultrasonography.[38] Diffusion-weighted echo-planar MRI techniques are helpful in differentiation of PAs and myoepithelial adenomas from parotid malignancies and other benign histologic subtypes.[39]

Morphologic distinction of PA from other benign salivary gland tumors can be difficult because of its varying histologic composition and significant morphologic overlap with other benign salivary entities. However, PAs demonstrate consistent expression of the *PLAG1* gene irrespective of other gene rearrangements; *PLAG1* likely plays a fundamental role in PA development and is a specific immunohistochemical marker that can confirm the diagnosis of PA.[40] In addition to *PLAG1* rearrangements, *HMGA2* translocations have also been found to be specific to PAs; thus, the detection of these specific gene rearrangements using either reverse transcriptase polymerase chain reactions or fluorescence in-site hybridization can aid in diagnosis.[41] PAs are also distinct from normal salivary tissue in terms of their microRNA profiles, and the interaction of microRNAs with the 3' *UTR* genes that normally inhibit translation may be a critical factor in PLAG1 dysregulation leading to PA tumorigenesis.[42]

Despite its standard classification and typical behavior as a "benign" neoplasm, PAs do feature a risk of malignant degeneration to carcinoma-ex pleomorphic adenoma (Ca-ex PA). Moreover, in a small set of subset of patients, PAs may feature metastatic potential in the absence of histopathologic or cytologic markers of malignancy. The actual rate of malignant degeneration of PAs is unknown, with a reported overall rate of 6.2%.[43] The likelihood of malignant degeneration is correlated to increasing duration of tumor presence, with rates of transformation to Ca-ex PA increasing from 1.6% in tumors present for less than 5 years to 9.6% among patients with PAs for more than 15 years.[44] The precise mechanism of malignant transformation has yet to be elaborated, but recent work has begun to elucidate the factors involved and holds the potential for the future development of molecular diagnostic and treatment modalities targeting progression to Ca-ex PA. Although focal capsular invasion or capsule absence has been implicated in the tendency of PAs to recur, such histologic features do not correlate with propensity for malignant degeneration. Transformation to Ca-ex PA involves overexpression of the p16 tumor suppressor protein in the cytoplasm with corresponding decreased nuclear and p16 promoter methylation.[45] Quantitative promoter methylation of *RASSF1* is a statistically significant epigenetic biomarker of malignant evolution of PAs.[46] The influence of fibroblast growth factor receptor 2 on myoepithelial cells has been linked to neoplastic progression of PAs to carcinoma.[47] The Wilms tumor 1 gene protein is also a reliable and specific marker for myoepithelial neoplasticity in PAs.[48] Additional events implicated in malignant transformation of PAs include overexpression of CDK4, HMGA2, and MDM2.[49,50] In addition to frank malignant transformation, PAs may also feature metastatic potential in the absence of histologic characteristics of malignancy. The histologic and molecular factors associated with nonmalignant metastatic PA are unknown, but this "submalignant" metastatic potential may be associated with a propensity for early vascular invasion in the setting of perlecan myxoid stroma facilitating hematogenous spread.[51,52]

Warthin Tumor

Warthin tumor is the second most common salivary gland neoplasm, representing approximately 4 to 11% of all salivary gland tumors.[53] It is also known as *papillary cystadenoma lymphomatosum* or *adenolymphoma*, and it occurs almost exclusively in the parotid gland. Patients tend to present in their sixth decade of life. A strong association with cigarette smoking has been demonstrated. Men have traditionally been affected more than women; however, recently the male-to-female ratio has decreased, possibly because of the increasing incidence of smoking in women.[54,55] Bilateral involvement occurs in 10% of cases and may either be synchronous or metachronous in nature.[56] Patients frequently present with an asymptomatic mass, but pain, swelling, and inflammatory changes can acutely manifest.

Grossly, Warthin tumors are encapsulated and have a smooth or lobulated surface. Sectioning reveals papillary cystic spaces with white nodules of lymphoid tissue occasionally visible on the cyst walls. Microscopically, Warthin tumor is characterized by bilayered oncocytic epithelial cells arranged as papillary projections lining cystic spaces. A defining feature is the presence of a prominent lymphoid stroma. The lymphoid component is polyclonal in nature, consisting of predominantly T lymphocytes with a smaller number of B lymphocytes. Follicles with germinal centers are also present. The pathogenesis is controversial; however, it is generally thought that the epithelial component of the tumor represents the neoplastic proliferation of salivary ducts that have been entrapped during the course of embryologic development.[57]

Imaging can be a useful adjunct in the preoperative work-up of suspected Warthin tumor, but no investigation is mandated. With US examination, these tumors appear rounded or lobulated and may demonstrate cystic change.[58] MRI and CT may both be used to define the tumor extent, although MRI is superior in differentiating soft tissue planes. On MRI, the cystic foci appear hyperintense on T2 weighting and the lesion does not enhance following injection of intravenous contrast.[59] Warthin tumor, as well as oncocytomas, demonstrate increased technetium-99m uptake, while most other salivary neoplasms are cold or show normal uptake.[60]

The recurrence rates reported in the literature ranges from 1 to 12%,[55,61,62] with superficial parotidectomy being the most common surgical approach. Incomplete excision and multicentricity have been identified as predictors of recurrence.[63] However, in some cases recurrent tumors simply represent residual multicentric foci of tumor. The role of radiation therapy in the treatment of salivary gland PAs is limited, but such treatment may be useful in the following circumstances: positive margin status at surgical resection, unresectability of primary tumor, or multifocal recurrence following surgical extirpation.[64]

Basal Cell Adenoma

Basal cell adenomas are benign salivary gland epithelial neoplasms accounting for roughly 1 to 2% of all salivary gland tumors.[65] These tumors are rarely found in minor salivary glands, with the majority occurring within the parotid gland. Clinically, basal cell adenomas present as firm, mobile, asymptomatic masses that slowly increase in size over a period of several months or years.

The excised tumors are solid and well-demarcated. Grossly, the cut surface is grayish-white to yellow-brown and frequently resembles an enlarged lymph node. Tumors found in the parotid gland often are encapsulated, whereas those originating from minor glands are not. Histologically, basal cell adenomas are composed of isomorphic basaloid cells and interlaced trabeculae with a well-defined, prominent basement membrane. These neoplasms can be subdivided according to their histopathological features into the following categories: solid, trabecular, tubular, or membranous. The solid pattern predominates, although individual tumors commonly display a combination of the previously mentioned growth patterns.[65]

Discrimination of basal cell adenoma from other salivary tumors, particularly PA, basal cell adenocarcinoma, and adenoid cystic carcinoma (ACC), can be difficult. An intact basement membrane and lack of a chondromyxoid stromal component help distinguish basal cell adenoma from PA. In addition, basal cell adenomas show uniform cellular arrangement without the loss of polarity typically observed in PAs.[66] The histologic features that are helpful in identifying malignant basal cell adenocarcinoma include cellular atypia, mitotic figures, perineural or vascular invasion, and a microinvasive growth pattern. Similarly, ACCs demonstrate cellular atypia, mitotic figures, perineural or vascular invasion, necrosis, and a finger-like matrix material while basal call adenomas lack these features.[67,68]

Oncocytoma

Oncocytomas, also known as oncocytic adenoma or oxyphilic adenoma, are uncommon, benign tumors that occur preferentially in the parotid gland and less frequently in the submandibular gland. Minor salivary gland oncocytoma is rare, accounting for less than 1% of all salivary gland tumors.[69] Most affected patients are older than 50 years, with a peak incidence reported between 60 and 80 years of age. No gender predilection for oncocytomas has been demonstrated.[70] These tumors usually appears as a painless, slow-growing mass in the affected gland.

Oncocytomas are well-circumscribed, encapsulated, firm nodules that rarely exceed 5 cm in size.[71] The cut surface has a tan-brown color and is usually solid in appearance; however, some tumors show areas of cyst formation. Parotid oncocytomas selectively incorporate technetium-99m pertechnetate and appear as hot spots on radionucleotide imaging.[72] The tumor is microscopically characterized by metabolically transformed large epithelial cells with vesicular nuclei and innumerable mitochondria. The abundant mitochondria result in a deeply eosinophilic, finely granular cytoplasm.[69] The oncocytic cells are arranged in solid nests of sheets.[71,73] Diagnosis can be challenging as other salivary gland tumors have the potential to undergo oncocytic metaplasia and mimic oncocytomas.

Cystadenoma

Cystadenomas are rare, benign epithelial neoplasms that occur predominantly in the minor salivary glands. The lip is the most commonly involved site, but cystadenomas can also develop in the minor salivary glands of the buccal mucosa, tongue, and palate.[74-76] Cystadenomas are classified into papillary and mucous subtypes, with the former being the most common.[77]

On pathologic examination, the tumors appear as smooth nodules that are well-circumscribed, or even encapsulated, by a rim of fibrous tissue.[74] Histologically, these lesions are characterized by unicystic or multicystic growth. The papillary subtype demonstrates intraluminal papillary projections lined by cuboidal to columnar cells with limited solid areas. Neoplastic proliferation with variable differentiation is noted in the epithelial layer lining the cysts. This tumor demonstrates microscopic similarities to Warthin tumor; however, papillary cystadenoma lacks the lymphocytic stroma and conspicuous lymphoid follicles observed in Warthin tumor.[75]

Canalicular Adenoma

Canalicular adenomas are rare neoplasms that occur almost exclusively in the intraoral minor salivary glands. These tumors demonstrate a predilection for the upper lip and are the second most frequent benign salivary gland tumor at this site, followed by PA. Roughly 70% of tumors can be localized to the upper lip, with the buccal mucosa and palate representing the other anatomic sites most frequently involved.[78,79] This tumor is usually present in older adults and demonstrates a slight female predominance.[77] It manifests similarly to other benign salivary neoplasms as a slow-growing, asymptomatic submucosal mass.

This lesion is usually well-circumscribed, but may appear unencapsulated if the tumor violates its capsule. The overlying mucosa is typically healthy, though ulceration has been reported.[80,81] On microscopic examination, canalicular adenomas consist of columnar epithelial cells that form branching, interconnecting cords of single- or double-cell layers. The stroma is loose, poorly collagenized, and highly vascular.[82]

Unlike most other salivary gland tumors, canalicular adenoma can be multifocal in nature. Multifocality can manifest clinically as distinct lesions or microscopically as foci of tumor cells with intervening, normal-appearing salivary gland tissue. Multifocal lesions have been reported to occur in approximately 20% of cases.[77] Despite the fact that this tumor can be characterized by multicentric foci of tumor cells, the recurrence rate remains low and the prognosis is excellent with complete surgical excision.[79] The multifocality of these tumors should not be misinterpreted as invasive carcinoma. Recurrent tumors may represent growth of residual microscopic islands of disease after removal of clinically evident masses.[83] For this reason, clinicians should consider prolonged postoperative follow-up for patients who have undergone resection of canalicular adenoma, particularly those who initially present with multiple lesions.

Myoepithelioma

Myoepitheliomas are rare, benign salivary gland neoplasms, accounting for less than 1% of all salivary gland tumors.[84] These tumors develop predominantly in the major salivary glands and less often in the minor salivary glands of the oral cavity. Patients suffering from benign myoepithelioma usually present with a painless mass of long duration. Those affected are typically older adults, with both sexes being equally represented.[85]

These tumors have a smooth external surface and are typically well-demarcated from surrounding tissue. Histologically, the tumor cells show wide morphologic variation and are composed of spindle, plasmacytoid, epithelioid, and clear cells exhibiting myoepithelial differentiation. The cell type does not appear to have any influence on biologic behavior patterns; however, it has been suggested that the clear-cell type should be regarded as potentially malignant.[84,86] Immunohistochemistry can be helpful in identifying tumors of myoepithelial origin. Vimentin and S-100 are sensitive but nonspecific markers for myoepithelial tumors. α-SMA or calponin plus vimentin represent the optimal staining protocol, as neoplastic myoepithelial cells are rarely fully differentiated.[87]

Differentiation of benign from malignant salivary gland myoepithelial tumors may be challenging. Malignant myoepitheliomas, also known as myoepithelial carcinomas, exhibit extensive local growth and infiltration of adjacent tissues. In contrast, benign myoepitheliomas are typically well-circumscribed and encapsulated. Further, cellular atypia, necrosis, and high counts of mitotic figures are histologic features suggestive of malignancy.[88] Malignant transformation is rare.[84]

Ductal Papilloma

Ductal papillomas are rare, benign tumors that predominantly occur in the minor salivary glands. Clinically, these tumors present as raised, submucosal masses most frequently localized to the lip and buccal mucosa.[89] While papillary characteristics can be a histologic feature of several other tumors of excretory duct origin, papillary growth of the ductal epithelium is the primary component of ductal papillomas. According to cell type, morphology, and location this tumor can be subdivided as follows: sialadenoma papilliferum, inverted papilloma, and intraductal papilloma.[90]

Lymphadenoma

Lymphadenomas are uncommon salivary epithelial tumors. The majority of these tumors originate in the major salivary glands. Adults above the age of 50 years are most commonly affected and typically present with an asymptomatic mass that has been present for a prolonged period with slow enlargement. Grossly, lymphadenomas tend to be well-circumscribed and encapsulated. On pathologic sectioning, they are homogenous and grossly cystic, with a gray-tan to yellow cut surface. While sebaceous glands do arise from intralobular ducts in normal salivary tissue, neoplastic proliferation is rare. Histologically, these tumors are usually characterized by an epithelial component with sebaceous differentiation and prominent, reactive lymphoid proliferation. The lymphocytic infiltrate is a defining feature composed of mixed T and B lymphocytes. Germinal centers may or may not be present in the lymphoid stroma.[91] Occasionally, tumors may lack epithelial sebaceous differentiation.[92,93] Interestingly, this subtype demonstrates a female predominance whereas tumors with sebaceous differentiation more commonly affect men. This may be attributed to the higher number of sebaceous glands associated with facial hair in men. Malignant transformation is rare but has been reported to occur in the epithelial component.[91]

Sebaceous Adenoma

Sebaceous adenomas are benign epithelial tumors that comprise roughly 0.1% of all salivary gland tumors.[94] Sebaceous adenomas are most common in adult males and preferentially affect the parotid gland.[95] Rarely, sebaceous adenoma originates from a minor salivary gland. As with most other benign salivary gland tumors, patients frequently note a slow-growing mass in the affected gland.

Sebaceous adenomas are typically well-circumscribed and sharply demarcated from surrounding, normal tissue. They can be either solid or cystic.[96] On microscopic examination, cells demonstrating sebaceous differentiation without atypia are arranged in nests forming acinar and duct-like structures with intervening fibrous stroma. Areas of squamous differentiation with minimal atypia and pleomorphism are often present.[97,98]

Oncocytic metaplasia has been reported, although the etiology is unclear.[98,99] Lipani et al proposed the following criteria for establishing the diagnosis of sebaceous adenoma: (1) a well-circumscribed tumor with organoid pattern, (2) differentiated sebaceous lobules demonstrating irregularity of size and shape, (3) lobules containing varying proportions of both mature sebaceous cells and small germinal cells that may be arranged in an irregular pattern, and (4) lack of dilated excretory ducts or a common excretory duct.[100]

Salivary Gland Cancer

Salivary gland cancers are relatively rare, accounting for only 20% of salivary gland tumors and 5% of head and neck malignancies.[1] The incidence rate is estimated to be three new cases per 100,000 people per year worldwide, with an average of 2500 new cases per year in the United States. The parotid gland is the most common site for salivary gland cancer; however, only 20 to 25% of parotid tumors are malignant compared with 40% of submandibular tumors, 50% of minor salivary gland tumors, and 90% of sublingual tumors.[101] Salivary gland cancer comprises the most heterogeneous group of cancers in the body, with up to 24 different cancer subtypes occurring within the glands.

The relative rarity and significant diversity of these cancers prevent broad application of standardized therapy; therefore, it requires multidisciplinary cooperation and decision making to individualize the best course of care for a given patient. Vander Poorten et al have developed a prognostic index for salivary gland malignancy based on a Cox regression analysis model; the most important predictive factors for malignancy are facial nerve paralysis (coefficient = 0.91), facial pain (0.62), and skin involvement (0.63) followed by T stage (0.44) and nodal involvement (0.45).[102] Overall, the most powerful determinant of survival across histologic subtypes is regional lymph node metastasis.[103] Rates of distant metastasis for salivary gland malignancies are quite high as compared with other types of head and neck cancer, varying from 20 to 50% based on histologic subtype and gland of origin.[104] Distant metastases are the most common cause of death in patients with salivary gland malignancies, most commonly occurring in the lungs (80%), bone (15%), and liver and others sites (5%).[105]

The risk of locoregional and distal recurrences of salivary gland cancer ranges from 15 to 80% at 5 years but is strongly influenced by the underlying tumor type and stage. Patients with recurrent salivary gland cancer can be successfully salvaged for cure with aggressive multimodality therapy in many cases or effectively palliated to improve locoregional control and provide symptomatic relief in the event of distant disease. A key feature distinguishing salivary gland malignancies from other malignant tumors of the head and neck is their propensity for late (more than 5-year posttreatment) recurrence, with more than 20% of patients experiencing late recurrence and the majority of those subsequently succumbing to their disease. This phenomenon is most commonly referenced in the context of ACC; however, a recent study demonstrated no statistically significant correlation between late salivary gland tumor recurrence and malignant subtype.[106] Because of the high risk of late recurrence, salivary gland malignancies necessitate lifelong follow-up by a head and neck surgeon. The appropriate role of chemotherapy and biologic agents for salivary gland cancers has yet to be comprehensively delineated. **Table 22.3** summarizes the management of primary salivary gland malignancies.

Surgical Management of Salivary Gland Cancer

Complete surgical excision with negative margins and without tumor spillage continues to be the primary therapy of choice for all salivary gland tumors. The likely extent of surgery can often be determined preoperatively if the tumor is classified as malignant by FNA and staged with physical examination and appropriate imaging. If preoperative FNA is indeterminate or benign, the surgeon should plan to fully excise the mass with a negative margin but be prepared to extend the surgery based on intraoperative findings. Findings such as nerve encasement, extensive soft tissue invasion, or adenopathy should alert the surgeon to the possibility of malignancy. Frozen section analysis of the mass can be done if there is no risk of spillage to help determine if nerve sacrifice and/or neck dissection is indicated.

The need for adjuvant therapy is largely dependent on the final pathology of the surgical specimen. Pathologic findings that suggest the need for adjuvant therapy include:

- Tumor grade: intermediate (mucoepidermoid carcinoma [MEC], ACC, Ca-ex PA) or high-grade (salivary duct carcinoma, adenocarcinoma) tumors that are T1 or greater
- Tumor size: T3 or greater for any grade tumor
- Extraparenchymal extension
- Neural/perineural invasion
- Multicentric tumor
- Lymph node metastasis
- Lymphovascular invasion
- Close (less than or equal to 1 mm) or positive margins

High-Risk Molecular Markers

Given the limited correlation between tumor grade and biologic behavior, a growing body of research has focused on whether molecular tumor markers have prognostic significance. While no salivary tumor marker is frequently used in clinical practice, the following are among the most studied and/or most promising:

1. K_i-67 is a cellular protein that is involved in cellular transcription and has been used as a marker of cell proliferation. It has been shown repeatedly that MECs and ACCs that express a higher level of K_i-67 have a worse 5-year survival, which has been validated in multivariate analysis.[107–109] However, one recent study failed to show that K_i-67 was an independent prognostic indicator in MEC when newer tumor markers, such as MEC translocated 1–mastermind-like 2 (MECT1-MAML2) (see below), were included in the analysis.[110] Various cutoffs for expression have been employed, with 5% expression being the most frequently employed. At this point, K_i-67 staining may be considered a useful tool in the evaluation of the aggressiveness of some salivary gland neoplasms.

2. p53 is a tumor suppressor protein that helps control the cell cycle whose mutation is widely implicated in a variety of human neoplasms. Despite this observation, and the fact that it is the most studied of the salivary gland tumor markers, p53 has not been consistently found to be altered in salivary malignancies, with the p53 staining ratio

Table 22.3 Management of Primary Salivary Gland Malignancies

Risk Category	Surgery		Radiation
Low • Stage T1, N0 (any pathology) • Acinic cell, myoepithelial, epithelial-myoepithelial, low-grade MEC, polymorphous low-grade AC, basal cell AC • Marker negative	Parotid	Partial parotidectomy with VII preservation; level-2 dissection	Not indicated unless • < 1 mm margin • Positive margin without ability to re-resect • Tumor spillage • Perineural spread
	SMG	Gland excision with level Ib dissection	
	Minor	Wide local excision only ± local flap; skin graft	
Moderate • T2 and/or N1 (any pathology) • Intermediate or high-grade MEC, ACC, Ca-ex PA • Marker positive	Parotid	Subtotal versus total parotidectomy sparing VII if possible; selective dissection of levels 1b, 2 a/b, 3; consider level 5 if ear canal or postauricular involvement	≥ 60 Gy to primary and involved neck; ≥ 44 Gy to uninvolved neck basins; Consider concurrent chemotherapy if close or positive margin or tumor spillage
	SMG	Wide gland excision with level 1b (including facial nodes), 2a/b, and 3 dissection	
	Minor	Wide local excision/ composite resection ± local flap, skin graft, free tissue transfer, or obturator	
High • T3/4, N2/3 (any pathology) • Salivary duct carcinoma, AC NOS, undifferentiated carcinoma • Marker positive	Parotid	Total versus radical parotidectomy with selective neck dissection (1b, 2a/b, 3, 5); temporal bone resection; ± facial nerve grafting v. static suspension; ± free tissue transfer	Consider concurrent chemoradiation therapy using platin-based regimen
	SMG	Wide gland excision with level 1b (including facial nodes), 2a/b, and 3 dissection; ± regional versus free tissue flap	
	Minor	Same as above	

SMG, submandibular gland; MEC, mucoepidermoid carcinoma; AC, adenocarcinoma; ACC, adenoid cystic carcinoma; Ca-ex PA, carcinoma-ex pleomorphic adenoma; AC NOS, adenocarcinoma not otherwise specified.

varying greatly among studies. Although p53 accumulation has been shown in some studies to be an independent prognostic indicator of 5-year survival in MEC, several other studies have been unable to corroborate this finding.[110–113] There have been similar incongruent findings in ACC and Ca-ex PA. At this point, there is no role for the use of p53 in the prognosis of salivary gland neoplasms.

3. Epidermal growth factor receptor (EGFR); EGF is expressed in the salivary gland where it plays a vital role in the normal development and differentiation of the acini and ductals. This is of interest because of the availability of an anti-EGFR antibody therapy (cetuximab) that could be employed against these tumors. The expression of EGFR in salivary gland cancer varies by histopathology with salivary duct carcinoma demonstrating the highest rate of expression (92%), followed by ACC (25 to 85%), and then MEC (25%). However, the prognostic significance of EGFR expression in salivary gland cancer has not been elucidated.[101]

4. HER2, also known as erbB2, is a member of the same transmembrane tyrosine kinase receptor family as EGFR. HER2 expression has been examined in salivary duct carcinoma, which histologically resembles breast carcinoma and frequently expresses HER2. However, only 17 of 66 (26%) tumors tested displayed significant HER2 expression.[114] The clinical implications of this expression have yet to be established.

5. MECT1-MAML2, also called CRTC1-MAML2, is a fusion gene that is specific to MECs and is thought to be associated with an improved prognosis. It has been found to be expressed on 38 to 60% of MECs, and its expression in MEC tumors has been shown to be an independent positive prognostic indicator, showing generally less aggressive behavior and better overall survival.[110,115–117] Additional studies have found that this tumor fusion gene is generally expressed in low- and intermediate-grade MECs but can be found expressed on high grade as well. Even within the histologically high-grade group, the expression of this

fusion gene creates a less aggressive tumor.[115] However, improved long-term survival in prospective studies has thus far not been corroborated; while this is a promising tumor marker, its use cannot yet be advocated in clinical practice.

6. p27 is a protein involved in the regulation of the cell cycle whose decreased expression has been shown to be an independent negative prognostic factor in overall and disease-free survival in MEC, which has thus far been corroborated in a few small studies.[110,118]

Radiation Therapy

Adjuvant radiation therapy is indicated for intermediate to high-risk disease.[1,101] In a meta-analysis of 19 studies of postoperative radiotherapy for salivary gland cancer, patients with advanced T3/4 disease, node positive disease, or high-grade histopathology demonstrated a threefold reduction in the odds of death compared with patients who did not receive radiation.[1] The standard and most widely available form is photon or photon/electron based radiotherapy delivered to a total dose more than or equal to 60 Gy (1.8 to 2.0 Gy/fraction) with an additional 44 to 64 Gy (1.6 to 2.0 Gy/fraction) to uninvolved nodal groups. Intensity-modulated radiotherapy has allowed sparing of critical structures within the field such as the spinal cord, inner ear, and adjacent salivary tissue.[119] Radiotherapy or concurrent chemoradiotherapy may be used as primary therapy in select cases that are deemed to be surgically unresectable because of advanced stage (T4b), significant medical comorbidities, or patient refusal to undergo surgical resection. Adjuvant radiotherapy can successfully control disease in cases where the postoperative pathology reveals close or microscopically positive margins preventing the need for immediate re-resection.[120] Re-resection should be considered if gross tumor remains in the field. Grade 3 radiotherapy-related acute toxicity of the skin and mucosa occur in 25% of patients, but late toxicity of the skin and soft tissues are rarely observed.[121] Neutron beam radiotherapy has demonstrated improved locoregional control over photon therapy for high-grade tumors in both randomized and nonrandomized series; however, no long-term survival advantage was observed in the neutron cohorts because of the high rate of distant metastasis in these patients.[1] In addition, neutron therapy is expensive, not widely available, and significantly more toxic to surrounding tissues, resulting in greater risk of complications when compared with photon and photon/electron-based radiotherapy.[119]

Chemotherapy

Chemotherapy as a single modality is generally ineffective in the treatment of salivary gland cancer.[122] As a result, chemotherapy is not indicated as an adjuvant therapy for salivary gland cancer except in select circumstances.

However, in a retrospective series of 255 patients with major salivary gland malignancy, 57 patients (22%) developed distant metastasis underscoring the need for better systemic therapy to address this problem.[123] The lungs were the most common metastatic site (65%) and ACC the most frequent histological type involved.[123] Determination of chemotherapy efficacy with clinical trials has been challenging because of the low incidence of salivary gland cancers, their diverse histopathology, and the lack of routine analysis of molecular markers. Chemotherapy is sometimes given concurrently with adjuvant radiotherapy in select high-grade tumors such as salivary duct carcinoma, high-grade adenocarcinoma, and solid-type ACC because of the higher than average risk of distant metastatic spread. Other indications for concurrent chemoradiotherapy include close or positive margins and/or tumor spillage of an intermediate or high-risk tumor, unresectable stage T4b disease, patient comorbidity preventing surgical resection, or patient refusal to undergo surgery. Cisplatin is first-line therapy when considering adjuvant chemoradiation therapy because it is the most extensively studied chemotherapy demonstrating effect across a broad range of salivary tumor types and is known to augment the local effect of radiation therapy.[101]

Salivary Gland Cancer—Types

Although a wide range of malignant salivary gland tumors exist, only five types are likely to be encountered in routine practice: MEC, ACC, Ca-ex PA, acinic cell carcinoma (AcCC), and polymorphous low-grade carcinoma.[124]

Mucoepidermoid Carcinomas

MEC is the most common subtype of salivary gland malignancy in both pediatric and adult patients. Typical presentation involves an asymptomatic, slow-growing mass. Intraoral MECs tend to feature a blue hue because of the presence of intracystic mucin. Histologically, MEC is composed of a combination of epithelial and mucin type cells in varying proportions. Prognosis for MEC varies considerably depending on both clinical and histopathologic staging. Although no universally accepted histopathologic staging system has been established, MEC tumors are generally classified as low-, intermediate-, or high-grade based on the relative predominance of mucous, intermediate, and squamous or epidermoid elements. Based primarily on the ratio of mucin to epithelial constituent cells, various histologic grading systems incorporate additional criteria including mitotic rate, perineural invasion, and anaplasia. To a greater degree than in any other salivary tumor subtype, histologic grading in MEC has direct prognostic implications. The 5-year survival exceeds 92% for low-grade MEC tumors, falling to 62 to 92% for intermediate-grade, and less than 43% for high-grade tumors.[44] In addition to histologic grade, decreased 5-year survival rates in MEC have been linked to the following clinical factors: (1) age above 40 years, (2) T stage T3 or greater, and (3) lymph node metastases.[125]

Treatment strategies for MEC vary in accordance with histologic grade. Conservative excision is generally considered sufficient for low-grade MECs, while high-grade tumors require more comprehensive treatment including possible selective neck dissection and adjuvant radiation therapy. Significant controversy exists with respect to the optimal management of intermediate-grade MEC, in part because of discrepancies in the major histopathologic grading systems.[126] Application of the two most commonly used grading indices, the Armed Forces Institute of Pathology (AFIP) and the Brandwein systems, frequently yields discordant results when applied to "intermediate" stage tumors, with the AFIP system tending to "downgrade" and the Brandwein system tending to "upgrade" grading of such tumors in a manner that has complicated classification of such lesions.[127] In terms of biomarkers, MECT-1-MAML2 expression has been demonstrated as inversely correlated with MEC aggressiveness, although survival implications remain unclear. Expression of the *MUC 19* gene has recently been described as a biomarker for MEC, and quantitative assessment of MUC 4 shows promise as a prognostic tool.[128] Aggressiveness of high-grade MEC is correlated with *EGFR* gene copy and pERK1/2 expression, suggesting a possible role for EGFR antagonists or MAPK pathway inhibitors as adjuvant therapies.[129]

Adenoid Cystic Carcinoma

ACC is a relatively common malignant salivary gland tumor, representing roughly 6% of all salivary gland neoplasms.[130] This tumor is highly invasive and is characterized by an infiltrative growth pattern, tendency for perineural invasion, and high recurrence rate. It is notoriously slow growing; thus, patients often suffer from a protracted, relentless course and may survive for years even in the presence of distant metastases. Patients typically present with a firm salivary gland tumors that has been present for years, and they may endorse pain characterized as a dull ache. The palate is the most commonly implicated intraoral site; however, involvement of the floor of mouth, tongue, and gingiva has also been reported.[131] The tumor has a peak incidence in the fifth and sixth decades of life and no clear sex predilection has been demonstrated.

Macroscopically, these lesions are firm, well-circumscribed, and tend to be either partially encapsulated or nonencapsulated. Microscopically, they are divided into three recognized morphologic patterns: tubular, cribiform, and solid. The cribiform pattern is the most recognizable pattern and characterized by basaloid epithelial cells that surround gland-like spaces. These central spaces consist of duplicated basement membrane and myxoid material, presumably produced by the tumor. The epithelial cells themselves are small and fairly uniform with deeply basophilic nuclei; mitotic activity is rarely seen.[132] ACC has a marked propensity for perineural invasion, which is reported to occur in approximately 75% of cases. Perineural

invasion can extend both centrally up through the skull base and peripherally. Nerve involvement can be particularly advanced at the time of surgical excision given that the tumor's slow growth often delays diagnosis. While spread to regional lymphatics is rare, the incidence of distant metastases is high, particularly to the lungs.

Szanto et al described a tumor-grading system taking into account both the predominant histologic pattern and percentage of solid component. This grading system can provide the treating clinician with useful prognostic information.[133,134] Grade 1 ACCs are well-differentiated and composed of tubular patterns, with or without cribiform patterns, and no solid component. Grade 2 ACCs consist of cribiform or mixed patterns, with less than 30% solid areas. Lastly, grade 3 ACCs display cribiform morphology with greater than 30% solid areas.[133] In addition to histopathologic grade, advanced clinical stage, positive surgical margins, and perineural invasion are considered poor prognostic factors in ACC.[135,136]

Acinic Cell Carcinoma

AcCC is a rare subtype of salivary gland malignancy, representing less than 5% of all salivary gland lesions. Initially discovered in the 1870s, the malignant and metastatic potential of AcCC was not recognized until the 1950s. Predominantly occurring in the parotid gland (80 to 90%) followed by the minor salivary glands, AcCC is also the salivary malignancy subtype most likely to involve bilateral lesions. AcCC typically presents as an indolent, solitary mass, with associated facial pain or tenderness present in up to 50% of cases.[137] Although generally considered to be a low-grade carcinoma, AcCC in fact demonstrates highly variable biological activity and poorly understood patterns of recurrence and metastasis.[138] A key factor distinguishing AcCC from other salivary malignancies is age of onset. Data from the Surveillance, Epidemiology, and End Results panel indicate that the median age for diagnosis of malignant AcCC is 50 years for males and 48 years for females as compared with above 72 years of age for other salivary gland carcinomas.[139] Overall, prognosis for AcCC is favorable as compared with other subtypes of salivary malignancy.[140] However, AcCC does feature a substantial rate of metastasis and late recurrence along with occasional high-grade transformation, with up to 25% of patients eventually succumbing to their disease.[141] Although specific histologic factors have been identified that correlate with adverse outcome, no formal grading system has been developed to guide the surgeon in clinical decision making.

Grossly, AcCC specimens typically involve a circumscribed nodular mass. Encapsulation is incomplete at the microscopic level and focal invasion is ubiquitous. Histologic characteristics include serous acinar differentiation, polygonal borders, eccentric nuclei with orientation toward the secretory lumen, and basophilic zymogene secretory granules. Despite the predominance of serous acinar cells, AcCC may incorporate a wide range of different cells types, complicating cytologic diagnosis; this diversity is thought to recapitulate the differentiation of pluripotent reserve cells to serious acinar morphology, and AcCC neoplasia appears to derive from pluripotent stems cells of the intercalated ducts.[142] AcCC can be definitively diagnosed based on the following constellation of cytopathologic features: (1) characteristic combination of solid, follicular, microcystic, and/or papillary-cystic elements, (2) zymogene granules on periodic acid-Schiff stain, and (3) negative p63 immunostain.[143]

Carcinoma-ex Pleomorphic Adenoma

Ca-ex PA is a malignant epithelial neoplasm that arises from a PA. The rate and mechanism of malignant degeneration of PA are discussed earlier in this chapter. Ca-ex PA is relatively uncommon despite being the most frequently encountered type of mixed malignant tumor. These tumors most frequently manifest in the major salivary glands, with the majority of cases noted in the parotid gland. They can also occur in the minor salivary glands of the oral cavity and tend to be smaller at these sites. Patients classically present with a long-standing history of a salivary gland gland that undergoes sudden, rapid growth. Pain may result from local extension into adjacent tissue. Ca-ex PA demonstrates a predilection for the female sex and occurs in patients who are, on average, 12 years older than patients with PA.[144,145]

Macroscopically, the tumor appearance depends on the relative presence of adenoma and carcinoma components. If the malignant component is dominant, the tumor will be tan-yellow, poorly defined, and widely infiltrative. Microscopically, the tumor is composed of both PA and carcinoma. The PA component is characterized by a mixture of epithelial cells and chondromyxoid stroma. The amount of epithelial versus mesenchymal matrix varies widely.[32] The carcinoma component typically consists of collagenous stromal hyalinization. Essentially any type of carcinoma can be found, but poorly differentiated adenocarcinoma and salivary duct carcinoma are most common.[144,145] It is important to keep in mind that the carcinoma component differs between tumors and may be low or high grade. Prognosis and management of Ca-ex PA is therefore greatly dependent on the histologic type and grade of the carcinoma identified.

Based on the extent of invasion of the carcinoma component, Ca-ex PA can be subclassified into the following groups: noninvasive, minimally invasive (less than 1.5 mm beyond the fibrous capsule), and invasive (more than 1.5 mm beyond the fibrous capsule). Cancers that fall into either the noninvasive or minimally invasive categories rarely behave in a malignant fashion.[146] Invasive tumors have been shown to have a poor prognosis with a reported overall 5-year survival of approximately 30%.[147] Tumor size, tumor grade, lymph node involvement, presence of local/distant metastasis, and completeness of tumor resection have also been identified as critical prognostic indicators.[16,43]

Clinical Pearls

- Salivary gland neoplasms, both benign and malignant, most commonly present as asymptomatic, slow-growing masses that increase in size over a period of several months to years. All salivary masses require comprehensive and timely evaluation.

- Imaging can be a useful adjunct in the preoperative workup of salivary gland tumors. Ultrasound is the preferred imaging modality for suspected benign submandibular, sublingual, and superficial parotid tumors. Magnetic resonance imaging with gadolinium is indicated in cases where salivary malignancy is suspected.

- The sensitivity of fine-needle aspiration for detection of salivary gland neoplasia is 90%, and accuracy in discriminating between benign and malignant salivary gland tumors is 80%.

- Exam findings suggestive of malignancy include cranial nerve VII paresis, facial pain, overlying skin changes, size more than 4 cm, and lymphadenopathy.

- Complete surgical excision is recommended for virtually all salivary tumors in suitable patients. In cases of malignancy, additional measures, such as lymphadenectomy or adjuvant radiation therapy, are variably required depending on tumor histology and other clinical features.

- In patients with high-risk tumor features, adjuvant radiation decreases the risk of death from salivary gland malignancy by threefold.

- Salivary glands demonstrate an extremely diverse array of tumor morphologies. Key features of the most important subtypes and treatment recommendations are presented in **Tables 22.1** (benign tumors) and **22.3** (malignant tumors).

Pitfalls

- The indolent growth rate and benign appearance of most salivary gland tumors should not cause delay in timely, appropriate assessment and treatment.

- The morphology of the most common benign salivary gland tumor subtype, pleomorphic adenoma, is highly variable, making cytologic or histopathologic diagnosis challenging.

- Distinguishing benign from malignant salivary gland tumors histologically can be difficult. Cellular atypia, necrosis, and high counts of mitotic figures are features suggestive of malignancy. Collaboration and effective communication with an experienced pathologist is paramount.

- A key feature distinguishing salivary gland malignancies from other head and neck cancers is a propensity for late recurrence.

- More than 20% of patients treated for malignant salivary gland tumors will experience recurrence at more than 5 years posttreatment. Because of the risk for late recurrence, all patients treated for salivary gland malignancy require lifelong follow-up.

- Optimal approaches for benign parotid lesions without deep lobe involvement are controversial and may vary depending on histology. **Table 22.2** presents an overview of surgical techniques.

- No imaging modality can accurately depict the relationship of a parotid tumor to cranial nerve VII, but the lateral border of the retromandibular vein serves as a useful proxy on preoperative imaging.

- In the setting of facial nerve sparing procedures, the effective surgical margin that can be achieved depends in most cases on the proximity of the tumor from the closest cranial nerve VII branch.

References

1. Jeannon JP, Calman F, Gleeson M, et al. Management of advanced parotid cancer. A systematic review. Eur J Surg Oncol 2009;35(9):908–915

2. Lingam RK, Daghir AA, Nigar E, Abbas SA, Kumar M. Pleomorphic adenoma (benign mixed tumour) of the salivary glands: its diverse clinical, radiological, and histopathological presentation. Br J Oral Maxillofac Surg 2011;49(1):14–20

3. Katz P, Hartl DM, Guerre A. Clinical ultrasound of the salivary glands. Otolaryngol Clin North Am 2009;42(6):973–1000 Table of Contents

4. Kraft M, Lang F, Mihaescu A, Wolfensberger M. Evaluation of clinician-operated sonography and fine-needle aspiration in the assessment of salivary gland tumours. Clin Otolaryngol 2008;33(1):18–24

5. Ahuja A, Evans R, Valantis A. Salivary gland cancer. In: Ahuja A, ed. Imaging in Head and Neck Cancer. London: Greenwich Medical; 2003

6. Shah GV. MR imaging of salivary glands. Magn Reson Imaging Clin N Am 2002;10(4):631–662

7. Keyes JW Jr, Harkness BA, Greven KM, Williams DW III, Watson NE Jr, McGuirt WF. Salivary gland tumors: pretherapy evaluation with PET. Radiology 1994;192(1):99–102

8. Viguer JM, Vicandi B, Jiménez-Heffernan JA, López-Ferrer P, González-Peramato P, Castillo C. Role of fine needle aspiration cytology in the diagnosis and management of Warthin's tumour of the salivary glands. Cytopathology 2010;21(3):164–169

9. Zhang S, Bao R, Bagby J, Abreo F. Fine needle aspiration of salivary glands: 5-year experience from a single academic center. Acta Cytol 2009;53(4):375–382

10. McIvor NP, Freeman JL, Salem S, Elden L, Noyek AM, Bedard YC. Ultrasonography and ultrasound-guided fine-needle aspiration biopsy of head and neck lesions: a surgical perspective. Laryngoscope 1994;104(6 Pt 1):669–674

11. Cohen EG, Patel SG, Lin O, et al. Fine-needle aspiration biopsy of salivary gland lesions in a selected patient population. Arch Otolaryngol Head Neck Surg 2004;130(6):773–778

12. Cho HW, Kim J, Choi J, et al. Sonographically guided fine-needle aspiration biopsy of major salivary gland masses: a review of 245 cases. AJR Am J Roentgenol 2011;196(5):1160–1163

13. Brennan PA, Davies B, Poller D, et al. Fine needle aspiration cytology (FNAC) of salivary gland tumours: repeat aspiration provides further information in cases with an unclear initial cytological diagnosis. Br J Oral Maxillofac Surg 2010;48(1):26–29

14. Ashraf A, Shaikh AS, Kamal F, Sarfraz R, Bukhari MH. Diagnostic reliability of FNAC for salivary gland swellings: a comparative study. Diagn Cytopathol 2010;38(7):499–504

15. Christensen RK, Bjørndal K, Godballe C, Krogdahl A. Value of fine-needle aspiration biopsy of salivary gland lesions. Head Neck 2010;32(1):104–108

16. Barnes LEJ, Reichart P, Sidransky D. World Health Organization Classification of Tumors. Lyon: IARC Press; 2005.

17. Patey DH, Thackray AC. The treatment of parotid tumours in the light of a pathological study of parotidectomy material. Br J Surg 1958;45(193):477–487

18. Iizuka K, Ishikawa K. Surgical techniques for benign parotid tumors: segmental resection vs extracapsular lumpectomy. Acta Otolaryngol Suppl 1998;537:75–81

19. Gleave EN, Whittaker JS, Nicholson A. Salivary tumours—experience over thirty years. Clin Otolaryngol Allied Sci 1979;4(4):247–257

20. Lin SD, Tsai CC, Lai CS, Lee SS, Chang KP. Endoscope-assisted parotidectomy for benign parotid tumors. Ann Plast Surg 2000;45(3):269–273

21. Piekarski J, Nejc D, Szymczak W, Wronski K, Jeziorski A. Results of extracapsular dissection of pleomorphic adenoma of parotid gland. J Oral Maxillofac Surg 2004;62(10):1198–1202

22. Riad MA, Abdel-Rahman H, Ezzat WF, Adly A, Dessouky O, Shehata M. Variables related to recurrence of pleomorphic adenomas: outcome of parotid surgery in 182 cases. Laryngoscope 2011;121(7):1467–1472

23. Witt RL. Minimally invasive surgery for parotid pleomorphic adenoma. Ear Nose Throat J 2005;84(308):310–311

24. Donovan DT, Conley JJ. Capsular significance in parotid tumor surgery: reality and myths of lateral lobectomy. Laryngoscope 1984;94(3):324–329

25. Hancock BD. Clinically benign parotid tumours: local dissection as an alternative to superficial parotidectomy in selected cases. Ann R Coll Surg Engl 1999;81(5):299–301

26. Smith SL, Komisar A. Limited parotidectomy: the role of extracapsular dissection in parotid gland neoplasms. Laryngoscope 2007;117(7):1163–1167

27. McGurk M, Thomas BL, Renehan AG. Extracapsular dissection for clinically benign parotid lumps: reduced morbidity without oncological compromise. Br J Cancer 2003;89(9):1610–1613

28. Speight PM, Barrett AW. Salivary gland tumours. Oral Dis 2002;8(5):229–240

29. Farina A, Pelucchi S, Carinci F. Evidence of bimodal distribution of age in patients affected by pleomorphic adenoma of the parotid gland. Oral Oncol 1997;33(4):288–289

30. Norberg L, Stratis M, Dardick I. Quantitation and localization of cycling tumor cells in pleomorphic adenomas and myoepitheliomas: an immunohistochemical analysis. J Oral Pathol Med 1997;26(3):124–128

31. Spiro RH. Salivary neoplasms: overview of a 35-year experience with 2,807 patients. Head Neck Surg 1986;8(3):177–184

32. Polat S, Serin GM, Öztürk O, Üneri C. Pleomorphic adenomas recurrences within the parapharyngeal space. J Craniofac Surg 2011;22(3):1124–1128

33. Handa U, Dhingra N, Chopra R, Mohan H. Pleomorphic adenoma: cytologic variations and potential diagnostic pitfalls. Diagn Cytopathol 2009;37(1):11–15

34. Kakimoto N, Gamoh S, Tamaki J, Kishino M, Murakami S, Furukawa S. CT and MR images of pleomorphic adenoma in major and minor salivary glands. Eur J Radiol 2009;69(3):464–472

35. Som PM, Biller HF. High-grade malignancies of the parotid gland: identification with MR imaging. Radiology 1989;173(3):823–826

36. Joe VQ, Westesson PL. Tumors of the parotid gland: MR imaging characteristics of various histologic types. AJR Am J Roentgenol 1994;163(2):433–438

37. Yuan WH, Hsu HC, Chou YH, Hsueh HC, Tseng TK, Tiu CM. Gray-scale and color Doppler ultrasonographic features of pleomorphic adenoma and Warthin's tumor in major salivary glands. Clin Imaging 2009;33(5):348–353

38. Dumitriu D, Dudea SM, Botar-Jid C, Băciuţ G. Ultrasonographic and sonoelastographic features of pleomorphic adenomas of the salivary glands. Med Ultrasound 2010;12(3):175–183

39. Habermann CR, Arndt C, Graessner J, et al. Diffusion-weighted echo-planar MR imaging of primary parotid gland tumors: is a prediction of different histologic subtypes possible? AJNR Am J Neuroradiol 2009;30(3):591–596

40. Matsuyama A, Hisaoka M, Nagao Y, Hashimoto H. Aberrant PLAG1 expression in pleomorphic adenomas of the salivary gland: a molecular genetic and immunohistochemical study. Virchows Arch 2011;458(5):583–592

41. Cheuk W, Chan JK. Advances in salivary gland pathology. Histopathology 2007;51(1):1–20

42. Zhang X, Cairns M, Rose B, et al. Alterations in miRNA processing and expression in pleomorphic adenomas of the salivary gland. Int J Cancer 2009;124(12):2855–2863

43. Gnepp DR. Malignant mixed tumors of the salivary glands: a review. Pathol Annu 1993;28(Pt 1):279–328

44. Ellis GAP. Malignant epithelial tumors. In: Ellis GAP, ed. Atlas of Tumor Pathology. Washington, DC: Armed Forces Institute of Pathology; 1996

45. Hu YH, Zhang CY, Tian Z, Wang LZ, Li J. Aberrant protein expression and promoter methylation of p16 gene are correlated with malignant transformation of salivary pleomorphic adenoma. Arch Pathol Lab Med 2011;135(7):882–889

46. Schache AG, Hall G, Woolgar JA, et al. Quantitative promoter methylation differentiates carcinoma ex pleomorphic adenoma from pleomorphic salivary adenoma. Br J Cancer 2010;103(12):1846–1851

47. Martinez EF, Demasi AP, Miguita L, Altemani A, Araújo NS, Araújo VC. FGF-2 is overexpressed in myoepithelial cells of carcinoma ex-pleomorphic adenoma in situ structures. Oncol Rep 2010;24(1):155–160

48. Langman G, Andrews CL, Weissferdt A. WT1 expression in salivary gland pleomorphic adenomas: a reliable marker of the neoplastic myoepithelium. Mod Pathol 2011;24(2):168–174

49. Rao PH, Murty VV, Louie DC, Chaganti RS. Nonsyntenic amplification of MYC with CDK4 and MDM2 in a malignant mixed tumor of salivary gland. Cancer Genet Cytogenet 1998;105(2):160–163

50. Röijer ENA, Nordkvist A, Ström AK, et al. Translocation, deletion/amplification, and expression of HMGIC and MDM2 in a carcinoma ex pleomorphic adenoma. Am J Pathol 2002;160(2):433–440

51. Maruyama S, Cheng J, Yamazaki M, Liu A, Saku T. Keratinocyte growth factor colocalized with perlecan at the site of capsular invasion and vascular involvement in salivary pleomorphic adenomas. J Oral Pathol Med 2009;38(4):377–385

52. Manucha V, Ioffe OB. Metastasizing pleomorphic adenoma of the salivary gland. Arch Pathol Lab Med 2008;132(9):1445–1447

53. Pinkston JA, Cole P. Incidence rates of salivary gland tumors: results from a population-based study. Otolaryngol Head Neck Surg 1999;120(6):834–840

54. Chapnik JS. The controversy of Warthin's tumor. Laryngoscope 1983;93(6):695–716

55. Yoo GH, Eisele DW, Askin FB, Driben JS, Johns ME. Warthin's tumor: a 40-year experience at The Johns Hopkins Hospital. Laryngoscope 1994;104(7):799–803

56. Teymoortash A, Krasnewicz Y, Werner JA. Clinical features of cystadenolymphoma (Warthin's tumor) of the parotid gland: a retrospective comparative study of 96 cases. Oral Oncol 2006;42(6):569–573

57. Aguirre JM, Echebarría MA, Martínez-Conde R, Rodriguez C, Burgos JJ, Rivera JM. Warthin tumor. A new hypothesis concerning its development. Oral Surg Oral Med Oral Pathol Oral Radiol Endod 1998;85(1):60–63

58. Howlett DC, Kesse KW, Hughes DV, Sallomi DF. The role of imaging in the evaluation of parotid disease. Clin Radiol 2002;57(8):692–701

59. Minami M, Tanioka H, Oyama K, et al. Warthin tumor of the parotid gland: MR-pathologic correlation. AJNR Am J Neuroradiol 1993;14(1):209–214

60. Higashi T, Murahashi H, Ikuta H, Mori Y, Watanabe Y. Identification of Warthin's tumor with technetium-99m pertechnetate. Clin Nucl Med 1987;12(10):796–800

61. Eveson JW, Cawson RA. Warthin's tumor (cystadenolymphoma) of salivary glands. A clinicopathologic investigation of 278 cases. Oral Surg Oral Med Oral Pathol 1986;61(3):256–262

62. Byrne MN, Spector JG. Parotid masses: evaluation, analysis, and current management. Laryngoscope 1988;98(1):99–105

63. Ethunandan M, Pratt CA, Higgins B, et al. Factors influencing the occurrence of multicentric and 'recurrent' Warthin's tumour: a cross sectional study. Int J Oral Maxillofac Surg 2008;37(9):831–834

64. Mendenhall WM, Mendenhall CM, Werning JW, Malyapa RS, Mendenhall NP. Salivary gland pleomorphic adenoma. Am J Clin Oncol 2008;31(1):95–99

65. Takeshita T, Tanaka H, Harasawa A, Kaminaga T, Imamura T, Furui S. CT and MR findings of basal cell adenoma of the parotid gland. Radiat Med 2004;22(4):260–264

66. Elsheikh TM, Bernacki EG. Fine needle aspiration cytology of cellular pleomorphic adenoma. Acta Cytol 1996;40(6):1165–1175

67. Klijanienko J, el-Naggar AK, Vielh P. Comparative cytologic and histologic study of fifteen salivary basal-cell tumors: differential diagnostic considerations. Diagn Cytopathol 1999;21(1):30–34

68. Klijanienko J, Vielh P. Fine-needle sampling of salivary gland lesions. III. Cytologic and histologic correlation of 75 cases of adenoid cystic carcinoma: review and experience at the Institut Curie with emphasis on cytologic pitfalls. Diagn Cytopathol 1997;17(1):36–41

69. Chang A, Harawi SJ. Oncocytes, oncocytosis, and oncocytic tumors. Pathol Annu 1992;27(Pt 1):263–304

70. Brandwein MS, Huvos AG. Oncocytic tumors of major salivary glands. A study of 68 cases with follow-up of 44 patients. Am J Surg Pathol 1991;15(6):514–528

71. Zhou CX, Gao Y. Oncocytoma of the salivary glands: a clinicopathologic and immunohistochemical study. Oral Oncol 2009;45(12):e232–e238

72. Sakai E, Yoda T, Shimamoto H, Hirano Y, Kusama M, Enomoto S. Pathologic and imaging findings of an oncocytoma in the deep lobe of the left parotid gland. Int J Oral Maxillofac Surg 2003;32(5): 563–565

73. Wakely PE Jr. Oncocytic and oncocyte-like lesions of the head and neck. Ann Diagn Pathol 2008;12(3):222–230

74. Tsurumi K, Kamiya H, Yokoi M, Kameyama Y. Papillary oncocytic cystadenoma of palatal minor salivary gland: a case report. J Oral Maxillofac Surg 2003;61(5):631–633

75. Kusafuka K, Ueno T, Kurihara K, et al. Cystadenoma of the palate: immunohistochemistry of mucins. Pathol Int 2008;58(8):524–528

76. Lim CS, Ngu I, Collins AP, McKellar GM. Papillary cystadenoma of a minor salivary gland: report of a case involving cytological analysis and review of the literature. Oral Surg Oral Med Oral Pathol Oral Radiol Endod 2008;105(1):e28–e33

77. Waldron CA, el-Mofty SK, Gnepp DR. Tumors of the intraoral minor salivary glands: a demographic and histologic study of 426 cases. Oral Surg Oral Med Oral Pathol 1988;66(3):323–333

78. Daley TD, Gardner DG, Smout MS. Canalicular adenoma: not a basal cell adenoma. Oral Surg Oral Med Oral Pathol 1984;57(2):181–188

79. Suarez P, Hammond HL, Luna MA, Stimson PG. Palatal canalicular adenoma: report of 12 cases and review of the literature. Ann Diagn Pathol 1998;2(4):224–228

80. Mintz GA, Abrams AM, Melrose RJ. Monomorphic adenomas of the major and minor salivary glands. Report of twenty-one cases and review of the literature. Oral Surg Oral Med Oral Pathol 1982;53(4):375–386

81. McCoy-Collins RC, Calhoun NR, Redman RS, Saini N. Monomorphic adenoma of the buccal mucosa. J Oral Maxillofac Surg 1985;43(8):644–648

82. Smullin SE, Fielding AF, Susarla SM, Pringle G, Eichstaedt R. Canalicular adenoma of the palate: case report and literature review. Oral Surg Oral Med Oral Pathol Oral Radiol Endod 2004;98(1):32–36

83. Rousseau A, Mock D, Dover DG, Jordan RC. Multiple canalicular adenomas: a case report and review of the literature. Oral Surg Oral Med Oral Pathol Oral Radiol Endod 1999;87(3):346–350

84. Nagao T, Sugano I, Ishida Y, et al. Salivary gland malignant myoepithelioma: a clinicopathologic and immunohistochemical study of ten cases. Cancer 1998;83(7):1292–1299

85. Bégin LR, Rochon L, Frenkiel S. Spindle cell myoepithelioma of the nasal cavity. Am J Surg Pathol 1991;15(2):184–190

86. Luna MA, Batsakis JG, Ordóñez NG, Mackay B, Tortoledo ME. Salivary gland adenocarcinomas: a clinicopathologic analysis of three distinctive types. Semin Diagn Pathol 1987;4(2):117–135

87. Barnes L, Appel BN, Perez H, El-Attar AM. Myoepithelioma of the head and neck: case report and review. J Surg Oncol 1985;28(1):21–28

88. Savera AT, Sloman A, Huvos AG, Klimstra DS. Myoepithelial carcinoma of the salivary glands: a clinicopathologic study of 25 patients. Am J Surg Pathol 2000;24(6):761–774

89. Chen YK, Chen JY, Hsu HR, Wang WC, Lin LM. Intraoral intraductal papilloma: a case report. Gerodontology 2008;25(4):258–260

90. Brannon RB, Sciubba JJ, Giulani M. Ductal papillomas of salivary gland origin: a report of 19 cases and a review of the literature. Oral Surg Oral Med Oral Pathol Oral Radiol Endod 2001;92(1):68–77

91. Seethala RR, Thompson LD, Gnepp DR, et al. Lymphadenoma of the salivary gland: clinicopathological and immunohistochemical analysis of 33 tumors. Mod Pathol 2012;25(1):26–35

92. Bos I, Meyer S, Merz H. [Lymphadenoma of the parotid gland without sebaceous differentiation. Immunohistochemical investigations]. Pathologe 2004;25(1):73–78

93. Ma J, Chan JK, Chow CW, Orell SR. Lymphadenoma: a report of three cases of an uncommon salivary gland neoplasm. Histopathology 2002;41(4):342–350

94. Ellis GL, Auclair PL, Gnepp DR. Surgical Pathology of the Salivary Glands. Philadelphia, PA: Saunders; 1991: 252–268

95. Gnepp DR, Brannon R. Sebaceous neoplasms of salivary gland origin. Report of 21 cases. Cancer 1984;53(10):2155–2170

96. Welch KC, Papadimitriou JC, Morales R, Wolf JS. Sebaceous adenoma of the parotid gland in a 2-year-old male. Otolaryngol Head Neck Surg 2007;136(4):672–673

97. Dent CD, Hunter WE, Svirsky JA. Sebaceous gland hyperplasia: case report and literature review. J Oral Maxillofac Surg 1995;53(8):936–938

98. Zare-Mahmoodabadi R, Salehinejad J, Saghafi S, Ghazi N, Mahmoudi P, Harraji A. Sebaceous adenoma of the submandibular gland: a case report. J Oral Sci 2009;51(4):641–644

99. Ribeiro KdeC, Dib LL, Curi MM, Santos GdaC. Sebaceous adenoma of the submandibular gland: a case report. Oral Surg Oral Med Oral Pathol Oral Radiol Endod 1996;82(2):200–203

100. Lipani C, Woytash JJ, Greene GW Jr. Sebaceous adenoma of the oral cavity. J Oral Maxillofac Surg 1983;41(1):56–60

101. Surakanti SG, Agulnik M. Salivary gland malignancies: the role for chemotherapy and molecular targeted agents. Semin Oncol 2008;35(3):309–319

102. Vander Poorten VL, Hart AA, van der Laan BF, et al. Prognostic index for patients with parotid carcinoma: external validation using the nationwide 1985-1994 Dutch Head and Neck Oncology Cooperative Group database. Cancer 2003;97(6):1453–1463

103. Bhattacharyya N, Fried MP. Determinants of survival in parotid gland carcinoma: a population-based study. Am J Otolaryngol 2005;26(1):39–44

104. Gallo O, Franchi A, Bottai GV, Fini-Storchi I, Tesi G, Boddi V. Risk factors for distant metastases from carcinoma of the parotid gland. Cancer 1997;80(5):844–851

105. Guzzo M, Locati LD, Prott FJ, Gatta G, McGurk M, Licitra L. Major and minor salivary gland tumors. Crit Rev Oncol Hematol 2010;74(2):134–148

106. Chen AM, Garcia J, Granchi PJ, Johnson J, Eisele DW. Late recurrence from salivary gland cancer: when does "cure" mean cure? Cancer 2008;112(2):340–344

107. Skalova A, Leivo I, Von Boguslawsky K, Saksela E. Cell proliferation correlates with prognosis in acinic cell carcinomas of salivary gland origin. Immunohistochemical study of 30 cases using the MIB 1 antibody in formalin-fixed paraffin sections. J Pathol 1994;173(1):13–21

108. Luukkaa H, Klemi P, Leivo I, Vahlberg T, Grénman R. Prognostic significance of Ki-67 and p53 as tumor markers in salivary gland malignancies in Finland: an evaluation of 212 cases. Acta Oncol 2006;45(6):669–675

109. Nordgård S, Franzén G, Boysen M, Halvorsen TB. Ki-67 as a prognostic marker in adenoid cystic carcinoma assessed with the monoclonal antibody MIB1 in paraffin sections. Laryngoscope 1997;107(4):531–536

110. Miyabe S, Okabe M, Nagatsuka H, et al. Prognostic significance of p27Kip1, Ki-67, and CRTC1-MAML2 fusion transcript in mucoepidermoid carcinoma: a molecular and clinicopathologic study of 101 cases. J Oral Maxillofac Surg 2009;67(7):1432–1441

111. Hoyek-Gebeily J, Nehmé E, Aftimos G, Sader-Ghorra C, Sargi Z, Haddad A. Prognostic significance of EGFR, p53 and E-cadherin in mucoepidermoid cancer of the salivary glands: a retrospective case series. J Med Liban 2007;55(2):83–88

112. Kärjä VJ, Syrjänen KJ, Kurvinen AK, Syrjänen SM. Expression and mutations of p53 in salivary gland tumours. J Oral Pathol Med 1997;26(5):217–223

113. Kiyoshima T, Shima K, Kobayashi I, et al. Expression of p53 tumor suppressor gene in adenoid cystic and mucoepidermoid carcinomas of the salivary glands. Oral Oncol 2001;37(3): 315–322

114. Williams MD, Roberts DB, Kies MS, Mao L, Weber RS, El-Naggar AK. Genetic and expression analysis of HER-2 and EGFR genes in salivary duct carcinoma: empirical and therapeutic significance. Clin Cancer Res 2010;16(8):2266–2274

115. Seethala RR, Dacic S, Cieply K, Kelly LM, Nikiforova MN. A reappraisal of the MECT1/MAML2 translocation in salivary mucoepidermoid carcinomas. Am J Surg Pathol 2010;34(8):1106–1121

116. Okabe M, Miyabe S, Nagatsuka H, et al. MECT1-MAML2 fusion transcript defines a favorable subset of mucoepidermoid carcinoma. Clin Cancer Res 2006;12(13):3902–3907

117. Okumura Y, Miyabe S, Nakayama T, et al. Impact of CRTC1/3-MAML2 fusions on histological classification and prognosis of mucoepidermoid carcinoma. Histopathology 2011;59(1): 90–97

118. Ben-Izhak O, Akrish S, Gan S, Nagler RM. p27 and salivary cancer. Cancer Immunol Immunother 2009;58(3):469–473

119. Terhaard CH. Postoperative and primary radiotherapy for salivary gland carcinomas: indications, techniques, and results. Int J Radiat Oncol Biol Phys 2007; 69(Suppl 2):S52–S55

120. Kaszuba SM, Zafereo ME, Rosenthal DI, El-Naggar AK, Weber RS. Effect of initial treatment on disease outcome for patients with submandibular gland carcinoma. Arch Otolaryngol Head Neck Surg 2007;133(6):546–550

121. Alterio D, Jereczek-Fossa BA, Griseri M, et al. Three-dimensional conformal postoperative radiotherapy in patients with parotid tumors: 10 years' experience at the European Institute of Oncology. Tumori 2011;97(3):328–334

122. Locati LD, Bossi P, Perrone F, et al. Cetuximab in recurrent and/or metastatic salivary gland carcinomas: a phase II study. Oral Oncol 2009;45(7):574–578

123. Mariano FV, da Silva SD, Chulan TC, de Almeida OP, Kowalski LP. Clinicopathological factors are predictors of distant metastasis from major salivary gland carcinomas. Int J Oral Maxillofac Surg 2011;40(5):504–509

124. Speight PM, Barrett AW. Prognostic factors in malignant tumours of the salivary glands. Br J Oral Maxillofac Surg 2009;47(8): 587–593

125. Pires FR, de Almeida OP, de Araújo VC, Kowalski LP. Prognostic factors in head and neck mucoepidermoid carcinoma. Arch Otolaryngol Head Neck Surg 2004;130(2):174–180

126. Seethala RR. Histologic grading and prognostic biomarkers in salivary gland carcinomas. Adv Anat Pathol 2011;18(1):29–45

127. Seethala RR, Hoschar AP, Bennett A. Reproducibility of grading in salivary gland mucoepidermoid carcinoma and correlation with outcome: does system really matter? Mod Pathol 2008; 21(S1):241A

128. Shemirani N, Osipov V, Kolker A, Khampang P, Kerschner JE. Expression of mucin (MUC) genes in mucoepidermoid carcinoma. Laryngoscope 2011;121(1):167–170

129. Lujan B, Hakim S, Moyano S, et al. Activation of the EGFR/ERK pathway in high-grade mucoepidermoid carcinomas of the salivary glands. Br J Cancer 2010;103(4):510–516

130. Gondivkar SM, Gadbail AR, Chole R, Parikh RV. Adenoid cystic carcinoma: a rare clinical entity and literature review. Oral Oncol 2011;47(4):231–236

131. Isacsson G, Shear M. Intraoral salivary gland tumors: a retrospective study of 201 cases. J Oral Pathol 1983;12(1):57–62

132. Neville BWDD, Allen CM, Bouquot JF. Salivary Gland Pathology. Philadelphia, PA: Saunders; 2002

133. da Cruz Perez DE, de Abreu Alves F, Nobuko Nishimoto I, de Almeida OP, Kowalski LP. Prognostic factors in head and neck adenoid cystic carcinoma. Oral Oncol 2006;42(2):139–146

134. Szanto PA, Luna MA, Tortoledo ME, White RA. Histologic grading of adenoid cystic carcinoma of the salivary glands. Cancer 1984;54(6):1062–1069

135. Huang M, Ma D, Sun K, Yu G, Guo C, Gao F. Factors influencing survival rate in adenoid cystic carcinoma of the salivary glands. Int J Oral Maxillofac Surg 1997;26(6):435–439

136. Spiro RH, Huvos AG, Strong EW. Adenoid cystic carcinoma: factors influencing survival. Am J Surg 1979;138(4):579–583

137. Thompson LD. Salivary gland acinic cell carcinoma. Ear Nose Throat J 2010;89(11):530–532

138. Timon CI, Dardick I. The importance of dedifferentiation in recurrent acinic cell carcinoma. J Laryngol Otol 2001;115(8):639–644

139. Boukheris H, Curtis RE, Land CE, Dores GM. Incidence of carcinoma of the major salivary glands according to the WHO classification, 1992 to 2006: a population-based study in the United States. Cancer Epidemiol Biomarkers Prev 2009;18(11):2899–2906

140. Wahlberg P, Anderson H, Biörklund A, Möller T, Perfekt R. Carcinoma of the parotid and submandibular glands—a study of survival in 2465 patients. Oral Oncol 2002;38(7):706–713

141. Lewis JE, Olsen KD, Weiland LH. Acinic cell carcinoma. Clinicopathologic review. Cancer 1991;67(1):172–179

142. Hall DA, Pu RT. Acinic cell carcinoma of the salivary gland: a continuing medical education case. Diagn Cytopathol 2008;36(6):379–385, quiz 386–387

143. Chiosea SI, Peel R, Barnes EL, Seethala RR. Salivary type tumors seen in consultation. Virchows Arch 2009;454(4):457–466

144. Lewis JE, Olsen KD, Sebo TJ. Carcinoma ex pleomorphic adenoma: pathologic analysis of 73 cases. Hum Pathol 2001;32(6):596–604

145. Ellis GAP. Carcinoma Ex Pleomorphic Adenoma. 4th ed. Washington, DC: ARP Press; 2008

146. Brandwein M, Huvos AG, Dardick I, Thomas MJ, Theise ND. Noninvasive and minimally invasive carcinoma ex mixed tumor: a clinicopathologic and ploidy study of 12 patients with major salivary tumors of low (or no?) malignant potential. Oral Surg Oral Med Oral Pathol Oral Radiol Endod 1996;81(6):655–664

147. Olsen KD, Lewis JE. Carcinoma ex pleomorphic adenoma: a clinicopathologic review. Head Neck 2001;23(9):705–712

D. Other Tumors of the Head and Neck

23 Lymphoma for the Head and Neck Surgeon

Emily Z. Stucken, Chaz L. Stucken, and David I. Kutler

Core Messages

- The most common presentation of lymphoma in the head and neck is painless cervical lymphadenopathy.

- Lymphomas are divided into Hodgkin and non-Hodgkin lymphomas. There are many extranodal sites of non-Hodgkin lymphoma within the head and neck, including the Waldeyer ring, the salivary glands, the nose and paranasal sinuses, the thyroid gland, the larynx and trachea, the orbit, the temporal bone, and the skin. Each site has a unique and characteristic clinicopathologic behavior, treatment, and prognosis.

- The head and neck surgeon plays an important role in providing a technically appropriate tissue specimen for diagnosis of lymphoma. Surgical specimens should be sent fresh for pathologic evaluation including immunophenotyping and flow cytometry.

- The mainstay for treatment of lymphoma consists of chemotherapy, radiation therapy, or combined modality treatment with chemotherapy and radiation therapy.

Lymphoma is commonly present in the head and neck region. It is the second most common head and neck malignancy after squamous cell carcinoma (SCC)[1] and is the most common nonepithelial tumor of the head and neck.[2] It is imperative for the head and neck surgeon to have a good working knowledge of the various head and neck manifestations of lymphoma as he or she will often play a pivotal role in obtaining the diagnosis. Lymphoma may have diverse presentations within the head and neck, and the head and neck surgeon may be the first physician that a patient sees at the onset of symptoms. Patients may present with cervical lymphadenopathy or with a mass in one of the many extranodal sites within the head and neck. In most instances, the role of the head and neck surgeon is to provide prompt and adequate tissue specimen for diagnosis, so that the patient may begin the appropriate therapy. The otolaryngologist may be called upon to provide tissue diagnosis when a primary lymphoma is suspected or to biopsy a clinically changing node in a patient with a known indolent lymphoma so as to rule out transformation to a high-grade lesion. Beyond establishing a tissue diagnosis, the management of head and neck lymphomas is primarily nonsurgical.

Lymphomas occurring in the head and neck can be divided broadly into two categories: primary nodal lymphomas and extranodal lymphomas. Primary nodal lymphomas include Hodgkin and non-Hodgkin lymphomas. Lymphomas that originate outside lymph nodes are termed extranodal lymphomas and are mainly non-Hodgkin type.

Primary Nodal Lymphoma

Primary nodal lymphoma is divided into two forms: Hodgkin lymphoma and non-Hodgkin lymphoma. Both present with painless cervical lymphadenopathy, often involving lower cervical or supraclavicular nodes.[3] The enlarged cervical nodes may wax and wane in size and appearance and may have been present for a variable amount of time. The involved nodes tend to be less firm and more mobile than metastatic lymph nodes from SCC. A complete history and physical examination is imperative in patients presenting with cervical lymphadenopathy, with careful attention to constitutional "B" symptoms such as fever, night sweats, fatigue, and weight loss. Physical examination should include a complete head and neck examination with special interest paid to all mucosal surfaces and particularly the lymphoid-rich region of the Waldeyer ring.

Any unexplained cervical lymphadenopathy warrants biopsy. Fine-needle aspiration (FNA) is usually the first step in obtaining a tissue specimen; this technique can help differentiate epithelial from nonepithelial neoplasms. In addition, cell blocks may allow for immunophenotypic and flow cytometric data to be obtained from FNA specimens. If FNA demonstrates a lymphoid tumor that cannot be further characterized, this should be followed by excisional or incisional biopsy of the mass. Excisional biopsy of an accessible cervical node is generally performed unless the complete removal would result in undue morbidity, in which case an incisional biopsy is acceptable. Often times this can be performed under local anesthesia or monitored anesthesia care. Ample tissue specimen should be provided to preserve the nodal architecture. All specimens should be sent fresh in saline rather than fixed in formalin or other preservatives. This is imperative to allow for the immunohistochemical and flow cytometric studies that are required to classify and prognosticate lymphoma subtypes.

Once the diagnosis of lymphoma has been established, further work-up is indicated to determine the patient's stage. This work-up includes hematologic studies as well as radiologic studies to determine the extent of disease. Often, the work-up will include computed tomography (CT) scans of the head and neck, the chest, the abdomen, and the pelvis. Additional suspicious lymphadenopathy or extranodal masses that are detected on radiographic images should be biopsied. Often, bone marrow biopsies from the iliac crest are performed early in the staging process, as involvement of the bone marrow is diagnostic of stage IV disease and thus can render unnecessary other invasive diagnostic procedures.[4] The Ann Arbor staging system (**Table 23.1**) was initially developed for Hodgkin lymphoma and is currently used for both Hodgkin and non-Hodgkin lymphoma.[5]

Non-Hodgkin Lymphoma

Non-Hodgkin lymphoma accounts for 5% of head and neck malignancies. Non-Hodgkin lymphoma is more prevalent than Hodgkin lymphoma, with an incidence of 16 cases per 100,000 people per year in the United States.[4] The incidence of non-Hodgkin lymphoma has been rising since the 1970s[6,7]; theoretical causes for this rise include the human immunodeficiency virus (HIV) epidemic,[8-10] *Helicobacter pylori* infection,[11] autoimmune disease,[12,13] transplant-related immunosupression,[14] and the increasing age of the U.S. population.[4] Non-Hodgkin lymphoma is diagnosed most commonly in the fifth, sixth, and seventh decades of life.[4]

Several classification systems have been developed to stratify and prognosticate different types of non-Hodgkin lymphoma. The most commonly used classification schemes for non-Hodgkin lymphoma include the National Cancer Institute's (NCI) working formulation,[15] the revised European American lymphoma (REAL) classification,[16] and the World Health Organization (WHO) classification.[17] The NCI working formulation divides non-Hodgkin lymphomas into low-, intermediate-, and high-grade lymphomas according to their clinical behavior. In contrast, the REAL classification groups lesions according to their histopathologic, immunophenotypic, and clinical features. In this classification system, lymphomas are identified according to their cell lineage as B-cell lymphomas, T-cell lymphomas, and natural killer (NK) lymphomas, with subtypes of each defined according to tumor histology. The WHO classification expands upon the REAL classification to include Hodgkin lymphoma and other lymphoproliferative lesions.

Treatment of non-Hodgkin lymphoma consists of chemotherapy and radiation therapy as determined by the clinical stage and tumor classification. Other important factors that determine treatment options include the patient's age, comorbidities, and degree of symptomatology.[4] Low-grade non-Hodgkin lymphomas tend to be widespread at the time of diagnosis. Though remission can be achieved, relapse is common.[18] The current recommendation is to delay treatment of low-grade non-Hodgkin lymphomas until the patient becomes symptomatic, as treatment provided at the time of diagnosis does not lengthen long-term survival compared with treatment started at the time of symptom onset.[19,20] Treatment consists of chemotherapy with a single agent.[19] Relapses can often be treated with the same regimen that induced initial remission.[4] The mean survival for patients diagnosed with low-grade lymphomas is 10 to 15 years.[21]

Intermediate- and high-grade aggressive lymphomas are treated with a goal of complete remission and cure.

Table 23.1 Ann Arbor Staging System for Lymphoma

Stage	Description
I	Involvement of a single lymph node region (I) or a single extralymphatic organ or site (I$_E$)
II	Involvement of two or more lymph node regions on the same side of the diaphragm (II) or localized involvement of extralymphatic organ or site and of one or more lymph node regions on the same side of the diaphragm (II$_E$)
III	Involvement of lymph node regions on both sides of the diaphragm (III), which may also be accompanied by localized involvement of extralymphatic organ or site (III$_E$) or by involvement of the spleen (III$_S$), or both (III$_{SE}$)
IV	Diffuse or disseminated involvement of one or more extralymphatic organs or tissues with or without associated lymph node enlargement
Symptom modifiers	
A	No constitutional symptoms
B	Unexplained weight loss of more than 10% of the body weight in the 6 mo previous to admission; unexplained fever with temperatures above 38°C; and night sweats

mo, months.

Localized lesions are treated with radiation alone, which can induce complete remission in more than 80% of patients.[22,23] Chemotherapy is integral in treating advanced stage disease or bulky localized disease. The most effective chemotherapy regimen is cyclophosphamide, doxorubicin, vincristine, and prednisone (CHOP).[4] Immunotherapy with monoclonal antibodies, such as rituximab, is currently evolving as adjuvant therapy.[24–28]

Hodgkin Lymphoma

Hodgkin lymphoma has an incidence of 3 cases per 100,000 people per year. Hodgkin lymphoma presents with a bimodal age distribution, peaking in the second and fifth decades of life. Hodgkin lymphoma is more likely to be accompanied by constitutional symptoms than non-Hodgkin lymphoma.[29] The majority of patients are male, and higher socioeconomic class has been associated with the development of Hodgkin lymphoma.[30,31]

The histopathological diagnosis of Hodgkin lymphoma is made by the presence of the classic Reed-Sternberg cells in a characteristic background of reactive lymphocytes, neutrophils, plasma cells, and eosinophils.[4] The WHO system is the most commonly used classification scheme; it categorizes Hodgkin lymphomas into six subtypes. Nodular sclerosing is the most common subtype, representing almost 80% of cases. The prognosis for nodular sclerosis is generally good. Mixed cellularity is the second most common subtype, accounting for 15 to 20% of cases. The mixed-cellularity subtype is the most commonly found type in HIV-positive patients. Lymphocyte-rich classic Hodgkin lymphoma accounts for approximately 6% of cases. The lymphocyte-predominant subtype is considered a nonclassical subtype of Hodgkin lymphoma. It makes up approximately 4 to 5% of Hodgkin lymphomas and has an excellent prognosis. The lymphocyte-depleted subtype is the least common, making up only 1% of the diagnoses of Hodgkin lymphoma. This subtype has the worst prognosis, often presenting at an advanced stage. The final subtype, unclassifiable Hodgkin lymphoma, includes lesions that do not otherwise fit into one of the aforementioned categories.[4,32]

Treatment of Hodgkin lymphomas consists of combined modality therapy including both chemotherapy and radiation therapy. The most commonly used chemotherapeutic regimen is doxorubicin, bleomycin, vinblastine, and dacarbazine. Radiation is given to the involved field only; doses are in the range of 3600 to 4000 cGy.[33] Survival outcomes are superior in Hodgkin lymphoma than in non-Hodgkin lymphoma. In one comparative study, 12% of patients with Hodgkin lymphoma died of their disease, contrasted with 41% of patients with non-Hodgkin lymphoma.[29] Unfortunately, many patients with Hodgkin lymphoma are young, and, in addition to the standard side effects and complications of chemotherapy and radiotherapy, up to 5% of patients may develop a secondary malignancy as the result of combined modality treatment.[34]

Primary Extranodal Head and Neck Lymphomas

Lymphoma arising primarily from a site other than a lymph node is a relatively common occurrence within the head and neck. One-third of extranodal lymphomas are localized to the head and neck region,[35] and 23 to 28.4% of all head and neck non-Hodgkin lymphomas are extranodal.[29,36] Extranodal lymphomas are almost exclusively non-Hodgkin type. Anatomic sites include the Waldeyer ring, the salivary glands, the nose and paranasal sinuses, the thyroid gland, the larynx and trachea, the orbit, the temporal bone, and the skin. Tumors tend to be submucosal rather than ulcerative.[37] The diagnosis may not be readily apparent at the time of initial evaluation, and, in children, extranodal tumors may mimic other disease processes such as inflammatory disease, Langerhans cell histiocytosis, or rhabdomyosarcoma.[38] It is therefore important that the head and neck surgeon maintains a good working knowledge of the diverse presentations of extranodal lymphomas. As a group, extranodal non-Hodgkin lymphomas have a better prognosis than their nodal counterparts, but tumors of each anatomic site have characteristic clinicopathological features and varying levels of aggressiveness and response to treatment.

Waldeyer Ring

The Waldeyer ring is an anatomic region of the oropharynx and nasopharynx that is heavily populated with lymphoid tissue. This area is composed of the palatine tonsil, the pharyngeal tonsil, the tubal tonsils of Gerlach, and the lingual tonsil on the base of tongue. The Waldeyer ring is the most common site of primary extranodal lymphoma in the head and neck, accounting for more than half of the cases.[39,40] The tonsil is the most common site of lymphoma within the Waldeyer ring and is the most common single anatomic site of primary extranodal non-Hodgkin lymphoma overall. Tonsillar lymphomas have been cited as comprising 40 to 79% of the Waldeyer ring lymphomas, with the next most frequent location being the nasopharynx, followed by the base of tongue and the soft palate.[39,41–46] Within the broader context of head and neck malignancies, however, tonsillar lymphoma is still relatively rare, representing less than 1% of head and neck cancers.[47]

The median age of patients diagnosed with primary lymphoma of the Waldeyer ring is 45 to 60 years,[35,39,41,42,44,45] and there is a slight male predominance of 1.3 males for every female affected.[35] The Waldeyer ring lymphomas may present with observable tonsillar enlargement, or they may present with symptoms of obstructive sleep apnea. Tonsillar lymphoma is a common presentation of posttransplant lymphoproliferative disorder (PTLD); this entity will be discussed in detail later in the chapter. The incidental diagnosis of tonsillar lymphoma is exceedingly rare in the absence of clinical suspicion. In a study examining the cost-effectiveness of routine pathologic evaluation of pediatric tonsillar specimens, zero cases of unsuspected pathology were found in 4186 routine tonsil specimens.[48]

The vast majority of primary Waldeyer ring lymphomas are B-cell lymphomas, with diffuse large B-cell lymphomas being the most common type.[35,39,47] In a recent literature review, B-cell lymphomas were found to make up 82% of tonsillar lymphomas. They are often of intermediate- to high-grade, but tend to be localized at the time of presentation.[35] Diagnosis is made by tissue biopsy, usually via tonsillectomy. Surgery does not play a role in the management of the Waldeyer ring lymphomas except in the rare incidence of upper airway obstruction from severe lymphoid hypertrophy necessitating surgical intervention.

The accepted treatment of primary lymphoma of the Waldeyer ring is combined chemotherapy and radiation therapy. In a randomized, prospective clinical trial of 316 patients with stage I primary lymphoma of the Waldeyer ring, combined modality treatment with chemotherapy and radiation therapy achieved superior failure-free survival and overall survival rates than the chemotherapy-alone and radiation therapy-alone study arms. Failure-free survival was 83% for patients treated with combined modality treatment compared with 48% for patients treated with radiation therapy alone and 45% for patients treated with chemotherapy alone. Overall survival was 90% for the combined-treatment arm compared with 56% in the radiation-only group and 58% in the chemotherapy-only group.[42] Other studies have similarly found an advantage with combined chemotherapy and radiation therapy over single-modality treatment.[35,39–41,49–53] Tonsillar lymphomas have a better prognosis than their analogs occurring in the nasopharynx or base of tongue.[39] Even though the Waldeyer ring lymphomas are often histologically intermediate- or high-grade tumors, the prognosis is generally favorable[35] and is better than for their more prevalent SCC counterparts.[54]

Salivary Gland Lymphoma

Primary lymphoma of the salivary glands is rare, accounting for only 1.7% of all salivary gland neoplasms.[55] Patients most commonly present with painless, firm enlargement of a salivary gland, although occasionally the lesion may be painful. Patients may have bilateral swelling and may give a history of relapsing and remitting swelling consistent with recurrent sialadenitis.[55,56] Often, patients will not have accompanying systemic symptoms.[57] The parotid gland is most frequently affected, occurring in 65% of cases. This is followed in descending order of frequency by the submandibular glands, the minor salivary glands, and the sublingual glands. The median age at diagnosis is 50 to 70 years, and there is a female predominance.[55–61]

The vast majority of salivary gland lymphomas are non-Hodgkin lymphomas, predominantly B-cell lymphomas. Approximately 60% of cases are mucosa-associated lymphoid tissue (MALT) lymphomas. Follicular lymphoma and diffuse

large B-cell lymphomas are next in order of frequency, with the remainder composed of mantle cell lymphoma, lymphoblastic lymphoma, peripheral T-cell lymphoma, and Hodgkin lymphoma.[55,57,58] MALT lymphomas tend to be low grade, though rare transformation to high-grade tumors has been described.[58,62] It is debated whether primary lymphomas of the salivary glands are truly extranodal lymphomas or if they arise from intraparenchymal or adjacent lymph nodes, as extranodal lymphoid tissue is not normally present in the salivary glands. It is proposed that chronic inflammation in the form of myoepithelial sialoadenitis leads to the reactive infiltration of the gland with lymphoid tissue, which has the potential to transform into MALT lymphoma.[62–64] Hyman and Wolff proposed three criteria to diagnose a primary salivary gland lymphoma; the lesion had to be confirmed histologically to be malignant and had to involve the gland parenchyma rather than only adjacent soft tissue or lymph nodes. In addition, the presentation in the salivary gland had to be the first clinical manifestation of the disease.[65]

Patients who carry the diagnosis of Sjögren syndrome deserve special mention. Sjögren syndrome is a chronic autoimmune disease whereby prolonged infiltration of salivary and lacrimal glands with lymphocytes and histiocytes leads to symptoms of xerostomia and keratoconjunctivitis sicca. Sjögren syndrome may be associated with other autoimmune phenomena in which case it is referred to as secondary Sjögren syndrome. Patients affected by Sjögren syndrome have a 6- to 44-fold increased risk of developing non-Hodgkin lymphoma compared with the general population.[66–68] About 4 to 10% of patients affected by Sjögren syndrome go on to develop non-Hodgkin lymphoma,[69–72] and approximately 20% of patients with primary salivary gland lymphoma have Sjögren syndrome.[57] The salivary glands are involved in 37% of these cases of non-Hodgkin lymphoma, and the majority are MALT lymphomas.[69] Tonami et al did not find an association between time of onset or severity of disease and the development of non-Hodgkin lymphoma.[69] Several studies have demonstrated a worse prognosis in patients with Sjögren syndrome who develop primary salivary gland lymphoma,[59,73] but others have not found this to be the case.[56]

A tissue sample should be obtained on any patient with a salivary gland mass. FNA cytology has a reported sensitivity of 73% for identifying specimens as benign or malignant in the salivary glands, though the accuracy of FNA for correctly identifying a specific pathologic diagnosis is as low as 48%. In a multi-institutional study of 6249 pathologic salivary specimens, the diagnosis of lymphoma on FNA had the highest false-negative rate of any malignancy at 57%.[74] The authors stress the importance of immunophenotyping studies with flow cytometry. If enough tissue for flow cytometry cannot be obtained by FNA, surgical biopsy should be considered to make the diagnosis. Excisional biopsy in the parotid gland often requires superficial parotidectomy.

Salivary gland lymphoma is believed to have a superior prognosis compared with lymphoma of other extranodal sites.[57,59,73,75] Tumors tend to remain localized with slow regional progression and low rates of local relapse.[58] The median survival is 49 months.[55] MALT lymphomas of the salivary gland have been found to have improved prognosis over other B-cell salivary gland lymphomas,[58,76] although follicular lymphoma of the salivary gland may have equally good prognosis to MALT.[57] Overall 5-year survival for salivary gland lymphoma has been quoted at 83%, with 5-year disease-free survival of 71.5%.[58] Recommended treatment is radiotherapy for stage I non-Hodgkin lymphomas and chemotherapy plus or minus radiotherapy for stage II through IV disease.[56,77] All patients with non-Hodgkin lymphomas other than MALT type should receive systemic chemotherapy.[58] Some advocate delaying treatment in the case of low-grade histology in an asymptomatic patient.[20,56] There is no role for definitive surgical management of salivary gland lymphomas after the diagnosis has been established.[56]

Nasal and Paranasal Sinus Lymphoma

Nasal and paranasal sinus lymphomas are a rare entity in Western populations, composing only 0.17% of all lymphomas.[78] Now collectively referred to as sinonasal lymphomas, they have previously been included under various nomenclatures such as lethal midline granuloma, midline malignant reticulosis, polymorphic reticulosis, and angiocentric immunoproliferative lesions.[16,79–89] Sinonasal lymphomas make up a diverse group of non-Hodgkin lymphomas and have been classified according to the WHO classification.[90] These malignancies are more prevalent in Asian populations and in certain regions of Central and South America.[89,91–96] B-cell lymphomas are more prevalent within the Western population, while Asian and South American populations have a higher incidence of T-cell and NK/T-cell lymphomas.[78,91–94,97–103] Sinonasal lymphomas are more common in males than in females[104] and commonly develop in the sixth to eighth decades of life, with slightly younger disease onset in T-cell lymphomas than in B-cell types.[80,93,94,105] These varying immunophenotypes have been shown to differ in their presentation, disease characteristics, prognosis, and response to treatment, with T-cell lymphomas having a poorer response to treatment than B-cell sinonasal lesions.[94,99,106–109]

B-cell sinonasal lymphomas more commonly originate in the paranasal sinuses than in the nasal cavity proper.[110,111] Patients often complain of a long history of sinonasal obstructive symptoms, and tumors often present with soft tissue expansion and invasion into the surrounding orbit, nasopharynx, and/or anterior cranial fossa. This may lead to osseous destruction and symptoms of mass effect such as proptosis.[88,104,112]

T-cell and NK/T-cell sinonasal lymphomas most often arise in the nasal cavity and present with aggressive local destruction within the nasal cavity and associated nasal septal perforation, extensive intranasal crusting, destruction of the external nose, and erosion through the palate.[88,89,94,104,110,111,113] T-cell and NK/T-cell lymphomas have a high association with Epstein-Barr virus (EBV) positivity.[16,78,88,89,92,97–100,108] Disease onset occurs at a younger age than in B-cell sinonasal lymphoma, with a median age near 50 years.[80,93,94,105]

Sinonasal lymphomas have a uniformly poor prognosis; outcomes are unfavorable when compared with other forms of non-Hodgkin lymphoma.[94,108,114] Most patients present with intermediate- and high-grade tumors.[93,94,104,115,116] The majority of patients are staged as IE at time of diagnosis.[96,111,115] Despite the preponderance of localized disease at the time of diagnosis, overall 5-year survival rates are poor, ranging from 36 to 52%.[108,110,114,115,117,118] This is reflected in the fact that though up to 81% of patients experience complete remission after initial therapy, up to 55% of these will experience treatment failure.[110,114] For early-stage lesions (Ann Arbor stage IE), radiotherapy remains the primary treatment.[108,119] Some studies have shown no survival benefit with the addition of chemotherapy in stage IE patients,[93,94,108,112,116,120–122] while others advocate combined modality treatment with chemotherapy and radiation therapy for these early-stage lesions.[103,109,115,123,124] For patients with extensive stage IE disease as well as all patients with stage II to IV disease, recommend therapy consists of combined chemotherapy and radiation.[112,115,116] Radiation should be delivered to the entire nasal cavity as well as to the ipsilateral maxillary and ethmoid sinuses; the nasopharynx can be included if the tumor approximates the nasopharynx.[116] Elective radiation to the ipsilateral neck is not recommended for limited stage IE disease, as the incidence of cervical lymphadenopathy is less than 20%.[110,116] Systemic therapy with CHOP is the most commonly employed chemotherapy regimen.[114]

Thyroid Lymphoma

Primary thyroid lymphoma is characterized by the presence of lymphoma within the thyroid gland with or without spread to its regional lymph nodes without evidence of contiguous spread from another site or metastatic spread from a distant source. Primary thyroid lymphoma is a rare disease that is estimated to account for 1 to 5% of all thyroid malignancies and only 2% of all extranodal lymphomas.[125] Thyroid lymphoma sometimes offers the clinician a diagnostic challenge; however, the early recognition of this disease is important because curative treatments are available and vary greatly from the management of other thyroid tumors.

A recent Surveillance, Epidemiology, and End Result (SEER) analysis comprising more than 1400 patients demonstrated that primary thyroid lymphoma most commonly occurs in Caucasian females in the seventh decade of life (93% Caucasian, 75% female, mean age at diagnosis = 66 years).[126] The association between Hashimoto thyroiditis (chronic lymphocytic thyroiditis) and thyroid lymphoma has been well-described, and the presence of thyroid nodules in the setting of Hashimoto thyroiditis should raise the clinician's index of suspicion for the development of malignancy. Patients with Hashimoto thyroiditis have a 67-fold increased relative risk of developing primary thyroid lymphoma,[127] and as high as 94% of patients with thyroid lymphoma have histologic evidence of lymphocytic thyroiditis.[128] Although there is a strong correlation between Hashimoto thyroiditis and the thyroid lymphoma, the pathophysiologic mechanism of oncogenesis is unclear. Researchers hypothesize that clonal immunoglobulin heavy chain variable region gene rearrangements in the setting of continuous lymphocytic stimulation lead to malignant transformation.[129,130]

The classically described presentation of patients with primary thyroid lymphoma is one of a rapidly enlarging thyroid mass with associated compressive symptoms. While thyroid lymphoma has historically presented with overt clinical signs and symptoms, Graff-Baker et al shows that patients are now presenting with earlier stage disease;[126] this may be related either to the increased use of screening ultrasonography or because of increased use of reportable databases such as the SEER database. The impact of earlier diagnosis on survival outcomes remains to be determined.

The most common subtype of primary thyroid lymphoma is diffuse large B-cell lymphoma, which accounts for 50 to 70% of all thyroid lymphomas. Other subtypes include MALT lymphoma (10 to 30%) and follicular lymphoma (10%). The remaining histologic subtypes of thyroid lymphoma each represent only 1 to 3% of cases; these subtypes include small lymphocytic, mixed diffuse B-cell, Hodgkin, mantle cell, and Burkitt lymphomas.[125,131] Staging criteria is based on the Ann Arbor staging system. Approximately 90% of patients present with stage IE or IIE disease.[128,131]

Imaging plays an important role in determining the stage of disease, with CT being the imaging modality of choice for both staging and disease surveillance. CT imaging of the chest, the abdomen, and the pelvis is recommended for evaluating disease on both sides of the diaphragm. The role of fluorodeoxyglucose positron emission tomography (FDG-PET) is currently under investigation. FDG-PET/CT is a highly sensitive modality for the detection and surveillance of diffuse large B-cell lymphoma, and Basu et al suggests that it may detect recurrences earlier than CT alone.[132] However, FDG-PET/CT has limited utility in cases of MALT lymphoma because the MALT subtype has a lower metabolic rate, and the higher incidence of coexistent Hashimoto thyroiditis causes increased FDG uptake in the thyroid gland.[133]

FNA plays an integral role in the diagnosis of thyroid lymphoma, though it has historically produced unpredictable results, with one study demonstrating accurate FNA results in only 20% of cases of thyroid lymphoma.[134] Newer techniques including flow cytometry for specific cell-surface markers have increased the diagnostic accuracy of FNA, with a recent study showing that FNA established a firm diagnosis of lymphoma in 65% of cases while missing only 12% of cases.[135] Although the accuracy of FNA has improved, open biopsy may be necessary in cases in which the FNA yields equivocal results, especially in the setting of Hashimoto thyroiditis.[136]

As is the case for nodal lymphomas, patients with primary thyroid lymphoma should undergo treatment based on the specific lymphoma subtype. The standard of care for diffuse large B-cell lymphoma of the thyroid is similar to its primary nodal disease correlate: multimodality therapy using a combination of locoregional radiotherapy and systemic chemotherapy with CHOP. Historically, patients were treated by surgery followed by radiotherapy, but survival rates were only 50%.[125] Doria et al showed the benefit of combined chemoradiotherapy for patients with stage IE and IIE disease.[137] In a retrospective review, they found overall relapse rates of 7.7, 37.1, and 43% and local relapse rates of 2.6, 12.6, and 23% for combined chemoradiotherapy, radiation therapy alone, and chemotherapy alone, respectively. Diffuse large B-cell lymphoma is the most aggressive form of thyroid lymphoma and has the worst prognosis, with a 5-year disease-specific survival of 75%.[126]

The treatment of MALT lymphomas is less aggressive because the disease is a low-grade, indolent malignancy. MALT lymphomas generally respond well to single-modality therapy by involved field radiation therapy (IFRT), with a 5-year disease-specific survival of 95%.[126] Tsang et al published their experience in treating 13 patients with stage IE and IIE thyroid MALT lymphomas using IFRT; their cohort had a 0% relapse rate after a median follow-up of 5.1 years.[138]

The role of surgery in treating MALT lymphomas of the thyroid is controversial. While some series have shown overall survival rates of 100%,[128,139] the use of surgery may be associated with increased morbidity without conferring a survival advantage. In an attempt to better understand the role of surgery in treating primary thyroid lymphoma, Pyke et al compared patients who received debulking surgery followed by radiation or biopsy alone followed by radiation.[140] They found that the remission and survival rates were the same in each group, but the patients who underwent debulking surgery experienced a 6.5% complication rate including recurrent laryngeal nerve paralysis and permanent hypoparathyroidism. Because of concerns related to surgical morbidity as well as strong evidence for the use of radiation therapy to treat MALT lymphomas, surgery is performed less frequently. Most commonly, a diagnosis of MALT lymphoma is made after a thyroidectomy has already been performed. In these cases completeness of the resection is the pivotal determinant; if the surgical resection is not deemed to be complete, then the patient should be referred for adjuvant radiotherapy.[141]

Laryngeal and Tracheal Manifestations of Lymphoma

Primary lymphoma of the larynx is an extremely rare disease that accounts for less than 1% of all laryngeal malignancies and has been reported in fewer than 100 cases in the English literature.[142] Most cases of laryngeal lymphoma are secondary lymphomas in which the larynx is affected by a systemic lymphoma. True cases of primary laryngeal lymphoma are rare and typically present with dysphonia, shortness of breath, dysphagia, and globus sensation. The tumors frequently arise as submucosal masses in the lymphoid-containing regions of the laryngeal supraglottis and ventricles. The majority of cases are diffuse large B-cell lymphomas, followed by MALT lymphomas, and NK/T cell lymphomas.[143]

The pathophysiology of laryngeal MALT lymphoma appears to be related to chronic inflammation, similar to the etiology of salivary gland MALT lymphoma in patients with Sjögren syndrome and thyroid MALT lymphoma in patients with Hashimono thyroiditis. Researchers have hypothesized that laryngeal MALT lymphoma may be related to chronic inflammation caused by laryngopharyngeal reflux.[144] The rarity of primary lymphoma of the subglottis and trachea (4:1 ratio of supraglottic:glottic manifestations of laryngeal lymphoma) further supports the notion that an inflammatory process is involved, as the glottis would act as a barrier to laryngopharyngeal reflux.[144,145]

Because laryngeal lymphoma is typically submucosal, it is important to obtain deep biopsies and to send fresh tissue for immunohistochemistry, flow cytometry, and immunophenotyping. After obtaining a diagnosis of laryngeal lymphoma, the complete staging work-up of the patient includes hematologic testing, bone marrow biopsy, and imaging.[143] The Ann Arbor staging system is used to classify the extent of disease.

Because of the rarity of this disease entity, there are no large studies comparing treatment modalities. Thus, cases are treated in accordance with accepted standards determined for other extranodal lymphomas of similar stage. The most commonly used modality is IFRT. Although radiation alone has shown promising results,[142] more recent literature has described the use of chemotherapy alone (R-CHOP) to treat laryngeal diffuse large B-cell lymphoma, and some reports demonstrate the use of combined modality treatment using chemotherapy and radiotherapy.[143,146] The utility of surgery in treating primary laryngeal lymphoma is limited to securing the airway by tracheotomy when indicated, and some reports have described debulking procedures using the CO_2 laser to open the airway and avoid the need for tracheotomy.[146]

Lymphoma in the Immunosuppressed Population

Immunosuppressed patients are at increased risk for developing lymphoma compared with the immunocompetent population. This risk applies regardless of whether the immunosuppression is acquired through infection as in the HIV or iatrogenic as in the case of solid organ transplant recipients. The most frequent type of lymphoma to develop in both patient populations is non-Hodgkin lymphoma, most commonly B-cell subtypes.[147] The risk of non-Hodgkin lymphoma in this population has been estimated at 50 times higher than in the general population.[148]

Human Immunodeficiency Virus

Non-Hodgkin lymphoma is considered an AIDS-defining illness. Non-Hodgkin lymphoma is the second most common malignancy in people with AIDS, after Kaposi sarcoma.[149] The relative risk for the development of non-Hodgkin lymphoma in human immunodeficiency virus (HIV) patients ranges from 15 for low-grade lesions to more than 400 for high-grade lymphomas. The risk of Hodgkin lymphoma is also increased, with about a 10-fold increased risk.[150] AIDS-related non-Hodgkin lymphoma tends to present at advanced stage, with 70 to 80% presenting with stage III or IV disease.[151,152] These patients are much more likely to experience systemic symptoms such as fever, weight loss, or night sweats.[152] A disproportionally high number of patients with AIDS-related non-Hodgkin lymphoma (68 to 98%) exhibit extranodal involvement.[10,153–156] Sixty-three percent of patients with AIDS-related non-Hodgkin lymphoma have head and neck manifestations of disease.[157] The HIV-positive population often displays diffuse cervical lymphadenopathy at baseline, and any change in nodal status should be viewed with suspicion and biopsied when clinically indicated. Treatment of AIDS-related lymphomas includes multiagent chemotherapy combined with highly active antiretroviral therapy (HAART).[158] Prognosis has improved since the development of HAART therapy, and remission rates approaching those of the general population have been reported.[159]

Organ Transplant Recipients

Solid organ transplant recipients are also at increased risk of development of lymphomas, specifically non-Hodgkin lymphoma. The risk of lymphoma correlates closely with the degree of immunosuppression and thus is highest in the first year after transplant when immunosuppression is greatest.[160] Recipients of heart, heart-lung, liver, and intestinal transplants have higher incidence of non-Hodgkin lymphoma, while the incidence in renal transplant patients is relatively lower.[160,161] These malignancies are often associated with EBV positivity, and patients who are EBV negative before transplantation are at greater risk.[162,163] Lymphoma in this population falls under the broader category of PTLD. This umbrella term includes early lymphoproliferative lesions, polymorphic PTLDs, monomorphic PTLDs such as B- and T-cell lymphomas, plasmacytomas, and Hodgkin lymphomas.[164] PTLD is the second most common malignancy to occur in patients undergoing immunosuppression after solid-organ transplant,[165] and head and neck primary sites occur in 50% of patients. This reflects a greater proportion of head and neck primary involvement than in the general population.[165,166] Patients often present with cervical lymphadenopathy or lymphoid hypertrophy in Waldeyer ring, and the head and neck surgeon plays an important role in establishing the diagnosis through tissue biopsy or tonsillectomy. Treatment is reduction or cessation of immunosuppressive therapy. Lymphomas that do not respond to reduction of immunosuppression are treated with combination chemotherapy, most commonly CHOP.[165]

Conclusion

Lymphoma is the second most common malignancy of the head and neck, after SCC. Lymphomas may present with both nodal and extranodal involvement. Common head and neck manifestations include painless cervical lymphadenopathy and localized lymphoid enlargement. Extranodal involvement in the upper aerodigestive tract may cause symptoms of airway obstruction. It is imperative for the head and neck surgeon to maintain a high level of suspicion for head and neck lymphomas, as he or she may be the first physician to evaluate the patient for their cardinal symptoms. The most important role of the head and neck surgeon is to obtain a technically appropriate tissue specimen for diagnosis when indicated. In the majority of cases, definitive management of head and neck lymphomas is nonsurgical.

References

1. DePeña CA, Van Tassel P, Lee YY. Lymphoma of the head and neck. Radiol Clin North Am 1990;28(4):723–743
2. Bragg DG. Radiology of the lymphomas. Curr Probl Diagn Radiol 1987;16(4):177–206
3. Zapater E, Bagán JV, Carbonell F, Basterra J. Malignant lymphoma of the head and neck. Oral Dis 2010;16(2):119–128
4. Nayak LM, Deschler DG. Lymphomas. Otolaryngol Clin North Am 2003;36(4):625–646
5. Carbone PP, Kaplan HS, Musshoff K, Smithers DW, Tubiana M. Report of the Committee on Hodgkin's Disease Staging Classification. Cancer Res 1971;31(11):1860–1861
6. Weisenburger DD. Epidemiology of non-Hodgkin's lymphoma: recent findings regarding an emerging epidemic. Ann Oncol 1994;5(Suppl 1):19–24
7. American Cancer Society. Non-Hodgkin's lymphoma. Available at: http://www.cancer.org. 2011. Accessed 2/10/11
8. Powles T, Matthews G, Bower M. AIDS related systemic non-Hodgkin's lymphoma. Sex Transm Infect 2000;76(5):335–341
9. Kaplan LD. HIV-associated lymphoma. AIDS Clin Rev 1993-1994:145–166
10. Kaplan LD, Abrams DI, Feigal E, et al. AIDS-associated non-Hodgkin's lymphoma in San Francisco. JAMA 1989;261(5):719–724
11. Kelly SM, Geraghty JM, Neale G. H pylori, gastric carcinoma, and MALT lymphoma. Lancet 1994;343(8894):418
12. Hyjek E, Isaacson PG. Primary B cell lymphoma of the thyroid and its relationship to Hashimoto's thyroiditis. Hum Pathol 1988;19(11):1315–1326
13. Hyjek E, Smith WJ, Isaacson PG. Primary B-cell lymphoma of salivary glands and its relationship to myoepithelial sialadenitis. Hum Pathol 1988;19(7):766–776
14. Penn I. The incidence of malignancies in transplant recipients. Transplant Proc 1975;7(2):323–326
15. National Cancer Institute sponsored study of classifications of non-Hodgkin's lymphomas: summary and description of a working formulation for clinical usage. The Non-Hodgkin's Lymphoma Pathologic Classification Project. Cancer 1982;49(10):2112–2135
16. Harris NL, Jaffe ES, Stein H, et al. A revised European-American classification of lymphoid neoplasms: a proposal from the International Lymphoma Study Group. Blood 1994;84(5):1361–1392
17. Harris NL, Jaffe ES, Diebold J, Flandrin G, Muller-Hermelink HK, Vardiman J. Lymphoma classification—from controversy to consensus: the R.E.A.L. and WHO Classification of lymphoid neoplasms. Ann Oncol 2000;11(Suppl 1):3–10
18. Marion J. Diagnosis and treatment of lymphomas. In: Thawley S, Panje W, Batskis J, eds. Comprehensive Management of Head and Neck Tumors. Philadelphia, PA: W.B. Saunders Co.; 1987: 1840–1853
19. Armitage JO. Treatment of non-Hodgkin's lymphoma. N Engl J Med 1993;328(14):1023–1030
20. Portlock CS, Rosenberg SA. No initial therapy for stage III and IV non-Hodgkin's lymphomas of favorable histologic types. Ann Intern Med 1979;90(1):10–13
21. Horning SJ, Rosenberg SA. The natural history of initially untreated low-grade non-Hodgkin's lymphomas. N Engl J Med 1984;311(23):1471–1475
22. Vaughan Hudson B, Vaughan Hudson G, MacLennan KA, Anderson L, Linch DC. Clinical stage 1 non-Hodgkin's lymphoma: long-term follow-up of patients treated by the British National Lymphoma Investigation with radiotherapy alone as initial therapy. Br J Cancer 1994;69(6):1088–1093
23. Ruijs CD, Dekker AW, van Kempen-Harteveld ML, van Baarlen J, Hordijk GJ. Treatment of localized non-Hodgkin's lymphomas of the head and neck. Cancer 1994;74(2):703–707
24. Czuczman MS. Immunochemotherapy in indolent non-Hodgkin's lymphoma. Semin Oncol 2002;29(2, Suppl 6):11–17
25. Coiffier B. Rituximab in combination with CHOP improves survival in elderly patients with aggressive non-Hodgkin's lymphoma. Semin Oncol 2002;29(2, Suppl 6):18–22
26. Press OW, Leonard JP, Coiffier B, Levy R, Timmerman J. Immunotherapy of Non-Hodgkin's lymphomas. Hematology (Am Soc Hematol Educ Program) 2001:221–240
27. Vose JM, Link BK, Grossbard ML, et al. Phase II study of rituximab in combination with chop chemotherapy in patients with previously untreated, aggressive non-Hodgkin's lymphoma. J Clin Oncol 2001;19(2):389–397
28. Kimby E. Beyond immunochemotherapy: combinations of rituximab with cytokines interferon-alpha2a and granulocyte colony stimulating factor [corrected]. Semin Oncol 2002;29(2, Suppl 6):7–10
29. Urquhart A, Berg R. Hodgkin's and non-Hodgkin's lymphoma of the head and neck. Laryngoscope 2001;111(9):1565–1569
30. Harris NL. Hodgkin's lymphomas: classification, diagnosis, and grading. Semin Hematol 1999;36(3):220–232
31. Urba WJ, Longo DL. Hodgkin's disease. N Engl J Med 1992;326(10):678–687
32. Pileri SA, Ascani S, Leoncini L, et al. Hodgkin's lymphoma: the pathologist's viewpoint. J Clin Pathol 2002;55(3):162–176
33. Fung HC, Nademanee AP. Approach to Hodgkin's lymphoma in the new millennium. Hematol Oncol 2002;20(1):1–15
34. Várady E, Deák B, Molnár ZS, et al. Second malignancies after treatment for Hodgkin's disease. Leuk Lymphoma 2001;42(6): 1275–1281
35. Mohammadianpanah M, Daneshbod Y, Ramzi M, et al. Primary tonsillar lymphomas according to the new World Health Organization classification: to report 87 cases and literature review and analysis. Ann Hematol 2010;89(10):993–1001
36. Artese L, Di Alberti L, Lombardo M, Liberatore E, Piattelli A. Head and neck non-Hodgkin's lymphomas. Eur J Cancer B Oral Oncol 1995;31B(5):299–300

37. Nathu RM, Mendenhall NP, Almasri NM, Lynch JW. Non-Hodgkin's lymphoma of the head and neck: a 30-year experience at the University of Florida. Head Neck 1999;21(3):247–254

38. La Quaglia MP. Non-Hodgkin's lymphoma of the head and neck in childhood. Semin Pediatr Surg 1994;3(3):207–215

39. Ezzat AA, Ibrahim EM, El Weshi AN, et al. Localized non-Hodgkin's lymphoma of Waldeyer's ring: clinical features, management, and prognosis of 130 adult patients. Head Neck 2001;23(7):547–558

40. Jacobs C, Hoppe RT. Non-Hodgkin's lymphomas of head and neck extranodal sites. Int J Radiat Oncol Biol Phys 1985;11(2):357–364

41. Saul SH, Kapadia SB. Primary lymphoma of Waldeyer's ring. Clinicopathologic study of 68 cases. Cancer 1985;56(1):157–166

42. Avilés A, Delgado S, Ruiz H, de la Torre A, Guzman R, Talavera A. Treatment of non-Hodgkin's lymphoma of Waldeyer's ring: radiotherapy versus chemotherapy versus combined therapy. Eur J Cancer B Oral Oncol 1996;32B(1):19–23

43. Zucca E, Roggero E, Bertoni F, Conconi A, Cavalli F. Primary extranodal non-Hodgkin's lymphomas. Part 2: Head and neck, central nervous system and other less common sites. Ann Oncol 1999;10(9):1023–1033

44. Liang R, Chiu E, Todd D, Chan TK, Choy D, Loke SL. Combined chemotherapy and radiotherapy for lymphomas of Waldeyer's ring. Oncology 1991;48(5):362–364

45. Harabuchi Y, Tsubota H, Ohguro S, et al. Prognostic factors and treatment outcome in non-Hodgkin's lymphoma of Waldeyer's ring. Acta Oncol 1997;36(4):413–420

46. Economopoulos T, Asprou N, Stathakis N, et al. Primary extranodal non-Hodgkin's lymphoma of the head and neck. Oncology 1992;49(6):484–488

47. Mohammadianpanah M, Omidvai S, Mosalei A, Ahmadloo N. Treatment results of tonsillar lymphoma: a 10-year experience. Ann Hematol 2005;84(4):223–226

48. Nelson ME, Gernon TJ, Taylor JC, McHugh JB, Thorne MC. Pathologic evaluation of routine pediatric tonsillectomy specimens: analysis of cost-effectiveness. Otolaryngol Head Neck Surg 2011;144(5):778–783

49. Gurkaynak M, Cengiz M, Akyurek S, Ozyar E, Atahan IL, Tekuzman G. Waldeyer's ring lymphomas: treatment results and prognostic factors. Am J Clin Oncol 2003;26(5):437–440

50. Yong W, Zhang Y, Zheng W, Wei Y. Prognostic factors and therapeutic efficacy of combined radio-chemotherapy in Waldeyer's ring non-Hodgkin lymphoma. Chin Med J (Engl) 2000;113(2):148–150

51. Laskar S, Bahl G, Muckaden MA, et al. Primary diffuse large B-cell lymphoma of the tonsil: is a higher radiotherapy dose required? Cancer 2007;110(4):816–823

52. Fujitani T, Takahara T, Hattori H, Imajo Y, Ogasawara H. Radiochemotherapy for non-Hodgkin's lymphoma in palatine tonsil. Cancer 1984;54(7):1288–1292

53. Shima N, Kobashi Y, Tsutsui K, et al. Extranodal non-Hodgkin's lymphoma of the head and neck. A clinicopathologic study in the Kyoto-Nara area of Japan. Cancer 1990;66(6):1190–1197

54. Rowley H, McRae RD, Cook JA, Helliwell TR, Husband D, Jones AS. Lymphoma presenting to a head and neck clinic. Clin Otolaryngol Allied Sci 1995;20(2):139–144

55. Gleeson MJ, Bennett MH, Cawson RA. Lymphomas of salivary glands. Cancer 1986;58(3):699–704

56. Mehle ME, Kraus DH, Wood BG, Tubbs R, Tucker HM, Lavertu P. Lymphoma of the parotid gland. Laryngoscope 1993;103(1 Pt 1):17–21

57. Kojima M, Shimizu K, Nishikawa M, et al. Primary salivary gland lymphoma among Japanese: A clinicopathological study of 30 cases. Leuk Lymphoma 2007;48(9):1793–1798

58. Roh JL, Huh J, Suh C. Primary non-Hodgkin's lymphomas of the major salivary glands. J Surg Oncol 2008;97(1):35–39

59. Batsakis JG. Primary lymphomas of the major salivary glands. Ann Otol Rhinol Laryngol 1986;95(1 Pt 1):107–108

60. Anacak Y, Miller RC, Constantinou N, et al. Primary mucosa-associated lymphoid tissue lymphoma of the salivary glands: a multicenter Rare Cancer Network study. Int J Radiat Oncol Biol Phys 2012;82(1):315–320

61. Kalpadakis C, Pangalis GA, Vassilakopoulos TP, et al. Non-gastric extra-nodal marginal zone lymphomas–a single centre experience on 76 patients. Leuk Lymphoma 2008;49:2308–2315

62. DiGiuseppe JA, Corio RL, Westra WH. Lymphoid infiltrates of the salivary glands: pathology, biology and clinical significance. Curr Opin Oncol 1996;8(3):232–237

63. Harris NL. Lymphoid proliferations of the salivary glands. Am J Clin Pathol 1999; 111(1, Suppl 1)S94–S103

64. Isaacson PG. Extranodal lymphomas: the MALT concept. Verh Dtsch Ges Pathol 1992;76:14–23

65. Hyman GA, Wolff M. Malignant lymphomas of the salivary glands. Review of the literature and report of 33 new cases, including four cases associated with the lymphoepithelial lesion. Am J Clin Pathol 1976;65(4):421–438

66. Smedby KE, Hjalgrim H, Askling J, et al. Autoimmune and chronic inflammatory disorders and risk of non-Hodgkin lymphoma by subtype. J Natl Cancer Inst 2006;98(1):51–60

67. Kassan SS, Thomas TL, Moutsopoulos HM, et al. Increased risk of lymphoma in sicca syndrome. Ann Intern Med 1978;89(6):888–892

68. Zintzaras E, Voulgarelis M, Moutsopoulos HM. The risk of lymphoma development in autoimmune diseases: a meta-analysis. Arch Intern Med 2005;165(20):2337–2344

69. Tonami H, Matoba M, Kuginuki Y, et al. Clinical and imaging findings of lymphoma in patients with Sjögren syndrome. J Comput Assist Tomogr 2003;27(4):517–524

70. Sutcliffe N, Inanc M, Speight P, Isenberg D. Predictors of lymphoma development in primary Sjögren's syndrome. Semin Arthritis Rheum 1998;28(2):80–87

71. Zufferey P, Meyer OC, Grossin M, Kahn MF. Primary Sjögren's syndrome (SS) and malignant lymphoma. A retrospective cohort study of 55 patients with SS. Scand J Rheumatol 1995;24(6):342–345

72. Theander E, Vasaitis L, Baecklund E, et al. Lymphoid organisation in labial salivary gland biopsies is a possible predictor for the development of malignant lymphoma in primary Sjögren's syndrome. Ann Rheum Dis 2011;70(8):1363–1368

73. Nime FA, Cooper HS, Eggleston JC. Primary malignant lymphomas of the salivary glands. Cancer 1976;37(2):906–912

74. Hughes JH, Volk EE, Wilbur DC; Cytopathology Resource Committee, College of American Pathologists. Pitfalls in salivary gland fine-needle aspiration cytology: lessons from the College of American Pathologists Interlaboratory Comparison Program in Nongynecologic Cytology. Arch Pathol Lab Med 2005;129(1):26–31

75. Freeman C, Berg JW, Cutler SJ. Occurrence and prognosis of extranodal lymphomas. Cancer 1972;29(1):252–260

76. Wolvius EB, van der Valk P, van der Wal JE, et al. Primary non-Hodgkin's lymphoma of the salivary glands. An analysis of 22 cases. J Oral Pathol Med 1996;25(4):177–181

77. Macht SD, Pett SD, Tsangaris NT. Non-Hodgkin lymphoma of the parotid gland: diagnosis, evaluation, and treatment. Ann Plast Surg 1979;2(1):37–41

78. Fellbaum C, Hansmann ML, Lennert K. Malignant lymphomas of the nasal cavity and paranasal sinuses. Virchows Arch A Pathol Anat Histopathol 1989;414(5):399–405

79. Eichel BS, Harrison EG Jr, Devine KD, Scanlon PW, Brown HA. Primary lymphoma of the nose including a relationship to lethal midline granuloma. Am J Surg 1966;112(4):597–605

80. Ho FC, Choy D, Loke SL, et al. Polymorphic reticulosis and conventional lymphomas of the nose and upper aerodigestive tract: a clinicopathologic study of 70 cases, and immunophenotypic studies of 16 cases. Hum Pathol 1990;21(10):1041–1050

81. Stamenkovic I, Toccanier MF, Kapanci Y. Polymorphic reticulosis (lethal midline granuloma) and lymphomatoid granulomatosis: identical or distinct entities? Virchows Arch A Pathol Anat Histol 1981;390(1):81–91

82. Burston HH. Lethal midline granuloma: is it a pathological entity. Laryngoscope 1959;69(1):1–43

83. Ishii Y, Yamanaka N, Ogawa K, et al. Nasal T-cell lymphoma as a type of so-called "lethal midline granuloma". Cancer 1982;50(11): 2336–2344

84. Michaels L, Gregory MM. Pathology of 'non-healing (midline) granuloma'. J Clin Pathol 1977;30(4):317–327

85. Ratech H, Burke JS, Blayney DW, Sheibani K, Rappaport H. A clinicopathologic study of malignant lymphomas of the nose, paranasal sinuses, and hard palate, including cases of lethal midline granuloma. Cancer 1989;64(12):2525–2531

86. Fechner RE, Lamppin DW. Midline malignant reticulosis. A clinicopathologic entity. Arch Otolaryngol 1972;95(5):467–476

87. Kassel SH, Echevarria RA, Guzzo FP. Midline malignant reticulosis (so-called lethal midline granuloma). Cancer 1969;23(4):920–935

88. Cleary KR, Batsakis JG. Sinonasal lymphomas. Ann Otol Rhinol Laryngol 1994;103(11):911–914

89. Jaffe ES, Chan JK, Su IJ, et al. Report of the Workshop on Nasal and Related Extranodal Angiocentric T/Natural Killer Cell Lymphomas. Definitions, differential diagnosis, and epidemiology. Am J Surg Pathol 1996;20(1):103–111

90. Harris NL, Jaffe ES, Diebold J, et al. World Health Organization classification of neoplastic diseases of the hematopoietic and lymphoid tissues: report of the Clinical Advisory Committee meeting-Airlie House, Virginia, November 1997. J Clin Oncol 1999;17(12):3835–3849

91. Ng CS, Chan JK, Lo ST, Poon YF. Immunophenotypic analysis of non-Hodgkin's lymphomas in Chinese. A study of 75 cases in Hong Kong. Pathology 1986;18(4):419–425

92. Arber DA, Weiss LM, Albújar PF, Chen YY, Jaffe ES. Nasal lymphomas in Peru. High incidence of T-cell immunophenotype and Epstein-Barr virus infection. Am J Surg Pathol 1993;17(4):392–399

93. Liang R, Todd D, Chan TK, et al. Nasal lymphoma. A retrospective analysis of 60 cases. Cancer 1990;66(10):2205–2209

94. Liang R, Todd D, Chan TK, et al. Treatment outcome and prognostic factors for primary nasal lymphoma. J Clin Oncol 1995;13(3): 666–670

95. Avilés A, Díaz NR, Neri N, Cleto S, Talavera A. Angiocentric nasal T/natural killer cell lymphoma: a single centre study of prognostic factors in 108 patients. Clin Lab Haematol 2000;22(4):215–220

96. Cheung MM, Chan JK, Lau WH, et al. Primary non-Hodgkin's lymphoma of the nose and nasopharynx: clinical features, tumor immunophenotype, and treatment outcome in 113 patients. J Clin Oncol 1998;16(1):70–77

97. Campo E, Cardesa A, Alos L, et al. Non-Hodgkin's lymphomas of nasal cavity and paranasal sinuses. An immunohistochemical study. Am J Clin Pathol 1991;96(2):184–190

98. Frierson HF Jr, Mills SE, Innes DJ Jr. Non-Hodgkin's lymphomas of the sinonasal region: histologic subtypes and their clinicopathologic features. Am J Clin Pathol 1984;81(6):721–727

99. Chan JK, Yip TT, Tsang WY, et al. Detection of Epstein-Barr viral RNA in malignant lymphomas of the upper aerodigestive tract. Am J Surg Pathol 1994;18(9):938–946

100. Harabuchi Y, Yamanaka N, Kataura A, et al. Epstein-Barr virus in nasal T-cell lymphomas in patients with lethal midline granuloma. Lancet 1990;335(8682):128–130

101. Frierson HF Jr, Innes DJ Jr, Mills SE, Wick MR. Immunophenotypic analysis of sinonasal non-Hodgkin's lymphomas. Hum Pathol 1989;20(7):636–642

102. Cuadra-Garcia I, Proulx GM, Wu CL, et al. Sinonasal lymphoma: a clinicopathologic analysis of 58 cases from the Massachusetts General Hospital. Am J Surg Pathol 1999;23(11):1356–1369

103. Proulx GM, Caudra-Garcia I, Ferry J, et al. Lymphoma of the nasal cavity and paranasal sinuses: treatment and outcome of early-stage disease. Am J Clin Oncol 2003;26(1):6–11

104. Abbondanzo SL, Wenig BM. Non-Hodgkin's lymphoma of the sinonasal tract. A clinicopathologic and immunophenotypic study of 120 cases. Cancer 1995;75(6):1281–1291

105. Chan JK, Ng CS, Lau WH, Lo ST. Most nasal/nasopharyngeal lymphomas are peripheral T-cell neoplasms. Am J Surg Pathol 1987;11(6):418–429

106. Lippman SM, Miller TP, Spier CM, Slymen DJ, Grogan TM. The prognostic significance of the immunotype in diffuse large-cell lymphoma: a comparative study of the T-cell and B-cell phenotype. Blood 1988;72(2):436–441

107. Stein RS, Greer JP, Flexner JM, et al. Large-cell lymphomas: clinical and prognostic features. J Clin Oncol 1990;8(8):1370–1379

108. Cheung MM, Chan JK, Lau WH, Ngan RK, Foo WW. Early stage nasal NK/T-cell lymphoma: clinical outcome, prognostic factors, and the effect of treatment modality. Int J Radiat Oncol Biol Phys 2002;54(1):182–190

109. Hausdorff J, Davis E, Long G, et al. Non-Hodgkin's lymphoma of the paranasal sinuses: clinical and pathological features, and response to combined-modality therapy. Cancer J Sci Am 1997;3(5):303–311

110. Kim GE, Koom WS, Yang WI, et al. Clinical relevance of three subtypes of primary sinonasal lymphoma characterized by immunophenotypic analysis. Head Neck 2004;26(7):584–593

111. Hatta C, Ogasawara H, Okita J, Kubota A, Ishida M, Sakagami M. Non-Hodgkin's malignant lymphoma of the sinonasal tract—treatment outcome for 53 patients according to REAL classification. Auris Nasus Larynx 2001;28(1):55–60

112. Robbins KT, Fuller LM, Vlasak M, et al. Primary lymphomas of the nasal cavity and paranasal sinuses. Cancer 1985;56(4):814–819

113. Yamanaka N, Harabuchi Y, Sambe S, et al. Non-Hodgkin's lymphoma of Waldeyer's ring and nasal cavity. Clinical and immunologic aspects. Cancer 1985;56(4):768–776

114. Li CC, Tien HF, Tang JL, et al. Treatment outcome and pattern of failure in 77 patients with sinonasal natural killer/T-cell or T-cell lymphoma. Cancer 2004;100(2):366–375

115. Logsdon MD, Ha CS, Kavadi VS, Cabanillas F, Hess MA, Cox JD. Lymphoma of the nasal cavity and paranasal sinuses: improved outcome and altered prognostic factors with combined modality therapy. Cancer 1997;80(3):477–488

116. Li YX, Coucke PA, Li JY, et al. Primary non-Hodgkin's lymphoma of the nasal cavity: prognostic significance of paranasal extension and the role of radiotherapy and chemotherapy. Cancer 1998;83(3):449–456

117. Kim TM, Park YH, Lee SY, et al. Local tumor invasiveness is more predictive of survival than International Prognostic Index in stage I(E)/II(E) extranodal NK/T-cell lymphoma, nasal type. Blood 2005;106(12):3785–3790

118. Lee J, Suh C, Park YH, et al. Extranodal natural killer T-cell lymphoma, nasal-type: a prognostic model from a retrospective multicenter study. J Clin Oncol 2006;24(4):612–618

119. You JY, Chi KH, Yang MH, et al. Radiation therapy versus chemotherapy as initial treatment for localized nasal natural killer (NK)/T-cell lymphoma: a single institute survey in Taiwan. Ann Oncol 2004;15(4):618–625

120. Li YX, Yao B, Jin J, et al. Radiotherapy as primary treatment for stage IE and IIE nasal natural killer/T-cell lymphoma. J Clin Oncol 2006;24(1):181–189

121. Kim GE, Lee SW, Chang SK, et al. Combined chemotherapy and radiation versus radiation alone in the management of localized angiocentric lymphoma of the head and neck. Radiother Oncol 2001;61(3):261–269

122. Kim K, Chie EK, Kim CW, Kim IH, Park CI. Treatment outcome of angiocentric T-cell and NK/T-cell lymphoma, nasal type: radiotherapy versus chemoradiotherapy. Jpn J Clin Oncol 2005;35(1):1–5

123. Miller TP, Dahlberg S, Cassady JR, et al. Chemotherapy alone compared with chemotherapy plus radiotherapy for localized intermediate- and high-grade non-Hodgkin's lymphoma. N Engl J Med 1998;339(1):21–26

124. Guo Y, Lu JJ, Ma X, et al. Combined chemoradiation for the management of nasal natural killer (NK)/T-cell lymphoma: elucidating the significance of systemic chemotherapy. Oral Oncol 2008;44(1):23–30

125. Widder S, Pasieka JL. Primary thyroid lymphomas. Curr Treat Options Oncol 2004;5(4):307–313

126. Graff-Baker A, Roman SA, Thomas DC, Udelsman R, Sosa JA. Prognosis of primary thyroid lymphoma: demographic, clinical, and pathologic predictors of survival in 1,408 cases. Surgery 2009;146(6):1105–1115

127. Holm LE, Blomgren H, Löwhagen T. Cancer risks in patients with chronic lymphocytic thyroiditis. N Engl J Med 1985;312(10):601–604

128. Derringer GA, Thompson LD, Frommelt RA, Bijwaard KE, Heffess CS, Abbondanzo SL. Malignant lymphoma of the thyroid gland: a clinicopathologic study of 108 cases. Am J Surg Pathol 2000;24(5):623–639

129. Kossev P, Livolsi V. Lymphoid lesions of the thyroid: review in light of the revised European-American lymphoma classification and upcoming World Health Organization classification. Thyroid 1999;9(12):1273–1280

130. Rossi D. Thyroid lymphoma: beyond antigen stimulation. Leuk Res 2009;33(5):607–609

131. Graff-Baker A, Sosa JA, Roman SA. Primary thyroid lymphoma: a review of recent developments in diagnosis and histology-driven treatment. Curr Opin Oncol 2010;22(1):17–22

132. Basu S, Li G, Bural G, Alavi A. Fluorodeoxyglucose positron emission tomography (FDG-PET) and PET/computed tomography imaging characteristics of thyroid lymphoma and their potential clinical utility. Acta Radiol 2009;50(2):201–204

133. Mikosch P, Würtz FG, Gallowitsch HJ, Kresnik E, Lind P. F-18-FDG-PET in a patient with Hashimoto's thyroiditis and MALT lymphoma recurrence of the thyroid. Wien Med Wochenschr 2003;153(3-4):89–92

134. Matsuda M, Sone H, Koyama H, Ishiguro S. Fine-needle aspiration cytology of malignant lymphoma of the thyroid. Diagn Cytopathol 1987;3(3):244–249

135. Morgen EK, Geddie W, Boerner S, Bailey D, Santos GdaC. The role of fine-needle aspiration in the diagnosis of thyroid lymphoma: a retrospective study of nine cases and review of published series. J Clin Pathol 2010;63(2):129–133

136. Cha C, Chen H, Westra WH, Udelsman R. Primary thyroid lymphoma: can the diagnosis be made solely by fine-needle aspiration? Ann Surg Oncol 2002;9(3):298–302

137. Doria R, Jekel JF, Cooper DL. Thyroid lymphoma. The case for combined modality therapy. Cancer 1994;73(1):200–206

138. Tsang RW, Gospodarowicz MK, Pintilie M, et al. Localized mucosa-associated lymphoid tissue lymphoma treated with radiation therapy has excellent clinical outcome. J Clin Oncol 2003;21(22):4157–4164

139. Thieblemont C, Mayer A, Dumontet C, et al. Primary thyroid lymphoma is a heterogeneous disease. J Clin Endocrinol Metab 2002;87(1):105–111

140. Pyke CM, Grant CS, Habermann TM, et al. Non-Hodgkin's lymphoma of the thyroid: is more than biopsy necessary? World J Surg 1992;16(4):604–609, discussion 609–610

141. Sakorafas GH, Kokkoris P, Farley DR. Primary thyroid lymphoma (correction of lympoma): diagnostic and therapeutic dilemmas. Surg Oncol 2010;19(4):e124–e129

142. Ansell SM, Habermann TM, Hoyer JD, Strickler JG, Chen MG, McDonald TJ. Primary laryngeal lymphoma. Laryngoscope 1997;107(11 Pt 1):1502–1506

143. Nayak JV, Cook JR, Molina JT, et al. Primary lymphoma of the larynx: new diagnostic and therapeutic approaches. ORL J Otorhinolaryngol Relat Spec 2003;65(6):321–326

144. Kania RE, Hartl DM, Badoual C, Le Maignan C, Brasnu DF. Primary mucosa-associated lymphoid tissue (MALT) lymphoma of the larynx. Head Neck 2005;27(3):258–262

145. Steffen A, Jafari C, Merz H, Galle J, Berger G. Subglottic MALT lymphoma of the larynx—more attention to the glottis. In Vivo 2007;21(4):695–698

146. Markou K, Goudakos J, Constantinidis J, Kostopoulos I, Vital V, Nikolaou A. Primary laryngeal lymphoma: report of 3 cases and review of the literature. Head Neck 2010;32(4):541–549

147. Cheung MC, Pantanowitz L, Dezube BJ. AIDS-related malignancies: emerging challenges in the era of highly active antiretroviral therapy. Oncologist 2005;10(6):412–426

148. Grulich AE, Vajdic CM, Cozen W. Altered immunity as a risk factor for non-Hodgkin lymphoma. Cancer Epidemiol Biomarkers Prev 2007;16(3):405–408

149. Dal Maso L, Serraino D, Franceschi S. Epidemiology of AIDS-related tumours in developed and developing countries. Eur J Cancer 2001;37(10):1188–1201

150. Dal Maso L, Franceschi S. Epidemiology of non-Hodgkin lymphomas and other haemolymphopoietic neoplasms in people with AIDS. Lancet Oncol 2003;4(2):110–119

151. Lim ST, Karim R, Tulpule A, Nathwani BN, Levine AM. Prognostic factors in HIV-related diffuse large-cell lymphoma: before versus after highly active antiretroviral therapy. J Clin Oncol 2005;23(33):8477–8482

152. Levine AM. Acquired immunodeficiency syndrome-related lymphoma. Blood 1992;80(1):8–20

153. Ziegler JL, Beckstead JA, Volberding PA, et al. Non-Hodgkin's lymphoma in 90 homosexual men. Relation to generalized lymphadenopathy and the acquired immunodeficiency syndrome. N Engl J Med 1984;311(9):565–570

154. Knowles DM, Chamulak GA, Subar M, et al. Lymphoid neoplasia associated with the acquired immunodeficiency syndrome (AIDS). The New York University Medical Center experience with 105 patients (1981-1986). Ann Intern Med 1988;108(5):744–753

155. Lowenthal DA, Straus DJ, Campbell SW, Gold JW, Clarkson BD, Koziner B. AIDS-related lymphoid neoplasia. The Memorial Hospital experience. Cancer 1988;61(11):2325–2337

156. Ioachim HL, Dorsett B, Cronin W, Maya M, Wahl S. Acquired immunodeficiency syndrome-associated lymphomas: clinical, pathologic, immunologic, and viral characteristics of 111 cases. Hum Pathol 1991;22(7):659–673

157. Singh B, Poluri A, Shaha AR, Michuart P, Har-El G, Lucente FE. Head and neck manifestations of non-Hodgkin's lymphoma in human immunodeficiency virus-infected patients. Am J Otolaryngol 2000;21(1):10–13

158. Mounier N, Spina M, Gisselbrecht C. Modern management of non-Hodgkin lymphoma in HIV-infected patients. Br J Haematol 2007;136(5):685–698

159. Palmieri C, Treibel T, Large O, Bower M. AIDS-related non-Hodgkin's lymphoma in the first decade of highly active antiretroviral therapy. QJM 2006;99(12):811–826

160. Opelz G, Döhler B. Lymphomas after solid organ transplantation: a collaborative transplant study report. Am J Transplant 2004;4(2):222–230

161. Nalesnik MA, Starzl TE. Epstein-Barr virus, infectious mononucleosis, and posttransplant lymphoproliferative disorders. Transplant Sci 1994;4(1):61–79

162. EBPG Expert Group on Renal Transplantation. European best practice guidelines for renal transplantation. Section IV: Long-term management of the transplant recipient. IV.6.1. Cancer risk after renal transplantation. Post-transplant lymphoproliferative disease (PTLD): prevention and treatment. Nephrol Dial Transplant 2002;17(Suppl 4):31–33, 35–36

163. Lim WH, Russ GR, Coates PT. Review of Epstein-Barr virus and post-transplant lymphoproliferative disorder post-solid organ transplantation. Nephrology (Carlton) 2006;11(4):355–366

164. Harris NL, Ferry JA, Swerdlow SH. Posttransplant lymphoproliferative disorders: summary of Society for Hematopathology Workshop. Semin Diagn Pathol 1997;14(1):8–14

165. Gourin CG, Terris DJ. Head and neck cancer in transplant recipients. Curr Opin Otolaryngol Head Neck Surg 2004;12(2):122–126

166. Pollard JD, Hanasono MM, Mikulec AA, Le QT, Terris DJ. Head and neck cancer in cardiothoracic transplant recipients. Laryngoscope 2000;110(8):1257–1261

24   Benign Aggressive Jaw Tumors

Eric R. Carlson and G. E. Ghali

Core Messages

- Although slow-growing, benign odontogenic tumors can be as destructive and life threatening as the more rapidly growing malignant tumors of the head and neck.

- Like other head and neck neoplasms, odontogenic tumors exhibit growth patterns and doubling times that are a function of the interaction of cytokines and tumor suppressor genes related to proliferation versus apoptosis.

- Langerhans cell histiocytosis represents a group of benign neoplastic processes comprising three morphologically similar lesions: eosinophilic granuloma, Hand-Schüller-Christian disease, and Letterer-Siwe disease.

- Fibro-osseous lesions frequently require the review of a radiograph of the pathologic process for proper diagnosis.

The designation of a benign or malignant classification to a pathologic process of the jaws is based on specific histologic criteria. These criteria include the histologic presence or absence of necrosis and mitotic figures as well as a basic understanding of the specific entity under consideration. The term *aggressive* has most commonly been used to describe malignant neoplasms because of their ability to grow quickly and invade surrounding structures that may result in significant local growth, metastatic disease, and death of the patient. This notwithstanding, the jaws are the site of many locally aggressive benign neoplasms that may also result in significant hard and soft tissue destruction and deformation of the patient (**Fig. 24.1**), with resultant loss of function and possible airway obstruction. Aggressive benign processes of the jaws may be distinguished from their malignant counterparts by the lack of skin invasion, the lack of epineural infiltration, and the observed enigma of aggressive growth despite slow growth as may occur in many of these benign processes. In some cases, benign tumors of the jaws may be more aggressive, destructive, and deforming than some of their malignant counterparts, despite the observation that the benign tumors grow more slowly than malignant tumors. This concept is not only a paradox but also highly controversial, poorly understood, and often disputed. In addition, the slow growth of many aggressive benign neoplasms of the jaws has often resulted in subtherapeutic conservative surgical treatment with the thought that a recurrence will be diagnosed in an early time frame with the performance of more radical surgery.

Benign neoplasms are dysmorphic tissue proliferations that have the capacity for persistent, autonomous growth. These tumors have the ability to progress unless completely removed. When completely removed, their reappearance is generally considered to not be possible, with a cure realized.

When benign jaw tumors reappear following surgical extirpation, they are often incorrectly described as recurrent when, in fact, they really represent persistent disease because of earlier incomplete removal. In addition, the mere mention of a metastatic benign tumor of the jaws is seemingly a contradiction of terms, despite being occasionally diagnosed. Malignant neoplasms, by distinction, are best described as dysmorphic proliferations of tissues that have the capacity for autonomous growth, and metastasis, as well. The genetic alterations present in malignant tumors allow for a change in doubling times and for the development of metastatic disease after showing no previous capability for metastasis.[1] The genetic alterations present in benign tumors are generally not susceptible to mutations, thereby conferring a relatively stable clinical course and prohibiting the development of metastatic disease. This genetic stability is what translates to relative consistency regarding fast versus slow growth, locally aggressive versus indolent infiltration of the surrounding tissues, and other clinical features of benign tumors. As mentioned earlier, a paradox exists with regard to the aggressive behavior of these benign processes and their rate of growth.

Growth of all pathologic lesions occurs in the cell cycle as a function of cell proliferation versus apoptosis (**Fig. 24.2**). Neoplasia is understood, therefore, as a cell cycle disease.[2] Alterations of genes that control the cell cycle are essential for the development of neoplastic disease. As such, neoplasia is characterized by a series of genetic alterations involving both oncogenes and tumor suppressor genes. Cell division comprises four phases including gap 1 (G1), DNA synthesis (S), gap 2 (G2), and mitosis (M). A major molecular event is the progression from the G1 to the S phase. Genetic alterations, if unrepaired in the G1 phase, may be carried into the S phase and perpetuated in subsequent cell divisions. This G1-S checkpoint is normally regulated by a well-coordinated and

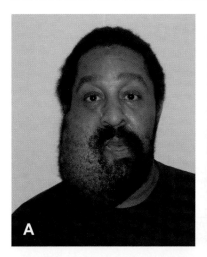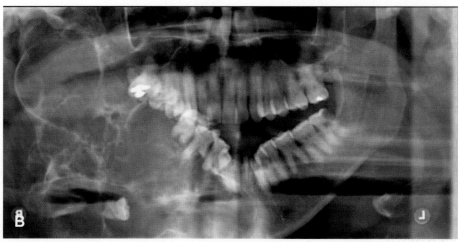

Figure 24.1 A very large ameloblastoma of the mandible exhibiting clinical signs of severe facial deformation (A) and radiographic evidence of significant bone destruction (B). This tumor had been present for at least 20 years according to the patient.

complex system of protein interactions whose balance and function are critical to normal cell division. Over production of inducing proteins or under production of inhibitor proteins may encourage the development of neoplastic disease. For example, *p53*, located on chromosome 17p13.1, is a tumor suppressor gene in its wild-type form. Normal *p53* acts as a "molecular policeman" in its monitoring of the integrity of the genome. If DNA is damaged, wild-type *p53* accumulates and inhibits replication to permit extra time for repair mechanisms to act. If repair fails, *p53* may trigger cell suicide by apoptosis.[3] As such, *p53* serves as a negative regulator at the G1-S checkpoint. A mutation of *p53*

can be expected to allow cells to proceed into the S phase of the cell cycle before DNA can be repaired, thus encouraging the development of a tumor.

The future understanding of the involvement of *p53* in tumor biology began in 1969 when Li et al reviewed medical records and death certificates of 648 childhood rhabdomyosarcoma patients and identified four families in which siblings or cousins had a childhood sarcoma.[4] These four families also had striking histories of breast cancer and other neoplasms, suggesting a new familial cancer syndrome of diverse tumors. This syndrome took the name of Li–Fraumeni syndrome. Since the original description of

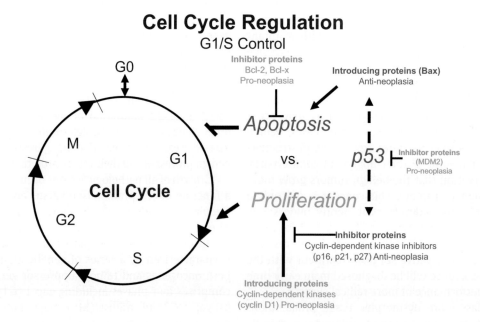

Figure 24.2 The cell cycle—a process of proliferation versus apoptosis (programmed cell death). A complex series of molecular events permits the proliferation of human tumors.

Reprinted with permission from: Guild for Scientific Advancement in Oral and Maxillofacial Surgery. Carlson ER, August M, Ruggiero SL. Locally aggressive benign processes of the oral and maxillofacial region. *Selected Readings in Oral and Maxillofacial Surgery* 2004.

the syndrome, systematic studies and anecdotal reports have confirmed its existence in various geographic and ethnic groups. The spectrum of cancers in this syndrome has been determined to include breast carcinomas, soft tissue sarcomas, brain tumors, osteosarcoma, leukemia, and adrenocortical carcinoma.[5] Possible component tumors of this syndrome include melanoma, gonadal germ cell tumors, and carcinomas of the lung, pancreas, and prostate. These diverse tumor types in family members characteristically develop at unusually early ages, and multiple primary tumors are frequent. The molecular etiology of this syndrome is now known to be related to a germ line mutation of one *p53* allele. Patients are therefore predisposed to develop malignant tumors as only one additional "hit" is required to inactivate the second, normal allele. Such individuals are said to have a 25-fold greater chance of developing a cancer by the of age 50 years compared with the general population.[6] Once believed to be very unique, the understanding of *p53* increased in 1997 with the discovery of another tumor suppressor gene called *p73*.[7,8] Located on chromosome 1p36, this gene encodes a protein that bears many similarities to *p53*. It has a DNA-binding domain that resembles the corresponding region of *p53*, and similar to the latter it can cause cell cycle arrest as well as apoptosis under appropriate conditions.[7,8]

As seen in **Fig. 24.2**, the expression of Bcl-2 and Bcl-x may also encourage neoplasia by inhibiting apoptosis, and MDM2 may directly inhibit p53. The *Bcl-2* proto-oncogene was initially discovered at the break point of the t(14;18) chromosomal translocation in follicular lymphomas.[9] *Bcl-2* gene product protects tumor cells by blocking postmitotic differentiation from apoptosis, thus maintaining a stem cell pool. *Bcl-x* gene, a *Bcl-2* homolog, encodes two proteins: a long form, Bcl-x$_L$, and a short form, Bcl-x$_S$.[10] Bcl-x$_L$ protein, structurally and functionally similar to Bcl-2, has antiapoptotic activity, while Bcl-x$_S$ protein promotes apoptosis by inhibiting Bcl-2. *Bax* gene, an additional Bcl-2 homolog, encodes a protein that induces apoptosis. Bax protein regulates apoptosis by interacting with Bcl-2 or Bcl-x$_L$ proteins. The *MDM2* oncogene on chromosome 12q13–14 encodes a nuclear phosphoprotein that interacts with both mutant and wild-type *p53*.[11] Its transcription is enhanced by wild-type *p53* through the existence of a *p53*-binding site in an intronic sequence in the *MDM2* gene. Both proteins regulate each other, forming an autoregulatory feedback loop that in turn regulates the transcriptional function of p53 protein and subsequent expression of the *MDM2* gene. The *MDM2* gene product can inhibit p53-mediated transactivation by masking the N-terminal acidic transactivation domain of p53 protein. High levels of MDM2 may inactivate the tumor suppressor activity of p53 by complexing to it. Therefore, deregulation of MDM2 function may be closely associated with tumorigenesis and/or tumor development. While the interaction of various cytokines with the cell cycle originally focused on malignant tumors, subsequent research identified that these cytokines and tumor suppressor genes are involved in molecular events related to benign tumor development, including many benign tumors of the jaws.

Proliferating cell nuclear antigen is a cell cycle related antigen and has been used for the evaluation of the proliferation ability of many types of tumors and their recurrences. The detection of Ki-67 antigen is also a means to assess tumor cell proliferation.[12] The monoclonal Ki-67 antibody was originally produced to a nuclear antigen in Hodgkin and Reed Sternberg cells, which was expressed in all proliferating cells during the G1, S, G2, and M phases of the cell cycle, but was absent in the G0 phase of the cell cycle.[13] The observation of low rates of proliferating cell nuclear antigen and Ki-67 positivity in nuclei of some locally aggressive benign tumors of the jaws supports the observation of their slow growth. This observation would also support the perceived paradox of slow yet aggressive growth.

Surgery for locally aggressive benign processes of the jaws is a function of the biologic behavior of the lesion. The principles of linear margins and anatomic barrier margins are important to consider. Linear margin principles refer to the inclusion of uninvolved soft and hard tissues surrounding the tumor specimen. Their inclusion occurs because of the understanding that tumors are not perfectly demarcated entities. Rather, tumors extend beyond their clinical and/or radiographic margins, such that inclusion of normal tissue assists in the likelihood of complete removal. Anatomic barriers are soft and hard tissues that surround a tumor and attempt to forestall its growth and infiltration of uninvolved tissues. The best known example is a capsule. Capsules surround some, but not all benign tumors. Unencapsulated benign neoplasms include the ameloblastoma and the pleomorphic adenoma. Other anatomic barriers include cortical bone, periosteum, muscle, mucosa, dermis, and skin. Locally aggressive benign tumors of the jaws often grow slowly such that violation of the skin does not occur (**Fig. 24.1**). Epidermal cells are thought to regenerate every 8 days, compared with a benign jaw tumor doubling time of several months or years. As such, the skin is able to maintain its integrity in the presence of the developing tumor and does not become violated by the tumor. True neoplasia is removed with attention to linear margins and anatomic barrier margins. The specific linear margin is a function of the histopathologic diagnosis of the neoplasm. Further, the removal of one uninvolved anatomic barrier margin with the tumor specimen seems to ensure complete removal (**Fig. 24.3**). An ameloblastoma that appears to be confined to the medullary component of the mandible, for example, may be able to be resected in a subperiosteal fashion. This notwithstanding, the surgeon may wish to proceed with a supraperiosteal dissection because of the fact that computed tomography (CT) scans may show intact cortical bone throughout, while the cortex may be perforated between CT cuts. The routine sacrifice of periosteum under such circumstances prevents entrance into tumor with inadvertent spilling.

Odontogenic Tumors

Odontogenic tumors represent a diverse group of pathologic entities that are of great interest to all surgeons of the head and neck. While a majority of these processes

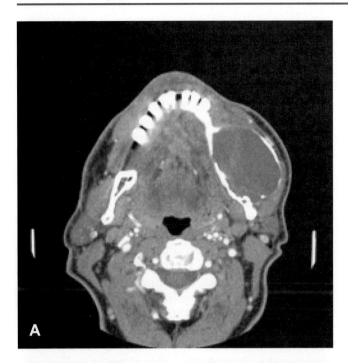

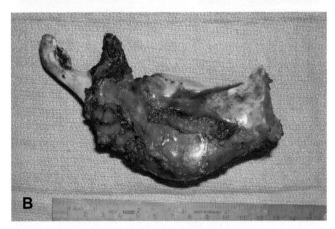

Figure 24.3 An ameloblastoma of the left mandible. The computed tomography scans show possible perforation of the lingual cortex of the mandible (A). As such, the anatomic barrier of periosteum and mylohyoid muscle was included on the medial aspect of the tumor specimen (B) so as to permit a clean margin in this area.

are centrally located neoplasms, some are believed to more accurately represent hamartomatous proliferations, and some may occur peripherally in soft tissue. True odontogenic neoplasms demonstrate varying inductive interactions between odontogenic epithelium and odontogenic ectomesenchyme. This ectomesenchyme was formerly referred to as mesenchyme as it was thought to be derived from the mesodermal layer of the embryo. It is now known and accepted that this tissue differentiates from the ectodermal layer in the cephalic portion of the embryo; hence, the designation ectomesenchyme.

Several of the aggressive odontogenic neoplasms represent prototypical examples of principles for benign tumor surgery of the jaws. These include the ameloblastoma,

odontogenic myxoma, and the Pindborg tumor. They are true neoplasms that require attention to detail regarding bony linear margins and the surrounding anatomic barriers when performing extirpative tumor surgery. They also exemplify the observed paradox of aggressive local growth despite slow growth.

Ameloblastoma

The ameloblastoma is a benign tumor of the jaws and surrounding soft tissues that is characteristically locally aggressive. The literature and our experience indicate that these neoplasms are capable of significant destruction and deformation of facial structures, and occasionally death.[14] The infiltration of surrounding soft and hard tissues of the face by the ameloblastoma is more outstanding than that accomplished by some malignant neoplasms of this anatomic area. In general terms, the aforementioned comments relate to the solid or multicystic variant of the ameloblastoma that requires a well-executed ablative surgery for cure. This notwithstanding, the unicystic ameloblastoma is, at times, also capable of significant destruction of the jaws. The unicystic ameloblastoma should not, therefore, be clinically underestimated and may require aggressive ablative surgery for cure. The peripheral ameloblastoma is, in contrast, innocuous and relatively indolent, thereby requiring relatively conservative surgery for cure. A review of 3677 cases of ameloblastoma found 2% to be peripheral, 6% to be unicystic, and the remaining 92% to be solid or multicystic.[15] Studies from North American authors find the ameloblastoma to comprise approximately 10% of all odontogenic tumors.[16,17]

Solid or Multicystic Ameloblastoma

The solid or multicystic ameloblastoma is the most common variant of ameloblastoma[15] and the most widely discussed.[18] It is also the variant whose treatment is perhaps the most controversial. As Regezi et al[2] and Gold[18] point out that this tumor was identified well more than a century ago, with either Cassock or Broca being credited with the first scientific report of the ameloblastoma in 1827 and 1868, respectively.[19]

Clinical and Radiographic Features
The solid or multicystic ameloblastoma is primarily a tumor of adults, occurring predominantly in the fourth and fifth decades, with an average age of occurrence of the early 30s[19]. While this variant of ameloblastoma is rare in children, studies document their existence.[20,21] These studies also point to the preponderance of the unicystic variant when a diagnosis of ameloblastoma in children is made. This variant of the ameloblastoma may occur throughout the maxilla or mandible, but has a predilection for the posterior mandible. In a study of 98 ameloblastomas by Mehlisch et al, 91 (93%) were located in the body or ramus of the mandible while 7% occurred in the symphysis.[22] Ueno et al reviewed their

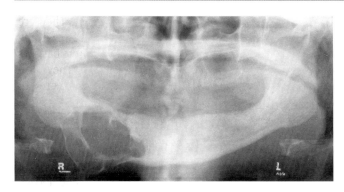

Figure 24.4 An ameloblastoma present in a 27-year-old male who presented with facial swelling. The panoramic radiograph shows a multilocular radiolucency.

findings with 104 ameloblastomas, of which 97 occurred in the mandible.[23] Of the mandibular ameloblastomas, 94 cases (97%) occurred in the molar region, 60 cases (62%) occurred in the ramus, while 28 cases (29%) occurred in the symphysis of the mandible. The maxilla is an infrequent site for the solid or multicystic variant of the ameloblastoma.[24–26] When this tumor involves the maxilla, approximately 90% occur in the posterior maxilla.[19]

The solid or multicystic ameloblastoma is most commonly asymptomatic, but may occasionally produce a painless mass. Pain, tooth mobility, and trismus are less common findings.[23] Radiographically, the solid or multicystic ameloblastoma most commonly appears as a multilocular radiolucency (**Fig. 24.4**). Because these processes are slow growing, the radiographic margins are usually well-defined and sclerotic.

Treatment and Prognosis

Treatment of the solid or multicystic ameloblastoma has been a source of contention in the oral and maxillofacial surgery literature for decades. While most would agree that this neoplasm is aggressive and deserves aggressive surgical management from the outset, there are several authors who advocate conservative treatment initially and reserve radical surgery for recurrences.[27–29] As pointed out previously, labeling tumors that reappear following conservative surgery as recurrences probably represents a misnomer, with persistent disease more accurately describing the clinical outcome. Conservative surgical management of this variant of the ameloblastoma has historically included enucleation and curettage, while aggressive or radical surgery has involved resection. Those who recommended curettage have relied on the belief that ameloblastoma invades cancellous bone but not cortical bone.[30] As pointed out by Carlson,[1] however, the cortical bone represents a competent anatomic barrier that may not be violated by a very small ameloblastoma. Larger tumors, however, show obvious clinical, radiographic, and histologic evidence of cortical bone invasion by the ameloblastoma. It should be clear that the advancing front of the tumor is beyond the radiographic or clinical margin, thereby requiring the inclusion of a linear margin of bone

in the tumor surgery. Other problems associated with curettage of this neoplasm include the violation of one of the first premises of tumor surgery that is to not spill tumor. An enucleation and curettage surgery, by definition, enters the tumor and likely predisposes the patient to persistent disease. It is our contention, therefore, that conservative measures have no role to play in the surgical management of the solid or multicystic ameloblastoma. Resection of the ameloblastoma with negative soft and hard tissue margins should be expected to result in cure of the patient.

In his review of patients with ameloblastoma treated in a variety of ways, Mehlisch et al revealed a "recurrence" rate of 90% for those patients treated with curettage, while infrequent "recurrence" for those patients treated with resection.[22] Sehdev et al reviewed 92 patients with ameloblastoma and noted curettage to be followed by "local recurrence" in 90% of mandibular ameloblastoma and 100% of maxillary ameloblastomas.[26] Equally worrisome was the finding that subsequent resection was able to control 80% of mandibular ameloblastomas and resection of "recurrent" maxillary ameloblastomas was ineffective in controlling the tumor.

In the final analysis, terms such as radical or conservative should probably not be used to describe the treatment of the ameloblastoma. A scientific understanding of this tumor is that it is a slow-growing, aggressive, benign neoplasm that is best controlled and cured with a resection with approximately 1.0 cm bony linear margins.[31] The surgeon may wish to verify the bony linear margin with an intraoperative specimen radiograph so as to provide security that a sufficient bone margin was sacrificed while the patient is still generally anesthetized (**Fig. 24.5**). Close bone margins noted on the specimen radiograph may be addressed with additional resection of bone. Cure of the patient should be realized if tumor is noted histologically to be well-contained within included anatomic barriers on the specimen. Under such circumstances, patients can be subsequently reconstructed and fully rehabilitated dentally. Attempts to control this tumor with more conservative measures compromise these objectives. Salvage with radiation therapy has been described for the management of ameloblastoma.[32,33] Once thought to be radioresistant, the ameloblastoma has been proved to respond to radiation therapy in limited series. The value of such therapy is realized in those cases where a full surgical excision would be technically difficult because of bulk and local invasion or where other medical factors, including age, would make radical surgery inappropriate. In the review by Atkinson et al,[32] 2 of the 10 patients underwent an attempt at surgical control of the tumors, yet with incomplete excision. As such, postoperative radiation therapy was offered, and the patients showed no evidence of disease at 30 and 60 months postoperatively. Of the remaining 8 patients, 6 showed no evidence of disease at a range of 1 to 10 years following the delivery of radiation therapy without surgical intervention. In 2 of these 8 patients, a residual mass was noted long after the conclusion of radiation therapy. We believe that radiation therapy should not be necessary as part of the therapy for ameloblastoma when primary surgery is executed properly. Radiation therapy may be considered for use, however, in the postoperative management of relatively nonresectable tumors that have previously been subtherapeutically managed with enucleation and curettage surgeries (**Fig. 24.6**).

Pathogenetic mechanisms of the solid or multicystic ameloblastoma include the expression of Bcl-2[10,34] and MDM2.[11] In their review of 25 surgical specimens of ameloblastoma by Mitsuyasu et al,[34] 12 of which were unicystic ameloblastomas, and 13 of which were solid or multicystic tumors, all were noted to express Bcl-2 protein, mainly in the outer layer of tumor cells. The stellate reticulum and squamoid cells were negative. In addition to inhibiting apoptosis, the Bcl-2 protein was felt to play a role in maintaining the stem-cell population in the peripheral layers of the tumor nests from which proliferating cells are recruited. Kumamoto and Ooya[10] studied the expression of Bcl-2 and Bax proteins in various types of ameloblastoma. The findings were the presence of Bcl-2 protein expression in ameloblastomas in the peripheral cells neighboring the basement membranes. Bcl-x protein was distributed similarly to Bcl-2 protein, but was expressed more extensively than Bcl-2 protein. Reactivity for bax protein was

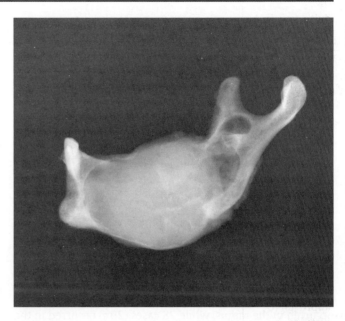

Figure 24.5   A specimen radiograph of an ameloblastoma resection showing at least 1 cm linear bony margins in the proximal and distal aspects of the resection. The specimen radiograph provides an intraoperative assessment of the adequacy of the specimen's bone margins.

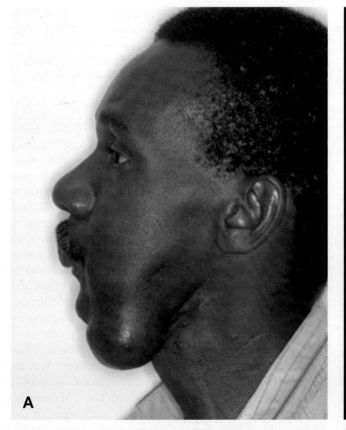

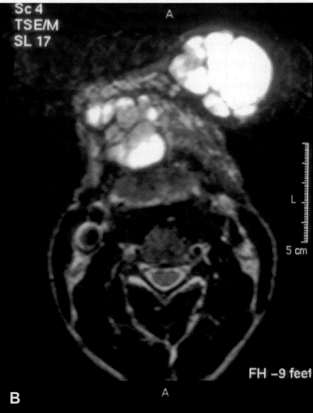

Figure 24.6   The clinical appearance (A) and magnetic resonance imaging (B) of a patient following two enucleation and curettage surgeries for ameloblastoma of the mandible. At this time, he displays soft tissue persistence of his tumor in the facial skin. In addition, substantial floor of mouth and pharyngeal extension of the tumor was noted. The patient underwent a skin sacrificing wide excision of this persistent tumor followed by the administration of postoperative radiation therapy.

quite low in ameloblastomas. Carvalhais et al[11] examined the expression of MDM2 in 13 ameloblastomas and a variety of other odontogenic lesions. These ameloblastomas showed higher MDM2 expression than radicular cysts, but lower than the two groups of odontogenic keratocysts. This notwithstanding, the presence of MDM2 gene expression by ameloblastomas supports their pathogenesis.

One very important question that has surfaced in the literature is whether or not the ameloblastoma is malignant. Discussions by Willis[35] and Carr and Halperin[36] exemplify this debate. Willis stated that attempts to distinguish between benign and malignant ameloblastoma are futile in that they are all malignant in that they are locally invasive and prone to recur. Carr and Halperin stated that malignant and benign are poor terms when applied generally to the ameloblastoma. Furthermore, they stated that the use of one term versus the other seems secondary to an understanding of how the tumor may behave and to an approach to treatment based upon this understanding. Gold justified his belief that all ameloblastomas are malignant in drawing an analogy between basal cell carcinoma of skin and the ameloblastoma.[37] He indicated that the basal cell carcinoma is slow growing, infiltrative, capable of great destruction of soft tissue and bone, recurrent when not completely eradicated, capable of invading vital structures, seldom metastatic but capable of metastasis, presenting several histologic patterns, and arising from the epithelial skin surface and skin adnexa. He rationalized that if one substitutes oral epithelium for skin surface and dental lamina/enamel organ for skin adnexa, one would be describing the ameloblastoma. Despite his argument, Gold lamented that the long-held traditional belief that the ameloblastoma is benign will be difficult to reverse. Finally, as agreed by most surgeons and pathologists, the ameloblastoma is distinctly aggressive, infiltrative, and unpredictable in its behavior.

Unicystic Ameloblastoma

In 1977, Robinson and Martinez reviewed 20 patients presenting with unilocular cystic lesions whose clinical, radiographic, and growth features were those of dentigerous or primordial cysts.[38] On the basis of morphology, the epithelial islands and portions of the lining epithelium seen in all of the 20 cases were indistinguishable from ameloblastic epithelium, the characteristics of which have been described by Vickers and Gorlin.[39] This feature of the unicystic ameloblastoma has been disputed by Gardner and Corio[40] who indicate that the basal cells are not remarkable and do not fulfill the criteria of Vickers and Gorlin for ameloblastoma.

Clinical and Radiographic Features

A review of the literature would suggest that the term unicystic developed from the observation that most of these lesions were, in fact, unilocular radiographically. Regezi et al[41] has recommended the term *cystic ameloblastoma*

because of the identification of an occasional multilocular lesion. In any event, three well-accepted histologic subtypes of this variant of the ameloblastoma have been noted, including the luminal, intraluminal, and mural subtypes. While the unicystic ameloblastoma in general can be treated conservatively with a high rate of cure, the mural subtype should be discussed separately, owing to its different biologic behavior.[42] With an inherently more aggressive behavior, it is considered one of the locally aggressive benign tumors of the jaws and ought to be treated similarly to the solid or multicystic ameloblastoma.[43]

The average age of occurrence for the unicystic ameloblastoma is the mid-twenties. In general, this is younger than that of the solid or multicystic ameloblastoma. In Robinson and Martinez's series of 20 patients, the mean age was 27.7 years. This finding has been confirmed by other authors.[40,41,44] The site of predilection for this variant of the ameloblastoma is the mandible, with the molar/ramus region being most commonly affected (**Fig. 24.7**). This tumor is frequently associated with an impacted tooth. Eversole found six radiographic patterns in his review of 31 cases of unicystic ameloblastoma.[45] In all six patterns, the lesions were radiolucent and well-defined. Three radiographic patterns were observed in cases where these lesions were associated with impacted third molars, and three radiographic patterns were seen in cases that were not associated with an impacted tooth. Four of the six patterns were distinctly unilocular. The author stressed that any large unilocular or multilocular radiolucency in a child, teenager, or young adult should develop suspicion for the presence of a unicystic ameloblastoma.

Treatment and Prognosis

Historically, the literature regarding the unicystic ameloblastoma has found a much lower rate of "recurrence" following curettage compared with that of the solid or multicystic ameloblastoma. The series by Robinson and Martinez[38] showed a 25% "recurrence" rate following curettage, and Gardner and Corio[41] reported a "recurrence" rate of 10.7% following curettage. In general, the luminal and intraluminal variants of the unicystic ameloblastoma are readily cured with an enucleation and curettage surgery

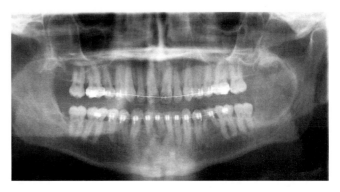

Figure 24.7 A unicystic ameloblastoma of the left mandible presenting as a unilocular radiolucency.

(**Fig. 24.8**). The mural variant of the unicystic ameloblastoma is, because of its anatomic location, less likely to be cured with this type of surgery. Most of the studies discussing the unicystic ameloblastoma do not separate the mural variant from the more favorable luminal and intraluminal variants. As such, we believe that the inclusion of the mural variant in discussion of cure rates negatively impacts the cure rates of the unicystic ameloblastoma as a whole. In other words, the luminal and intraluminal variants of the unicystic ameloblastoma are highly curable lesions when performing an enucleation and curettage surgery. The mural variant of the unicystic ameloblastoma, however, is truly a locally aggressive benign neoplasm of the jaws whose biologic behavior parallels that of the solid or multicystic ameloblastoma. As such, the mural subtype of the unicystic ameloblastoma should be treated with resection[34,43] (**Fig. 24.9**). As has been pointed out, a definitive diagnosis of the mural subtype of the unicystic ameloblastoma may occasionally be made following an enucleation and curettage surgery, under which circumstances the surgeon may wish to adopt close follow-up rather than committing the patient to a return to the operating room for resection. Serial panoramic radiographs should be obtained at regular intervals so as to promptly diagnose the presence of persistent disease with subsequent resection. If the diagnosis of a mural subtype of the unicystic ameloblastoma is made based on incisional biopsy, we recommend primary aggressive management with resection.

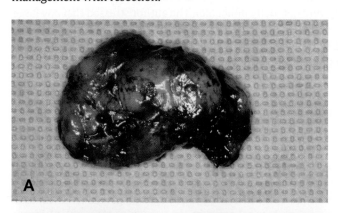

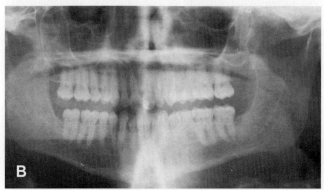

Figure 24.8   The tumor depicted in **Fig. 24.7** was treated with enucleation and curettage (A). The 3-year postoperative radiograph demonstrates bone regeneration without signs of persistent disease (B).

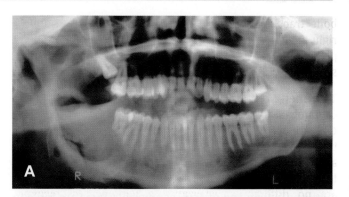

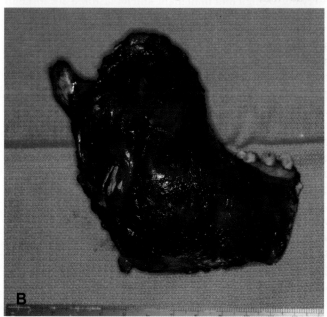

Figure 24.9   A unicystic ameloblastoma, mural subtype, of the mandible. The panoramic radiograph (A) shows a destructive, expansile process of the right mandible. A disarticulation resection was required for curative therapy (B).

Odontogenic Myxoma

The odontogenic myxoma is the second broad category of odontogenic tumor that exemplifies the locally aggressive benign tumor classification. This uncommon benign neoplasm is thought to be derived from ectomesenchyme and histologically resembles the dental papilla of the developing tooth. These tumors represent between 3 and 5% of all odontogenic tumors.[16,17]

Clinical and Radiographic Features

Odontogenic myxomas are most common in the second and third decades, with a range of approximately 5 to 72 years of age.[46] One very unusual case, however, has been reported in a 17-month-old child.[47] The odontogenic myxoma may occur in any area of the jaws with some studies identifying more tumors located in the maxilla, and some reporting more tumors located in the mandible.[46] From a radiographic standpoint, large, multilocular tumors are commonly reported, with a characteristic pattern of very fine or wispy bone trabeculae within the radiolucent defects, often at right angles to one another (**Fig. 24.10**). This feature is not pathognomonic for the odontogenic myxoma, but highly suggestive of this diagnosis.

Treatment and Prognosis

Odontogenic myxomas should be placed in the same category of aggressiveness, ability to infiltrate normal, surrounding tissues, and the ability to persist if treated conservatively as occurs with the solid or multicystic ameloblastoma. In so far as these characteristics are concerned, there are no differences between the odontogenic myxoma and the solid or multicystic ameloblastoma. As such, we recommend identical treatment, with resection including a 1-cm linear bone margin, confirmed by intraoperative specimen radiographs (**Fig. 24.10**). This notwithstanding, the treatment of the odontogenic myxoma has been recommended to be conservative curettage when the tumor is small, with resection reserved for larger tumors. This recommendation for treatment based on size of a tumor is a misconception of tumor surgery. Treatment should be based on the known biologic behavior of a tumor, a genetically determined attribute. A small tumor has the same potential biologic behavior as a large tumor. The difference is only time. As such, treating a small odontogenic myxoma with a conservative surgery while treating a larger tumor with resection fails to appreciate the biologic behavior of such a tumor. Resection of a small tumor is prudent as it provides curative therapy for the patient, while committing that patient to a smaller reconstruction, either on an immediate or a delayed basis.

The pathogenetic mechanisms of the odontogenic myxoma have not been reported on as extensively as that of the ameloblastoma. One study assessed the overexpression of apoptotic proteins and matrix metalloproteinases in the

odontogenic myxoma.[48] A total of 26 odontogenic myxomas were studied. Specimen slides showed an increase in cells staining positively for antiapoptotic proteins Bcl-2 and Bcl-x. An average of 6.5% of specimen cells was positive for Bcl-2 and 10.4% for Bcl-x. Control tissue showed only 1.1% of cells to be positive for Bcl-2 and 1.2% for Bcl-x. Proapoptotic proteins including Bak and Bax were not detected in tumor or control cells. Ninety percent of tumor cells stained positively for MMP-2 compared with 10% of controls. Specimen and control tissues were negative for MMP-3 and MMP-9.

Pindborg Tumor

The calcifying epithelial odontogenic tumor, or Pindborg tumor, after the oral pathologist who first described the neoplasm, shares numerous features in common with the ameloblastoma and odontogenic myxoma. The tumor is distinctly locally aggressive, and accounts for approximately 1% of all odontogenic tumors.[16,17] Microscopically, there are unique features to the Pindborg tumor, with no resemblance to either the ameloblastoma or odontogenic myxoma.

Clinical and Radiographic Features

The Pindborg tumor is seen in patients ranging in age from the second to the tenth decade with a mean age of approximately 40 years.[2] There appears to be no gender predilection, and the mandible is affected about twice as often as the maxilla. As with the ameloblastoma, the molar/ramus region is the most common site of occurrence of this tumor. Painless expansion of the jaws, often noted serendipitously, is most common. Radiographically, the tumors are often associated with impacted teeth, and may be unilocular or multilocular. A mixed radio-opaque/radiolucent pattern is most typical (**Fig. 24.11**).

Treatment and Prognosis

Treatment recommendations for the Pindborg tumor have ranged from simple enucleation and curettage surgeries to resection, not unlike those for the ameloblastoma and odontogenic myxoma. In 1976, Franklin and Pindborg reported on 113 cases of this tumor.[49] Follow-up information was available for 79 cases. Sixteen recurrences were noted, most commonly in those patients who were treated conservatively with curettage only, enucleation only, or incomplete removal. More aggressive removal with resection resulted in infrequent recurrence.

Langerhans Cell Histiocytosis

Langerhans cell histiocytosis (LCH) is a rare disorder in which lesions contain cells with features similar to the LC of the epidermis. Formerly referred to as histiocytosis X, LCH comprises three morphologically similar lesions: eosinophilic granuloma, Hand-Schüller-Christian disease, and Letterer-Siwe disease. The term *histiocyte* refers to two groups of immune cells: (1) macrophages, the primary

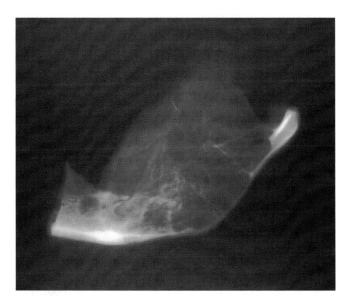

Figure 24.10 A specimen radiograph of a segmental resection of the mandible for odontogenic myxoma. The characteristic radiographic pattern of bone trabeculae at right angles to one another is noted.

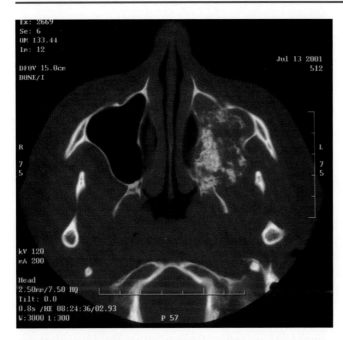

Figure 24.11 The typical mixed radiolucent-radiopaque pattern of the Pindborg tumor. These tumors are destructive and expansile as noted on this computed tomography scan.

antigen-processing cells and (2) dendritic cells, the primary antigen-presenting cells, each of which contributes to an immunocytologic continuum.[50] Recent nosology of the histiocytic disorders places LCH in the category of dendritic cell-related diseases of varied biologic behavior together with juvenile xanthogranuloma and the histiocytomas. Although there are rare malignancies featuring cells with the LC phenotype, malignant LCH is not recognized.[51] The extraordinarily rare malignant disorders are referred to as dendritic cell-related histiocytic sarcomas, LC type.[50] Clinical and radiographic assessment of patients with LCH allows for classification of the disease as follows:

- Eosinophilic granuloma–monostotic or polyostotic involvement without visceral involvement.
- Hand-Schüller-Christian disease–involvement of bone, skin, and viscera.
- Letterer-Siwe disease–prominent cutaneous, visceral, and bone marrow involvement occurring mainly in infants.

Letter-Siwe disease is a highly lethal form of LCH that affects young children and has a rapidly declining course. Its cardinal clinical features include hepatosplenomegaly and anemia. Head and neck manifestations are less common than those noted in eosinophilic granuloma and Hand-Schüller-Christian disease, so Letterer-Siwe disease will not be reviewed in this chapter. Furthermore, because eosinophilic granuloma represents the prototypical form of LC disease in the jaws, only this variant will be discussed in this chapter.

The etiology of LCH is somewhat obscure. Some recent studies have demonstrated a clonal proliferation of LCs, supporting the concept of a neoplastic process.[52] It has also been suggested that the disease may result from exuberant reactions to an unknown antigenic challenge. Evidence is emerging that some patients with LCH may exhibit defects in certain aspects of the cell-mediated arm of the immune system. A deficiency of suppressor T lymphocytes, as well as low levels of serum thymic factor, suggest the presence of a thymic abnormality in this disease.

Eosinophilic Granuloma

Clinical and Radiographic Features

Eosinophilic granuloma of bone is a disease with an incidence of one new case per 350,000 to 2 million per year.[51] Most patients are younger than 20 years of age when the diagnosis is made.[53] Common locations are the ribs, the spine, and the skull. Tenderness, pain, and swelling are common patient complaints. Loosening of teeth in the affected alveolar bone is commonly noted. Radiographically, the jaws may exhibit solitary or multiple radiolucent, destructive lesions (**Fig. 24.12**). The lesions generally affect alveolar bone, giving the appearance of teeth floating in air. Jaw lesions may be accompanied by bone involvement elsewhere in the skeleton.

Although LCH may be encountered in patients over a wide age range, more than 50% of cases are seen in patients under the age of 10 years.[52] There seems to be a definite male predilection. Children younger than 10 years of age most often have skull and femoral lesions, while patients older than 20 years of age more often have lesions in the ribs, shoulder girdle, and mandible.

Work-Up, Treatment, and Prognosis

The microscopic confirmation of LCH in the jaws requires examination of the biopsy specimen with hematoxylin-eosin stains and supplementation with confirmatory S-100 and CD1a immunohistochemical stains for definitive diagnosis. Staging of patients with a skeletal radiographic series is also required that serves to differentiate monostotic from

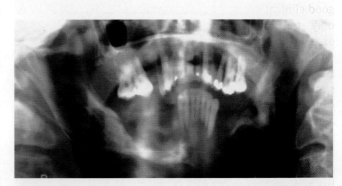

Figure 24.12 Eosinophilic granuloma of the mandible. Note the destructive process of the mandible, with teeth floating in air.

Reprinted with permission from: Guild for Scientific Advancement in Oral and Maxillofacial Surgery. Carlson ER, August M, Ruggiero SL. Locally aggressive benign processes of the oral and maxillofacial region. *Selected Readings in Oral and Maxillofacial Surgery* 2004.

polyostotic involvement of the skeleton. Additional work-up of LCH is specifically based on the results of the physical examination. For example, the observation of exophthalmos in a patient with a biopsy proved LCH might lead to the acquisition of a CT or a magnetic resonance imaging in such a patient for the purpose of identifying calvarial involvement as might occur in patients with Hand–Schüller–Christian disease that would be treated very differently than a monostotic eosinophilic granuloma of the jaws.

Once definitively diagnosed and staged, LCH lesions of the maxilla and mandible are usually treated with surgical curettage where sufficient bone remains to permit bony regeneration postoperatively.[53] Extensive disease of the maxilla and mandible might have to be treated with resection for effective surgical management. Low doses of radiation therapy may be employed for inaccessible lesions, incompletely removed lesions in bone, or recurrent lesions. The potential for induction of malignant disease secondary to radiation therapy is a concern in younger patients and may be avoided as a result. As such, its use should be recommended with caution. Intralesional corticosteroid administration has also been reported to be effective in some patients with localized bone lesions. Long-term follow-up is essential to rule out recurrent disease. Monostotic disease without visceral involvement generally responds well to curettage with or without postoperative radiation therapy.[53] Patients with polyostotic disease without visceral involvement are at much higher risk of recurrent disease.

Fibro-Osseous Lesions of the Facial Bones

The nomenclature of fibro-osseous lesions (FOLs) of the jaws can be confusing, so oral pathologists often rely upon radiological and clinical information in addition to histologic material in rendering a definitive diagnosis of a FOL of the jaws. Charles Waldron once stated that "in the absence of good clinical and radiologic information, a pathologist can only state that a given biopsy is consistent with a fibro-osseous lesion."[54] He also indicated that the radiograph would provide the best information for diagnosis of a FOL of the jaws because the histology of these lesions can be quite similar in appearance. In general terms, these lesions are composed of fibrous connective tissue of varying cellularity admixed with osteoid, mature bone, and/or cementum-like structures in combination. When discussing FOLs, dysplastic and hamartomatous processes such as fibrous dysplasia and cemento-osseous dysplasia are part of an inclusive list and are generally less aggressive. On occasion, fibrous dysplasia may present in a destructive fashion and will be included in this discussion. The cemento-ossifying fibroma (COF) and its variants, including the more aggressive juvenile and psammomatoid types, as well as the desmoplastic fibroma will be included in this discussion as well.

Fibrous Dysplasia

Patients with fibrous dysplasia exhibit slow, asymptomatic enlargement of either one (monostotic) or multiple bones (polyostotic). The enlargement is because of replacement of medullary bone with fibrous connective tissue proliferation containing variable amounts of osseous matrix that do not mature to lamellar bone. The cause of fibrous dysplasia is unknown; however, the presence of an activating mutation of Gs α gene in osteoblastic progenitor cells has been proposed to lead to increased proliferation and abnormal differentiation of bone.[55] Fibrous dysplasia can be a component of multiple syndromes. The combination of polyostotic fibrous dysplasia, café-au-lait spots, and endocrine abnormalities including precocious sexual development, acromegaly, hyperthyroidism, hyperparathyroidism, and hyperprolactinemia is McCune-Albright syndrome. The combination of cutaneous melanotic pigmentation and multiple skeletal lesions consisting of fibrous dysplasia is known as Jaffe–Lichtenstein syndrome.

Clinical and Radiographic Features

Monostotic fibrous dysplasia commonly involves the jaws, skull, long bones, pelvis, and ribs. Jaw involvement involves the maxilla more commonly than the mandible; the premolar region is most commonly involved in the former and the body region in the latter. Patients usually notice slow, asymptomatic enlargement.[56] Whereas displacement of teeth commonly occurs, mobility of teeth is uncommon. A key clinical and radiographic feature for diagnosing fibrous dysplasia is the lack of a clear margin between the affected bone and the normal bone. The histologic features of fibrous dysplasia consist of fibroblasts within a background of collagen.

Treatment and Prognosis

Treatment for fibrous dysplasia is necessary only when patients develop functional or cosmetic disturbances as a result of the expansion and should be delayed until adulthood if possible (**Fig. 24.13**). Lesion expansion will typically stabilize after puberty. A skeletal survey can be used to determine whether the patient has polyostotic or monostotic fibrous dysplasia. Clinical and radiographic examination can be used to follow the extent and progression of disease. When the maxilla or mandible is affected, bone recontouring can be performed transorally. Resection has been recommended in cases in which hearing, vision, swallowing, or breathing was threatened; however, prophylactic decompression is not recommended.[57,58] Spontaneous sarcomatous degeneration of fibrous dysplasia is a rare phenomenon in adolescence.[59]

Cemento-Ossifying Fibroma

Clinical and Radiographic Features

COF is the most common fibro-osseous neoplasm diagnosed in the jaws. It is essentially identical to lesions designated

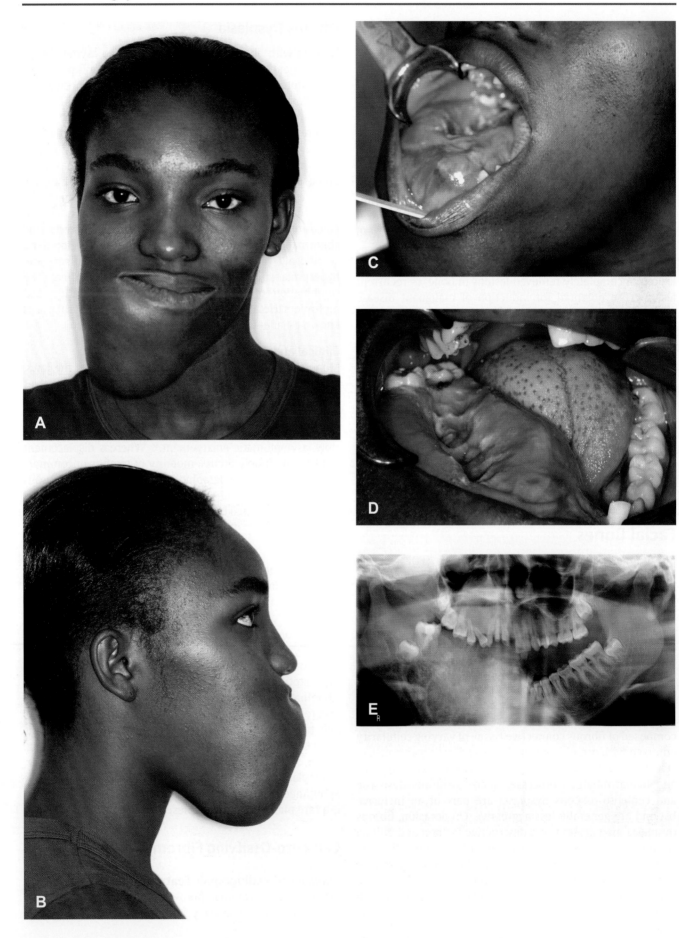

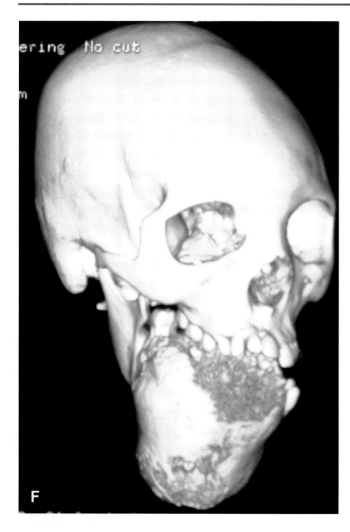

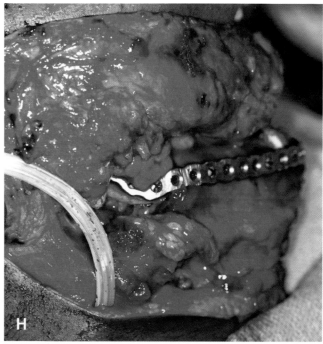

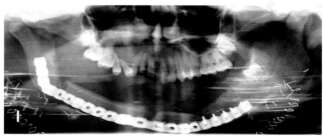

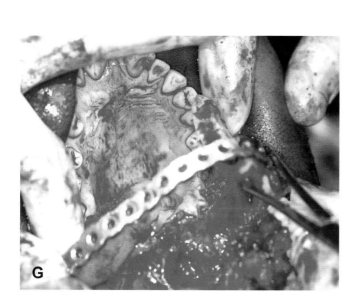

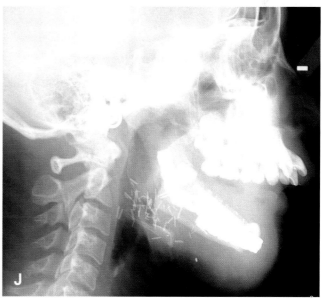

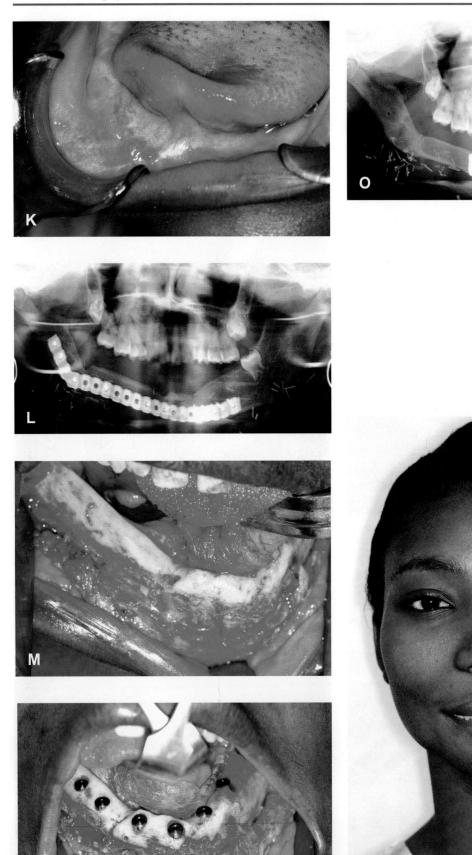

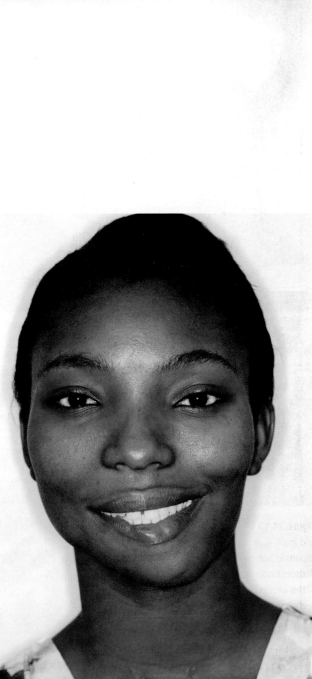

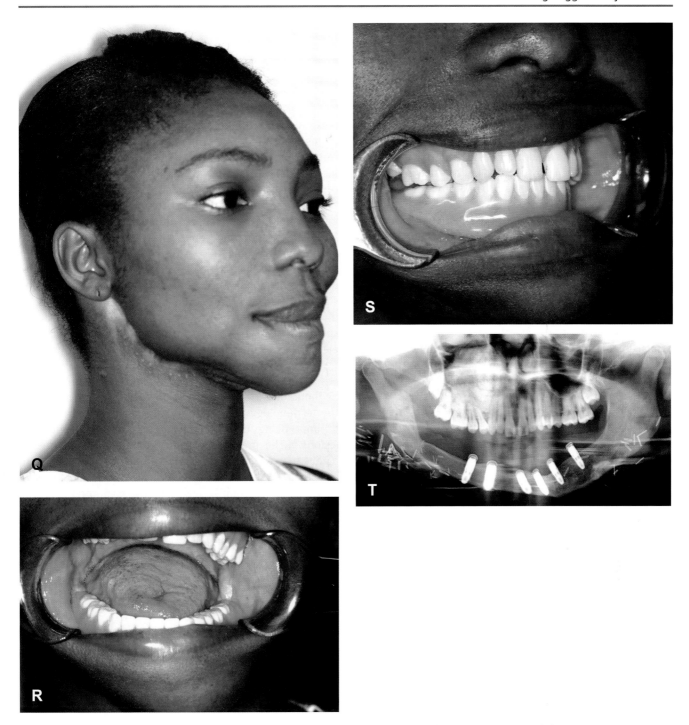

Figure 24.13 An 18-year-old with biopsy-proven craniofacial fibrous dysplasia desires comprehensive treatment to include resection, reconstruction, and implant rehabilitation. (A) Preoperative frontal facial view. (B) Preoperative right lateral facial view. (C) Preoperative intraoral view demonstrating expansile nature of the mass. (D) Preoperative intraoral view demonstrating significant tongue displacement. (E) Preoperative panoramic radiograph demonstrating extent of destruction and confines beyond that of the film borders. (F) 3-D computed tomography scan demonstrates destructive nature of this extensive lesion. (G) Following a combined intraoral and transcutaneous approach, the patient underwent a segmental subtotal mandibulectomy and placement of a locking reconstruction plate. (H) Immediate osseous reconstruction is achieved with a microvascular free tissue transfer (MFTT) of a fibula flap secured to the plate. (I) Immediate postoperative panoramic radiograph. Note the removal of both coronoid processes to facilitate rehabilitation. (J) Immediate postoperative lateral cephalogram demonstrating adequate relationship with maxilla for dental rehabilitation. (K) Postoperative intraoral view at the 1 year following resection. (L) Postoperative panoramic radiograph at the 1-year mark demonstrating osseous healing at the osteotomy and fixation sites. (M) Intraoperative view following transoral plate removal demonstrating appearance of "neo-mandible." (N) Following plate removal immediate placement of six dental implants. (O) Postoperative panoramic radiograph demonstrating plate removal and implant placement. (P) Final postoperative frontal facial view 2 years after initial resection and MFTT reconstruction. (Q) Final postoperative three-quarter facial view 2 year after initial resection and MFTT reconstruction. (R) Final prosthesis viewed from an open mouth view. (S) Final prosthesis viewed from a closed mouth view. (T) Final postoperative panoramic radiograph demonstrating implant attachments.

as cementifying fibroma and ossifying fibroma, so the nomenclature is identical for those tumors of the jaws. It is a benign intraosseous lesion and is characterized radiographically and microscopically as being sharply demarcated from the surrounding uninvolved bone. In its nonaggressive form, it may be treated conservatively with enucleation and curettage with minimal likelihood of recurrence.[60] Histologically, the lesion can look identical to fibrous dysplasia; thus, the clinical and radiologic features are critical to the rendering of a correct diagnosis.[61] A review by Voytek et al demonstrated isolated jaw lesions that showed components of both fibrous dysplasia and COF within the same lesion.[62]

The radiologic appearance of the COF depends upon its stage at diagnosis.[63] Early lesions may be primarily lucent and misdiagnosed as an odontogenic cyst or ameloblastoma (**Fig. 24.14**). They are frequently unilocular and associated with a smooth and corticated border. With maturation, a mixed radiolucent/radio-opaque pattern is common (**Fig. 24.15**). The borders in both cases are distinct and growth appears symmetrical and concentric. Tooth displacement and root resorption are commonly found and there often exists a thin lucent rim surrounding the mass. In the mandible, a characteristic downward bowing of the inferior border is often noted.

COFs occur most frequently in the mandible but other sites in the craniofacial skeleton may be involved.[64] A female preponderance is reported, with peak incidence during the third and fourth decades of life. Most lesions are slow growing and are rarely associated with pain or paresthesia. Involvement in and around the paranasal sinuses and orbits is described and the clinical behavior of these lesions is often reported as being more expansile and aggressive.[65] In these sites, the lesion is more likely to contain cementum-like (psammomatoid) bodies within a fibrous stroma that may be highly cellular. Several investigators have recommended reservation of the term "cementum" only for the bone-like substance attached to tooth roots and consider these cementum-like bodies to derive from bone.[66,67] Jaw COFs are thought to arise from cellular elements within the periodontal ligament space, although similar lesions are found in extragnathic bones, and therefore other cellular sources are probable.[68]

A variety of histologic patterns are found in COFs.[69] The microscopic appearance is largely dependent upon the stage at diagnosis. Most commonly, the lesion is composed of a cellular, relatively avascular stroma characterized by spindle-shaped cells with bland nuclei. Focal multinucleated giant cells are often found. The calcified tissue consists of trabeculae of woven and occasionally lamellar bone. Deposits of basophilic calcifications resembling cementum can also be found. It is the presence of these bodies that has led to the terminology COF, ossifying fibroma, and cementifying fibroma being used synonymously in describing these lesions.[70] The presence of these identical cementum-like bodies in extragnathic sites makes these bodies unlikely to be cemental in nature.[71]

Hyperparathyroidism-jaw tumor syndrome is an autosomal dominant disorder characterized by multiple well-circumscribed ossifying fibromas. Renal anomalies and other tumors are found in these patients.[72] Another unusual

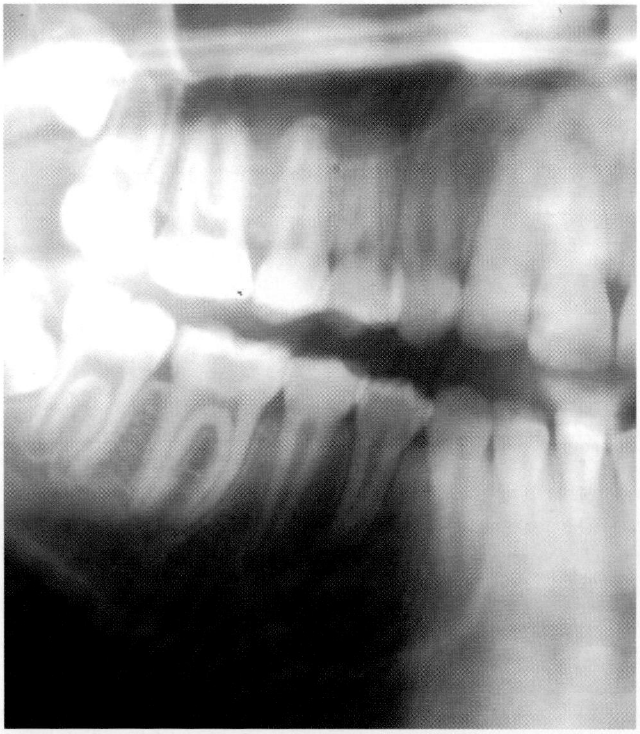

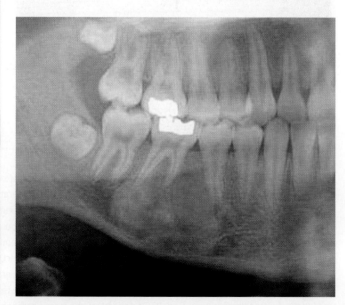

Figure 24.14 A unilocular radiolucency of the right mandible in a 9-year-old girl. The differential diagnosis should include odontogenic cysts, adenomatoid odontogenic tumor, ameloblastic fibroma, and cemento-ossifying fibroma.

Figure 24.15 An opaque mass of the right mandible that is well-demarcated, heterogenous, and highly suggestive of cemento-ossifying fibroma. The tumor has resulted in divergence of the second premolar and first molar roots.

manifestation of the COF is its occurrence in multiple quadrants within the jaws. These lesions may mimic polyostotic fibrous dysplasia both clinically and radiographically. Both familial and nonfamilial cases have been reported.[73]

Treatment and Prognosis
Treatment of COFs is dependent upon their size, clinical behavior, radiographic appearance, and associated symptoms.[74] Radiolucent tumors that are well-demarcated from the surrounding bone are removed with enucleation and curettage surgeries (**Fig. 24.16**). Often, the lesion shells out intact or in large fragments from the surrounding bone. However, incomplete removal is associated with a variable rate of recurrence. Those lesions demonstrating aggressive features (a history of rapid growth, multiple episodes of recurrence, problematic anatomic location), and a radio-opaque radiographic character typically are resected for complete removal (**Fig. 24.17**).

Juvenile Ossifying Fibroma

Clinical and Radiographic Features
This relatively uncommon lesion may be distinguished from other FOLs of the jaws by the age of the patient at time of diagnosis, clinical presentation, and potentially aggressive behavior.[75] The term was coined in 1952 by Johnson and further established as additional cases were reported and described. In 1991, a review of 112 cases collected at the Armed Forces Institute of Pathology over a 45-year time period further codified the nomenclature, although a plethora of synonymous terms certainly adds to the diagnostic confusion the juvenile ossifying fibroma (JOF) has generated.[76]

JOF is most often diagnosed before the age of 15 years and tends to show a male predilection.[77] Because of rapid proliferation, associated facial swelling is common. Localization to the facial bones is reported in 85%, the calvarium in 12%, and noncraniofacial sites in 4%.[78] The facial bony lesions most commonly arise in areas contiguous with the paranasal sinuses (90%) but jaw lesions have been described in 10%. Johnson et al hypothesized that the JOF arises from an overproduction of the myxofibrous cellular stroma normally involved in the development of the nasal septum and the sinuses as they enlarge.[76] Similarly, such overproduction in sutural lines in the skull may also account for the tumor's localization to these sites. The etiology of the jaw lesions is less clear, but some authors speculate that maldevelopment of tissue septa between the roots of teeth may be of etiologic significance.[79]

Common presenting complaints, in addition to facial swelling, can include nasal obstruction, proptosis, and rarely, intracranial extension. The tumor frequently erodes the bony septa of the sinuses and leads to encroachment upon the orbit, nose, and skull. Impaired sinus drainage with associated mucocele formation is common. Visual loss from optic nerve compression has also been reported. Because the dura is an effective barrier to brain invasion, other neurologic signs are uncommon.[80]

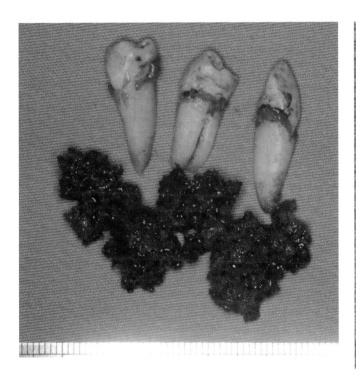

Figure 24.16 Enucleation and curettage is the preferred surgical technique for cemento-ossifying fibromas that present as radiolucent tumors. This specimen resulted from the surgery of the patient whose radiograph is shown in **Fig. 24.14**.

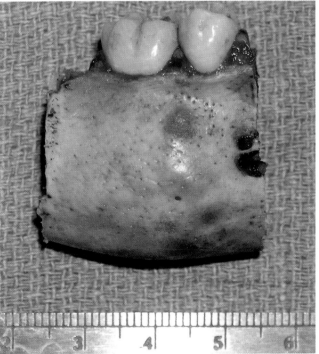

Figure 24.17 Resection of a cemento-ossifying fibroma is required when the mass is calcified. This specimen resulted from the surgery of the patient whose radiograph is shown in **Fig. 24.15**.

Radiographically, the features of JOF are relatively nonspecific. The lesions may be uni- or multilocular and generally have irregular borders. Cortical thinning and perforation are frequently identified. Maxillary tumors tend to obliterate the sinuses.[81] CT scans often show these lesions widening and filling the medullary space of bone. The degree of associated ossification is variable.[82] Magnetic resonance images are hypointense on both T1 and T2 weighted sequences. If cystic spaces are present within the tumor, these will image as hyperintense on T2. The tumor will enhance with the use of gadolinium contrast.[83]

Two variants of JOF (trabecular and psammomatoid) are recognized, although controversy still exists as to whether the latter should be considered a COF.[84] Both variants occur most frequently during the first and second decades of life. Approximately 75% of the psammomatoid variants develop in the orbits, paranasal sinus region, and the skull.[85] They are less common in the jaws where the trabecular variant predominates.[86] Some authors prefer to restrict the designation JOF to those lesions characterized by the presence of osteoid strands (the trabecular variant) and consider the psammomatoid variant to be a COF.

The growth pattern of JOF can be variable and the clinical signs depend upon the anatomic site of origin. Because of the clinical presentation and radiographic findings, these lesions must be distinguished from craniofacial malignancies such as osteosarcoma, fibrosarcoma, and Ewing sarcoma.[87] In addition, benign jaw neoplasms (both odontogenic and nonodontogenic) with aggressive behavior should also be included in the differential diagnosis.

On gross examination, these tumors are whitish in coloration and often have a gritty consistency. Within the gross tumor itself, cystic spaces with blood breakdown products are often found. Histologically, these lesions may closely resemble the COF and there is an overlap between the trabecular and psammomatoid variants.[88] These tumors are characterized by a highly cellular stroma without notable mitotic activity. Embedded within the stroma are numerous mineralized structures (ossicles, chondricles, and cementicles). Vascularity is prominent at the periphery of the tumor only. Reactive bone may also be found at the periphery and the lesion often infiltrates the surrounding normal bone, making complete removal difficult.[89] Distinguishing features of JOF may include the following: morphologic heterogeneity as compared with the generally uniform pattern describe for the COF; areas of dense cellularity within a myxomatous stroma; and uneven distribution of bone and calcified structures within the tumor.

Treatment and Prognosis

Treatment of the JOF is controversial. The recurrence rate for JOF treated with local excision or curettage is reported between 30 and 58%.[60] Thus, if this treatment is selected, careful longitudinal follow-up is imperative. Local excision is not recommended in cases of cortical expansion, periosteal elevation, and frank bony perforation. Wide resection with complete surgical resection is associated with a lower rate of recurrence. Despite the aggressive nature of JOF, malignant transformation over time has not been described.

Desmoplastic Fibroma (Aggressive Fibromatosis; Central Fibroma, Desmoid Type)

Clinical and Radiographic Features

Desmoplastic fibroma is an unusual benign tumor of connective tissue origin that has most commonly been described in the metaphyseal region of the long bones.[90] Its name derives from the fact that, histologically, it closely resembles desmoid tumors of the abdominal soft tissue.[91] This entity within the soft tissue has also been referred to as aggressive fibromatosis.[92] First recognized by Jaffe in 1958, isolated cases within the jaws and paraoral soft tissue have been reported. The ramus-angle region of the mandible appears to be the most common site of involvement (**Fig. 24.18**). The tumor is typically locally aggressive and destructive.

Clinically, the tumor presents with bony expansion and extension into the surrounding soft tissue. For those lesions predominantly involving soft tissue, surface resorption of the underlying bone is a common feature. The majority of patients are younger than 30 years with an average age of onset of 14 years.[93] Radiographically, the desmoplastic fibroma may be unilocular or multilocular and the mandible is most commonly involved (**Fig. 24.18**). Cortical perforation and root resorption are seen in larger tumors. The etiology is unknown, although authors have suggested an association with previous trauma, endocrine abnormalities, and genetic factors.

Histologically, the lesion is composed of thick bundles of collagenized fibrous tissue and aggregates of elongated, spindle-shaped cells with hyperchromatic nuclei. Little or no mitotic activity is noted. However, the clinically aggressive nature of this tumor, coupled with the fact that it is nonencapsulated and poorly demarcated from the surrounding bone, make it imperative to distinguish it from a well-differentiated fibrosarcoma.

Treatment and Prognosis

Although benign, this tumor is locally aggressive and conservative therapy with curettage is associated with a reported recurrence rate as high as 35%.[94] Because of this high recurrence rate, wide surgical excision is the recommended treatment (**Fig. 24.19**). Many authors describe the difficulty in obtaining adequate margins because of the invasion of the tumor into surrounding bone.[95,96] If the tumor has eroded the bone and extends into the surrounding soft tissue, even wider resection will be required. Radiation therapy and chemotherapy appear to have little role in primary treatment, as effective surgical treatment offers the best opportunity for tumor control and minimal disruption of growth of the patient.[97]

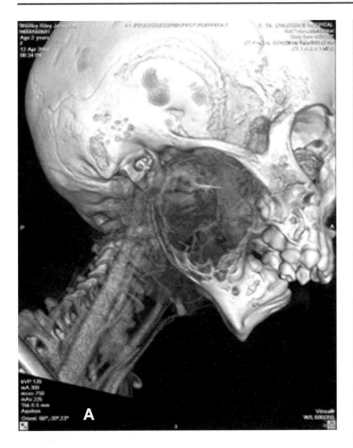

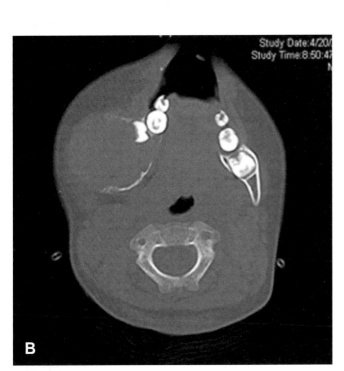

Figure 24.18   A desmoplastic fibroma of the mandible in a 2-year-old girl. The 3-D computed tomography (CT) scan (A) and the axial CT scan (B) show that the tumor had completely destroyed the bone of the mandibular angle and ramus, including the condyle.

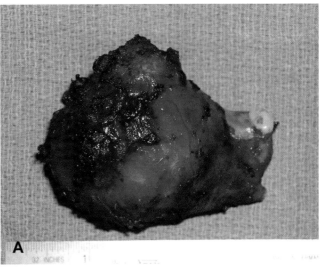

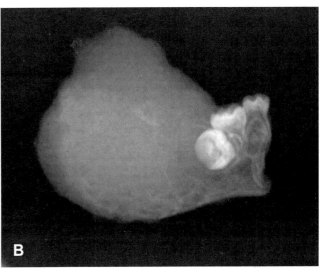

Figure 24.19   The desmoplastic fibroma illustrated in **Fig. 24.18** was treated with a disarticulation resection of the right mandible (A). The specimen radiograph (B) from that resection demonstrates significant destruction of bone of the mandible.

References

1. Carlson ER. Pathologic facial asymmetries. In: Lew D, ed. Management of Facial Asymmetry. Atlas of the Oral and Maxillofacial Surgery Clinics of North America. Philadelphia, PA: WB Saunders; 1996:19–35

2. Regezi JA, Sciubba JJ, Jordan RCK. Ulcerative conditions. In: Regezi JA, Sciubba JJ, Jordan RCK, eds. Oral Pathology. Clinical Pathologic Correlations. 4th ed. St. Louis, MO: Elsevier Science; 2003:54–55

3. Lane DP. Cancer. p53, guardian of the genome. Nature 1992;358(6381):15–16

4. Li FP, Fraumeni JF Jr, Mulvihill JJ, et al. A cancer family syndrome in twenty-four kindreds. Cancer Res 1988;48(18):5358–5362

5. Malkin D, Li FP, Strong LC, et al. Germ line p53 mutations in a familial syndrome of breast cancer, sarcomas, and other neoplasms. Science 1990;250(4985):1233–1238

6. Cotran RS, Kumar V, Collins T. Neoplasia. Cotran RS, Kumar V, Collins T, eds. Robbins Pathologic Basis of Disease. 6th ed. Philadelphia, PA: WB Saunders Co.; 1999:260–327

7. Jost CA, Marin MC, Kaelin WG. p73 is a human p53-related protein that can induce apoptosis. Nature 1997;389:191–194

8. Oren M. Lonely no more: p53 finds its kin in a tumor suppressor haven. Cell 1997;90(5):829–832

9. Carson DA, Ribeiro JM. Apoptosis and disease. Lancet 1993;341(8855):1251–1254

10. Kumamoto H, Ooya K. Immunohistochemical analysis of bcl-2 family proteins in benign and malignant ameloblastomas. J Oral Pathol Med 1999;28(8):343–349

11. Carvalhais JN, Aguiar M, Araújo V, Araújo N, Gomez R. p53 and MDM2 expression in odontogenic cysts and tumours. Oral Dis 1999;5(3):218–222

12. Ong'uti MN, Cruchley AT, Howells GL, Williams DM. Ki-67 antigen in ameloblastomas: correlation with clinical and histological parameters in 54 cases from Kenya. Int J Oral Maxillofac Surg 1997;26(5):376–379

13. Gerdes J, Lemke H, Baisch H, Wacker HH, Schwab U, Stein H. Cell cycle analysis of a cell proliferation-associated human nuclear antigen defined by the monoclonal antibody Ki-67. J Immunol 1984;133(4):1710–1715

14. Oka K, Fukui M, Yamashita M, et al. Mandibular ameloblastoma with intracranial extension and distant metastasis. Clin Neurol Neurosurg 1986;88(4):303–309

15. Reichart PA, Philipsen HP, Sonner S. Ameloblastoma: biological profile of 3677 cases. Eur J Cancer B Oral Oncol 1995;31B(2):86–99

16. Regezi JA, Kerr DA, Courtney RM. Odontogenic tumors: analysis of 706 cases. J Oral Surg 1978;36(10):771–778

17. Daley TD, Wysocki GP, Pringle GA. Relative incidence of odontogenic tumors and oral and jaw cysts in a Canadian population. Oral Surg Oral Med Oral Pathol 1994;77(3):276–280

18. Gold L. Biologic behavior of ameloblastoma. In: Assael L, ed. Benign Lesions of the Jaws. Oral and Maxillofacial Surgery Clinics of North America. Philadelphia, PA: WB Saunders; 1991:21–71

19. Williams T. The ameloblastoma: a review of the literature. Selected readings oral maxillofacial surgery. 2nd ed. Dallas: The Guild for Scientific Advancement in Oral and Maxiloacial Surgery; 1992:1–17

20. Ord RA, Blanchaert RH Jr, Nikitakis NG, Sauk JJ. Ameloblastoma in children. J Oral Maxillofac Surg 2002;60(7):762–770, discussion 770–771

21. Takahashi K, Miyauchi K, Sato K. Treatment of ameloblastoma in children. Br J Oral Maxillofac Surg 1998;36(6):453–456

22. Mehlisch DR, Dahlin DC, Masson JK. Ameloblastoma: a clinicopathologic report. J Oral Surg 1972;30(1):9–22

23. Ueno S, Nakamura S, Mushimoto K, Shirasu R. A clinicopathologic study of ameloblastoma. J Oral Maxillofac Surg 1986;44(5):361–365

24. Nastri AL, Wiesenfeld D, Radden BG, Eveson J, Scully C. Maxillary ameloblastoma: a retrospective study of 13 cases. Br J Oral Maxillofac Surg 1995;33(1):28–32

25. Jackson IT, Callan PP, Forté RA. An anatomical classification of maxillary ameloblastoma as an aid to surgical treatment. J Craniomaxillofac Surg 1996;24(4):230–236

26. Sehdev MK, Huvos AG, Strong EW, Gerold FP, Willis GW. Proceedings: ameloblastoma of maxilla and mandible. Cancer 1974;33(2):324–333

27. Huffman GG, Thatcher JW. Ameloblastoma—the conservative surgical approach to treatment: report of four cases. J Oral Surg 1974;32(11):850–854

28. Vedtofte P, Hjorting-Hansen E, Jensen BN, Roed-Peterson B. Conservative surgical treatment of mandibular ameloblastomas. Int J Oral Surg 1978;7(3):156–161

29. Müller H, Slootweg PJ. The ameloblastoma, the controversial approach to therapy. J Maxillofac Surg 1985;13(2):79–84

30. Gardner DG. A pathologist's approach to the treatment of ameloblastoma. J Oral Maxillofac Surg 1984;42(3):161–166

31. Carlson ER, Marx RE. The ameloblastoma: primary, curative surgical management. J Oral Maxillofac Surg 2006;64(3):484–494

32. Atkinson CH, Harwood AR, Cummings BJ. Ameloblastoma of the jaw. A reappraisal of the role of megavoltage irradiation. Cancer 1984;53(4):869–873

33. Gardner DG. Radiotherapy in the treatment of ameloblastoma. Int J Oral Maxillofac Surg 1988;17(3):201–205

34. Mitsuyasu T, Harada H, Higuchi Y, et al. Immunohistochemical demonstration of bcl-2 protein in ameloblastoma. J Oral Pathol Med 1997;26(8):345–348

35. Willis RA. Pathology of Tumors. St. Louis, MO: CV Mosby; 1948

36. Carr RF, Halperin V. Malignant ameloblastomas from 1953 to 1966. Review of the literature and report of a case. Oral Surg Oral Med Oral Pathol 1968;26(4):514–522

37. Gold L, Williams TP. Odontogenic tumors: surgical pathology and management. In: Fonseca R, Marciani R, Turvey T, eds. Oral and Maxillofacial Surgery. 2nd ed. St. Louis: Elsevier;466–538.

38. Robinson L, Martinez MG. Unicystic ameloblastoma: a prognostically distinct entity. Cancer 1977;40(5):2278–2285

39. Vickers RA, Gorlin RJ. Ameloblastoma: delineation of early histopathologic features of neoplasia. Cancer 1970;26(3):699–710

40. Gardner DG, Corio RL. The relationship of plexiform unicystic ameloblastoma to conventional ameloblastoma. Oral Surg Oral Med Oral Pathol 1983;56(1):54–60

41. Regezi JA, Sciubba JJ, Jordan RCK. Odontogenic tumors. In: Regezi JA, Sciubba JJ, Jordan RCK, eds. Oral Pathology Clinical Pathologic Correlations. 4th ed. St. Louis, MO: Elsevier; 2003:267–288

42. Gardner DG, Corio RL. Plexiform unicystic ameloblastoma. A variant of ameloblastoma with a low-recurrence rate after enucleation. Cancer 1984;53(8):1730–1735

43. Carlson ER. Odontogenic cysts and tumors. In: Miloro, ed. Peterson's Principles of Oral and Maxillofacial Surgery. Hamilton, ON: BC Decker; 2004

44. Gardner DG. Plexiform unicystic ameloblastoma: a diagnostic problem in dentigerous cysts. Cancer 1981;47(6):1358–1363

45. Eversole LR, Leider AS, Strub D. Radiographic characteristics of cystogenic ameloblastoma. Oral Surg Oral Med Oral Pathol 1984;57(5):572–577

46. Barker BF. Odontogenic myxoma. Semin Diagn Pathol 1999;16(4):297–301

47. Fenton S, Slootweg PJ, Dunnebier EA, Mourits MP. Odontogenic myxoma in a 17-month-old child: a case report. J Oral Maxillofac Surg 2003;61(6):734–736

48. Bast BT, Pogrel MA, Regezi JA. The expression of apoptotic proteins and matrix metalloproteinases in odontogenic myxomas. J Oral Maxillofac Surg 2003;61(12):1463–1466

49. Franklin CD, Pindborg JJ. The calcifying epithelial odontogenic tumor. A review and analysis of 113 cases. Oral Surg Oral Med Oral Pathol 1976;42(6):753–765

50. Schmitz L, Favara BE. Nosology and pathology of Langerhans cell histiocytosis. Hematol Oncol Clin North Am 1998;12(2):221–246

51. Eckardt A, Schultze A. Maxillofacial manifestations of Langerhans cell histiocytosis: a clinical and therapeutic analysis of 10 patients. Oral Oncol 2003;39(7):687–694

52. Regezi J, Sciubba J, Jordan RCK, eds. Oral Pathology: Clinical Pathologic Correlations. 4th ed. Philadelphia, PA: WB Saunders Co.; 2003:303

53. Carlson ER, Campbell JA. Langerhans cell histiocytosis. In: Fonseca R, Marciani R, Turvey T, eds. Oral and Maxillofacial Surgery. 2nd ed. St. Louis, MO: Saunders Elsevier; 2009

54. Neville BW, Damm DD, Allen CM, Bouquot JE. Hematologic disorders. In: Neville BW, Damm DD, Allen CM, Bouquot JE, eds. Oral and Maxillofacial Pathology. 2nd ed. Philadelphia, PA: WB Saunders Co.;2002:497–531

55. Shenker A, Weinstein LS, Sweet DE, Spiegel AM. An activating Gs alpha mutation is present in fibrous dysplasia of bone in the McCune-Albright syndrome. J Clin Endocrinol Metab 1994;79(3):750–755

56. MacDonald-Jankowski D. Fibrous dysplasia: a systematic review. Dentomaxillofac Radiol 2009;38(4):196–215

57. Lee JS, FitzGibbon E, Butman JA, et al. Normal vision despite narrowing of the optic canal in fibrous dysplasia. N Engl J Med 2002;347(21):1670–1676

58. Kim DD, Ghali GE, Wright JM, Edwards SP. Surgical treatment of giant fibrous dysplasia of the mandible with concomitant craniofacial involvement. J Oral Maxillofac Surg 2012;70(1):102–118

59. Sadeghi SM, Hosseini SN. Spontaneous conversion of fibrous dysplasia into osteosarcoma. J Craniofac Surg 2011;22(3):959–961

60. Waldron CA. Fibro-osseous lesions of the jaws. J Oral Maxillofac Surg 1993;51:823–835

61. Waldron CA, Giansanti JS. Benign fibro-osseous lesions of the jaws: a clinico-radiologic-histologic review of sixty-five cases. Oral Surg Oral Med Oral Pathol 1973;35(2):190–201

62. Voytek TM, Ro JY, Edeiken J, Ayala AG. Fibrous dysplasia and cemento-ossifying fibroma. A histologic spectrum. Am J Surg Pathol 1995;19(7):775–781

63. Eversole LR, Merrell PW, Strub D. Radiographic characteristics of central ossifying fibroma. Oral Surg Oral Med Oral Pathol 1985;59(5):522–527

64. Fechner RE. Problematic lesions of the craniofacial bones. Am J Surg Pathol 1989;13(Suppl 1):17–30

65. Boysen ME, Olving JH, Vatne K, Koppang HS. Fibro-osseous lesions of the cranio-facial bones. J Laryngol Otol 1979;93(8):793–807

66. Margo CE, Ragsdale BD, Perman KI, Zimmerman LE, Sweet DE. Psammomatoid (juvenile) ossifying fibroma of the orbit. Ophthalmology 1985;92(1):150–159

67. Slootweg PJ. Maxillofacial fibro-osseous lesions: classification and differential diagnosis. Semin Diagn Pathol 1996;13(2):104–112

68. Brannon RB, Fowler CB. Benign fibro-osseous lesions: a review of current concepts. Adv Anat Pathol 2001;8(3):126–143

69. Su L, Weathers DR, Waldron CA. Distinguishing features of focal cemento-osseous dysplasias and cemento-ossifying fibromas: I. A pathologic spectrum of 316 cases. Oral Surg Oral Med Oral Pathol Oral Radiol Endod 1997;84(3):301–309

70. Craig RG. Cementum vs. bone: an experimental perspective. Oral Maxillofac Surg Clin North Am 1997;9(4):581–595.

71. Mirra JM, Bernard GW, Bullough PG, Johnston W, Mink G. Cementum-like production in solitary bone cysts (so-called "cementoma" of long bones). Report of three cases. Electron microscopic observations supporting a synovial origin to the simple bone cyst. Clin Orthop Relat Res 1978;135:295–307

72. Warnakulasuriya S, Markwell BD, Williams DM. Familial hyperparathyroidism associated with cementifying fibromas of the jaws in two siblings. Oral Surg Oral Med Oral Pathol 1985;59(3):269–274

73. Bertolini F, Caradonna L, Binachi B, et al.Multiple ossifying fibromas of the jaws: a case report. J Oral Maxillofac Surg 2002;60:225

74. Eversole LR, Leider AS, Nelson K. Ossifying fibroma: a clinicopathologic study of sixty-four cases. Oral Surg Oral Med Oral Pathol 1985;60(5):505–511

75. Slootweg PJ, Müller H. Juvenile ossifying fibroma. Report of four cases. J Craniomaxillofac Surg 1990;18(3):125–129

76. Johnson LC, Yousefi M, Vinh TN, Heffner DK, Hyams VJ, Hartman KS. Juvenile active ossifying fibroma. Its nature, dynamics and origin. Acta Otolaryngol Suppl 1991;488:1–40

77. Lawton MT, Heiserman JE, Coons SW, Ragsdale BD, Spetzler RF. Juvenile active ossifying fibroma. Report of four cases. J Neurosurg 1997;86(2):279–285

78. Janecka IP, Housepian E. Craniofacial approach to ossifying fibromas. Laryngoscope 1985;95:305–306

79. Noffke CEE. Juvenile ossifying fibroma of the mandible. An 8 year radiological follow-up. Dentomaxillofac Radiol 1998;27(6):363–366

80. Som PM, Lidov M. The benign fibroosseous lesion: its association with paranasal sinus mucoceles and its MR appearance. J Comput Assist Tomogr 1992;16(6):871–876

81. Slootweg PJ, Panders AK, Koopmans R, Nikkels PGJ. Juvenile ossifying fibroma. An analysis of 33 cases with emphasis on histopathological aspects. J Oral Pathol Med 1994;23(9):385–388

82. Dehner LP. Tumors of the mandible and maxilla in children. I. Clinicopathologic study of 46 histologically benign lesions. Cancer 1973;31(2):364–384

83. Sciubba JJ, Younai F. Ossifying fibroma of the mandible and maxilla: review of 18 cases. J Oral Pathol Med 1989;18(6):315–321

84. El-Mofty S. Psammomatoid and trabecular juvenile ossifying fibroma of the craniofacial skeleton: two distinct clinicopathologic entities. Oral Surg Oral Med Oral Pathol Oral Radiol Endod 2002;93(3):296–304

85. Alawi F. Benign fibro-osseous diseases of the maxillofacial bones. A review and differential diagnosis. Am J Clin Pathol 2002;118(Suppl):S50–S70

86. Rinaggio J, Land M, Cleveland DB. Juvenile ossifying fibroma of the mandible. J Pediatr Surg 2003;38(4):648–650

87. Batsakis JG. Tumors of the Head and Neck: Clinical and Pathological Considerations. 2nd ed. Baltimore, MD: Williams and Wilkins; 1984:410

88. Williams HK, Mangham C, Speight PM. Juvenile ossifying fibroma. An analysis of eight cases and a comparison with other fibro-osseous lesions. J Oral Pathol Med 2000;29(1):13–18

89. Macintosh RB. Juvenile ossifying fibroma. Oral Maxillofac Surg Clin North Am 1997;9(4):713

90. Inwards CY, Unni KK, Beabout JW, Sim FH. Desmoplastic fibroma of bone. Cancer 1991;68(9):1978–1983

91. Fowler CB, Hartman KS, Brannon RB. Fibromatosis of the oral and paraoral region. Oral Surg Oral Med Oral Pathol 1994;77(4):373–386

92. Jaffe HL. Tumors and Tumorous Conditions of the Bones and Joints. Philadelphia, PA: Lea and Febiger; 1958:298

93. Hopkins KM, Huttula CS, Kahn MA, Albright JE. Desmoplastic fibroma of the mandible: review and report of two cases. J Oral Maxillofac Surg 1996;54(10):1249–1254

94. Kwon PH, Horswell BB, Gatto DJ. Desmoplastic fibroma of the jaws: surgical management and review of the literature. Head Neck 1989;11(1):67–75

95. Green MF, Sirikumara M. Desmoplastic fibroma of the mandible. Ann Plast Surg 1987;19(3):284–290

96. Vally IM, Altini M. Fibromatoses of the oral and paraoral soft tissues and jaws. Review of the literature and report of 12 new cases. Oral Surg Oral Med Oral Pathol 1990;69(2):191–198

97. Schmidt BL. Benign nonodontogenic tumors. In: Fonseca R, Marciani R, Turvey T, eds. Oral and Maxillofacial Surgery. 2nd ed. St. Louis, MO: Saunders Elsevier; 2009

E. Rehabilitation of Patients with Head and Neck Cancer

25 Swallowing

Boban M. Erovic, Rosemary Martino, and Jonathan Irish

Core Messages

- Effective swallowing requires a highly complex net of interactions between the central nervous system, peripheral nerves, and the muscles that they innervate. In patients with head and neck cancer (HNC), alteration from either the tumor itself or the tumor treatment can result in dysphagia and subsequently lead to pneumonia, malnutrition, and a poor quality of life. Accurate knowledge of the anatomy and physiology of the swallowing mechanism is essential for optimal management of dysphagia following treatment of HNC patients. While local and regional tumor control is paramount, cancer treatment planning should always include considerations about functional outcomes that include swallowing function. Every patient is unique; therefore, there can be significant variability in swallowing ability from patient factors such as age and other medical comorbidities.

- Treatment of HNC can include surgery, radiation, or chemotherapy. Increasingly, combined modality treatment approaches are being applied. In the past two decades, so-called organ preservation protocols have been implemented. However, "organ preservation" treatment approaches do not necessarily mean that a more "functional" swallow may be the end result after completion of these treatments.

- The extent of surgery, with resultant resection of the nerves and muscles responsible for mastication and swallowing, is an important factor, which will affect posttreatment swallowing physiology. Careful surgical reconstruction can mitigate some of these effects, and thereby reduce the negative impact of ablation on the swallow. Small defects can heal by secondary intention or be reconstructed by primary closure or skin grafts, while more radical resections require regional flap or microvascular free flap reconstruction.

Radiotherapy can be administered to head and neck cancer (HNC) patients postoperatively to control microscopic disease or as primary therapy. As a consequence, it too may induce damage in normal tissue increasing the incidence of swallowing dysfunction. The introduction of intensity-modulated radiation therapy (IMRT) has allowed improved tumor volume targeting and reduction in collateral surrounding tissue toxicity, but at the same time dose escalation may negate some of these benefits.

Regardless of how the tumor is treated, the best chance of successful rehabilitation of the HNC patient requires a team approach that includes a speech–language pathologist with strong clinical expertise in swallowing rehabilitation.

The patient with HNC is at high risk for impaired swallowing because of either the cancer itself or secondary to cancer treatment. Swallowing can be further complicated by tumor recurrence. The resulting impaired swallow, or dysphagia, can lead to devastating complications such as pneumonia, malnutrition, and poor quality of life for these patients.

Normal Swallow Physiology and Central Control

To diagnose and treat dysphagia it is important to understand the normal swallowing mechanism. Under normal physiological conditions, humans swallow 1000 to 3000 times daily and significantly less during the night. Swallowing includes not only eating and drinking but also clearing of the esophagus. Normal swallow physiology is a highly complex mechanism originating in the medulla oblongata where there is a network of sensory and motor nuclei and interneurons that form the "swallowing center." This area coordinates muscle function in the oral cavity, pharynx, larynx, and esophagus via cranial nerves V, VII to X, and XII along with peripheral nerves C1 to C3. Normal swallowing involves four sequential phases: oral preparation, oral transport, pharyngeal transport, and esophageal transport.

Oral Preparatory Phase

Food is cut and chewed by movements of the dentate mandible and afterward intermixed with saliva to form a cohesive bolus. The tongue is constantly moving the bolus toward the occlusal surface of the teeth. The lips and buccal muscles of the oral cavity help keep the bolus within the oral cavity. At the same time, the tongue and the soft palate create a seal serving to prevent the newly formulated bolus from spilling into the pharynx prematurely (**Fig. 25.1A**).

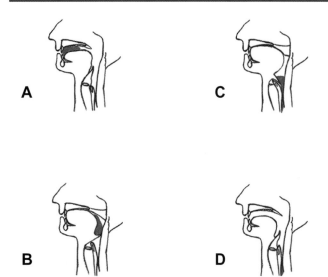

Figure 25.1 Bolus is cut, chewed, and maintained within the oral cavity (A). Tongue is pressing against the hard palate, the nasopharynx is closed by the soft palate and the bolus is transported toward the pharynx (B). To prevent aspiration the larynx is elevated and closed by the true and false cords, the epiglottis, and the aryepiglottic folds (C). Relaxation of the cricopharyngeus muscle enables the transport of the bolus into the esophagus (D).

Oral Transport Phase

In this phase the lips close the mouth to prevent escape of saliva and excess intake of air. Simultaneously, the tongue sequentially presses against the hard palate in a posterior direction serving to propel the newly formulated bolus toward the oropharynx. This process takes about 1 second.

Pharyngeal Transport Phase

The trigger of the pharyngeal swallow is initiated through sensory information traveling to the medulla via the ninth and tenth cranial nerves. This trigger is activated when the bolus reaches the oropharynx. The duration of the normal pharyngeal transport lasts for about 1 second. During a short phase of apnea during the early stage of expiration, the nasopharynx is closed by the soft palate and the pharyngeal constrictors contract while the cricopharyngeal muscle relaxes (**Fig. 25.1B**). To prevent aspiration of food or liquids, the larynx is elevated by contraction of the suprahyoid musculature and closed by adduction of the true and false cords, epiglottic deflection, and approximation of the arytenoids to the base of the epiglottis (**Fig. 25.1C**). The actions of laryngeal elevation, along with relaxation of the cricopharyngeus muscle, lead to a negative pressure in the esophagus that enables the movement of the bolus from the hypopharynx to the esophagus (**Fig. 25.1D**).

Esophageal Phase

Through peristaltic contractions of the esophageal musculature, traveling approximately 3 to 4 cm/s, the bolus is transported into the stomach. These wave-like contractions serve to clear the residue of food from the esophagus and limit gastric reflux for approximately 1 hour after intake. In contrast to both the oral transport and pharyngeal phase, the esophageal phase is longer in duration, lasting between 8 and 20 seconds. With advancing age, the decreased amplitude of these peristaltic waves in the esophagus may contribute to reflux disease.

Dysphagia and Aspiration

Dysphagia derives from the Greek word *dysphagein* and describes a delay or even obstruction of fluid and solid food during swallowing. As a consequence of dysphagia, food and liquid may spill into the respiratory tract and cause aspiration. Aspiration can be divided as occurring before, during, or after the trigger of the pharyngeal swallow. Reduced oral motor control and delayed or even absent trigger of the pharyngeal swallow can lead to aspiration before swallowing. Reduced laryngeal closure, decreased epiglottic deflection, or reduced laryngeal elevation may result in aspiration during swallowing. Structural abnormalities, dysfunction of pharyngeal peristalsis and/or the cricopharyngeus muscle, or reduced laryngeal elevation can cause aspiration after the swallow.

Iatrogenic Causes of Dysphagia Following Treatment of Head and Neck Cancer

Treatment of malignant tumors of the head and neck may include surgery, radiotherapy, and chemotherapy either as single modalities or in combination. These treatments, while treating the cancer, may, in turn, cause or exacerbate dysphagia in the HNC patient.

Resection of Malignant Tumors of the Skin, Lips, and Salivary Glands

Facial Nerve Paralysis
Facial nerve paralysis is a significant factor for patients with HNC, leading to a variety of aesthetic and functional problems including dysphagia. A common functional disability related to dysphagia is the loss of oral sphincter function often leading to drooling of food and liquids and even saliva.

Treatment of facial nerve paralysis in HNC patients depends on the cause of the paralysis. Peripheral facial nerve paralysis can be caused by the presence of malignant tumors of the temporal bone, major salivary glands, skin, and lip. Where resection or transection of the facial nerve occurs after surgical procedures the preferred treatment is primary repair of the facial nerve or an interposition graft from either the greater auricular nerve or sural nerve. These interventions can result in functional and dynamic reconstruction by maintaining good facial movement and muscular tone. Static options include suspension of facial soft tissue and muscles using the palmaris longus tendon or fascia lata slings, or Gore-Tex or AlloDerm.[1] Dynamic surgical procedures that target facial reamination use temporalis muscle transfer or the gracilis muscle free flap with cross-face nerve grafting.[2]

Lip Cancer

Before resection of malignant tumors of the facial skin or lips, it is critical to meticulously plan the reconstruction of oral sphincter function. Resection of small lesions around the mouth–lip–nose unit can be reconstructed simply with advancement or rotation flaps to achieve the best functional and cosmetic results.[3] Although lower lip defects (up to 80% of total lower lip) can be reconstructed with local flaps, microstomia and nonfunctional lip are still major challenges and usually require secondary procedures to maximize function and cosmetic outcome. Studies show that lip reconstruction with local flaps can result in minimal functional compromise in terms of oral competence, facial expression, diet, denture and cutlery usage, and sensation despite reduced circumference of the oral stoma.[4] Reconstruction of defects larger than 80% of the lower lip, especially with the resection of chin or cheek tissue, requires reconstruction with regional flaps or free flaps.

Oral and Oropharyngeal Surgery

Reconstructing the oral cavity and the oropharynx to achieve a satisfactory functional outcome after ablative surgery is one of the most challenging problems in head and neck surgery. Depending on the size small defects may heal by secondary intention, with other small defects being amenable to reconstruction by primary closure or skin grafting, whereas advanced tumor resections require reconstruction with pedicled or free flaps. Nevertheless, the surgeon should be ready to use a variety of techniques for reconstruction because the extent of the resection is not always predictable. In general, the likelihood of dysphagia depends on the site of resection and the extent of the resection, with the quality of the reconstruction being a determinant of the final functional outcome. McConnel et al[5] have shown that small resections of the oral tongue (smaller than 30%) and tongue base (smaller than 60%) reconstructed with free flaps show no significant improvement in swallowing efficiency compared with primary closure. Moreover, patients with primary closure had better swallowing results on liquids than the patient group with free flaps. The authors speculated that the free flap acts as an adynamic segment that impairs the driving force of the remaining tongue, thereby reducing the swallowing efficiency.[5] In an earlier publication it was demonstrated that skin grafts gave better functional results than pedicled distal flaps.[6] Many of these studies are hampered by the fact that heterogeneous groups are compared with differing extents of resection and different modalities of reconstruction.

Sessions et al[7] determined that it was not the size but the location of the ablation that is best predictive for dysphagia. In particular, dysphagia is worse in patients suffering from tumors in the tongue base compared with patients with anterior floor of mouth tumors. Seikaly et al[8] prospectively examined swallowing outcome in 27 patients with soft palate, lateral pharyngeal wall, or base of tongue involvement. All defects were reconstructed with a radial artery forearm free flap. Swallowing data were collected preoperatively and before and after radiation therapy. Patients with resections of half or more of the soft palate had significantly higher nasalance values and larger velopharyngeal orifice areas than individuals who had less than a half of the soft palate resected (**Fig. 25.2**). A majority (94%) of the patients were able to resume a normal or soft diet. There was a 6% incidence of aspiration in 128 swallows that were analyzed. In 44 patients the effect of sensory reinnervation with reanastomosis of the lingual and/or hypoglossal nerves was prospectively investigated.[9] Videofluoroscopic swallowing studies were performed preoperatively and 12 months postoperatively to record the oral residue, bolus oral transit time, and aspiration for all patients. The authors showed that the oral transit time and oral residue score were the poorest in patients where both the lingual and hypoglossal nerves were resected. The most interesting finding of this study was that oral swallowing efficiency was preserved if one or both of the lingual and hypoglossal nerves were preserved or reconstructed following cancer resection. Most (91%) of these patients swallowed safely at 12 months postoperatively.[9] Another step forward in oral cancer reconstruction was the introduction of the anterolateral thigh flap by Song in 1984. de Vicente et al[10] compared the functional outcome in 20 patients undergoing hemiglossectomy. In this study, 10 patients had primary reconstruction with a forearm free flap and 10 with an anterolateral thigh flap. The patients' functional outcome was assessed after 6 months, and it was seen that there was no significant difference in the mean scores for deglutition between the two groups. However, in this study a significant

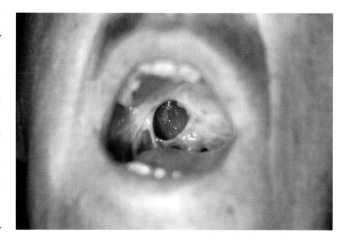

Figure 25.2 Laser resection of a squamous cell carcinoma of the soft palate resulted in a large velopharyngeal orifice that lead to significant dysphagia.

difference in the donor site morbidity was observed where the harvest site was closed primarily in the anterolateral thigh flap group but skin grafts were used for closure in the forearm group. In 4 out of 10 patients, a partial skin graft failure was observed with donor sites healing by secondary intention.[10] In more advanced disease, a total glossectomy has been associated with the risk of aspiration; therefore, simultaneous total laryngectomy is often performed prophylactically. Several studies show that the rectus abdominis musculocutaneous free flap is a valuable option for tongue reconstruction after total glossectomy. Yun et al[11] described 14 patients who were able to eat a soft diet and resume verbal communication after reconstruction with the rectus abdominis musculocutaneous or anterolateral thigh free flap. In this study, the rectus abdominis musculocutaneous flap had better speech and swallowing outcomes. This success might be because the rectus abdominis musculocutaneous free flap produced a reconstructed tongue with a significantly greater volume than the anterolateral thigh free flap.[11] It was also shown that deglutition was significantly poorer in patients with flat or depressed tongues in comparison with patients with protuberant or semiprotuberant tongues. The authors suggested that wider and thicker flaps, such as the rectus abdominis musculocutaneous flap, should be used for reconstruction of the tongue.

Advanced oral cavity tumors may infiltrate the mandible requiring bone resection. In those patients requiring mandibular resection the functional outcome is poor unless reconstitution of a stable mandibular skeleton is performed. The fibula free flap is a widely used reconstruction technique following mandibular resection. Studies comparing different free flaps, such as the osseocutaneous radial forearm free flap with free-fibular and scapular flaps,[12] show that there is no difference in the functional outcome.

Maxillectomy

Tumors involving the palate and maxillary sinus that are treated by surgical extirpation often result in oronasal and oromaxillary fistulae with loss of dentition. Adequate restoration of the three-dimensional maxillary structure is required to replace form and function of the native tissue.

Obturators

In patients who undergo a partial maxillectomy the use of a maxillectomy obturator that can be fabricated preoperatively or immediately postoperatively is an effective reconstruction option. Preoperatively fitted obturators are intended to provide temporary closure; therefore, the fit is not usually ideal and adjustment is required to optimize the function. Another option is to fabricate obturators immediately after surgery. Such hollow-type obturators are very light and provide reasonable levels of swallowing and mastication.[13] In a 2009 published study of 42 patients who underwent partial maxillectomies and had reconstruction of the defect with postoral obturators showed a generally good overall quality of life and oral function.[14] Postoperative quality of life

questionnaires showed that chewing difficulties in general and oral leakage during swallowing foods (29%, n = 12) were the most frequently reported problems.

Free Flap Reconstruction

To optimize reconstruction of larger volume maxillectomies or in patients who do not have stable dentition to support an obturator after ablative surgery, several different options are proposed. The choice of reconstruction depends on size and localization of the defect. Small defects can be covered by local flaps, whereas large defects involving soft tissue and bone need composite flap reconstruction.[15] Triana et al[16] evaluated the functional outcome in 55 patients with palatal defects after composite flap reconstruction with fibula, rectus abdominis, scapular, radial forearm, and latissimus dorsi flaps. Thirty-eight patients (69%) were on a regular diet and the remaining patients maintained a soft diet.[16] In a retrospective series of 14 patients who underwent maxillectomy and reconstruction with scapular angle flap showed acceptable functional outcomes.[17] In particular, with a range of 4 to 29 days postoperatively five patients were able to maintain a normal diet and nine were able to tolerate a soft-to-firm diet. None of the patients required nutritional supplementation.[17]

Larynx Surgery

The goal of treatment for larynx cancer is to achieve cure and to preserve laryngeal function as much as possible.

Endoscopic Laser Surgery on the Larynx

Laser surgery for HNC patients has been introduced in 1972 by Jako in Boston and popularized in Europe by Burian in Vienna, Austria, and Steiner in Goettingen, Germany.

Glottic Cancer

To date the largest study comparing functional outcomes in patients with glottic T1a and T1b glottic cancer has shown that the transoral endoscopic laser approach is superior compared with open functional procedures when comparing the rate of aspiration and tracheotomy requirement. Swallowing after endoscopic resections tends to be restored more quickly because the laser denervates only tumor tissue keeping the innervation of healthy tissue intact. Transsection of the superior laryngeal nerves during the transcervical approach leads to a sensory field defect that interferes with bolus detection and recognition, and to a weakening of the glottic closure response. Analyzing this factor, Sasaki et al[18] demonstrated that the glottic closure reflex remained intact 48 to 72 hours after endoscopic laser surgery compared with 3 weeks to 12 years after open supraglottic laryngectomy. The authors concluded that the sensory field defect caused by superior laryngeal nerve section is largely irreversible. Indeed, preservation of the glottic closure response appears to enhance recovery of swallowing following laser surgery, while compensatory mechanisms are learned.

Supraglottic Cancer

Agrawal et al[19] reported that 24 (70.5%) of 34 patients with supraglottic cancer subjects achieved fully adequate oral nutrition before discharge from the hospital, 7 subjects (21%) required prolonged use of feeding tubes (2 weeks postoperatively) and 3 patients (9%) did not achieve recovery of oral alimentation after laser resection of stage I–III supraglottic larynx. Hinni et al[20] performed laser surgery for advanced larynx cancer in 117 patients. They observed that out of the 68 patients alive on follow-up, only 7% were feeding tube-dependent. Thirty patients were evaluated and showed normal swallowing function with no episodic or daily symptoms of dysphagia.[20,21] Steiner[22] has shown that airway closure at the laryngeal entrance and the movement of the tongue base to make complete contact with the posterior pharyngeal wall can be preserved with laser surgery[22,23]

Tumor stage is a significant clinical predictor for dysphagia. Patients with T3/4 tumors are more at risk of poor functional outcome than are those requiring simple epiglottectomy or resection of only one vestibular fold.[24] Controversy still exists about management of recurrent laryngeal carcinomas after primary radiotherapy. Piazza et al[25] published recently their experience with laser treatment of 22 patients with rT2-rT4 larynx carcinomas. All patients had a good functional result in terms of swallowing with lower complication rates and shorter hospitalization times.[25]

Base of Tongue Cancer

Transoral laser resections have excellent functional and comparable oncological outcome in patients with malignant tumors of the base of the tongue. Steiner[26] has shown that in 20 patients with T2–4 base of tongue carcinomas treated with transoral laser surgery that 92% had normal diet intake. Camp et al[27] reported transoral laser resections in 67 patients with oropharyngeal tumors. Quality of life data were collected from 46 patients and out of them 45 patients had only minimally impaired to normal swallowing.[27]

Open Functional Surgery on the Larynx

The development and improvement of transoral endoscopic laser surgery technique has replaced the previously standard techniques of open partial laryngectomy for early cancer stages. Implementation of new technology using robotic manipulation coupled with a flexible CO_2 laser arm has the unique advantage of cutting tissue very precisely in a variety of angles with minimal peripheral thermal injury. Recently published studies show that transoral robotic surgery provides a significant emerging alternative for selected primary and salvage head and neck tumors with low morbidity and acceptable functional outcomes.[28]

Partial Laryngectomy

Partial laryngectomy is divided into vertical and horizontal partial laryngectomies. Vertical partial laryngectomy was first described by Som in 1951 and includes laryngofissure with cordectomy, extended hemilaryngectomies with cricoid excision, and epiglottic reconstruction. The procedures require a vertical transection of the thyroid cartilage and a glottic resection extending into the paraglottic space. A study found that 12 of 25 total laryngectomy patients and 1 of 11 frontolateral laryngectomy patients had significant dysphagia, with an overall incidence of 36% ($n = 13$) in all treated patients.[29] In another study, functional outcome was significantly worse in patients who underwent open surgery compared with patients with a simple cordectomy.[30]

Horizontal Partial Laryngectomies

Supraglottic laryngectomy was originally described by Alonso in 1947. Supraglottic laryngectomy spares the true vocal cords, arytenoids, tongue base, and the hyoid. Peretti et al[31] compared supraglottic laryngectomy versus laser resection in selected T1 to T3 larynx cancer patients. Fourteen patients treated with endoscopic laser surgery were compared with 14 patients matched for T category treated with open functional supraglottic laryngectomy. Aspiration rates showed no statistically significant differences; however, significant better outcome was found for swallowing, feeding tube duration, and tracheotomy duration in the transoral laser group. From the oncological point of view Cabanillas et al[32] have shown that the oncologic result of endoscopic laser approach is equivalent to those of the classic open surgery. In summary, both the endoscopic transoral laser resection and the functional open supraglottic laryngectomy should be considered as established therapeutic modalities. However, tumor extent, the technical skill of the surgeon, surgical experience, and the feasibility to perform an endoscopic procedure will determine the surgical approach in each patient.

Supracricoid Laryngectomy

Supracricoid partial laryngectomy (SCPL) was first reported in Vienna, in 1959, by Meyer and Rieder. This surgery consists of removing of the entire supraglottis, the false and true vocal folds, and the thyroid cartilage including the paraglottic and pre-epiglottic spaces. The cricoid cartilage, hyoid bone, and at least one arytenoid are preserved. Phonatory and swallowing functions are maintained by the movement of the spared arytenoid to the tongue base. There are two types of reconstruction techniques: SCPL cricohyoidopexy and SCPL cricohyoidoepiglottopexy.

In summary, the functional results of transoral laser resection are superior to those of the conventional open approach in terms of the time required to restore swallowing, tracheotomy rate, incidence of pharyngocutaneous fistulae, and shorter hospital stay. These functional advantages can be attributed to the more conservative nature of the endoscopic procedure, because normal tissues are not disrupted during the operation. However, it must be recognized that most studies that compare the outcomes of patients with an endoscopic versus conservative or radical open approaches are selected; therefore, it is difficult to definitively compare patient outcomes. Clearly, however, therapeutic decision making must balance maximizing local and regional disease control versus minimizing collateral damage to normal tissue that presumably translates to improved postoperative function.

Hypopharyngectomy–Laryngectomy

Hypopharynx

Because of the overall poor prognosis of patients with hypopharyngeal carcinomas, the aim of hypopharyngeal resections is to minimize morbidity and mortality, shorten hospital stay, and restore swallowing function as soon as possible. Depending on the localization and tumor size a partial pharyngectomy can be performed. Defects of the lateral pharyngeal wall have been reconstructed with radial forearm free flaps and the functional outcome regarding swallowing is satisfactory.[33]

Laser treatment of patients with hypopharyngeal carcinomas showed that 27% of patients achieved oral intake on the first postoperative day without nasogastric feeding tube. The median duration of nasogastric feeding in the remaining 94 (72.9%) patients was 7 days.[22] Kutter et al[34] found that feeding tubes were necessary in 67% (n = 37) of the 55 patients following transoral laser resections of pharyngeal cancer compared with 100% (n = 100) of the patients in the open surgery group. The feeding tubes remained in place for a shorter period in the transoral group than in patients who underwent open surgery and radiotherapy.[34]

Near-Total Laryngectomy

Oysu and Aslan[35] compared patients' functional outcome with T1b glottic cancer. Seventeen patients were treated by cricohyoidoepiglottopexy and 21 patients underwent near-total laryngectomy with epiglottic reconstruction (NTLER). The time of removal of the nasogastric tubes was shorter in the NTLER group; however, on long-term follow-up swallow function was good in both groups.[35] In another prospectively conducted study 28 patients with laryngeal cancer were treated with NTLER.[36] Five patients (18%) developed fistulas and that was subsequently associated with increased likelihood of aspiration.

Laryngectomy

Patients who require a total laryngectomy for local disease control can also experience postoperative dysphagia. Studies could show that dysphagia may result from tumor recurrence or even a second primary stricture or because of the loss of the pharyngeal constrictor function. Early radiographic studies defined the mucosal fold at the junction between the base of the tongue and the reconstructed circumferential pharynx as a "pseudo-epiglottis."[37] This area is particularly prone to collapsing against the tongue base to form a pocket. This pocket can accumulate food and cause dysphagia.

In 2009, one published study analyzed swallowing function after total laryngectomy and laryngopharyngectomy and found that dysphagia was observed in 18 (64%) of 28 patients,[38] with two-thirds of this group having mild

dysphagia. Comparing the swallowing function of patients who had a laryngectomy and either a T- or vertical closure it was observed that patients who had a T-closure had better swallowing functions than the vertical closure group.[39]

Laryngopharyngectomy

In general, the prognosis of advanced hypopharyngeal carcinomas is still dismal. Therefore, it is of extreme importance that after treatment patients remain with satisfying swallowing functions and thus with good quality of life. Resections of the whole circumference of the pharynx and esophagus require reconstruction with visceral transpositions or tubed free flaps (anterolateral thigh, radial forearm, omental or jejunal free flaps) or myocutaneous flaps.[40] The pectoralis major flap for circumferential reconstruction represents a viable second option with satisfying functional results after total pharyngolaryngectomy.[41] Recently published studies could show that the use of the pectoralis major flap can also be performed in combination with a jejunal free flap.[42] In a study of 55 patients who underwent total laryngectomy and 37 who underwent laryngopharyngectomy with jejunal reconstruction, it was observed that 15 (27%) patients of the laryngectomy group and 24 (65%) patients of the laryngopharyngectomy group developed swallowing-related complications[43] (**Fig. 25.3**). Circumferential reconstruction is particularly prone to stenosis. Varvares et al[44] employed the use of salivary tubes to stent the tubed radial forearm free flap. In a study of 20 patients postoperative stricture was observed in 2 (10%) patients. However, 17 (85%) patients were able to take a normal diet whereas 3 (15%) patients remained G-tube dependent. The anterolateral thigh flap has also been used for circumferential reconstruction with excellent functional outcome. In a study of 114 patients, Yu et al[45] reported that pharyngocutaneous strictures occurred in 6% (n = 7) of patients and 91% (n = 104) of patients tolerated an oral diet without the need for tube feeding.

Radiotherapy

One of the cornerstones of treatment of HNC patients is radiation therapy. The radiation fields often include critical structures necessary for normal deglutition, including the oral mucosa, tongue, larynx, pharynx, and pharyngeal muscles. One of the major acute and long-term side effects of radiation therapy is dysphagia.[46] In addition to dysphagia, other chronic side effects include trismus, stenosis of the pharynx, larynx, and esophagus, and damage to the laryngeal skeleton. In particular, radiation therapy can lead to significant impairment of the oropharyngeal phase, including insufficient velopharyngeal closure, reduced pharyngeal contraction, reduced hyoid and laryngeal motion, and reduced opening of the upper esophageal sphincter.[47]

On average, 3 months after patients finish their treatment, acute dysphagia symptoms, that is, mucositis, edema, erythema, and desquamation of the skin, resolve and

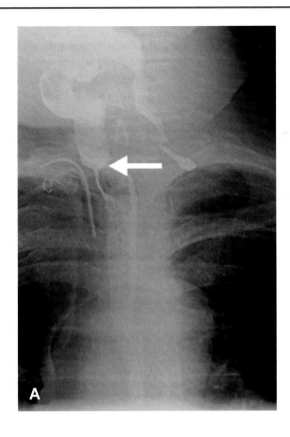

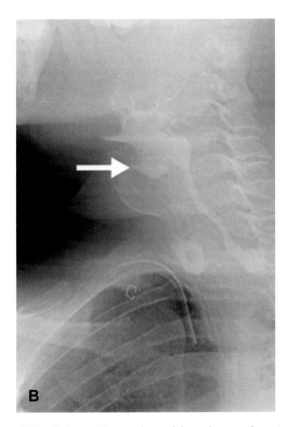

Figure 25.3 Patient with an advanced hypopharyngeal carcinoma underwent a pharyngolaryngeal resection and reconstruction with a jejunal free flap. (A) Anteroposterior and (B) lateral views show a complete obstruction of the jejunum after modified barium swallow test.

the normal swallowing function improves in most patients. Unfortunately, continuous activation of cytokines, ongoing hypoxia, and hyperactivation through hydroxyl radicals of transforming growth factor-b1 may perpetuate tissue damage. Contractility of soft tissues and muscles decreases over time because of fibrosis and lymphedema. Abnormal motility of deglutition muscles can lead to impaired pharyngeal contraction[48] and impaired laryngeal elevation causing dysphagia and aspiration.[49]

Conventional Radiotherapy and Dysphagia

Rubira et al[50] conducted a study to evaluate the oral sequelae in 100 patients with HNC treated by conventional radiotherapy. Patients were evaluated on average 28 months after completing treatment. It was observed that 30% of the patients had dysgeusia, 38% had dysphagia, and 68% had xerostomia. The authors concluded that the postradiotherapy sequelae are dependent on radiation field, radiation dose, use of antixerostomic medication, and postradiotherapy time. Another study including 100 patients with nasopharyngeal carcinoma showed that radiotherapy alone affected 93% of patients with impaired pharyngeal contraction, 74% with aspiration, and 87% with laryngeal penetration.[48]

Hyperfractionated Radiotherapy and Dysphagia

To maximize local and regional disease control rates, treatment of HNC has increasingly moved to employing combined modality approaches with radiation in combination with chemotherapy and with altered fractionation (hyperfractionation, accelerated fractionation) techniques. While the intent is to improve survival the benefits must ultimately be weighed against short-term and long-term toxicity. The European Organisation for Research and Treatment of Cancer protocol 22791 compared daily fractionation to pure hyperfractionation of 80.5 Gy in 70 fractions in 7 weeks using 3 fractions of 1.15 Gy per day in advanced oropharyngeal carcinoma.[51] All patients were followed for at least 2 years. There was an improved locoregional control noted in the hyperfractionation schedule but acute mucosal reactions were more severe compared with the convential group. Interestingly, there was no difference in the late normal tissue damage between the two groups. Another study showed the outcome of 70 patients with squamous cell carcinoma of the oral cavity, larynx, and hypopharynx.[52] Patients underwent postoperative accelerated hyperfractionation radiation versus conventional fractionation. The 3-year locoregional control rate was significantly better in the accelerated hyperfractionation compared with the conventional group, but not in survival. Xerostomia, early mucositis, fibrosis, and edema progressed more rapidly and to a more severe level in the accelerated hyperfractionation group.

Intensity-Modulated Radiation Therapy and Dysphagia

In recent years, there have been favorable results reported with the introduction of conformal three-dimensional radiotherapy techniques and, in particular, with the introduction of intensity modulated radiation therapy techniques. This technique allows for radiation to be more accurately delivered to the tumor volume while sparing surrounding healthy tissues. However, the benefits of this technique may be negated by the fact that there may be a tendency to dose escalation and increasing local toxicity. In one 2010 published study 83 patients underwent definitive IMRT for squamous cell carcinoma of the head and neck.[53] Patients who received a mean dose greater than 41 Gy or when more than 24% of the volume of the larynx received greater than 60 Gy were significantly more likely to be percutaneous endoscopic gastrostomy (PEG) tube dependent because of high risk of aspiration. In addition, patients who received 60 Gy to more than 12% of the inferior pharyngeal constrictor were also significantly at risk for PEG tube dependence and aspiration. Those patients who received 65 Gy to more than 33% to the superior pharyngeal constrictor or to more than 75% to the middle pharyngeal constrictor were at risk for the development of a pharyngoesophageal stricture. Chen et al[54] comparing conventional radiotherapy and IMRT showed that both therapeutic regimens are equally effective in terms of tumor control for locally advanced oral cavity cancer, but patients who received IMRT had significantly less late toxicity.

Chemoradiation Therapy

Over the past two decades combined chemotherapy and radiation treatment protocols have been developed to enhance locoregional disease control, reduce the likelihood of distant metastases, and preserve anatomic function in HNC patients. However, as disease control and overall survival continue to improve in patients with advanced HNC, functional and quality-of-life issues become more important.

Studies looking at functional outcomes of patients after concurrent therapies have correlated the use of cytostatic agents with dysfunction of the base of the tongue, larynx, and pharyngeal muscles. Subsequently, this leads to vallecular residue, epiglottic dysmotility, and aspiration. In combination with neutropenia arising from chemotherapy, aspiration may lead to aspiration pneumonia, sepsis, and respiratory failure. Mucositis is a significant problem in patients receiving concurrent chemoradiation treatment for HNC. The incidence and prevalence of oral mucositis in 2047 HNC patients treated with chemoradiation in 55 Spanish hospitals was reviewed.[55] Data were collected and recorded on a Radiation Therapy Oncology Group and pain scale (**Table 25.1**). The prevalence of oral mucositis was 26.4%, whereas 95.7% of the patients had grade 3 mucositis and 4.3% of patients had grade 4 mucositis. Oral mucositis resolved in 62.3% of patients after 2 months follow-up. In the same study, 96% of patients had significant pain, but after 2 months only 39.8% of patients complained about pain. The authors conclude that pain because of mucositis is a common side effect of chemotherapy and radiation and that the decreases of nutritional intake and oral function are significant.[55]

Tracheotomy

Swallowing and respiration are highly complex, coordinated, and interdependent functions. When one of these processes is impaired, the consequences may be negative for the other. Tracheotomy may be used as a short- or long-term intervention for several reasons, namely airway obstruction because of tumor bulk, postoperative edema, or where supraglottic and glottic edema may occur during chemoradiation. Tracheotomy may also be indicated because of significant physiological impairment affecting laryngeal competence, thereby increasing aspiration risk.

To complicate matters, the tracheotomy itself can also impair the swallow significantly and lead to an increased risk for aspiration[56] (**Fig. 25.4**). Causes for aspiration from a tracheotomy can be because of either mechanical or neurological factors. Fixation of the trachea and larynx by the tracheotomy tube leads to reduced laryngeal elevation and closure, reduced laryngeal sensitivity, and altered coughing response. Pressure in the upper esophagus may be increased because of high tracheotomy tube cuff pressure. Low volume, low pressure cuffs significantly decrease this risk of aspiration.[57] It is reported that the presence of an inflated cuff may negatively impact on the range of laryngeal motion and, thus, interfere with airway protection and cricopharyngeal opening. Dysphagia management in the patient with a tracheotomy tube should be approached from a multidisciplinary point of view so that appropriate decisions can be made regarding management and the decannulation process.

Feeding Tubes: Percutaneous Gastrostomy and Nasogastric Tubes

Oral intake in patients who suffer from HNC may lead to inadequate nutritional support during treatment, resulting in a need for enteral feeding. Enteral feeding may be delivered via a nasogastric or a gastrostomy tube. Over the late 1980s and early 1990s, the PEG was popularized and became widely accepted by most HNC centers allowing convenient access for nutritional support and for medication administration. Another advantage of PEG tube is that the incidence of aspiration seems to be lower in patients with PEG tubes compared with patients with nasogastric feeding tubes.[58] Insertion of the PEG tubes requires general anesthesia,

Table 25.1 Radiation Therapy Oncology Group Scale for Oral Mucositis

Grade 0	Normal oral mucosa
Grade 1	Erythema of the mucosa
Grade 2	Patchy reaction < 1.5 cm, noncontiguous
Grade 3	Confluent reaction > 1.5 cm, contiguous
Grade 4	Necrosis or deep ulceration, ± bleeding

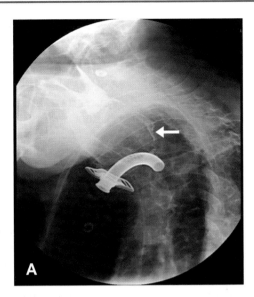

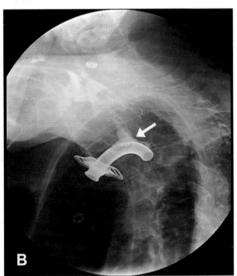

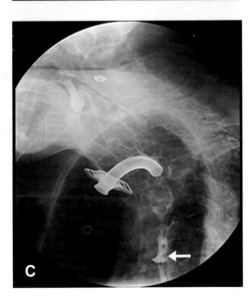

Figure 25.4 Tracheotomy was performed to secure the airway in a patient with an oropharynx cancer. (A) Oropharyngeal phase, (B) penetration through the glottis, and (C) aspiration.

whereas nasogastric tubes can be placed in an outpatient setting without using any anesthesia. Sequelae of the PEG are pain, infection around the insertion, malposition,[59] and blockage of the tube. Sequelae of nasogastric tubes are discomfort and foreign body sensation in the nose and pharynx. However, it has been shown that patients with nasogastric feeding tubes continue to swallow more frequently during the time that they require the enteral nutrition and that this improves rehabilitation of swallowing after surgery or radiochemotherapy treatment.[60]

Clinical studies comparing nasogastric versus PEG feeding tubes show that 32 patients with PEG had less initial weight loss but a higher insertion infection rate, longer duration of use, and more severe dysphagia compared with patients with nasogastric tubes.[61] Kutter et al[34] advocates that PEG feeding tubes should be used only in patients with severe swallowing dysfunction. Regardless of tube, active swallowing rehabilitation should be continued even when a gastrostomy tube is placed.

Age: A Noniatrogenic Factor Causing Dysphagia

When considering the therapeutic options for cancer treatment and the resultant toxicity of that treatment, it is important to consider that the swallow is also affected by advancing age. Recent studies show that there is a significant difference between swallowing function of healthy young and older individuals. Sarcopenia is defined as the age-related reduction of muscle fibers and results in a significantly reduced static tongue pressure and slower swallowing compared with younger healthy volunteers.[62] This slowness can impair bolus penetration and lead to aspiration. With age, there is also a decrease of sensory discrimination in the oral cavity, pharynx, and larynx. It has been shown that a disruption of the sensory–cortical–motor feedback loop may cause improper bolus formation and discoordination of the swallowing motor sequence that leads to impaired swallowing.[63]

Another factor affecting swallowing function in the aging patient is the significant decrease in number of saliva-producing acinar cells in the salivary glands. Older individuals produce the same amount of saliva; however, their saliva reserve is significantly lower than in younger volunteers. This means that radiation therapy is more likely to induce more severe xerostomia than in younger patients by further reducing saliva production. This reduced available saliva, along with reduced esophageal peristalsis, during radiation therapy can cause significant difficulties in swallowing in older patients who are less able to compensate for the alterations in their swallowing mechanism.

Evaluation of Swallowing

Swallowing assessment and therapy of HNC patients is of enormous importance and should be considered as an integral part of the management of all patients with HNC. Ideally, speech–language pathologists should be involved in pretreatment assessment whenever possible, and a routine follow-up should be provided to ensure intervention is prescribed whenever necessary.

Evaluation of a patients' medical history followed by a clinical evaluation of the head and neck and swallowing ability is mandatory. Clinical evaluation of swallowing aims at determining whether there are any pretreatment swallowing difficulties and, if present, generating a treatment plan that includes patient education and swallow therapy to ensure adequate and safe nutrition. It is of significant importance to identify patients with a risk for dysphagia.

The most common and widely used method for evaluation of swallowing is the modified barium swallow study. This is a videofluoroscopic examination of swallowing that allows dynamic evaluation of swallowing function from the oral preparatory phase to the upper esophageal phase. This method allows the radiologist, the head and neck surgeon,

and the speech–language pathologist to diagnose the impaired swallow physiology, including the risk for or actual aspiration, and design an appropriate treatment regime to address these impairments. The procedure includes standardized barium contrast containing liquids and foods of varying mouthful sizes and consistencies (**Fig. 25.5A**).

In addition to the modified barium swallow, clinicians also use flexible endoscopic evaluation of swallowing to assess the swallow physiology. This method uses direct visualization of the nasopharynx, base of tongue, hypopharynx, larynx, and vocal folds. In practice, the patient is fed with liquids and foods of varying consistencies that have been stained with blue food dye for easier visualization against the pharyngeal mucosa. The consistencies evaluated are thin liquid (milk), thick liquid (i.e., milkshake), pureed solid (i.e., applesauce), soft solid (i.e., chopped fruits), and hard solid (i.e., biscuit) (**Fig. 25.5B**). The main criteria used to evaluate swallowing are delay, multiple swallows, pooling, residue, penetration, and aspiration.[64] In 1998 a

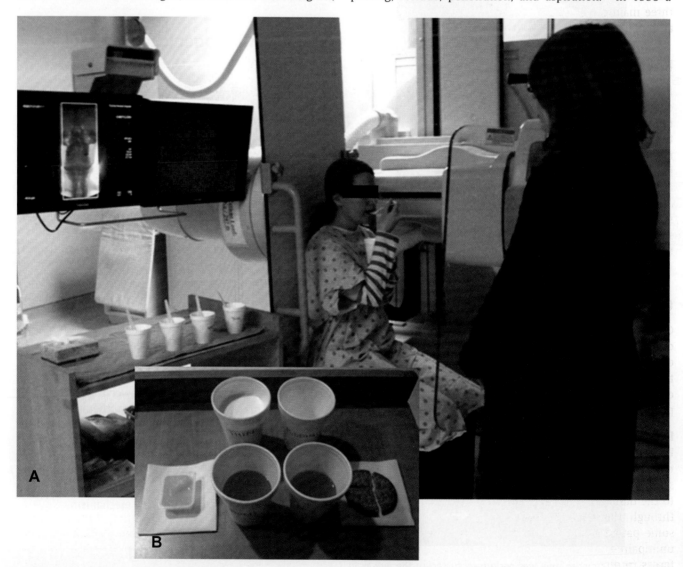

Figure 25.5 Videofluoroscopic assessment shows (A) patient positioned in an anterior-posterior view. (B) Variety of textures are mixed with barium sulfate and taken orally by the patient.

new method of bedside assessment of both the motor and sensory components of swallowing was introduced called fiberoptic endoscopic evaluation of swallowing with sensory testing.[65] This technique allows for objective determination of laryngopharyngeal sensory discrimination thresholds by delivering air pulse stimuli to the mucosa innervated by the superior laryngeal nerve via a flexible endoscope. These thresholds provide information regarding the timing of the pharyngeal swallow trigger.

Rehabilitation

Swallowing disorders arising as a result of HNC can significantly impair the patients' quality of life. The optimal rehabilitation of HNC patients starts with pretreatment assessment by the speech–language pathologist, radiologist, dietician, and clinical treatment team. Following treatment, or in the case of radiation or chemotherapy also during treatment, rehabilitation of dysphagia can be divided into three main categories: (1) preventative, (2) compensatory, and (3) physical exercises and maneuvers.

Preventative Measures

Emerging evidence suggests prophylactic swallowing exercises before commencing radiotherapy help maintain functional swallowing physiology during and after treatment outcome.[66] Implementation of IMRT technique is shown to reduce the radiation-induced salivary gland hypofunction compared with conventional radiotherapy and is being considered a preventative measure for dysphagia.[54] Additionally, salivary loss can be prevented by the use of sialogogues, such as pilocarpine or amifostine.[67] Pilocarpine stimulates minor salivary glands, which are more resistant to the effects of radiation than the parotid glands, and amifostine reduces xerostomia during and after radiation therapy.

Compensatory Measures

Compensatory approaches should be introduced early during swallowing to redirect or improve bolus flow and/or eliminate patient symptoms.[23] This includes posturing of the head and neck, improvement of oral sensory awareness, diet modification, swallowing maneuvers, and intraoral prosthetics.

Postural Techniques
Patients who can follow instructions and have good movement of the head and neck are candidates for these strategies. A common technique is rotation of the head to the damaged or weakened pharynx to direct the bolus through the healthy pharynx (**Fig. 25.6**). In contrast, some patients compensate better with a head tilt to the unimpaired oral cavity, thereby utilizing gravitational forces to direct the bolus through the health side. Other posture techniques include chin tuck, head back, and upper torso tilt.

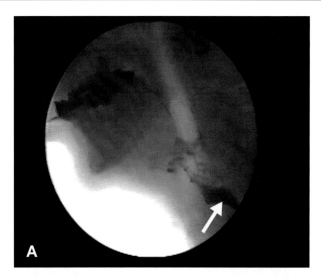

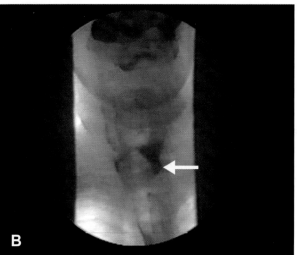

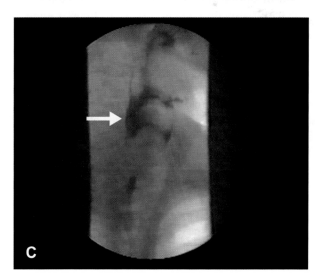

Figure 25.6 Videofluoroscopic images of the oropharyngeal swallow for a patient with paralysis of the left cranial nerves IX and X. (A) Lateral view identifying residue in the pyriform sinus. (B) Anterior-posterior view confirming residue in mainly the left pyriform sinus. (C) Anterior-posterior view depicting benefit from a left head turn to direct the bolus down the more functional right pharynx.

Techniques to Improve Sensory Awareness

Sensory feedback can be prescribed with food intake. The aim is to increase bolus awareness and thus decrease any delays in bolus transit times or trigger of the pharyngeal swallow. Common techniques include downward pressure of the spoon against the tongue, alteration of food consistency, taste (chilled or sour), and size (larger bolus volumes). Encouraging patients to feed themselves can at times serve to increase sensory feedback as well.

Food Consistency Changes

Thickening liquids lead to a slower passage through the oral cavity and pharynx, thereby compensating for delays in oral transport and trigger of the pharyngeal swallow. Patients with trismus or limited mastication ability can be assisted with pureeing solids. Diet texture restrictions should be the last compensatory strategy considered because it can have serious negative side effects for the patient.[23] These side effects include dehydration and malnutrition as well as depression and anxiety.[68] Pretreatment counseling and psychosocial support and motivation can be especially helpful in the social and physical rehabilitation of these patients.

Swallowing Maneuvers

Based on normal physiology, swallow maneuvers intend to compensate for the impaired coordination of swallowing and respiration. The supraglottic swallow maneuver aims to duplicate a functional swallow by adducting the vocal folds to intentionally cease respiration during the entire swallow. The Mendelsohn maneuver is used in patients with impaired upper esophageal sphincter opening. This maneuver facilitates greater anterior and superior hyolaryngeal movement during the swallow, which often compensates by increasing the duration and range of upper esophageal sphincter opening.

Intraoral Prosthetics

An effective intervention to compensate for dysphagia after surgical treatment is the use of prosthetic devices. Prostheses can improve mastication and close palatal defects, subsequently improving the efficiency of the swallow mechanism. A palatal lift, for example, serves to lift the existing velum toward the posterior pharyngeal wall preventing nasal regurgitation. Obturators serve to fill the palatal defects in patients with a resected velum. In patients where surgical ablation includes the tongue, the maxilla can be lowered or reshaped to allow for a better contact with the tongue during oral bolus transport.

Physical Exercises

In addition to compensatory strategies, active therapy strategies aim to facilitate remediation of the impaired swallow physiology. This includes a range of motion and resistance exercises targeting specific muscles or muscle groups of the jaw, lips, and tongue. These exercises should be introduced before the start of chemoradiation treatment to prevent or decrease the severity of the swallowing impairment before they even develop. Oral movements should be encouraged at all times either in a structured active oral exercise regime or simply during normal intake of food and liquids. Therefore, a nil-per-os strategy is discouraged for patients undergoing particularly radiation therapy or chemoradiotherapy. During these treatments, patients should instead be encouraged to maintain oral intake for as long and as much as they can tolerate. The premise is that neural circuits that do not actively engage in tasks for an extended period of time begin to degrade. This is more commonly referred to as the "use it or lose it" principle of physical rehabilitation.[69]

Clinical Pearls

- Pretreatment evaluation, planning, and assessment are critical to identify the patient who may be at risk for developing dysphagia during and after treatment.

- Balancing the oncological and swallowing outcomes between different treatment options is crucial for ensuring a successful patient outcome.

- Every patient is different and should carefully be evaluated regarding risk factors for dysphagia and aspiration.

- Advancing age is a further risk factor.

- Management of head and neck cancer patients, including diagnosis, therapy, and rehabilitation, requires a team of speech language pathologists, radiologists, radiation oncologists, and surgeons.

- To prevent dysphagia, patients should be instructed and encouraged to perform swallowing exercises and oral movements before and during chemoradiation treatment.

References

1. Mehta RP. Surgical treatment of facial paralysis. Clin Exp Otorhinolaryngol 2009;2(1):1–5
2. Faria JC, Scopel GP, Alonso N, Ferreira MC. Muscle transplants for facial reanimation: rationale and results of insertion technique using the palmaris longus tendon. Ann Plast Surg 2009;63(2):148–152
3. Anvar BA, Evans BC, Evans GR. Lip reconstruction. Plast Reconstr Surg 2007;120(4):57e–64e
4. Ethunandan M, Macpherson DW, Santhanam V. Karapandzic flap for reconstruction of lip defects. J Oral Maxillofac Surg 2007;65(12):2512–2517
5. McConnel FM, Pauloski BR, Logemann JA, et al. Functional results of primary closure vs flaps in oropharyngeal reconstruction: a prospective study of speech and swallowing. Arch Otolaryngol Head Neck Surg 1998;124(6):625–630
6. McConnel FM, Teichgraeber JF, Adler RK. A comparison of three methods of oral reconstruction. Arch Otolaryngol Head Neck Surg 1987;113(5):496–500

7. Sessions DG, Zill R, Schwartz SL. Deglutition after conservation surgery for cancer of the larynx and hypopharynx. Otolaryngol Head Neck Surg (1979) 1979;87(6):779–796

8. Seikaly H, Rieger J, Wolfaardt J, Moysa G, Harris J, Jha N. Functional outcomes after primary oropharyngeal cancer resection and reconstruction with the radial forearm free flap. Laryngoscope 2003;113(5):897–904

9. O'Connell DA, Reiger J, Dziegielewski PT, et al. Effect of lingual and hypoglossal nerve reconstruction on swallowing function in head and neck surgery: prospective functional outcomes study. J Otolaryngol Head Neck Surg 2009;38(2):246–254

10. de Vicente JC, de Villalaín L, Torre A, Peña I. Microvascular free tissue transfer for tongue reconstruction after hemiglossectomy: a functional assessment of radial forearm versus anterolateral thigh flap. J Oral Maxillofac Surg 2008;66(11):2270–2275

11. Yun IS, Lee DW, Lee WJ, Lew DH, Choi EC, Rah DK. Correlation of neotongue volume changes with functional outcomes after long-term follow-up of total glossectomy. J Craniofac Surg 2010;21(1):111–116

12. Seikaly H, Maharaj M, Rieger J, Harris J. Functional outcomes after primary mandibular resection and reconstruction with the fibular free flap. J Otolaryngol 2005;34(1):25–28

13. Shimizu H, Yoshida K, Mori N, Takahashi Y. An alternative procedure for fabricating a hollow interim obturator for a partial maxillectomy patient. J Prosthodont 2009;18(3):276–278

14. Irish J, Sandhu N, Simpson C, et al. Quality of life in patients with maxillectomy prostheses. Head Neck 2009;31(6):813–821

15. Shrime MG, Gilbert RW. Reconstruction of the midface and maxilla. Facial Plast Surg Clin North Am 2009;17(2):211–223

16. Triana RJ Jr, Uglesic V, Virag M, et al. Microvascular free flap reconstructive options in patients with partial and total maxillectomy defects. Arch Facial Plast Surg 2000;2(2):91–101

17. Clark JR, Vesely M, Gilbert R. Scapular angle osteomyogenous flap in postmaxillectomy reconstruction: defect, reconstruction, shoulder function, and harvest technique. Head Neck 2008;30(1):10–20

18. Sasaki CT, Leder SB, Acton LM, Maune S. Comparison of the glottic closure reflex in traditional "open" versus endoscopic laser supraglottic laryngectomy. Ann Otol Rhinol Laryngol 2006;115(2):93–96

19. Agrawal A, Moon J, Davis RK, et al; Southwest Oncology Group. Transoral carbon dioxide laser supraglottic laryngectomy and irradiation in stage I, II, and III squamous cell carcinoma of the supraglottic larynx: report of Southwest Oncology Group Phase 2 Trial S9709. Arch Otolaryngol Head Neck Surg 2007;133(10):1044–1050

20. Hinni ML, Salassa JR, Grant DG, et al. Transoral laser microsurgery for advanced laryngeal cancer. Arch Otolaryngol Head Neck Surg 2007;133(12):1198–1204

21. Salassa JR. A functional outcome swallowing scale for staging oropharyngeal dysphagia. Dig Dis 1999;17(4):230–234

22. Steiner W, Ambrosch P, Hess CF, Kron M. Organ preservation by transoral laser microsurgery in piriform sinus carcinoma. Otolaryngol Head Neck Surg 2001;124(1):58–67

23. Logemann JA, Bytell DE. Swallowing disorders in three types of head and neck surgical patients. Cancer 1979;44(3):1095–1105

24. Roh JL, Yoon YH. Prevention of hypopharyngeal stenosis with silastic sheeting following transoral resection. Dysphagia 2006;21(2):112–115

25. Piazza C, Peretti G, Cattaneo A, Garrubba F, De Zinis LO, Nicolai P. Salvage surgery after radiotherapy for laryngeal cancer: from endoscopic resections to open-neck partial and total laryngectomies. Arch Otolaryngol Head Neck Surg 2007;133(10):1037–1043

26. Steiner W, Fierek O, Ambrosch P, Hommerich CP, Kron M. Transoral laser microsurgery for squamous cell carcinoma of the base of the tongue. Arch Otolaryngol Head Neck Surg 2003;129(1):36–43

27. Camp AA, Fundakowski C, Petruzzelli GJ, Emami B. Functional and oncologic results following transoral laser microsurgical excision of base of tongue carcinoma. Otolaryngol Head Neck Surg 2009;141(1):66–69

28. Iseli TA, Kulbersh BD, Iseli CE, Carroll WR, Rosenthal EL, Magnuson JS. Functional outcomes after transoral robotic surgery for head and neck cancer. Otolaryngol Head Neck Surg 2009;141(2):166–171

29. Pillon J, Gonçalves MI, De Biase NG. Changes in eating habits following total and frontolateral laryngectomy. Sao Paulo Med J 2004;122(5):195–199

30. Kandogan T, Sanal A. Quality of life, functional outcome, and voice handicap index in partial laryngectomy patients for early glottic cancer. BMC Ear Nose Throat Disord 2005;5(1):3

31. Peretti G, Piazza C, Cattaneo A, De Benedetto L, Martin E, Nicolai P. Comparison of functional outcomes after endoscopic versus open-neck supraglottic laryngectomies. Ann Otol Rhinol Laryngol 2006;115(11):827–832

32. Cabanillas R, Rodrigo JP, Llorente JL, Suárez C. Oncologic outcomes of transoral laser surgery of supraglottic carcinoma compared with a transcervical approach. Head Neck 2008;30(6):750–755

33. Azizzadeh B, Yafai S, Rawnsley JD, et al. Radial forearm free flap pharyngoesophageal reconstruction. Laryngoscope 2001;111(5):807–810

34. Kutter J, Lang F, Monnier P, Pasche P. Transoral laser surgery for pharyngeal and pharyngolaryngeal carcinomas. Arch Otolaryngol Head Neck Surg 2007;133(2):139–144

35. Oysu C, Aslan I. Cricohyoidoepiglottopexy vs near-total laryngectomy with epiglottic reconstruction in the treatment of early glottic carcinoma. Arch Otolaryngol Head Neck Surg 2006;132(10):1065–1068

36. Thakar A, Bahadur S, Toran KC, Mohanti BK, Julka PK. Analysis of oncological and functional failures following near-total laryngectomy. J Laryngol Otol 2009;123(3):327–332

37. Balfe DM, Koehler RE, Setzen M, Weyman PJ, Baron RL, Ogura JH. Barium examination of the esophagus after total laryngectomy. Radiology 1982;143(2):501–508

38. Queija DdosS, Portas JG, Dedivitis RA, Lehn CN, Barros AP. Swallowing and quality of life after total laryngectomy and pharyngolaryngectomy. Braz J Otorhinolaryngol 2009;75(4):556–564

39. Davis RK, Vincent ME, Shapshay SM, Strong MS. The anatomy and complications of "T" versus vertical closure of the hypopharynx after laryngectomy. Laryngoscope 1982;92(1):16–22

40. Patel RS, Goldstein DP, Brown D, Irish J, Gullane PJ, Gilbert RW. Circumferential pharyngeal reconstruction: history, critical analysis of techniques, and current therapeutic recommendations. Head Neck 2010;32(1):109–120

41. Morshed K, Szymański M, Gołąbek W. Reconstruction of the hypopharynx with U-shaped pectoralis major myocutaneous flap after total pharyngo-laryngectomy. Eur Arch Otorhinolaryngol 2005;262(4):259–262

42. Dubsky PC, Stift A, Rath T, Kornfehl J. Salvage surgery for recurrent carcinoma of the hypopharynx and reconstruction using jejunal free tissue transfer and pectoralis major muscle pedicled flap. Arch Otolaryngol Head Neck Surg 2007;133(6):551–555

43. Ward EC, Bishop B, Frisby J, Stevens M. Swallowing outcomes following laryngectomy and pharyngolaryngectomy. Arch Otolaryngol Head Neck Surg 2002;128(2):181–186

44. Varvares MA, Cheney ML, Gliklich RE, et al. Use of the radial forearm fasciocutaneous free flap and montgomery salivary bypass tube for pharyngoesophageal reconstruction. Head Neck 2000;22(5):463–468

45. Yu P, Hanasono MM, Skoracki RJ, et al. Pharyngoesophageal reconstruction with the anterolateral thigh flap after total laryngopharyngectomy. Cancer 2010;116(7):1718–1724

46. Rancati T, Schwarz M, Allen AM, et al. Radiation dose-volume effects in the larynx and pharynx. Int J Radiat Oncol Biol Phys 2010;76(3, Suppl)S64–S69

47. Murphy BA, Gilbert J. Dysphagia in head and neck cancer patients treated with radiation: assessment, sequelae, and rehabilitation. Semin Radiat Oncol 2009;19(1):35–42

48. Ku PK, Vlantis AC, Leung SF, et al. Laryngopharyngeal sensory deficits and impaired pharyngeal motor function predict aspiration in patients irradiated for nasopharyngeal carcinoma. Laryngoscope 2010;120(2):223–228

49. Popovtzer A, Cao Y, Feng FY, Eisbruch A. Anatomical changes in the pharyngeal constrictors after chemo-irradiation of head and neck cancer and their dose-effect relationships: MRI-based study. Radiother Oncol 2009;93(3):510–515

50. Rubira CM, Devides NJ, Ubeda LT, et al. Evaluation of some oral postradiotherapy sequelae in patients treated for head and neck tumors. Braz Oral Res 2007;21(3):272–277

51. Horiot JC, Le Fur R, N'Guyen T, et al. Hyperfractionation versus conventional fractionation in oropharyngeal carcinoma: final analysis of a randomized trial of the EORTC cooperative group of radiotherapy. Radiother Oncol 1992;25(4):231–241

52. Awwad HK, Lotayef M, Shouman T, et al. Accelerated hyperfractionation (AHF) compared to conventional fractionation (CF) in the postoperative radiotherapy of locally advanced head and neck cancer: influence of proliferation. Br J Cancer 2002;86(4):517–523

53. Caudell JJ, Schaner PE, Desmond RA, Meredith RF, Spencer SA, Bonner JA. Dosimetric factors associated with long-term dysphagia after definitive radiotherapy for squamous cell carcinoma of the head and neck. Int J Radiat Oncol Biol Phys 2010;76(2):403–409

54. Chen WC, Hwang TZ, Wang WH, et al. Comparison between conventional and intensity-modulated post-operative radiotherapy for stage III and IV oral cavity cancer in terms of treatment results and toxicity. Oral Oncol 2009;45(6):505–510

55. Mañas A, Palacios A, Contreras J, Sánchez-Magro I, Blanco P, Fernández-Pérez C. Incidence of oral mucositis, its treatment and pain management in patients receiving cancer treatment at Radiation Oncology Departments in Spanish hospitals (MUCODOL Study). Clin Transl Oncol 2009;11(10):669–676

56. Ding R, Logemann JA. Swallow physiology in patients with trach cuff inflated or deflated: a retrospective study. Head Neck 2005;27(9):809–813

57. Young PJ, Pakeerathan S, Blunt MC, Subramanya S. A low-volume, low-pressure tracheal tube cuff reduces pulmonary aspiration. Crit Care Med 2006;34(3):632–639

58. Attanasio A, Bedin M, Stocco S, et al. Clinical outcomes and complications of enteral nutrition among older adults. Minerva Med 2009;100(2):159–166

59. Metheny NA, Meert KL, Clouse RE. Complications related to feeding tube placement. Curr Opin Gastroenterol 2007;23(2):178–182

60. Mekhail TM, Adelstein DJ, Rybicki LA, Larto MA, Saxton JP, Lavertu P. Enteral nutrition during the treatment of head and neck carcinoma: is a percutaneous endoscopic gastrostomy tube preferable to a nasogastric tube? Cancer 2001;91(9):1785–1790

61. Corry J, Poon W, McPhee N, et al. Prospective study of percutaneous endoscopic gastrostomy tubes versus nasogastric tubes for enteral feeding in patients with head and neck cancer undergoing (chemo) radiation. Head Neck 2009;31(7):867–876

62. Robbins J, Levine R, Wood J, Roecker EB, Luschei E. Age effects on lingual pressure generation as a risk factor for dysphagia. J Gerontol A Biol Sci Med Sci 1995;50(5):M257–M262

63. Ney DM, Weiss JM, Kind AJ, Robbins J. Senescent swallowing: impact, strategies, and interventions. Nutr Clin Pract 2009;24(3):395–413

64. Langmore SE, Schatz K, Olson N. Endoscopic and videofluoroscopic evaluations of swallowing and aspiration. Ann Otol Rhinol Laryngol 1991;100(8):678–681

65. Aviv JE, Kim T, Thomson JE, Sunshine S, Kaplan S, Close LG. Fiberoptic endoscopic evaluation of swallowing with sensory testing (FEESST) in healthy controls. Dysphagia 1998;13(2):87–92

66. Lazarus CL. Effects of chemoradiotherapy on voice and swallowing. Curr Opin Otolaryngol Head Neck Surg 2009;17(3):172–178

67. Brosky ME. The role of saliva in oral health: strategies for prevention and management of xerostomia. J Support Oncol 2007;5(5):215–225

68. Martino R, Beaton D, Diamant NE. Perceptions of psychological issues related to dysphagia differ in acute and chronic patients. Dysphagia 2010;25(1):26–34

69. Robbins J, Butler SG, Daniels SK, et al. Swallowing and dysphagia rehabilitation: translating principles of neural plasticity into clinically oriented evidence. J Speech Lang Hear Res 2008;51(1):S276–S300

26 Dental Oncology

David J. Reisberg and Joel B. Epstein

Core Messages

- Surgery, radiation therapy, and chemotherapy are common modalities used in the treatment of head and neck cancer. Combination therapy is required with advanced disease.

- Each treatment modality has adverse side effects on normal oral tissues.

- These side effects should be minimized for patient comfort, function, and overall health and quality of life.

- Pretreatment oral evaluation is critical to manage acute oral conditions and to minimize acute and chronic side effects.

- Management of oral side effects is important during and after treatment.

- Management of oral conditions and prevention of oral complications is best provided by integrated multidisciplinary health care teams.

Surgery, radiation therapy, and chemotherapy are common modalities used to treat head and neck cancer (HNC). Depending on the type, size, stage, and location of the tumor, it may be treated with single or multimodality therapy. The intensity of the side effects is usually less if these modalities are used concomitantly.

Each type of treatment strives for a selective effect where there is a maximum therapeutic dose delivered to the tumor with minimal side effects to normal tissues. As these therapies have advanced, there have been more tumor-specific techniques and agents developed towards this end. However, unfavorable side effects still do occur and new side effects are being identified with new therapies. By minimizing and managing these effects, therapy may be made more effective and patient comfort, level of function, and overall quality of life will be improved and cost of care reduced.[1]

Radiation Effects and Management

Radiation therapy may affect the oral mucosa (epithelial and connective tissues), salivary glands, muscles, blood vessels, lymphatics, nerves, teeth, and bones. Side effects include mucositis, hyposalivation, dental caries, changes in oral flora, infection, loss of taste, neuropathy, muscle fibrosis and trismus, and soft tissue and bone necrosis. Severity is not uniform or consistent but depends upon the surgery performed, radiation therapy (fields, fractionation, total dose), and individual patient variability. The introduction of intensity-modulated radiation therapy (IMRT) has decreased the severity of some side effects, but not eliminated them.

Proper management dictates that all patients receive a comprehensive oral evaluation before commencement of cancer treatment, be monitored during therapy, and then be periodically followed for oral management once therapy has been completed. Oral management is best accomplished by experienced dental providers working as part of an oncology team. Some undesirable side effects of radiation and chemotherapy may improve once cancer treatment is complete while others linger on indefinitely and new, late complications may arise.

Mucositis

Mucositis appears early and intensifies as treatment progresses. Within the first 2 weeks, erythema is noted followed by desquamation and ulceration as treatment proceeds (**Fig. 26.1**). Changes are caused by a direct effect of radiation on epithelial and connective components of the mucosa as well as a change in the oral flora that may result in a shift in oral bacterial and fungal colonization. In patients who continue to use tobacco or alcohol, who suffer comorbidities such as diabetes, or who undergo concomitant chemotherapy, these mucosal changes may be intensified in severity and extended in duration. In the most severe cases, treatment may have to be delayed, interrupted, or discontinued to allow the mucosa to recover. Once radiation therapy is completed, the mucosa will return to a clinically normal appearance over a period of a few weeks to months; however, vascular and neurologic changes and mucosal atrophy may persist. Although the skin is similarly sensitive, we see less severe changes because of "skin-sparing" sources of irradiation and improved techniques such as IMRT.

Pain because of mucositis is a significant source of complaint for patients receiving HNC therapy. Oral prophylaxis may achieve a reduction in duration and

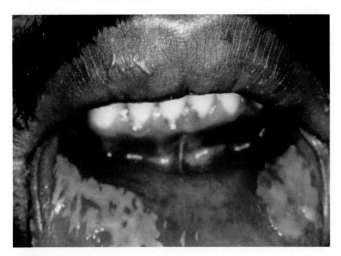

Figure 26.1 Mucositis.

severity of mucosal damage. Good oral hygiene, an atraumatic diet, and oral rinsing with saline are basic oral care recommendations. Food and Drug Administration–cleared devices for mucositis include coating agents such as sodium hyaluronate topical (Gelclair), mucoadhesive oral protectants (MuGard), and artificial saliva (Caphosol). Oral cooling with ice chips has been shown useful in short-acting, bolus chemotherapy, but not investigated in radiation therapy. Benzydamine (not available in the United States) has shown a preventive effect. Pain management should be provided as needed. Continuing studies provide reason for optimism for future advances in prevention and treatment of mucositis.[2]

Salivary Gland

After radiation of major salivary glands, reduced volume, increased viscosity, and changes in pH and inorganic and organic constituents of the saliva occur.[3] Saliva becomes more viscous and sticky and decreases in amount, leading to xerostomia (**Fig. 26.2A, B**). Radiation causes vascular damage, loss of acinar cells, and may lead to fibrosis of the salivary glands. This may contribute to not only discomfort and intensified mucositis but also persisting changes and

symptoms. Hyposalivation predisposes the patient to dental caries. It may also contribute to changes in taste, difficulty in swallowing, and the ability to wear a removable dental prosthesis as well as make the performance of routine oral hygiene tasks more difficult. Radiation-induced xerostomia may persist indefinitely. Patients may not report persisting dry mouth because of an acquired tolerance. Salivary changes after chemotherapy most often return to pretherapy baseline.

After radiation therapy, there may be recovery of some acinar cells depending on the radiation dose and schedule.[4] It is not likely that salivary gland tissue recovers from tumoricidal doses of radiation. The use of IMRT increases the potential for stimulation of residual function by reducing the volume of damage in the head and neck by sparing normal tissues. Lin et al[5] have demonstrated the regeneration of salivary gland tissue in laboratory animals, but this has not yet been tried in humans.

Minimizing exposure of the salivary glands and other critical anatomic structures is a goal of treatment planning. IMRT may have the effect of wider field/lower dose radiation exposure, which may result in increased responsiveness to systemic sialogogues if dry mouth persists. Amifostine is a salivary gland protector, indicated for use in patients with HNC receiving radiation therapy. Diagnosis of hyposalivation may be based on history and clinical observation. However, in persistent dry mouth, patients may accommodate over time and not report it while the conditions favor oral disease. Assessment of salivary flow is valuable in diagnosis and evaluating the response to treatment.

Treatment of hyposalivation should focus first on stimulating residual function. Systemic agents may be used to achieve an increase in volume and salivary constituents and may be documented with sialography. There are several choleretic medications such as pilocarpine (Salagen) and cevimeline (Evoxac) that are approved for this indication. Bethanechol (Urecholine) has been studied off-label. Other approaches have included acupuncture and nerve stimulation. If salivary flow cannot be improved, there are numerous mouth-wetting agents to consider, and treatment trials to identify the most helpful product should be conducted.

Jha et al[6] have described a technique for surgically transplanting the submandibular salivary glands to remove

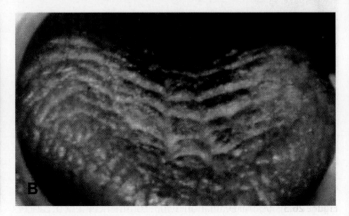

Figure 26.2 (A) Viscous saliva. (B) Severe xerostomia.

them from the field of radiation. The advent of IMRT may limit further study of this approach.

Teeth

It is unclear whether radiation has a direct effect on the enamel, dentin, and cementum of teeth. There have been conflicting reports regarding the changes in these structures caused by radiation and whether their solubility is affected.[7] It does appear that the dental pulp is significantly affected by tumoricidal doses of radiation. The vascular elements of the pulp fibrose and atrophy and sensory innervation may be affected. This may lead to an altered response to infection but may also decrease the degree of pulpal pain, even in the case of severe dental decay.

An indirect effect on the dentition is decay secondary to hyposalivation, a change in saliva consistency and pH, and a decrease in the mineralizing constituents in the saliva. These carious lesions begin as demineralized sites on the teeth involving the incisal edges of teeth and at the gingival margins, especially interproximally, sites where decay is not usually seen. These lesions may progress to the extent that the entire crown of the tooth may be lost (**Fig. 26.3A, B**).

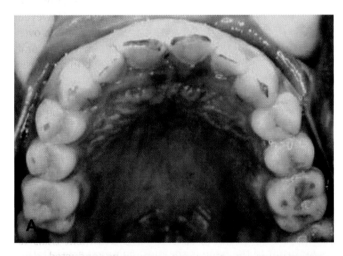

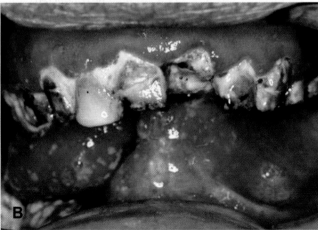

Figure 26.3 (A) Incipient radiation-induced dental caries. (B) Severe radiation-induced dental caries.

Changes in the oral flora are thought to be an indirect result of hyposalivation. An increase in cariogenic bacteria, such as *Streptococcus mutans* and *Lactobacillus*, predisposes to dental decay. A marked increase in the fungal population, most notably *Candida albicans*, may lead to an increase in oral infections.

Underlying risk factors should be addressed, including diet history, oral hygiene, and dry mouth. Dental structures may be better maintained with regular fluoride applications such as a daily fluoride rinse (ACT), a high-potency fluoride dentifrice, fluoride gel in a custom carrier, and/or fluoride varnishes. There are no studies documenting the most effective means of fluoride application. In patients with dry mouth, calcium and phosphate supplementation should be provided and management of hyposalivation should be attempted. Antimicrobials for the treatment of a shift to cariogenic oral flora should also be considered. The oral environment, the tooth structure, and the bacterial component must all be addressed in addition to strict oral hygiene and diet instruction. Candidiasis is a frequent oral infection and increases during and persists after cancer therapy (**Fig. 26.4**). Risk factors should be addressed. Reduction of antibiotics, steroids, and hyposalivation-inducing medications should be considered. The care provider may choose between topical and systemic antifungals, depending on circumstances and preference. It should be recognized that nystatin (Mycostatin and Nystan) suspension is sucrose sweetened, and in a patient with dry mouth, it may increase the caries risk dramatically.

Taste

Most patients who undergo radiation therapy experience a loss of taste. It is unclear whether this is due to a direct effect of the radiation on the taste buds or related to neural changes that affect them. In addition, salivary changes play a role, as loss of saliva may decrease both the number and the function of the remaining taste buds and limit the delivery of taste stimulants in solution to taste receptors. Loss of taste usually begins after the second week of therapy. In most cases, taste returns several weeks to months after the completion of therapy. In some cases, patients report a failure of taste to completely return, resulting in reduced or altered taste. This may be related to the total dose and ports of radiation. The loss of taste is significant aside from patient comfort. Patients report less desire to eat, and this may affect the body's ability to take nourishment to repair the damage to normal tissues injured by the radiation. Patients who experience altered or loss of taste will need to experiment with alternative diet choices. It is unlikely that those with normal taste experience can make appropriate recommendations.

Chronic taste alteration may be less common in those treated with IMRT. If dry mouth can be managed, it may assist in improving taste. Local oral, dental, and upper respiratory infection may affect taste and can be managed.

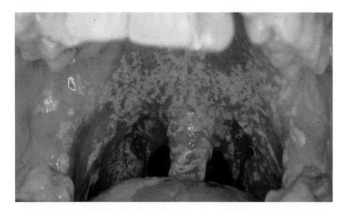

Figure 26.4   Candidiasis infection.

Effective management of persisting taste changes is not well documented. Zinc supplementation has shown conflicting results in trials to date. Clonazepam (Klonopin) has been considered in some cases and has been shown to be helpful in altered olfactory sensation.

Trismus

Many patients who complain of an inability to masticate food because of loss of teeth or saliva are, in fact, compromised by a reduced ability to swallow. Radiation affecting the pharynx results in a loss of elasticity and fibrosis that may lead to narrowing of the pharynx and limitation of movement, thus complicating deglutition.

Some surgical resections of tumors will involve the pterygoid space or the muscles of mastication. Muscle scarring as the result of wound healing may contribute to decreased oral opening. When the muscles of mastication are in the field of radiation, trismus or limitation of oral opening is a common side effect leading to disability. This is most often seen with tumors of the nasopharynx, soft palate, or parotid gland because of their location relative to these functional muscle groups. If the radiation is administered bilaterally or if in conjunction with surgery, the effects may be more severe.

Radiation causes fibrosis or scarring of the muscle fibers, limiting their ability to stretch and function normally. The limitation of oral opening will affect patient comfort and the ability to eat. Trismus may also limit the ability to have preventative and restorative dental procedures performed including fabrication of an obturator to restore speech and feeding. It may also limit the patient's ability to perform home hygiene procedures such as tooth brushing, dental flossing, and fluoride applications to the teeth. This may contribute to a rapid demise of the dentition.

Once it has occurred, trismus is permanent and patients do not recover fully. The most effective course in management is to minimize its occurrence by initiating a physical therapy program at the start of radiation and to continue it for 3 months after radiation therapy is completed. The use of IMRT in HNC is associated with lower risk of trismus. Several mechanical devices have gained popularity in managing trismus. Therabite (Atos Medical, West Allis, Wisconsin, United States) and Dynasplint (Dynasplint Systems, Severna Park, Maryland, United States) are two of the most popular devices. A comprehensive, active home exercise program has also been shown to be effective. In any case, patient compliance seems to be the key factor in success. If trismus is severe or long-standing, a little permanent, significant improvement in the range of opening is expected.

Bone

Tumoricidal radiation therapy has a significant effect on bone. Radiation-induced endarteritis causes a decrease in the size of the lumen of blood vessels and may cause total occlusion of fine vasculature within the bone. Bone that has been irradiated to tumoricidal doses may become acellular, avascular tissue, showing signs of fatty degeneration. The dynamic balance of osteoblastic and osteoclastic activity is interrupted and renders the bone a nonvital entity.[8-10] The mandible is denser than the maxilla and has less vascularity, which may explain the increased risk of necrosis compared with the maxilla. High-speed radiation and IMRT have helped to diminish these changes in recent years, but postradiation osteonecrosis (ORN) remains a serious side effect of radiation therapy (**Fig. 26.5**). It is a nonhealing wound in nonvital bone. It is not primarily an infection of bone, although the lesion may become secondarily infected. Pain associated with ORN varies widely from none to severe, often related to the presence of any secondary infection or to the presence of a pathologic fracture. Injury to overlying soft tissue alone may not cause ORN, but may result in bone exposure. If the injury extends through to expose bone or if the mucosa necroses, osteoradionecrosis may develop. The effects of radiation on bone are thought to be permanent. However, angiogenesis and collateral circulation may improve blood flow in irradiated bone over time. Still, most clinicians approach the oral treatment of patients who have had radiation therapy with great caution.

An insult to the bone is the most common precipitating factor in the development of ORN. Most often this is due to a dental extraction, but this may also be due to a periodontal or pulp infection, irritation from a removable dental prosthesis, or bone exposure may occur spontaneously followed by lack of healing of exposed bone. If a small sequestrum mobilizes sufficiently, it may be removed atraumatically. A more extensive surgical resection with bone reconstruction may be required for a larger necrotic area. Cronje described a protocal developed by Marx for the treatment of ORN that involves the use of hyperbaric oxygen (HBO) therapy and surgery. A controlled study of HBO alone did not show benefit in the recovery of ORN after radiation therapy. Many feel that surgical resection is an overly aggressive approach, but those who use it believe that it is the best way to treat the problem. Other approaches to management include the use of pentoxifylline (Trental) and vitamin E, which affect

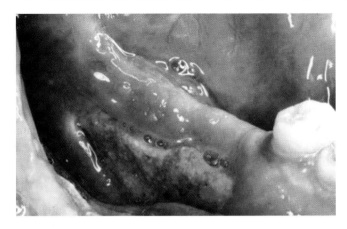

Figure 26.5 Osteoradionecrosis of the mandible.

fibrosis and blood flow and reduce tumor necrosis factor in the tissue. Prevention is paramount. Dental care before cancer therapy, an ongoing preventive program, and close follow-up are critical to minimizing the risk of ORN.

Chemotherapy Effects and Management

In the last 10 years, chemotherapy has become common in treating HNC. It may be used alone for induction therapy before combined chemotherapy and radiotherapy, as an adjunct to surgery and radiation, as a palliative measure, and most recently for control of persisting disease after standard therapy with a "curative intent." Many chemotherapeutic agents have toxicity profiles that result in oral side effects. Chemotherapy is used to treat non-HNCs such as breast, colon, and lung cancer; lymphoma; or leukemia, and adverse oral effects may occur.

Common side effects include nausea, vomiting, and diarrhea. The most common oral side effects associated with chemotherapy are mucositis, xerostomia, hemorrhage, and infection. Unlike radiation therapy where some side effects will linger indefinitely beyond the completion of treatment, the adverse side effects because of chemotherapy are more transient and resolve soon after therapy is completed and blood values return to normal. With today's more common chemoradiation protocols, each individual therapeutic modality potentiates the side effects of the other and may increase the severity and duration of both acute and chronic side effects.

There are several categories of agents used for chemotherapy that destroy or slow the growth of rapidly dividing tumor cells. These categories include both cell-cycle–specific and cell-cycle–nonspecific agents.[12] The most commonly used chemotherapy agents used to treat HNC are platinum derivatives, fluorouracil, taxanes, and epidermal growth factor antagonists. Unfortunately, normal cells may also be affected, most commonly those with a higher rate of proliferation including the oral cavity, digestive tract, and bone marrow.

Mucositis

Mucositis is the most common acute side effect of chemotherapy.[13,14] There is damage to mucosal vasculature, connective tissue, and epithelial compartments that result in erythema, thinning and loss of the epithelium, and degeneration of collagen. This process may initially appear with white changes in the mucosa but over a 2-week period progresses to erythema and ulceration. Although the etiology may differ, the associated oral pain is like that because of radiation therapy. Speaking, eating, taking oral medication, and performing oral hygiene may be difficult. In severe situations, ulcerative lesions may become secondarily infected, leading to a systemic infection that could be life-threatening. Sonis et al[15] developed the oral mucositis assessment scale to grade severity. It is based on subjective complaints, functional performance, and objective changes.

Effects on Salivary Glands

Chemotherapy is thought to have a direct, systemic effect on major and minor salivary glands.[16] It tends to be less severe and more transient than that induced by radiation therapy. Hyposalivation may increase pain and discomfort associated with mucositis and may lead to taste changes. In addition to the discomfort associated with decreased salivary flow, there is reduction of the protective constituents in saliva that may contribute to dental decay and secondary infection.

Oral Hemorrhage

The potential for oral hemorrhage is directly related to thrombocytopenia, liver function, and mucosal damage. Hemorrhagic mucositis is seen with reactivation of herpes viruses. In addition to being caused by the chemotherapeutic agents that are used to treat HNC, this condition may be manifested by other systemic cancers, such as leukemia, lymphoma, and Hodgkin disease, whereas myelosuppression occurs because of the agents used to treat them. When the platelet levels drop below 25,000 cells/mm³, there is a risk of induced or spontaneous, uncontrolled hemorrhage. During chemotherapy, the platelet levels must be monitored to avoid such dangers and platelet transfusions may be necessary before any necessary traumatic procedures such as an emergency dental extraction are performed.

Clinical signs of hemorrhage within the oral cavity include petechiae, ecchymosis, gingival oozing, hematoma, or frank bleeding. These may occur because of unintentional traumatic injuries from toothbrushing, wearing a removable dental prosthesis, or eating coarse foods. These may occur at the site of an existing oral ulceration. Spontaneous intraoral bleeding occurs most commonly from the gingival sulcus (**Fig. 26.6**). The epithelium is only a few cells thick, and it is not uncommon to have inflammation present because of gingival or periodontal disease that may be preexisting or may have developed as the result of the patient's

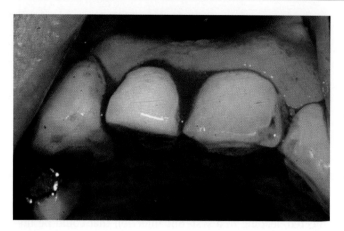

Figure 26.6 Gingival hemorrhage induced by chemotherapy and decreased platelet count.

compromised ability or desire to perform daily oral hygiene procedures.

Infection

Chemotherapy-induced immunosuppression related to the treatment of cancer (head and neck or other) increases the risk of serious infections that may ordinarily be controlled. Opportunistic microorganisms that normally inhabit the oral cavity may colonize, invade, and cause systemic infection because of neutropenia and loss of mucosal barriers.

A common site is the gingival sulcus where microorganisms normally tend to aggregate. A daily hygiene regimen that removes plaque from around teeth is important but must be carefully tempered by the consideration for inducing oral hemorrhage. Ulcerations present from mucositis are also common sites for secondary infection. If not controlled, these infections may be life-threatening.

Pretreatment Oral Management

All patients who are to undergo radiation and/or chemotherapy should receive a complete oral evaluation before treatment.[17] This should be completed as soon as possible after diagnosis, followed by a review once the oncologic treatment plan has been established. There may be significant oral discoveries made at the oral/dental examination that may affect oncologic treatment planning. In any event, the complete oral examination should be conducted at least 2 weeks before the initiation of therapy. This allows time for healing should any oral surgical procedures be necessary. This period also permits time for any restorative or hygiene procedures that need to be completed. The overall goals are to eliminate existing and potential sources of infection, stabilize the dentition, and to project future dental needs.

This evaluation should be performed by a dentist who has experience in managing patients with HNC—preferably one who is part of the HNC team. The evaluation should include complete head and neck, intraoral soft tissue, and dental examinations. Ideally, a complete dental radiographic examination should be included as part of the evaluation, but a panoramic radiograph may provide sufficient information. Standard intraoral photographs of the maxillary and mandibular dentitions are a useful supplement to any written record. This pretreatment evaluation should be required of all patients whether they have natural dentition or are edentulous. Areas of denture sores, retained roots, or affected teeth, bone cysts, abscesses, or other lesions should be identified to determine the need for removal before the initiation of therapy.

As a general rule, all teeth with severe decay or advanced periodontal disease should be extracted. Within the high-dose radiation field, those with moderate or severe dental caries or periodontal disease should be removed before therapy. The goal is to eliminate all symptomatic oral disease and potential sites of later infections or that would require future surgical intervention. Healthy teeth may be retained, even if in the direct site of the radiation, if maintenance of oral health and function is projected. Routine procedures such as dental restorations for moderate caries control, oral prophylaxis, and even endodontic therapy (root canal) may be performed. Extensive periodontal therapy or complex dental restorations should be avoided if they may delay the beginning of therapy. Any teeth that cannot be maintained for a lifetime should be deemed hopeless and be extracted.

Any planned removable partial or complete dentures should be deferred until after the oral soft tissues have recovered from the side effects of therapy. Preprosthetic surgery such as tori removal, smoothing of sharp bony areas, or tuberosity reductions should be performed before radiation therapy. This pretreatment planning is essential to avoid later prosthesis compromise and potential failure. If placement of a feeding tube or port is planned, any oral surgical procedures may be coupled with these procedures to limit the number of general anesthetics required.

If the patient is already wearing removable partial or complete dentures, these must be evaluated to determine whether they are a potential source of tissue trauma. If so, they must be adjusted or not worn during cancer treatment as they pose a potential for soft tissue irritation. If natural teeth remain, the patient must adhere to a strict regimen of oral home care that includes proper brushing, flossing, and daily application of fluoride to the teeth. Impressions for custom fluoride applicators should be made by the dentist before commencement of therapy.

Oral Management during Therapy

During therapy, prevention and management of acute oral complications are facilitated by experienced providers working on the oncology team. Oral evaluations should be conducted weekly or when symptoms develop. During therapy, only emergency dental care should be performed.

Proper pretreatment management should have eliminated the need for all but most emergent, unforeseen care.

As previously mentioned, the most common acute complaint is pain related to oral mucositis. Pain may be so severe as to interfere with normal oral care where even toothbrushing is too painful. Daily application of a chlorhexidine (Peridex) with an oral swab, such as a Toothetten (Sage Products, Cary, Illinois, United States), will decrease inflammation and make oral hygiene easier, whereas use of a sponge brush alone has been shown to have no effect on gingival health.

Taste change and alteration in saliva consistency and volume are anticipated. Dysphagia and odynophagia are problems associated with mucositis and may make eating difficult. Proper nutritional intake is important to combat the stress and demands placed on the body by radiation, chemotherapy, or both. Nutritional counseling should be provided by the oncology team to establish a comfortable, balanced diet. If mucositis is severe and oral intake is greatly reduced, a gastric feeding tube is used. Because of the toxicity of chemoradiation, placement of such a tube is often a part of the pretreatment protocol.

Posttreatment Oral Management

Having completed cancer therapy, patients should be placed on a 3-month dental recall until the oral status has stabilized adequately to resume regular 6-month evaluations. Routine dental procedures, such as oral prophylaxis, dental restorations, and endodontic therapy, may be performed. Some recommend prophylactic antibiotic therapy for endodontia in case of over instrumentation of the root canal with a possibility of infection, but this has not been borne out in any scientific studies.

After the completion of oncologic therapy, oral surgical procedures, such as dental extractions, periodontal surgery, and placement of osseointegrated dental implants, should be avoided within the high-dose radiation field. The lasting effects of radiation in bone makes it a subject of risk for healing following such procedures. The concern for ORN is greater with these procedures but may also occur spontaneously or at the site of a denture irritation or a pretreatment extraction site.

Removable partial and complete dentures may be fabricated, but these must be monitored closely to ensure that they do not cause soft tissue irritation that could contribute to ulcerations, soft tissue necrosis, and bone exposure.

To minimize posttreatment oral complications, standard oral hygiene procedures including proper brushing and flossing are recommended. The use of antiseptic mouthwashes to reduce the biofilm burden (e.g., chlorhexidine) has been suggested.

While an established and long accepted protocol[7] includes HBO therapy to promote vascularization, recent randomized trials have not shown benefit. In addition, there is a concern that HBO may provide increased oxygenation increasing tumor cell proliferation. Vascularized bone and soft tissue free flaps have been used for the management of localized defects. More recently, treatment aimed at elevated tumor necrosis factor and limited vascularization and fibrosis have been managed by using pentoxifylline and vitamin E. It is possible to extract a tooth after radiation therapy, but the protocol for doing this is not unanimous. Some dentists will do so without the benefit of prophylactic HBO but will opt for its use if postoperative healing is compromised and depending on the extent of surgery required. Other considerations for its use are total dose and fields of radiation, time because radiation has been completed, the cost of HBO, and access to it.

Survivorship issues (**Table 26.1**) are common and require assessment, diagnosis, and management, whenever possible. After therapy, all routine general dental procedures may be performed including dental prophylaxis, endodontic therapy, and restorative procedures such as fillings and crowns. Removable partial and complete dentures may also be made but must be monitored closely to make sure they do not cause soft tissue irritation that could lead to more serious consequences. Surgical and invasive procedures can be conducted out of the high-dose field of radiation therapy. Therefore, treatment planning must

Table 26.1 Survivorship and Chronic Oral Complications

Hyposalivation
- Mucosal infection
- Caries risk
- Periodontal disease
- Taste
- Dysphagia
- Speech
- Mucosal sensitivity

Neurologic
- Neuropathy
- Taste
- Speech
- Dysphagia
- Mucosal sensitivity

Fibrosis
- Trismus
- Limited soft tissue movement

Vascular change
- Soft tissue, bone necrosis risk

Recurrent cancer, second cancer

include details of the earlier treatment and prognosis of the treatment.

The background of many of the most reported complications is hyposalivation. If hyposalivation persists, oral functions of taste, speech, retention of prostheses (if present); formation of a food bolus; and swallowing are affected. The nutritional compromise may relate to weight increase, nutrient availability, and systemic health. Hyposalivation is associated with the risk of infection including candidiasis and dental caries and periodontal health. Mucosal sensitivity because of neuropathic changes or chronic infection and mucosal atrophy may contribute to adverse quality of life and also lead to dietary change. Postsurgical and radiotherapy fibrosis may affect range of movement of the jaw, oral aperture, tongue mobility, and dysphagia. All these aspects of chronic complications affect cost of care and quality of life, and prevention or management is needed.

Conclusions

Radiation and chemotherapy, either alone or in combination, are effective modalities used to treat HNC. Each has its side effects that may pose discomfort and even danger to the patient. A qualified dentist should be part of the management team and should evaluate, manage, and follow the patient before, during, and after cancer therapy to minimize the side effects.

Tips to Avoid Complications

- All patients should be seen by an oncologic dentist before cancer therapy begins.

- A dentist with experience managing the side effects of radiation and chemotherapy should be part of the cancer treatment team.

Clinical Pearls

- Radiation therapy and chemotherapy are common modalities used to treat head and neck cancer.

- Both acute and chronic side effects are inevitable.

- Some effects may be profound and chronic.

- Management by a qualified dental specialist is important to minimize these adverse effects and maintain a patient's quality of life.

References

1. Davies AN, Epstein JB, eds. Oral Complications of Cancer and its Management. Oxford: Oxford University Press; 2010
2. Peterson DE. New strategies for management of oral mucositis in cancer patients. J Support Oncol 2006;4(2, Suppl 1):9–13
3. Beumer J, Curtis TA, Marunick MT, eds. Maxillofacial Rehabilitation: Prosthodontic and Surgical Considerations. St. Louis, MO: Ishiyaku EuroAmerica; 1996:43–109
4. Konings AW, Coppes RP, Vissink A. On the mechanism of salivary gland radiosensitivity. Int J Radiat Orcal Biol Phys 2005;62:1187–1194
5. Lin CY, Chang FH, Chen CY, et al. Cell therapy for salivary gland regeneration. J Dent Res 2011;90(3):341–346
6. Jha N, Seikaly H, Harris J, et al. Phase III randomized study: oral pilocarpine versus submandibular salivary gland transfer protocol for the management of radiation-induced xerostomia. Head Neck 2009;31(2):234–243
7. Kielbasse AM. In situ induced demineralization in irradiated and non-irradiated human dentin. Eur J Oral Sci 2000;108(3):214–221
8. Marx RE. A new concept in the treatment of osteoradionecrosis. J Oral Maxillofac Surg 1983;41(6):351–357
9. Marx RE. Osteoradionecrosis: a new concept of its pathophysiology. J Oral Maxillofac Surg 1983;41(5):283–288
10. Jacobson AS, Buchbinder D, Hu K, Urken ML. Paradigm shifts in the management of osteoradionecrosis of the mandible. Oral Oncol 2010;46(11):795–801
11. Cronje FJ. A review of the Marx protocols: prevention and management of osteoradionecrosis by combining surgery and hyperbaric oxygen therapy. SADJ 1998;53(10):469–471
12. Chung EM, Sung EC. Oral management of chemotherapy patients. In: Beumer J, Marunick MT, Esposito SJ, eds. Maxillofacial Rehabilitation: Prosthodontic + Surgical Management of Cancer-related, Acquired, and Congenital Defects of the Head and Neck. Chicago, IL: Quintessence; 2011:425
13. Lockhart PB, Sonis ST. Alterations in the oral mucosa caused by chemotherapeutic agents. A histologic study. J Dermatol Surg Oncol 1981;7(12):1019–1025
14. Mosel DD, Bauer RL, Lynch DP, Hwang ST. Oral complications in the treatment of cancer patients. Oral Dis 2011;17(6):550–559 epub ahead of print
15. Sonis ST, Eilers JP, Epstein JB, et al; Mucositis Study Group. Validation of a new scoring system for the assessment of clinical trial research of oral mucositis induced by radiation or chemotherapy. Cancer 1999;85(10):2103–2113
16. Jensen SB, Pedersen AM, Vissink A, et al; Salivary Gland Hypofunction/Xerostomia Section, Oral Care Study Group, Multinational Association of Supportive Care in Cancer (MASCC)/International Society of Oral Oncology (ISOO). A systematic review of salivary gland hypofunction and xerostomia induced by cancer therapies: prevalence, severity and impact on quality of life. Support Care Cancer 2010;18(8):1039–1060
17. Chung EM, Sung EC. Dental management of chemoradiation patients. J Calif Dent Assoc 2006;34(9):735–742

Bibliography

- Bensadoun R-J, Riesenbeck D, Lockhart PB, Elting LS, Spijkervet FK, Brennan MT; Trismus Section, Oral Care Study Group, Multinational Association for Supportive Care in Cancer (MASCC)/International Society of Oral Oncology (ISOO). A systematic review of trismus induced by cancer therapies in head and neck cancer patients. Support Care Cancer 2010;18(8):1033–1038
- Elad S, Zadik Y, Hewson I, et al; Viral Infections Section, Oral Care Study Group, Multinational Association of Supportive Care in Cancer (MASCC)/International Society of Oral Oncology (ISOO). A systematic review of viral infections associated with oral

involvement in cancer patients: a spotlight on Herpesviridae. Support Care Cancer 2010;18(8):993–1006

- Epstein JB, Hong C, Logan RM, et al. A systematic review of orofacial pain in patients receiving cancer therapy. Support Care Cancer 2010;18(8):1023–1031
- Epstein JB, Murphy BA. Late effects of cancer and cancer therapy on oral health and quality of life. J Mass Dent Soc 2010;59(3):22–27
- Hong CHL, Napeñas JJ, Hodgson BD, et al; Dental Disease Section, Oral Care Study Group, Multi-national Association of Supportive Care in Cancer (MASCC)/International Society of Oral Oncology (ISOO). A systematic review of dental disease in patients undergoing cancer therapy. Support Care Cancer 2010;18(8):1007–1021
- Hovan AJ, Williams PM, Stevenson-Moore P, et al; Dysgeusia Section, Oral Care Study Group, Multinational Association of Supportive Care in Cancer (MASCC)/International Society of Oral Oncology (ISOO). A systematic review of dysgeusia induced by cancer therapies. Support Care Cancer 2010;18(8):1081–1087
- Jensen SB, Pedersen AML, Vissink A, et al; Salivary Gland Hypofunction/Xerostomia Section, Oral Care Study Group, Multinational Association of Supportive Care in Cancer (MASCC)/ International Society of Oral Oncology (ISOO). A systematic review of salivary gland hypofunction and xerostomia induced by cancer therapies: prevalence, severity and impact on quality of life. Support Care Cancer 2010a;18(8):1039–1060
- Jensen SB, Pedersen AML, Vissink A, et al; Salivary Gland Hypofunction/Xerostomia Section; Oral Care Study Group; Multinational Association of Supportive Care in Cancer (MASCC)/ International Society of Oral Oncology (ISOO). A systematic review of salivary gland hypofunction and xerostomia induced by cancer therapies: management strategies and economic impact. Support Care Cancer 2010b;18(8):1061–1079
- Lalla RV, Latortue MC, Hong CH, et al; Fungal Infections Section, Oral Care Study Group, Multinational Association of Supportive Care in Cancer (MASCC)/International Society of Oral Oncology (ISOO). A systematic review of oral fungal infections in patients receiving cancer therapy. Support Care Cancer 2010;18(8):985–992
- Migliorati CA, Woo S-B, Hewson I, et al; Bisphosphonate Osteonecrosis Section, Oral Care Study Group, Multinational Association of Supportive Care in Cancer (MASCC)/International Society of Oral Oncology (ISOO). A systematic review of bisphosphonate osteonecrosis (BON) in cancer. Support Care Cancer 2010;18(8):1099–1106
- Olver IN, ed. The MASCC Textbook of Cancer Supportive Care and Survivorship. New York, NY: Springer; 2010
- Peterson DE, Doerr W, Hovan A, et al. Osteoradionecrosis in cancer patients: the evidence base for treatment-dependent frequency, current management strategies, and future studies. Support Care Cancer 2010;18(8):1089–1098
- Rankin KV, Epstein J, Hubber MA, et al. Oral health in cancer therapy. Todays FDA 2009;21(8):37, 39–45
- Sonis ST. Mucositis: The impact, biology and therapeutic opportunities of oral mucositis. Oral Oncol 2009;45(12):1015–1020
- Sonis ST. Regimen-related gastrointestinal toxicities in cancer patients. Curr Opin Support Palliat Care 2010;4(1):26–30

27 Xerostomia and Hyposalivation in Patients with Cancer

Crispian Scully and Joel B. Epstein

Core Messages

- Hyposalivation has a major effect on patients with head and neck cancer during and after therapy.

- Hyposalivation affects quality of life and all aspects of oral function.

- Multiple factors in addition to radiotherapy may affect salivary gland function; these include chemotherapy, chronic comorbidities, such as diabetes, and commonly prescribed medications such as opioid analgesics, antihypertensives, anxiolytics, and antidepressants.

- Prevention and early intervention of hyposalivation and related complications are critical.

- The integrated multidisciplinary team has a critical role before, during, and after cancer treatment in promoting prevention, early detection of complications of hyposalivation, and management of saliva as well as complications that may follow for oral and dental health and oropharyngeal function.

Saliva is essential to oral health, and low salivary flow rates (hyposalivation) cause lack of mucosal wetting and oral lubrication, which affect many functions, and may predispose to infections as a consequence of reduced oral defenses. Hyposalivation is the objective measure of reduced saliva secretion.

Dry mouth (xerostomia) is a common symptomatic salivary complaint—not a disease, but a symptom arising from a wide range of triggering factors.

Definitions

Xerostomia is not synonymous with hyposalivation.

- Xerostomia: subjective complaint of oral dryness.

- Hyposalivation (hyposialia): reduction in saliva production.

Physiology of Saliva

Salivary tissue consists of the following:

- Acinar tissue: It contains serous or mucous cells or a combination and produces the initial secretion of fluid, with an electrolyte composition similar to that of plasma. Secretion appears to be dependent on several modulatory influences that act via either a cyclic adenosine monophospate or a calcium-dependent pathway.
- Duct cells: They specialize both in function and in structure. Striated duct cells selectively reabsorb

certain electrolytes and contain numerous peptides such as epidermal growth factor (EGF) and nerve growth factor.
- Myoepithelial cells: They are around acini and extend down the ducts, have contractile properties, and assist in saliva secretion.

Salivary Glands

Salivary glands are classified as follows:

- Major glands:
  - Parotid glands: They are principally serous with a "watery" secretion, primarily producing saliva upon physical or taste stimulation.
  - Submandibular and sublingual glands: They are largely mucous, secrete mucins that give saliva a more viscous, sticky nature, and provide much of the resting/basal saliva volume.
- Minor glands: They are scattered across the oral mucosa but are especially common in lips, soft palate, and the ventrum of the tongue; they are mainly mucous in type.

Control of Salivary Gland Secretion

Salivary gland secretion is controlled via neurotransmitters under the influence of the autonomic nervous system, although various hormones may also modulate salivary composition. In general, parasympathetic stimulation increases fluid secretion as a result of the activation of M3 muscarinic receptors on acinar cells; sympathetic stimulation via alpha-1-adrenergic receptors also produces more saliva, though much less than that occurs after muscarinic stimulation; and stimulation via beta-adrenergic receptors stimulates salivary protein release from acinar cells via fusion of zymogen granules. Neuropeptides (substance P and vasoactive intestinal peptide) and autacoids (histamine and bradykinin) may also influence salivary secretion. Water-specific channels or aquaporins facilitate water movement across acinar cell plasma membranes and provide the only source of fluid secretion in salivary glands.

Composition and Functions of Saliva

The most obvious function of saliva water, mucins, and proline-rich glycoproteins is to lubricate food and mucosa and help taste perception and swallowing, but other functions include the following (**Table 27.1**):

- Digestive: Salivary amylase has a very minor role in humans in the conversion of starch to maltose. Salivary lipase may assist fat digestion.
- Excretory: Some drugs, such as alcohol, are excreted in saliva. Secreted cancer chemotherapy agents may lead to mucosal toxicity, and some may result in altered taste.
- Maintenance of tooth integrity: The buffering capacity and supersaturated calcium and phosphate are important in maintaining tooth integrity.
- Hormonal: EGF (urogastrone), a polypeptide from submandibular glands (SMGs), may play a role in wound healing. Homeostatic proteases, such as kallikrein, renin, and tonin, may control local vascularity and water/electrolyte transport.
- Protective: The lubricative and mechanical washing effects of saliva as well as nonspecific and specific immune-protective mechanisms protect the host. Saliva is inhibitory to various microbial agents, including human immunodeficiency virus (HIV).

These mechanisms include the following:

- Mucins that aid lubrication, aggregate bacteria, are antiviral, and limit mucosal permeability to various toxins.

Table 27.1 Functions of Saliva

Maintaining mucosal barrier
Lubrication, speech, and deglutition
Allowing tastants to contact taste receptors
Regulating pH; hypotonic environment
Mineralization: supersaturated $CaPO_4$
Antimicrobial: lysozyme, lactoferrin, sIgA
Digestion: amylase

- Inhibitors of proteolytic enzymes, such as cysteine-containing phosphoproteins and antileukoproteases that are, with mucins, protective against proteolytic enzymes from bacteria and leukocytes.
- Bacterial aggregators that can aggregate bacteria and prevent their attachment to oral surfaces, such as mucins, some glycoproteins, and lysozyme.
- Direct nonimmune antimicrobial mechanisms, such as defensins,
  - Lysozyme interacts with anions such as thiocyanate to lyse gram-positive bacteria.
  - Defensins and histidine-rich peptides in parotid saliva also suppress oral bacteria and fungi.
  - Lactoferrin chelates iron and deprives bacteria of an essential factor.
  - Peroxidase with thiocyanate and hydrogen peroxidase acts against some gram-positive and gram-negative bacteria and yeasts.
  - Amylase may, for example, protect against *Neisseria gonorrhoeae*.
- Immune protection—principally via secretory immunoglobulin A antibodies.

Etiology of Hyposalivation

Treatment of head and neck cancer (HNC) and bone marrow (hematopoietic stem cell) transplants may especially be associated with xerostomia[1,2]; in patients with cancer, xerostomia has independent negative influences on the quality of life (QoL).[3,4] This also applies to children with malignant disease[5] and in patients who receive chemotherapy for solid tumors.[6] Furthermore, patients with advanced cancer frequently have xerostomia and dry mouth, which is commonly associated with oral discomfort and dysphagia.[7] This chapter summarizes the area and highlight recent advances and future directions: several recent reviews have covered this field comprehensively.[8]

The other main causes of hyposalivation are drugs (those with anticholinergic or sympathomimetic activity), irradiation of the major salivary glands, Sjögren syndrome, diabetes, HIV infection, sarcoidosis, and dehydration (**Table 27.2**).

Cancer Therapy Effects on Salivation

While the direct effects of some cancer therapies on salivary function frequently cause hyposalivation, 18 to 19% of both hospitalized patients with cancer and patients without cancer may suffer from dry mouth,[9] suggesting a strong role of medications and anxiety and/or depression in hospitalized patients.

Effects of Cancer Therapy

In addition to saliva production, the quality of saliva is frequently affected. Increased viscosity produces symptoms during cancer therapy, which may become a chronic complaint. The mucous acini of salivary glands have a reduced sensitivity to toxicity, and as serous secretions decline, they may retain function for some time. The production of excessively thickened secretions affects the flow of the secretion and may lead to nausea and vomiting, particularly in patients receiving chemotherapy that places them at increased risk for nausea.

Irradiation of the major salivary glands is common in the treatment of cancers of the head and neck (H&N), thyroid, and lymphomas. In HNC, when the salivary glands and bilateral neck irradiation is required, hyposalivation occurs. Hematopoietic stem cell transplantation also involves damage to salivary function,[10] particularly when total body irradiation is part of the conditioning protocol and if graft-versus-host disease develops and involves the salivary glands.[11]

Radiotherapy (RT) causes acinar cell apoptosis, leading to a change in saliva quantity and quality in approximately 1 to 2 weeks of beginning RT at a cumulative dose of approximately 10 Gy; salivary function falls as the RT dose increases, and at a total dose of more than 50 Gy, virtually complete hyposalivation can follow when all glands are in the RT field.[12,13] Salivary flow rates fall dramatically during the first 2 weeks of RT, and both the parotid and submandibular/sublingual glands can be similarly affected.[14]

Patients with HNC treated with RT either alone or in combination with chemotherapy or surgery report xerostomia as one of the most frequent complaints, and this has a significant effect on the more general dimensions of health-related QoL.[15] In HNC, xerostomia increases from 19% pretreatment to 62.6% during RT and 53.2% after RT.[16] In patients treated for nasopharyngeal carcinoma, xerostomia persisted at the last follow-up (24 months).[17]

Salivary function recovery may occur within 1 year after RT[18]; however, little improvement can be expected after 1 year following cancer treatment, and dry mouth is the most common chronic complaint of patients after HNC therapy that includes radiation therapy.

Diffusion-weighted magnetic resonance imaging allows noninvasive evaluation of functional changes in the major salivary glands after RT and is a promising tool for investigating RT-induced xerostomia.[19]

Effects on Quality of Life

The assessment of QoL in HNC includes the Head and Neck Symptom Scale of the University of Washington Quality of Life (UW-QoL) questionnaire, which includes items related to saliva amount and consistency (**Table 27.3**).[20]

The University of Michigan Xerostomia-Related Quality of Life Scale[21] is a 15-question survey, with each

Table 27.2 Causes of Xerostomia

Interference with neural transmission
- Medications/drugs
  - Drugs with anticholinergic or sympathomimetic effects
  - Drugs that directly damage salivary glands: antineoplastic agents
  - Drugs with anticholinergic activity: atropine, scopolamine
  - Antireflux agents: proton-pump inhibitors
  - Antidepressants
- Tricyclic antidepressants
- Selective serotonin reuptake inhibitors
  - Phenothiazines
  - Benzodiazepines
  - Opioids
  - Antihistamines
  - Drugs acting on sympathetic system: ephedrine
  - Antihypertensives

Autonomic dysfunction
Conditions affecting the central nervous system
Dehydration
- Diabetes mellitus
- Diabetes insipidus
- Diarrhea and vomiting
- Hypercalcemia
- Renal disease
- Severe hemorrhage

Starvation
Cancer therapy
- Irradiation (radiotherapy or radioactive iodine)
- Chemotherapy

Targeted therapy
- Chemoradiotherapy
- Hematopoietic stem cell transplantation/bone marrow transplantation/chronic graft- versus-host disease

Salivary gland aplasia
Systemic conditions affecting salivary glands
- Autoimmune conditions
- Sarcoidosis
- Cystic fibrosis
- Ectodermal dysplasia
- Viral infections
- Deposits

Table 27.3 Scoring Salivary Function

Saliva Amount	Saliva Consistency
10: I have a normal amount of saliva.	10: My saliva has normal consistency.
20: I have a mild loss of saliva.	20: My saliva is slightly thicker.
30: I have a moderate loss of saliva.	30: My saliva is moderately thicker.
40: I have a severe loss of saliva.	40: My saliva is extremely thicker.
50: I have no saliva.	50: I have saliva that dries in my mouth and/or on my lips.

response based on a 5-point severity response. Others have used broad QoL questionnaires with modifications or additional sections. Dry mouth has a significant effect on overall QoL.[22] Two hundred and eighty eight patients with all stages of HNC were assessed by using the European Organization for Research and Treatment Core QoL Questionnaire (EORTC QLQ-C30) and Radiation Therapy Oncology Group (RTOG) toxicity criteria up to 24 months after cancer therapy.

Xerostomia was found to have a significant effect on overall QoL ($p < 0.001$) and the effect on QoL increased over time.[22] One hundred and forty nine patients with stage III or IV HNC were assessed pretreatment and at 1 year after treatment by using EORTC QLQ-C30 and EORTC H&N35. The primary complaints were dysphagia, dry mouth, and thick saliva ($p < 0.05$), and patients with oral cancer had limited improvement at the last follow-up.[23]

A study of 65 patients with HNC who had completed RT more than 6 months earlier showed the most common chronic symptoms—dry mouth (92%), change in taste (75%), difficulty in swallowing (63%), moderate to severe difficulty in chewing (43%), and sore mouth when eating (40%).[24] A prospective study of 357 patients with HNC identified chronic oral symptoms—dental problems, trismus, xerostomia, and sticky saliva that persisted or increased over time after 1 year and persisted for 5 years.[25]

EORTC QLQ-C30 has been used for the assessment of QoL, and specific addenda addressing oral symptoms and effect on QoL have been used in several studies.[26]

Other tools have been assessed, including a visual analogue scale (VAS) for subjective assessment of saliva and a reliability of seven of eight VAS responses, which were found to predict changes in saliva flow induced by xerostomic medications.[27]

A prospective, multicenter study of QoL conducted in 122 patients with oral cancer (62% man, mean age 61 years) with patient reported outcomes completed pretreatment, and at 1 and 5 years after treatment,[28] it found oral complaints to include dry mouth, sticky saliva, speech changes, dental problems, and sleep disturbance. Symptom burden remained significant at 5 years after treatment in patients who were treated with RT, and these complaints were associated with decreased QoL ($p < 0.01$). In another study, 107 patients completed QoL surveys before and 6, 12, 24, and 36 months after HNC treatment.[29] Most short-term morbidity resolved in 1 year of cancer treatment. At the end of follow-up, physical functioning, taste/smell, dry mouth, and sticky saliva were significantly worse compared with those at baseline.

Several studies assessing chronic symptoms more than 6 months to 5 years following Tradiotherapy for HNC have shown that dry mouth, thick saliva, and dysphagia are the most common and troubling persisting complaints.[28,30,31] Most short-term morbidity resolved in 1 year of cancer treatment. At the end of follow-up physical functioning, taste/smell, dry mouth and sticky saliva were significantly worse compared with baseline.

Minimizing Radiation-Induced Xerostomia

Several strategies are available to minimize radiation damage to salivary glands (**Table 27.4**).

Table 27.4 Strategies to Minimize Radiation-Induced Xerostomia

Minimizing radiation field/volume
Using positioning devices, shielding, and conformational field planning
Using intensity-modulated radiation therapy, image-guided radiation therapy, or tomotherapy
Minimizing the exposure doses
Using radiation-protective agents
Repositioning of surgical salivary gland

Minimizing Radiation Exposure Doses

Minimizing salivary gland radiation exposure is one effective strategy to minimize radiation-induced xerostomia. For example, in selected patients with early and moderate stages, well-lateralized oral and oropharyngeal carcinomas, ipsilateral irradiation treatment of the primary site, and ipsilateral neck spares salivary gland function on the uninvolved side, without compromising locoregional control.[32]

In conventional RT, reducing the mean dose to the contralateral SMG below 40 Gy is possible with a reasonable dose coverage.[33] Limiting the mean parotid dose to 31 Gy or less and mean minor salivary gland dose to 11 Gy or less in patients with lymphoma having RT to the H&N reduces the risk of xerostomia.[34]

Using Positioning Devices, Shielding, and Conformational Field Planning

Positioning devices, shielding, and conformational field planning may also minimize salivary damage. The use of computed tomography (CT)-based delineation guidelines for organs at risk in the H&N should reduce inter- and intraobserver variability and therefore unambiguous reporting of possible dose-volume-effect relationships.[35]

Intensity-modulated radiotherapy (IMRT) reduces doses when compared with standard three-dimensional conformal radiotherapy (CRT)[36,37] and reduces xerostomia.[38]

Parotid gland sparing IMRT for patients with HNC improves xerostomia-related QoL compared with CRT both at rest and during meals: patients with laryngeal cancer had fewer complaints but benefited equally from IMRT compared with patients with oropharyngeal cancer.[39] IMRT in the treatment of nasopharyngeal carcinoma produced significant reductions in the occurrence rates and severity of acute skin reaction, neck fibrosis, trismus, and xerostomia.[40]

SMG dose reduction to less than 39 Gy and without target underdosing is feasible in some patients at the expense of modestly higher doses to some other organs.[41] Stimulated SMG flow rates decrease exponentially by 1.2% as mean doses increased up to 39 Gy threshold and then plateau near zero. At mean doses of 39 Gy or less, but not higher, flow rates recover over time at 2.2% a month. Similarly, the unstimulated salivary flow rates (USFRs) decrease exponentially by 3% as the mean dose increases and recovers over time if the mean dose was less than 39 Gy. IMRT replanning reduces mean contralateral SMG dose by an average of 12 Gy, achieving 39 Gy or less in five of eight patients, without target underdosing, and increasing the mean doses to the parotid glands and swallowing structures by an average of 2 to 3 Gy.

However, others have found that by 1 year after RT, normal tissue complication probability curves for IMRT and CRT were comparable with a median toxic dose (uniform dose leading to a 50% complication probability) of 38 and 40 Gy, respectively.[42] Helical tomotherapy (TomoTherapy Hi-Art System; Accuracy, Sunnyvale, California, United States) of the parotid gland seems to largely preserve the function.[43]

Using Radiation-Protective Agents

Radiation-protective agents can protect salivary glands in animal models, but translation of agents from animal testing to be used as prophylactic adjuncts or postexposure treatments in RT has been slow. Agents approved for the purpose by the U.S. Food and Drug Administration include amifostine (Ethyol, Ethiofos, WR-2721), an organic thiophosphate prodrug for alleviating xerostomia associated with RT. Amifostine is a free-radical scavenger, and it also accelerates DNA repair.[44] The selective protection of certain tissues of the body by amifostine is believed to be due to higher alkaline phosphatase activity, higher pH, and vascular permeation of normal tissues.

Acute xerostomia was significantly lessened in intravenous (IV) amifostine-treated patients with HNC (51%) compared with controls (78%).[45] Salivary output was significantly raised above that that for untreated controls 1 year after RT,[45] and xerostomia was reduced at 2-year follow-up.[46] Xerostomia after RT in a study by another group was similarly lower in amifostine-treated patients (57.5%) with HNC compared with controls (70%).[47] Amifostine was initially administered intravenously before chemotherapy or RT, but because of adverse effects and the cost of delivery, it is now provided through the subcutaneous (SC) route.[48] A study of 20 patients with HNC having RT-CT examined SC amifostine versus historical data of IV amifostine found outcomes from SC similar to those from IV but with reduced nausea/vomiting and hypotension after SC administration and showed xerostomia with SC drug as 42% (12 months) and 29% (18 months).[49] The Groupe d'Oncologie Radiothérapie Tête Et Cou study compared IV (200 mg/m²) versus SC (500 mg/d) amifostine in HNC and found less hypotension with SC amifostine,[50] which is virtually identical with other results.[51]

Both amifostine and IMRT are able to partially preserve parotid function after RT, although the effect of IMRT appears greater.[52]

However, amifostine has not been shown to provide significant radioprotective effects on salivary glands in high-dose radioactive iodine–treated patients with differentiated thyroid cancer.[53]

Pilocarpine (Salagen) is a slowly hydrolyzed muscarinic agonist with no nicotinic effects, which can increase secretion by the exocrine glands. The salivary, sweat, lacrimal, gastric, pancreatic, and intestinal glands and the mucous cells of the respiratory tract may be stimulated. In animal models, preirradiation treatment with pilocarpine induces a compensatory response at lower doses in the irradiated gland and at higher doses in the nonirradiated gland, reducing late damage, because of stimulation of unirradiated or surviving cells to divide.[54,55] A prospective, double-blind, placebo-controlled, randomized trial by the same authors in patients with HNC having RT showed that the concomitant administration of pilocarpine have no effect on parotid flow rate complications; however, patient-rated xerostomia scores showed trends toward less dryness-related complaints and there was reduced loss of parotid flow 1 year after RT in those patients who received pilocarpine and a mean parotid dose of more than 40 Gy.[56]

In patients with HNC treated with bilateral RT in a double-blind, placebo-controlled, randomized trial using 5 mg of pilocarpine five times a day during RT, there was an improved overall QoL and less oral discomfort.[57] Others have also found some improvements,[58] although the clinical impact of the effect on salivation is not well defined.

The use of pilocarpine both during and after RT is also beneficial.[59]

Repositioning of Surgical Salivary Gland

Surgical repositioning of the SMG out of the planned RT field to the submental space can protect the gland.[60] One study suggested that SMG transfer procedure is superior to pilocarpine in the management of RT-induced xerostomia.[61]

However, as RT is now delivered to the H&N with conformal fields/IMRT and tomotherapy, the reduction in the volume of high-dose radiation allows sparing of high-dose exposure to all salivary glands in many cases, with the increased potential for residual gland function and stimulation with sialogogues.

Management of the Patient with Cancer Liable to Hyposalivation

Recent recommendations for the management of patients with cancer liable to hyposalivation are as follows[62]:

- Patients with cancer should be regularly assessed for salivary gland dysfunction (SGD);

- The management of SGD should be individualized;
- Consideration should be given to strategies to prevent the development of RT-induced SGD;
- Consideration should be given to the treatment of the cause(s) of SGD;
- The treatment of choice for the symptomatic management of SGD is use of an appropriate saliva stimulant;
- Strategies to prevent the complications of SGD should be in place;
- Early diagnosis and treatment of the complications of SGD should be conducted; and
- Patients with SGD should be regularly reassessed.

Treatment is largely palliative and preventative in nature. Because oral dryness is a subjective complaint, it is not surprising that there is a great variation in the patient's threshold of discomfort or other symptoms and it is also affected by tolerance and adaptation over time.[63-65]

Clinical Features

Oral complaints (often the presenting features) can include

- Xerostomia;
- Oral soreness or burning sensation;
- Difficulty in eating dry foods;
- Difficulty in speaking for long periods of time, the development of hoarseness, or there may be a clicking quality of the speech as the tongue tends to stick to the palate;
- Difficulty in swallowing;
- Difficulty in controlling dentures;
- Need of putting up a glass of water at night (and, sometimes, resulting nocturia); and
- Complications such as unpleasant taste or loss of sense of taste, oral malodor, caries, candidosis, and sialadenitis.

Common Terminology Criteria for Adverse Events (CTCAE v3.0) are as in **Table 27.5**.[67]

A positive response to the questions in **Table 27.6** is significantly associated with reduced salivary output.[68]

Table 27.5 Common Terminology Criteria for Adverse Events

Symptomatic (dry or thick saliva) without significant dietary alteration; unstimulated saliva more than 0.2 mL/min.
Symptomatic and significant change in oral intake (e.g., copious water, other lubricants, diet limited to soft, moist foods); unstimulated saliva 0.1 to 0.2 mL/min.
Symptoms leading to inability to take oral nutrition; use of intravenous fluids, tube feedings, or total parenteral nutrition indicated; unstimulated saliva less than 0.1 mL/min.

Table 27.6 Features of Hyposalivation: Questions and Responses

Do you have difficulty in swallowing any food? Yes/No
Does your mouth feel dry while eating a meal? Yes/No
Do you sip liquids to aid swallowing dry food? Yes/No
Does the amount of saliva in your mouth seems to be too little, too much, or never noticed it?

Chronic Complications

Chronic complications of hyposalivation may include the following (**Table 27.7**):

- Shift in the oral microflora and risk of oral infection (caries, candidosis, bacterial sialadenitis) (**Figs. 27.1** to **27.4**);
- Oral malodor;
- Altered/reduced taste;
- Mucosal dryness and sensitivity;
- Impaired chewing: patients with reduced or increased salivary flow, however, may not present measurable alterations in masticatory efficiency[69];
- Difficulty in swallowing;
- Difficulty in denture use and function, but there are few clinical research studies on the effect of hyposalivation on denture retention and mucosal trauma[70];
- Nutritional defects; and
- Altered speech.

Table 27.7 Clinical Symptoms of Xerostomia

Dryness
Discomfort
Taste reduction
Speech and deglutition affected
Denture use and function affected
Compromised diet/nutrition

Quality of Life Scales Focused on Xerostomia

Scales focused on xerostomia are shown in **Table 27.8**. The UW-QoL saliva domain seems to be a suitable means of screening for dry mouth in head-and-neck clinics and can be used to trigger interventions.[71]

Patient self-reported, rather than physician-assessed, scores should be the main end points in evaluating xerostomia because correlations between RTOG/EORTC grades and salivary flow rates are poor; in contrast, significant correlations are found between the patient self-reported scores and nonstimulated or stimulated salivary flow rates. No significant correlation was found between the

Table 27.8 Quality of Life Scales

Xerostomia-Related Quality of Life Scale
The University of Washington Quality of Life questionnaire (Version 4; dry mouth item)
Vanderbilt Head and Neck Symptom Surgery ECOG QLQC30; HN35.

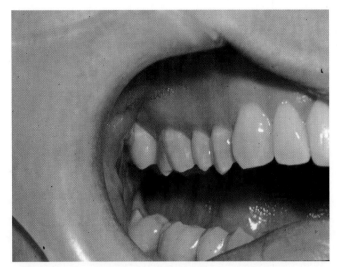

Figure 27.1   Early decalcification of teeth.

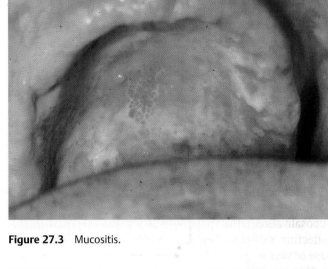

Figure 27.3   Mucositis.

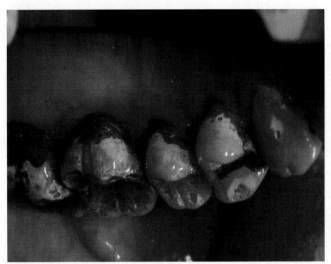

Figure 27.2   Dental caries (radiation caries).

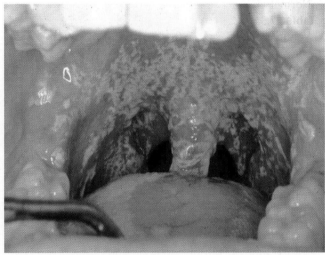

Figure 27.4   Candidosis.

RTOG/EORTC grades and the Xerostomia-Related Quality of Life Scale scores.[72–74]

Clinical Signs of Hyposalivation

The dry mucosa may become tacky and mucosal surfaces, including the lips, can adhere one to another. There may be saliva flowing poorly, if at all, from the ducts of the major glands on stimulation or palpation. The following signs may also be present:

- Tendency of the mucosa to stick to a dental mirror or tongue spatula.
- Food residues in the mouth after eating.
- Lack of sublingual salivary pooling.
- Frothiness of saliva, particularly in the lower sulcular reflection, and absence of frank salivation from major gland duct orifices.
- A change in tongue appearance—lobulated, usually red, surface with partial or complete depapillation.

- In advanced cases, clinically dry and glazed oral mucosae can be observed.

Examination

The patient should be examined

- Through inspecting.
- Through facial symmetry.
- For evidence of enlarged glands.
- Through salivary ducts for evidence of salivary or pus flow.
- Through saliva.
- By palpating the glands.
- Through parotids.
- By using fingers placed over the glands in front of the ears to detect pain or swelling.
- Through submandibulars.
- Through bimanual palpation between fingers inside the mouth and extraorally.

- Through the mucosa; note particularly mucositis, angular cheilitis, dryness, and lingual depapillation or erythema and masses in the immovable soft palate and posterior aspect of the hard palate.

Objective Determination of Hyposalivation

Because baseline salivary flow rates for individual patients with cancer are generally unknown, unless this is assessed before beginning cancer therapy, it is rarely possible to determine whether there has been a reduction in salivary flow. The normal salivary flow rate also varies by the time of day (diurnal variation) and varies widely from person to person.

The USFR of whole saliva is generally determined. The USFR uses a simple draining test for 5 minutes at rest: If USFR is less than or equal to 0.1 mL/min, the patient has hyposalivation. Stimulated saliva flow can be assessed by collecting saliva while chewing unflavored chewing gum base or wax for 5 minutes.

Normal and reference values for salivary flow are given in **Table 27.9**.

Volume of saliva can be measured, or the saliva collected can be weighed. The Saxon test is a simple, reproducible, and low-cost test for xerostomia, which involves chewing on a folded sterile sponge for 2 minutes. Saliva production is quantified by weighing the sponge before and after chewing. Normal control subjects produced 2.75 g or less of saliva in 2 minutes.[75]

Instruments to measure moisture include Moisture Checker (MucusIII; MCM; Life Co., Ltd., Saitama, Japan), a device for measuring moisture of the oral submucosa,[76] and the capacitance method Moisture Checker for Mucus (Life Co., Ltd., Saitama, Japan).[77]

Therapy

As noted, there may be little correlation between patient symptoms and objective tests of salivary flow. Clinical management may be based on the symptoms; however, as the effect on oral health depends on salivation, this should be considered in all patients as some may have symptomatically accommodated to their dry mouth.

Management is multidisciplinary and multimodal, and treatment essentially involves use of salivary stimulants and/or salivary substitutes and begins with simple measures such as the following:

Table 27.9 Whole Saliva Flow Rates

	Flow rate (mL/min)	
	Normal	**Hyposalivation**
Unstimulated (resting)	0.3–0.4	< 0.1
Stimulated	1–2	< 0.5

Note: Whole saliva is the total output from the major and minor salivary glands.

- Sipping water or other fluids throughout the day, protecting the lips with nonpetroleum-based lip applications, and modifying the eating behavior (e.g., small bites of food, eating slowly) and diet (moist, creamy foods [casseroles, soups] or cool foods with a high liquid content [melon, ice cream]) as well as moistening foods with water, gravies, sauces, extra oil, dressings, sour cream, mayonnaise, or yoghurt are advantageous.
- Avoiding mouth breathing, drugs that may produce xerostomia (e.g., tricyclic antidepressants), alcohol (including in mouthwashes), smoking, caffeine (coffee, some soft drinks), dry foods such as biscuits (or moisten in liquid first), spicy foods, and oral health care products containing sodium lauryl sulfate, which may irritate the mucosa. There is good evidence to support that xerostomia is commonly associated with anticholinergic and opioid drugs, and altering such agents, when possible, can be important in the management after RT.[78,79]

In patients with residual salivary gland function, salivary stimulants (**Table 27.10**) appear to be more beneficial than the simple use of salivary substitutes and should be considered before palliation of symptoms.[80]

Table 27.10 Stimulation of Salivation

Local/topical
• Taste stimulation
• Masticatory stimulation
• Oral rinses, gels, mouthwashes
• Acupuncture
Systemic sialogogues

Sialogogues

Salivation may be stimulated by using chewing gums (containing xylitol or sorbitol, not sucrose), sugar-free (diabetic) candies, or other topical agents that stimulate salivation (sialogogues) (**Table 27.11**).

Table 27.11 Gustatory/Mechanical Stimulation of Salivation

United States	**United Kingdom**
Sugar-free gum/candy	Sugar-free gum/candy
Salese Lozenge (Nuvora Inc.)	Salivix (KoGEN) Pastilles
Oramoist Lozenge (Quantum Inc.)	SST (Medac) tablets

If these fail to give satisfactory benefit, cholinergic sialogogues, such as pilocarpine, cevimeline, or bethanechol (Urecholine) may help, as may other agents (**Table 27.12**). Salivary stimulant medication may be needed indefinitely for maintenance of saliva flow.

Pilocarpine

Pilocarpine used after RT can increase salivation by 64.5%.[81] In controlled trials, pilocarpine used after RT increased

Table 27.12 Systemic Sialogogues

Cholinergic Agents[a]	Other Agents
Pilocarpine (Salagen)	Anetholetrithione (Sialor)[b]
Cevimeline (Evoxac)	
Bethanechol (Urecholine)	
Physostigmine	

See text for newer agents.

[a]May require several months to determine effectiveness; avoid in patients with narrow-angle glaucoma and uncontrolled asthma; caution in hypertensive patients using beta-blocker.

[b]Not available worldwide.

whole resting saliva (69 vs. 43% in controls), unstimulated parotid saliva (30 vs. 3%), and stimulated parotid saliva (45 vs. 28%).[82] A double-blind, placebo-controlled trial of pilocarpine (3 or 5 mg) versus placebo in patients with HNC after RT showed a significant increase in the unstimulated whole saliva flow rate.[83] Pilocarpine may also ameliorate xerostomia induced by opioid drugs[84] and likely other medications.

Adverse effects of pilocarpine include sweating, nausea, palpitation, and tearing, with sweating as the most common side effect.[85]

Pilocarpine is contraindicated in patients with uncontrolled asthma, narrow-angle glaucoma, and acute iritis and should be used with caution in patients with cardiovascular disease.[86] Pilocarpine produces maximum saliva stimulation after 1 hour, and the effect continues for 2 to 3 hours. Five milligrams of pilocarpine three times a day may cause a high incidence of unacceptable adverse effects in Japanese patients for whom a lower dose of pilocarpine should be considered.[87]

Cevimeline

Cevimeline is a parasympathomimetic agent with the pharmacologic profile similar to that of pilocarpine, a cholinergic agonist with the effect on M3 receptors located in smooth muscles and glands and endothelium.[88] In patients with HNC having xerostomia after RT, 30 mg of cevimeline (Evoxac) three times a day improved oral dryness and significantly increased unstimulated saliva flow.[89,90]

Bethanechol

Bethanechol used during RT may result in increased unstimulated whole salivary flow.[91]

Physostigmine

Application of physostigmine to the oromucosal surface produced long-lasting (120 minutes) relief in the feeling of dryness, which was six times greater than that to placebo. The volume of saliva collected in response to physostigmine was also five times higher over 180 minutes than that collected in response to placebo.[92]

Comparative Studies of Sialogogues

Forty-two patients with HNC having xerostomia after RT were randomized to pilocarpine or bethanechol. All subjects reported improved symptoms, but only minimal measurable increase in saliva volume. In 27 patients who completed the crossover, the possible increase in saliva suggested that an increased duration of sialogogues may improve the outcome.[93] Another study assessed 20 patients in a crossover design by using pilocarpine, cevimeline, or bethanechol, and all sialogogues increased saliva, but bethanechol increased saliva more than did pilocarpine ($p = 0.0272$); pilocarpine was more associated with increased sweating compared with both bethanechol ($p = 0.0588$) and cevimeline ($p = 0.0143$).[94]

Mouth-Wetting Agents (Saliva Substitutes)

Mouth-wetting agents may help symptomatically relieve xerostomia after RT.[95] Many of these agents are available (**Table 27.13**) with differences in their performance and patient acceptance. These topically applied products can be assessed in individual patients and the preferred agent determined.

Table 27.13 Mouth-Wetting Agents and Local Stimulants

United States	United Kingdom
Entertainer's Secret (KLI Corp) spray	AS Saliva Orthana (AS Pharma) spray
Glandosane (Fresenius Kabi) spray available unflavored, lemon, mint	Biotene Oralbalance (Anglican) gel
Moi-Stir (Kingswood Laboratories)	BioXtra (RIS products) gel
Mouth-Kote[a] (Parnell Pharmaceuticals)	Glandosane Frenius Kabl) spray
Oasis Mouthwash and Mouth Spray (GlaxoSmithKline) and liquid	Luborant (Goldshield) spray
Oral Balance (Laclede Professional Products) gel	Salinum (Crawford) liquid
Oramoist Lozenge (Quantum, Inc.) lozenges	Saliveze (Wyvern) spray
Salese Lozenge (Nuvora, Inc.) lozenges	Xerotin (SpePharm) spray
Saliva Substitute (Roxane Laboratories) liquid	
Salivart (Xenex Laboratories, Inc.)	
SalivaSure (Scandinavian Natural Health & Beauty) tablets	

[a]Contains citric acid.

Apart from water, various saliva substitutes are available, including those based on carboxymethylcellulose (CMC) (some are particularly useful because they contain fluoride and are thus caries protective). CMC-based saliva replacements have moderate effects on reducing dry mouth–related symptoms and behaviors, with more significant effects on patients whose residual secretory potency was severely compromised.[96]

In a sample of older adults with dry mouth, a mouthwash and oral gel containing the antimicrobial proteins lactoperoxidase, lactoferrin, and lysozyme improved some subjective and clinical aspects, though a placebo effect cannot be discarded.[97,98] Oral care using such a moisturizing gel might also have other benefits because it may contribute to preventing respiratory tract infections from oral contamination in patients with cerebrovascular disease.[99]

Other wetting agents are based on animal mucin, but there may be religious or cultural objections to the use of mucin.

Quality and Control of Saliva

Viscosity of oral secretions may be a considerable problem for patients with cancer during therapy and thereafter it may be a chronic problem. There has been limited study of approaches to management. Possible interventions include trials of systemic sialogogues that may increase residual serous saliva production; however, if serous function cannot be stimulated, they may serve to increase mucous secretions that increase patient symptoms. Mucolytic agents such as *N*-acetylcysteine (Acetadote) and guaifenesin (Duratuss G) have been considered, but no significant benefits have been demonstrated.

Management of oral secretions can be affected by diminished lip competence and tongue mobility, dysphagia, and fistulae.[100]

Management may include physical therapies (suction, frequent changes of dressing, pressure dressings, fibrin glue, aspiration of sialoceles), pharmacologic therapy (anticholinergics, xerogenic medications, botulinum toxoid),[101] or surgical approaches (gland removal, duct ligation, duct repositioning, chorda tympanectomy, tympanic neuroectomy).[102]

Management of Complications of Hyposalivation

Complications of hyposalivation should be managed by

- Avoiding sucrose-sweetened foods;
- Maintaining good oral hygiene and plaque control;
- Using fluorides and remineralizing products; and
- Using mouthwashes with chlorhexidine.

Dental Caries

Dental caries may be prevented as shown in **Table 27.14**.

Dietary control of sucrose intake, the daily use of fluoride toothpastes, and other fluoride applications are essential.

Table 27.14 Caries Prevention and Control after Radiotherapy

Caries risk assessment/diet assessment
Early detection of caries and prevention of demineralization
Remineralization
- Sodium fluoride: 1.1% neutral gel, lozenges, 0.05% rinse, 5% varnish
- Fluoride varnish: 1% difluorosilane varnish
- Calcium/phosphate: calcium and phosphate are essential components of the enamel and dentine and form highly insoluble complexes, but, in the presence of casein phosphopeptide (CPP), they remain soluble and biologically available as amorphous calcium phosphate (ACP). The CPP-ACP complex can be applied to teeth by means of chewing gum, toothpaste, lozenges, mouth rinses, sprays, and so on.

Recaldent-containing chewing gum
Artificial saliva (Caphosol)

Management of Cariogenic Flora

Cariogenic flora can be managed through

- Oral hygiene;
- Chlorhexidine; and
- Xylitol-containing products.

ACP can aid remineralization of white spot lesions in a similar effect to self-applied fluorides, which also reduces the appearance of new caries lesions.[103] One therapeutic approach is the daily use of a supersaturated calcium phosphate rinse in conjunction with 1.1% NaF.[104]

Candidosis

Candidosis may cause soreness or burning and thus should be treated with antifungals until symptoms and signs resolve. Risk factors must be addressed or infection will recur and prophylaxis should then be considered (**Table 27.15**).

Topical antifungal drugs in liquid form, such as nystatin, are effective and most acceptable because the mouth is

Table 27.15 Prevention and Management of Candidosis after Radiotherapy

Topical antifungal drug with lowest risk for dental caries
Nystatin (Mycostatin and Nystan) vaginal tablets three times a day
Clotrimazole (FungiCURE Pump Spray) five times a day
Compounded fluconazole (Diflucan) rinse
Sips of water as necessary to dissolve antifungal tablets
Dentures and mucosa require antifungal treatment
Topical antifungal creams applied to denture surface
Systemic antifungals are more effective with salivary stimulation
Continue antifungal drug until signs and symptoms resolve (4 to 10 weeks)
Consider maintenance dose of the antifungal drug

dry. However, the sucrose content of the product must be considered because of the effect of sucrose on dental caries, the risk of which is already increased in patients with dry mouth. Nystatin suspension has a high sucrose content (and a small level of alcohol). Fluconazole suspension also has a high sucrose content. Other preparations such as miconazole (Monistat; cream, adhesive tablet, or gel may be available), clotrimazole (not available in the United Kingdom), or amphotericin suspension (not available in the United States) are also effective.

Acrylic surfaces of prostheses are frequently infected, and so dentures and other removable appliances should be left out of the mouth at night and stored in antifungals such as sodium hypochlorite solution, chlorhexidine, or benzalkonium chloride to disinfect. An antifungal such as miconazole (cream or gel) or amphotericin or nystatin (cream or ointment) should be spread on the prosthesis fitting surface before reinserting it in the mouth.

Bacterial Sialadenitis

Mouth-wetting agents such as lactoperoxidase gel may reduce both periodontal-associated bacterial pathogens and *Candida* species.[105] Stimulation of salivation and antibacterial agents such as 0.12 or 0.2% chlorhexidine gluconate mouthrinse and xylitol (in sugar-free gums and mints) may also have utility. Bacterial sialadenitis may best be treated with a penicillinase-resistant antibiotic such as flucloxacillin.

Therapeutic Modalities in Trial Stages

Several therapeutic modalities for hyposalivation in trial stages are shown in **Table 27.16**.

Key Web Sites

Listed below are Web sites that provide information related to xerostomia and hyposalivation (accessed December 19, 2011).
- http://cancer.gov/cancertopics/pdq
- http://www.drymouth.info/practitioner/sources.asp
- http://mascc.org

Table 27.16 Therapeutic Modalities in Trial Stages

Modalities
• *Capparis masaikai Levl*
• Nizatidine
• Rebamipide
• Xialine
• Salivary irrigation
• Acupuncture
• Hypnosis
• Electrostimulation
• Stem cell therapy
• Gene therapy

Dilemmas

- Limited approaches to manage viscous/mucous secretions.
- Limited oral medications that are sucrose-free.
- Limited contact time of topical products in the oropharynx.
- Limited information on the pH of mouth-wetting agents.
- Limited data on remineralizing products.

Clinical Pearls

- To avoid tooth demineralization and caries, minimize or avoid refined carbohydrates or topical agents sweetened with sucrose.
- Topically applied mouth-wetting agents can be assessed in individual patients and the preferred agent determined.
- Where systemic sialogogues are considered, measure saliva production at rest and upon stimulation: if saliva is produced, anticipate beneficial effects. Challenge the patient with 5 mg of pilocarpine and assess salivary flow; if it increases, prescribe sialogogue. Reevaluate the patient after three consecutive months of treatment with 5 mg of pilocarpine three or four times per day.
- Dental providers should be involved as part of the multidisciplinary health care team.

References

1. Goldstein NE, Genden E, Morrison RS. Palliative care for patients with head and neck cancer: "I would like a quick return to a normal lifestyle". JAMA 2008;299(15):1818–1825
2. Jensen SB, Mouridsen HT, Reibel J, Brünner N, Nauntofte B. Adjuvant chemotherapy in breast cancer patients induces temporary salivary gland hypofunction. Oral Oncol 2008;44(2):162–173
3. van den Beuken-van Everdingen MH, de Rijke JM, Kessels AG, Schouten HC, van Kleef M, Patijn J. Quality of life and non-pain symptoms in patients with cancer. J Pain Symptom Manage 2009;38(2):216–233
4. Murphy BA, Dietrich MS, Wells N, et al. Reliability and validity of the Vanderbilt Head and Neck Symptom Survey: a tool to assess symptom burden in patients treated with chemoradiation. Head Neck 2010;32(1):26–37
5. Kaste SC, Goodman P, Leisenring W, et al. Impact of radiation and chemotherapy on risk of dental abnormalities: a report from the Childhood Cancer Survivor Study. Cancer 2009;115(24):5817–5827 epub ahead of print
6. Jensen SB, Mouridsen HT, Reibel J, Brünner N, Nauntofte B. Adjuvant chemotherapy in breast cancer patients induces temporary salivary gland hypofunction. Oral Oncol 2008;44(2):162–173

7. Davies AN, Broadley K, Beighton D. Salivary gland hypofunction in patients with advanced cancer. Oral Oncol 2002;38(7):680–685

8. Rankin KV, Epstein J, Huber MA, et al. Oral health in cancer therapy. Tex Dent J 2009;126(5):389–397, 406–419, 422–437

9. Fujisawa D, Park S, Kimura R, et al. Unmet supportive needs of cancer patients in an acute care hospital in Japan—a census study. Support Care Cancer 2010;18(11):1393–1403

10. Brand HS, Bots CP, Raber-Durlacher JE. Xerostomia and chronic oral complications among patients treated with haematopoietic stem cell transplantation. Br Dent J 2009;207(9):E17, discussion 428–429

11. Epstein JB, Raber-Durlacher JE, Wilkins A, Chavarria MG, Myint H. Advances in hematologic stem cell transplant: an update for oral health care providers. Oral Surg Oral Med Oral Pathol Oral Radiol Endod 2009;107(3):301–312

12. Münter MW, Karger CP, Hoffner SG, et al. Evaluation of salivary gland function after treatment of head-and-neck tumors with intensity-modulated radiotherapy by quantitative pertechnetate scintigraphy. Int J Radiat Oncol Biol Phys 2004;58(1):175–184

13. Eisbruch A, Dawson LA, Kim HM, et al. Conformal and intensity modulated irradiation of head and neck cancer: the potential for improved target irradiation, salivary gland function, and quality of life. Acta Otorhinolaryngol Belg 1999;53(3):271–275

14. Burlage FR, Coppes RP, Meertens H, Stokman MA, Vissink A. Parotid and submandibular/sublingual salivary flow during high dose radiotherapy. Radiother Oncol 2001;61(3):271–274

15. Langendijk JA, Doornaert P, Verdonck-de Leeuw IM, Leemans CR, Aaronson NK, Slotman BJ. Impact of late treatment-related toxicity on quality of life among patients with head and neck cancer treated with radiotherapy. J Clin Oncol 2008;26(22):3770–3776

16. Jham BC, Reis PM, Miranda EL, et al. Oral health status of 207 head and neck cancer patients before, during and after radiotherapy. Clin Oral Investig 2008;12(1):19–24

17. Oates JE, Clark JR, Read J, et al. Prospective evaluation of quality of life and nutrition before and after treatment for nasopharyngeal carcinoma. Arch Otolaryngol Head Neck Surg 2007;133(6):533–540

18. Marzi S, Iaccarino G, Pasciuti K, et al. Analysis of salivary flow and dose-volume modeling of complication incidence in patients with head-and-neck cancer receiving intensity-modulated radiotherapy. Int J Radiat Oncol Biol Phys 2009;73(4):1252–1259

19. Dirix P, De Keyzer F, Vandecaveye V, Stroobants S, Hermans R, Nuyts S. Diffusion-weighted magnetic resonance imaging to evaluate major salivary gland function before and after radiotherapy. Int J Radiat Oncol Biol Phys 2008;71(5):1365–1371

20. Hassan SJ, Weymuller EA Jr. Assessment of quality of life in head and neck cancer patients. Head Neck 1993;15(6):485–496

21. Henson BS, Inglehart MR, Eisbruch A, Ship JA. Preserved salivary output and xerostomia-related quality of life in head and neck cancer patients receiving parotid-sparing radiotherapy. Oral Oncol 2001;37(1):84–93

22. Jellema AP, Slotman BJ, Doornaert P, Leemans CR, Langendijk JA. Impact of radiation-induced xerostomia on quality of life after primary radiotherapy among patients with head and neck cancer. Int J Radiat Oncol Biol Phys 2007;69(3):751–760

23. Fang F-M, Tsai WL, Chien CY, et al. Changing quality of life in patients with advanced head and neck cancer after primary radiotherapy or chemoradiation. Oncology 2005;68(4-6):405–413

24. Epstein JB, Emerton S, Kolbinson DA, et al. Quality of life and oral function following radiotherapy for head and neck cancer. Head Neck 1999;21(1):1–11

25. Abendstein H, Nordgren M, Boysen M, et al. Quality of life and head and neck cancer: a 5 year prospective study. Laryngoscope 2005;115(12):2183–2192

26. Epstein JB, Murphy BM. Late Effects of Radiation Treatment on Oral Health for Patients with Head and Neck Cancer. Chicago, IL: American Society of Clinical Oncology Educational Book; 2009:312–319

27. Pai S, Ghezzi EM, Ship JA. Development of a Visual Analogue Scale questionnaire for subjective assessment of salivary dysfunction. Oral Surg Oral Med Oral Pathol Oral Radiol Endod 2001;91(3):311–316

28. Nordgren M, Hammerlid E, Bjordal K, Ahlner-Elmqvist M, Boysen M, Jannert M. Quality of life in oral carcinoma: a 5-year prospective study. Head Neck 2008;30(4):461–470

29. de Graeff A, de Leeuw JR, Ros WJ, Hordijk GJ, Blijham GH, Winnubst JA. Long-term quality of life of patients with head and neck cancer. Laryngoscope 2000;110(1):98–106

30. Epstein JB, Emerton S, Kolbinson DA, et al. Quality of life and oral function following radiotherapy for head and neck cancer. Head Neck 1999;21(1):1–11

31. Martino R, Ringash J. Evaluation of quality of life and organ function in head and neck squamous cell carcinoma. Hematol Oncol Clin North Am 2008;22(6):1239–1256, x

32. Cerezo L, Martín M, López M, Marín A, Gómez A. Ipsilateral irradiation for well lateralized carcinomas of the oral cavity and oropharynx: results on tumor control and xerostomia. Radiat Oncol 2009;4:33

33. Houweling AC, Dijkema T, Roesink JM, Terhaard CH, Raaijmakers CP. Sparing the contralateral submandibular gland in oropharyngeal cancer patients: a planning study. Radiother Oncol 2008;89(1):64–70

34. Rodrigues NA, Killion L, Hickey G, et al. A prospective study of salivary gland function in lymphoma patients receiving head and neck irradiation. Int J Radiat Oncol Biol Phys 2009;75(4):1079–1083

35. van de Water TA, Bijl HP, Westerlaan HE, Langendijk JA. Delineation guidelines for organs at risk involved in radiation-induced salivary dysfunction and xerostomia. Radiother Oncol 2009;93(3):545–552

36. Ahmed M, Hansen VN, Harrington KJ, Nutting CM. Reducing the risk of xerostomia and mandibular osteoradionecrosis: the potential benefits of intensity modulated radiotherapy in advanced oral cavity carcinoma. Med Dosim 2009;34(3):217–224

37. Vergeer MR, Doornaert PA, Rietveld DH, Leemans CR, Slotman BJ, Langendijk JA. Intensity-modulated radiotherapy reduces radiation-induced morbidity and improves health-related quality of life: results of a nonrandomized prospective study using a standardized follow-up program. Int J Radiat Oncol Biol Phys 2009;74(1):1–8

38. Eisbruch A. Radiotherapy: IMRT reduces xerostomia and potentially improves QoL. Nat Rev Clin Oncol 2009;6(10):567–568

39. van Rij CM, Oughlane-Heemsbergen WD, Ackerstaff AH, Lamers EA, Balm AJ, Rasch CR. Parotid gland sparing IMRT for head and neck cancer improves xerostomia related quality of life. Radiat Oncol 2008;3:41

40. Zhang Y, Lin ZA, Pan JJ, et al. [Concurrent control study of different radiotherapy for primary nasopharyngeal carcinoma: intensity-modulated radiotherapy versus conventional radiotherapy]. Ai Zheng 2009;28(11):1143–1148

41. Murdoch-Kinch CA, Kim HM, Vineberg KA, Ship JA, Eisbruch A. Dose-effect relationships for the submandibular salivary glands and implications for their sparing by intensity modulated radiotherapy. Int J Radiat Oncol Biol Phys 2008;72(2):373–382

42. Dijkema T, Terhaard CH, Roesink JM, et al. Large cohort dose-volume response analysis of parotid gland function after radiotherapy: intensity-modulated versus conventional radiotherapy. Int J Radiat Oncol Biol Phys 2008;72(4):1101–1109

43. Voordeckers M, Everaert H, Tournel K, et al. Longitudinal assessment of parotid function in patients receiving tomotherapy for head-and-neck cancer. Strahlenther Onkol 2008;184(8):400–405

44. Kouvaris JR, Kouloulias VE, Vlahos LJ. Amifostine: the first selective-target and broad-spectrum radioprotector. Oncologist 2007;12(6):738–747

45. Brizel DM, Wasserman TH, Henke M, et al. Phase III randomized trial of amifostine as a radioprotector in head and neck cancer. J Clin Oncol 2000;18(19):3339–3349

46. Wasserman TH, Brizel DM, Henke M, et al. Influence of intravenous amifostine on xerostomia, tumor control, and survival after radiotherapy for head-and- neck cancer: 2-year follow-up of a prospective, randomized, phase III trial. Int J Radiat Oncol Biol Phys 2005;63(4):985–990

47. Karacetin D, Yücel B, Leblebicioğlu B, Aksakal O, Maral O, Incekara O. A randomized trial of amifostine as radioprotector in the radiotherapy of head and neck cancer. J BUON 2004;9(1):23–26

48. Praetorius NP, Mandal TK. Alternate delivery route for amifostine as a radio-/chemo-protecting agent. J Pharm Pharmacol 2008;60(7):809–815

49. Law A, Kennedy T, Pellitteri P, Wood C, Christie D, Yumen O. Efficacy and safety of subcutaneous amifostine in minimizing radiation-induced toxicities in patients receiving combined-modality treatment for squamous cell carcinoma of the head and neck. Int J Radiat Oncol Biol Phys 2007;69(5):1361–1368

50. Bardet E, Martin L, Calais G, et al. Preliminary data of the GORTEC 2000-02 phase III trial comparing intravenous and subcutaneous administration of amifostine for head and neck tumors treated by external radiotherapy. Semin Oncol 2002;**29**(6, Suppl 19)57–60

51. Ozsahin M, Betz M, Matzinger O, et al. Feasibility and efficacy of subcutaneous amifostine therapy in patients with head and neck cancer treated with curative accelerated concomitant-boost radiation therapy. Arch Otolaryngol Head Neck Surg 2006;132(2):141–145

52. Rudat V, Münter M, Rades D, et al. The effect of amifostine or IMRT to preserve the parotid function after radiotherapy of the head and neck region measured by quantitative salivary gland scintigraphy. Radiother Oncol 2008;89(1):71–80

53. Ma C, Xie J, Chen Q, Wang G, Zuo S. Amifostine for salivary glands in high-dose radioactive iodine treated differentiated thyroid cancer. Cochrane Database Syst Rev 2009;(4):CD007956

54. Burlage FR, Faber H, Kampinga HH, Langendijk JA, Vissink A, Coppes RP. Enhanced proliferation of acinar and progenitor cells by prophylactic pilocarpine treatment underlies the observed amelioration of radiation injury to parotid glands. Radiother Oncol 2009;90(2):253–256

55. Burlage FR, Roesink JM, Faber H, et al. Optimum dose range for the amelioration of long term radiation-induced hyposalivation using prophylactic pilocarpine treatment. Radiother Oncol 2008;86(3):347–353

56. Burlage FR, Roesink JM, Kampinga HH, et al. Protection of salivary function by concomitant pilocarpine during radiotherapy: a double-blind, randomized, placebo-controlled study. Int J Radiat Oncol Biol Phys 2008;70(1):14–22

57. Gornitsky M, Shenouda G, Sultanem K, et al. Double-blind randomized, placebo-controlled study of pilocarpine to salvage salivary gland function during radiotherapy of patients with head and neck cancer. Oral Surg Oral Med Oral Pathol Oral Radiol Endod 2004;98(1):45–52

58. Scarpace SL, Brodzik FA, Mehdi S, Belgam R. Treatment of head and neck cancers: issues for clinical pharmacists. Pharmacotherapy 2009;29(5):578–592

59. Scarantino C, LeVeque F, Swann RS, et al. Effect of pilocarpine during radiation therapy: results of RTOG 97-99, a phase III randomized study in head and neck cancer patients. J Support Oncol 2006;4(5):252–258

60. Nyárády Z, Németh A, Bán A, et al. A randomized study to assess the effectiveness of orally administered pilocarpine during and after radiotherapy of head and neck cancer. Anticancer Res 2006;26(2B):1557–1562

61. Jha N, Seikaly H, Harris J, et al. Phase III randomized study: oral pilocarpine versus submandibular salivary gland transfer protocol for the management of radiation-induced xerostomia. Head Neck 2009;31(2):234–243

62. Davies A, Bagg J, Laverty D, et al. Salivary gland dysfunction ('dry mouth') in patients with cancer: a consensus statement. Eur J Cancer Care (Engl) 2010;19(2):172–177

63. Eisbruch A, Kim HM, Terrell JE, Marsh LH, Dawson LA, Ship JA. Xerostomia and its predictors following parotid-sparing irradiation of head-and-neck cancer. Int J Radiat Oncol Biol Phys 2001;50(3):695–704

64. Maes A, Weltens C, Flamen P, et al. Preservation of parotid function with uncomplicated conformal radiotherapy. Radiother Oncol 2002;63(2):203–211

65. Gorsky M, Epstein JB, Parry J, Epstein MS, Le ND, Silverman S. Jr. The efficacy of pilocarpine and bethanechol upon saliva production in cancer patients with hyposalivation following radiation therapy. Oral Surg Oral Med Oral Pathol Oral Radiol Endod 2004;97(2):190–195

66. Jellema AP, Slotman BJ, Doornaert P, Leemans CR, Langendijk JA. Impact of radiation-induced xerostomia on quality of life after primary radiotherapy among patients with head and neck cancer. Int J Radiat Oncol Biol Phys 2007;69(3):751–760

67. https://webapps.ctep.nci.nih.gov/webobjs/ctc/webhelp/Welcome_to_CTCAE_1.htm

68. Fox PC, Busch KA, Baum BJ. Subjective reports of xerostomia and objective measures of salivary gland performance. J Am Dent Assoc 1987;115(4):581–584

69. Gomes SG, Custódio W, Cury AA, Garcia RC. Effect of salivary flow rate on masticatory efficiency. Int J Prosthodont 2009;22(2):168–172

70. Turner M, Jahangiri L, Ship JA. Hyposalivation, xerostomia and the complete denture: a systematic review. J Am Dent Assoc 2008;139(2):146–150

71. Rogers SN, Johnson IA, Lowe D. Xerostomia after treatment for oral and oropharyngeal cancer using the University of Washington saliva domain and a Xerostomia-Related Quality-of-Life Scale. Int J Radiat Oncol Biol Phys 2010;77(1):16–23

72. Meirovitz A, Murdoch-Kinch CA, Schipper M, Pan C, Eisbruch A. Grading xerostomia by physicians or by patients after intensity-modulated radiotherapy of head-and-neck cancer. Int J Radiat Oncol Biol Phys 2006;66(2):445–453

73. http://www.rtog.org/members/protocols/0244/main.html#eleven

74. Al-Nawas B, Al-Nawas K, Kunkel M, Knut A, Grötz KA. Quantifying radioxerostomia: salivary flow rate, examiner's score, and quality of life questionnaire. Strahlenther Onkol 2006;182(6):336–341

75. Kohler PF, Winter ME. A quantitative test for xerostomia. The Saxon test, an oral equivalent of the Schirmer test. Arthritis Rheum 1985;28(10):1128–1132

76. Ishimoto S, Tsunoda K, Fujimaki Y, et al. Objective and non-invasive evaluation of dry mouth. Auris Nasus Larynx 2008;35(1):89–93

77. Sugiura Y, Soga Y, Nishide S, et al. Evaluation of xerostomia in hematopoietic cell transplantation by a simple capacitance method device. Support Care Cancer 2008;16(10):1197–1200

78. Bomeli SR, Desai SC, Johnson JT, Walvekar RR. Management of salivary flow in head and neck cancer patients—a systematic review. Oral Oncol 2008;44(11):1000–1008

79. Nieuw Amerongen AV, Veerman EC. Current therapies for xerostomia and salivary gland hypofunction associated with cancer therapies. Support Care Cancer 2003;11(4):226–231

80. Visvanathan V, Nix P. Managing the patient presenting with xerostomia: a review. Int J Clin Pract 2010;64(3):404–407

81. Mosqueda-Taylor A, Luna-Ortiz K, Irigoyen-Camacho ME, Díaz-Franco MA, Coll-Muñoz AM. Effect of pilocarpine hydrochloride on salivary production in previously irradiated head and neck cancer patients. Med Oral 2004;9(3):204–211

82. LeVeque FG, Montgomery M, Potter D, et al. A multicenter, randomized, double-blind, placebo-controlled, dose-titration study of oral pilocarpine for treatment of radiation-induced xerostomia in head and neck cancer patients. J Clin Oncol 1993;11(6):1124–1131

83. Taweechaisupapong S, Pesee M, Aromdee C, Laopaiboon M, Khunkitti W. Efficacy of pilocarpine lozenge for post-radiation xerostomia in patients with head and neck cancer. Aust Dent J 2006;51(4):333–337

84. Götrick B, Akerman S, Ericson D, Torstenson R, Tobin G. Oral pilocarpine for treatment of opioid-induced oral dryness in healthy adults. J Dent Res 2004;83(5):393–397

85. Chitapanarux I, Kamnerdsupaphon P, Tharavichitkul E, et al. Effect of oral pilocarpine on post-irradiation xerostomia in head and neck cancer patients: a single-center, single-blind clinical trial. J Med Assoc Thai 2008;91(9):1410–1415

86. Fox PC, Atkinson JC, Macynski AA, et al. Pilocarpine treatment of salivary gland hypofunction and dry mouth (xerostomia). Arch Intern Med 1991;151(6):1149–1152

87. Nakamura N, Sasano N, Yamashita H, et al. Oral pilocarpine (5 mg t.i.d.) used for xerostomia causes adverse effects in Japanese. Auris Nasus Larynx 2009;36(3):310–313

88. Weber J, Keating GM. Cevimeline. Drugs 2008;68(12):1691–1698

89. Chambers MS, Posner M, Jones CU, et al. Cevimeline for the treatment of postirradiation xerostomia in patients with head and neck cancer. Int J Radiat Oncol Biol Phys 2007;68(4):1102–1109

90. Chambers MS, Jones CU, Biel MA, et al. Open-label, long-term safety study of cevimeline in the treatment of postirradiation xerostomia. Int J Radiat Oncol Biol Phys 2007;69(5):1369–1376

91. Jham BC, Teixeira IV, Aboud CG, Carvalho AL, Coelho MdeM, Freire AR. A randomized phase III prospective trial of bethanechol to prevent radiotherapy-induced salivary gland damage in patients with head and neck cancer. Oral Oncol 2007;43(2):137–142

92. Khosravani N, Birkhed D, Ekström J. The cholinesterase inhibitor physostigmine for the local treatment of dry mouth: a randomized study. Eur J Oral Sci 2009;117(3):209–217

93. Gorsky M, Epstein JB, Parry J, Epstein MS, Le ND, Silverman S Jr. The efficacy of pilocarpine and bethanechol upon saliva production in cancer patients with hyposalivation following radiation therapy. Oral Surg Oral Med Oral Pathol Oral Radiol Endod 2004;97(2):190–195

94. Chainani-Wu N, Gorsky M, Mayer P, Bostrom A, Epstein JB, Silverman S Jr. Assessment of the use of sialogogues in the clinical management of patients with xerostomia. Spec Care Dentist 2006;26(4):164–170

95. Hahnel S, Behr M, Handel G, Bürgers R. Saliva substitutes for the treatment of radiation-induced xerostomia—a review. Support Care Cancer 2009;17(11):1331–1343

96. Oh DJ, Lee JY, Kim YK, Kho HS. Effects of carboxymethylcellulose (CMC)-based artificial saliva in patients with xerostomia. Int J Oral Maxillofac Surg 2008;37(11):1027–1031

97. Epstein JB, Emerton S, Le ND, Stevenson-Moore P. A double-blind crossover trial of Oral Balance gel and Biotene toothpaste versus placebo in patients with xerostomia following radiation therapy. Oral Oncol 1999;35(2):132–137

98. Gil-Montoya JA, Guardia-López I, González-Moles MA. Evaluation of the clinical efficacy of a mouthwash and oral gel containing the antimicrobial proteins lactoperoxidase, lysozyme and lactoferrin in elderly patients with dry mouth—a pilot study. Gerodontology 2008;25(1):3–9

99. Sudo E, Maejima I. [The effects of moisturizing gel to prevent dry mouth in patients with cerebrovascular disease]. Nippon Ronen Igakkai Zasshi 2008;45(2):196–201

100. Scully C, Limeres J, Gleeson M, Tomás I, Diz P. Drooling. J Oral Pathol Med 2009;38(4):321–327

101. Shiboski CH, Hodgson TA, Ship JA, Schiødt M. Management of salivary hypofunction during and after radiotherapy. Oral Surg Oral Med Oral Pathol Oral Radiol Endod 2007;103(Suppl):S66, e1–e19

102. Bomeli SR, Desai SC, Johnson JT, Walvekar RR. Management of salivary flow in head and neck cancer patients—a systematic review. Oral Oncol 2008;44(11):1000–1008

103. Llena C, Forner L, Baca P. Anticariogenicity of casein phosphopeptide-amorphous calcium phosphate: a review of the literature. J Contemp Dent Pract 2009;10(3):1–9

104. Singh ML, Papas AS. Long-term clinical observation of dental caries in salivary hypofunction patients using a supersaturated calcium-phosphate remineralizing rinse. J Clin Dent 2009;20(3):87–92

105. Nagy K, Urban E, Fazekas O, Thurzo L, Nagy E. Controlled study of lactoperoxidase gel on oral flora and saliva in irradiated patients with oral cancer. J Craniofac Surg 2007;18(5):1157–1164

28 Mucositis

Madhup Rastogi, Raghav C. Dwivedi, Kundan S. Chufal, and Rehan A. Kazi

Core Messages

- Oral mucositis (OM) is a major problem for patients with cancer receiving head and neck radiotherapy, stem cell transplantation, and myelosuppressive chemotherapy for solid tumors.

- Poorly managed OM is one of the leading causes for unplanned treatment interruptions, which are responsible for increased cost and time in delivering optimal treatment to the patients with head and neck cancer.

- Well-timed intervention and effective treatment is required to prevent or reduce the incidence and severity of mucositis.

- The better understanding of its pathologic basis has led to the development of targeted agents to combat mucositis.

- The Multinational Association of Supportive Care in Cancer and the International Society for Oral Oncology advocate guidelines for the prevention and treatment of mucositis.

Significant advancements have been made in the management of patients undergoing cancer chemotherapy (CT) and radiotherapy (RT). However, many debilitating side effects, such as nausea, vomiting, diarrhea, and mucositis, remain critical issues that often delay or restrict the therapy and impede recovery. Mounting evidence indicates that more aggressive regimens improve locoregional tumor control and survival in patients with head and neck cancer (HNC). The better treatment outcome, however, has come at the expense of increased patient morbidity, notably, an increase in severe (grades 3 to 4) mucositis that causes substantial pain, interferes with the patient's ability to chew and swallow, and worsens the patient's quality of life. Virtually all patients with HNC develop some degree of mucositis during their treatment by either RT or CT. Nowadays; a majority of patients with HNC are being treated by concurrent chemoradiotherapy (CRT) as radical or adjuvant management, which in turn increases the probability of flaring up of mucosal inflammation.

In general terms, mucositis is the inflammation of the mucous membrane lining of the digestive tract from the mouth on down to the anus. When it involves the mucous membrane of oral and oropharyngeal region, it is termed as oral mucositis (OM). It is due to systemic effects of chemotherapeutic agents and the local effects of radiation on the oral mucous membrane. Thus, OM, if not detected or treated adequately, can lead to pain, discomfort, and inability to tolerate food or fluids, with increased propensity for opportunistic infections in the mouth. Poorly managed OM is one of the leading causes for unplanned treatment interruptions[1] and therefore increases the overall treatment time. Prolongation of overall treatment time adversely affects the tumor control probability.[2] It also increases the overall cost of treatment.

Incidence

Trotti et al[3] studied more than 6000 patients with squamous cell cancers of the head and neck who received RT with or without CT. The overall incidence of OM in this patient population was 80%, with 39% of the cases being grade 3/4 (**Table 28.1**), which limited or prevented alimentation. Patients who received altered fractionation RT (AF-RT) were particularly at risk; all patients in this subgroup experienced OM, with 57% scored as grade 3/4.[3]

A smaller, but still significant proportion (approximately 40%) of patients who receive standard-dose CT also develop OM as a result of therapy, with the lowest risk occurring by "gentler" chemotherapeutics, such as gemcitabine, and the higher risk occurring with more aggressive agents such as 5-fluorouracil (5-FU) and cisplatin.

Higher OM incidence rates of 60% are seen in the stem cell transplantation setting, with reported incidence rates of up to 78% for ulcerative mucositis as a result of high-dose CT or total body irradiation. The severity of OM may be higher with allogeneic transplants than with autologous transplants.[4]

Predictive Indices/Risk Factors

The potential for developing OM after RT or CT is influenced by a variety of patient- and treatment-related risk factors (**Table 28.2**).[5]

Table 28.1 Incidence of Oral Mucositis among Cancer Patients[3]

	Incidence (%)	Grade 3/4 (%)
Radiotherapy for head and neck cancer	85–100	25–45
Stem-cell transplantation	75–100	25–60
Solid tumors with myelosuppression	5–40	5–15

Adapted from reference 3.

Patient-Related Risks

Numerous patient-related factors appear to increase the frequency and severity of OM after CT or RT, including gender, age of the patient, type of malignancy, pretreatment oral condition, oral care during treatment, nutritional status, and pretreatment neutrophil counts (**Table 28.2**). Disagreement exists relating to the effects of age and the development of OM. Younger individuals (< 20 years) are more susceptible because of the more rapid epithelial mitotic rate or the presence of more epidermal growth factor receptors in the epithelium. On the contrary, decline in renal function associated with aging is the possible reason of increased incidence of OM in older patients. (> 65 years) Poor oral hygiene, chronic periodontal disease, smoking, alcoholism, and oropharyngeal infection may contribute significantly to the development of OM. Decrease in neutrophil count results in an impaired ability to mount an adequate inflammatory response, leading to increased probability of OM.

Treatment-Related Risks

Treatment-related factors consist of specific chemotherapeutic drug, dose, schedule, whether continuous or bolus, and use of radiation therapy.[6] All these factors are summarized in **Table 28.2**.

Pathogenesis

The pathogenesis of cancer treatment–related OM is not fully elucidated. Recent advances in molecular cellular biology and translational research propose a complex multistep process taking place in the development of OM. Healthy oropharyngeal mucosa has a rapid cell turnover with a renewal period of 7 to 14 days, and it serves as a barrier to infections. Soon after CT or RT administration, acute inflammatory/vascular changes occur. Sonis[7] has described a five-phase model to characterize the major steps in the development and resolution of OM:

1. Initiation: Reactive oxygen species generated by exposure to CT or RT result in DNA strand breaks and damage to cells, tissues, and blood vessels, which ultimately cause apoptosis.

Table 28.2 Risk Factors for Oral Mucositis

Patient-related
- Gender
- Age older than 65 y or younger than 20 y
- Inadequate oral hygiene
- Periodontal diseases
- Chronic low-grade oral infections
- Salivary gland secretory dysfunction
- Herpes simplex virus infection
- Inborn inability to metabolize chemotherapeutic agents effectively
- Poor nutritional status
- Exposure to oral stressors including alcohol and smoking
- Ill-fitting dental prostheses

Treatment-related
- Radiation therapy: dose, schedule, and type such as conformal or intensity-modulated radiation therapy
- Chemotherapy: agent, dose, and schedule
- Myelosuppression
- Neutropenia
- Anemia
- Immunosuppression
- Reduced secretory immunoglobulin A
- Insufficient oral care during treatment
- Infections of bacterial, viral, and fungal origin
- Use of drugs such as antidepressants, opiates, antihypertensive, antihistamines, diuretics, and sedatives
- Deranged renal and/or hepatic function
- Protein or calorie malnutrition
- Dehydration

Adapted from reference 5.

y, year.

2. Message generation: Such damage triggers the activation of transcription factors such as nuclear factor kappa B, which in turn causes increased production of proinflammatory cytokines such as interleukin (IL)-1β and IL-6. These increased levels of cytokines trigger the initiation of various pathways that damage epithelial cells and surrounding fibroblasts, causing tissue injury and apoptosis.

3. Signaling and amplification: Proinflammatory cytokines, such as tumor necrosis factor α (TNF-α), activate ceramide and caspase pathways; these signals further increase the production of TNF-α, IL-1β, and IL-6, thus causing an amplification effect.

4. Ulceration and inflammation: Inflammatory infiltrate composed of polymorphonuclear and round inflammatory cells is found in the mucosa. As there is a breach in the mucosal barrier, penetration of the epithelium into the submucosa can occur and the mucosa is prone to bacterial infections, which further lead to an increase in the production of TNF-α, IL-1β, and IL-6. This further enhances the mucosal injury, thus causing more severe OM in the form of

ulceration, allowing colonization by oral bacteria and increasing the risk of sepsis. It is likely that in each of these OM stages, pathogenesis occurs in a continuous, overlapping manner.

5. Healing: Healing of oral lesions starts with a signal from the extracellular matrix in the nonmyelosuppressed patient within 2 to 3 weeks after cancer treatment. Mechanisms of healing include renewal of epithelial proliferation and differentiation in parallel with white blood cell recovery and reestablishment of normal local microbial flora.

Pathogenesis of OM has suggested a variety of potential therapeutic targets, which have resulted in the development of agents that can prevent or ameliorate associated symptoms. Several such compounds are thought to inhibit one or more steps in these pathways, thus enhancing their effectiveness. Because some agents act to downregulate nuclear factor kappa B activation, which is involved in upregulating numerous genes encoding proinflammatory cytokines, the resulting inhibition may be greatly enhanced.

Diagnosis

OM is typically diagnosed on the basis of the clinical appearance, location, timing of oral lesions, and use of certain types of therapies known to be associated with OM. Consistent and frequent oral cavity assessment under intense white light is needed to visualize all soft and hard tissues and dentition before, during, and after the treatment time course. Systematic assessment of the oral cavity permits early identification of the lesion. All assessors should have a thorough familiarity regarding clinical signs and symptoms of oral complications. Systemic effects of OM may result in the symptom complex, characterized by fatigue, taste alterations, anemia, anorexia, cachexia, neurocognitive alterations, and depression, which may often be termed as "sickness syndrome."[8] Mucosal damage by CT or RT results in the release of inflammatory mediators and the activation of biologic processes, which result in systemic effects. Several scoring systems have been defined to assess the severity of OM (**Table 28.3**), but no one scale is uniformly used. These evaluative tools vary in complexity. Some established guidelines are those proposed by the World Health Organization[9] and the National Cancer Institute's Common Toxicity Criteria.[10,11] In the World Health Organization scale, both objective mucosal changes (redness, ulceration) and functional outcomes (ability to eat) have been integrated. In contrast, National Cancer Institute's Common Toxicity Criteria have been developed to classify OM in patients receiving radiation therapy, CT, and conditioning regimens for bone marrow transplantation.[10,11] On clinical examination, four distinct stages/grades can be identified (**Fig. 28.1**). Patients are able to maintain oral intake in grade 1, oral intake is compromised in grade 2, patients are unable to take anything (food or liquids) in grade 3, and grade 4 is life-threatening.

In addition, Sonis et al[12] have devised an Oral Mucositis Assessment Scale. This scale separates objective and subjective findings. Degrees of ulceration and redness measured in specific sites in the mouth were primary indicators of OM, while oral pain, difficulty in swallowing, and the ability to eat were taken as secondary indicators. A single score is not produced from this scale, rather a score for ulceration and redness based on different locations in the mouth are used. This scale is more quantitative for clinical research but may be difficult to use in routine clinical care.

Other scoring systems by Radiation Therapy Oncology Group have been proposed,[13] but the lack of standardization has hampered their acceptance.

Other common conditions that may confuse OM include oral candidiasis (thrush), herpes simplex virus (HSV), and graft-versus-host disease (GVHD) in patients with transplant. Candidal overgrowth (candidiasis), which occurs in response to RT or CT, usually responds well to systemic antifungal medication. HSV is frequently seen in patients with immunocompromised cancer receiving CT, with lesions appearing on the lips (cold sores) or intraoral mucosa. Initiation of antiviral therapy may ameliorate HSV-associated OM and reduce symptoms. OM can also occur in patients receiving myeloablative conditioning regimens for allogeneic hematopoietic stem cell transplantation and in those with GVHD, affecting the oral mucosa. Consequently, an accurate diagnosis of OM is critical to ensure selection and timely initiation of optimal therapy.

Management Guidelines

A standardized approach for the prevention and treatment of CT- and RT-induced OM is essential. Numerous agents and protocols have been developed for the management or prevention of OM, but the most widely accepted guidelines were issued in 2004[14] and were updated by the Multinational Association of Supportive Care in Cancer and International Society for Oral Oncology (MASCC/ISOO).[15] These guidelines are based on a comprehensive review of more than 8000 English-language publications (1966 to 2001). Discussions by the panel resulted in the development of a set of recommendations for the prevention and treatment of OM. Guidelines that are relevant to the care of patients with HNC are discussed here (**Table 28.4**). The MASCC/ISOO Mucositis Study Group has continued to monitor the literature and in 2007 updated OM management guidelines.[16]

These guidelines emphasize multiprofessional interventions for appropriate management of OM. An interdisciplinary approach to oral care, routine assessment of oral cavity, pain management using validated instruments, and regular dental assessment and dental care before the start of cancer therapy is the foundation of care. The panel stressed the need for education of staff as well as patients and their families on proper oral care and the importance of outcome assessment using quality-improvement processes.

Currently, there is insufficient high-level evidence to recommend the use of bland and/or medicated oral rinses for the treatment of OM, although they may help reduce the degree of gingivitis and plaque as well as the risk of caries. OM-related pain should be carefully managed through the use of topical analgesics and nonsteroidal agents and patient-controlled analgesia (opioids) for severe pain, when necessary.

Treatment Options

Although several approaches to OM management have been advocated, a single efficacious intervention or agent for the prophylaxis or management of RT- or CT-induced OM has not yet been identified. Many different treatments are used to prevent or treat OM, and these interventions have been categorized under the following headings, though in the absence of double-blind and placebo-controlled clinical trials, many of the management recommendations are only subjective.

Basic Oral Care

Poor oral hygiene along with associated dental and periodontal pathology, such as dental caries, ill-fitting prostheses, and orthodontic appliances leads to a greater risk for OM in the course of RT or CT. The MASCC/ISOO recommends "basic oral care" as a standard practice to prevent and alleviate mucosal symptoms.[16] The "basic oral care" typically includes careful inspection of the oral cavity, evaluation by dental specialists, and dental work to eliminate caries and existing gum disease before beginning cancer treatment and should be repeated in the course of treatment.[15] Such practice not only helps in the differentiation of OM from preexisting changes, such as pemphigoid, lichen planus, leukoplakia, and GVHD, but also permits the identification and elimination of preexisting potential sources of infection that may affect the severity of the OM.

Table 28.3 Scales Used to Asses Oral Mucositis

	Grade 0	Grade 1	Grade 2	Grade 3	Grade 4
WHO[9]	None	Soreness with erythema	Erythema, ulcers, can eat solids	Ulcers, only liquid diet	Alimentation not possible
RTOG[13]	No change over baseline	Injection/may experience mild pain not requiring analgesic	Patchy mucositis that may produce an inflammatory serosanguinous discharge/may experience moderate pain requiring analgesia	Confluent fibrinous mucositis/may include severe pain requiring narcotic	Ulceration, hemorrhage, or necrosis
OMAS[12] Ulceration/ erythema	Normal Normal	Not severe < 1 cm²	Severe 1–3 cm²	NA > 3 cm²	NA NA
NCI-CTCAE v3.0[11] Clinical criteria Functional criteria	None	Erythema of the mucosa	Patchy ulcerations or pseudomembranes	Confluent ulcerations or pseudomembranes: bleeding with minor trauma	Tissue necrosis: significant spontaneous bleeding: life-threatening consequences
	None	Minimal symptoms, normal diet	Symptomatic but can eat and swallow modified diet	Symptomatic and unable to adequately aliment or hydrate orally	Symptoms associated with life-threatening consequences
NCI-CTCAE v4.0[10]	None	Asymptomatic or mild symptoms; intervention not indicated	Moderate pain; not interfering with oral intake; modified diet indicated	Severe pain; interfering with oral intake	Life-threatening consequences; urgent intervention indicated

WHO, World Health Organization; RTOG, Radiation Therapy Oncology Group; OMAS, Oral Mucositis Assessment Scale; NCI-CTCAE, National Cancer Institute Common Toxicity Criteria for Adverse Events.

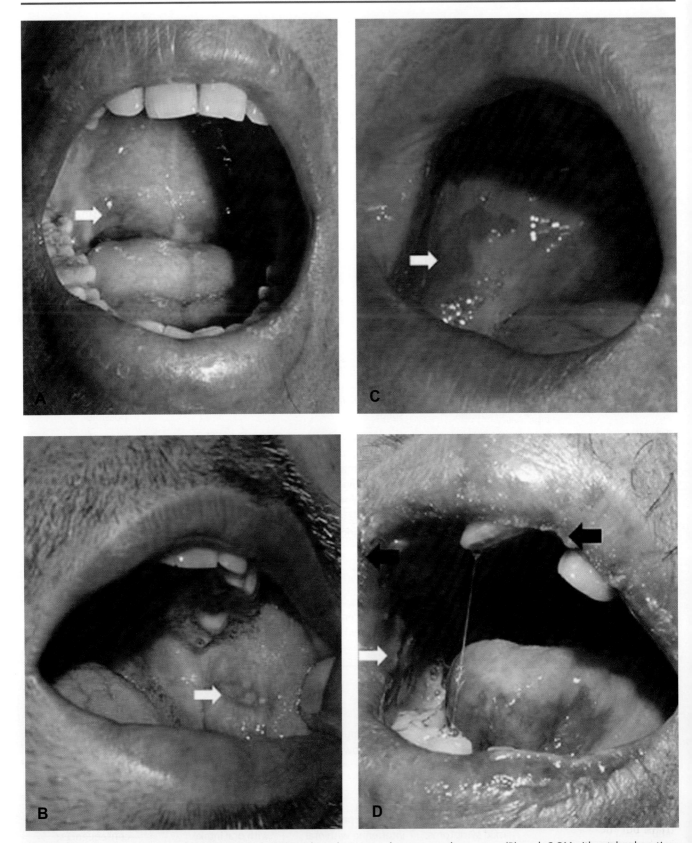

Figure 28.1   Grades of oral mucositis (OM): (A) grade 1 OM with erythematous changes over the mucosa; (B) grade 2 OM with patchy ulcerations or pseudo membrane; (C) grade 3 OM with confluent ulcerations or bleeding ulcers; (D) grade 4 OM with tissue necrosis, bleeding ulcers (white arrow), and crusting as a result of dehydration (black arrows).

Table 28.4   MASCC/ISOO Oral Mucositis Management Guidelines

Summary of Evidence-Based Clinical Practice Guidelines for Care of Patients with Oral and Gastrointestinal Mucositis (2005 Update)

Foundations of care

- Multidisciplinary development and evaluation of oral care protocols that include frequent use of nonmedicated oral rinses (e.g., saline mouth rinses four to six times daily) is recommended.
- Patient and staff education in the use of such protocols to reduce the severity of OM from CT and/or RT.
- As part of the protocols, the use of a soft toothbrush that is replaced on a regular basis is recommended.
- Elements of good clinical practice should include the use of validated tools to regularly assess oral pain and oral cavity health. The inclusion of dental professionals is vital throughout the treatment and follow-up phases.
- Patient-controlled analgesia with morphine as the treatment of choice for OM pain in patients undergoing hematopoietic stem cell transplantation.
- Regular oral pain assessment using validated instruments for self-reporting is essential.

RT–prevention	
Recommended	• Use of midline radiation blocks and three-dimensional radiation treatment to reduce mucosal injury • Benzydamine hydrochloride oral rinse for prevention of radiation-induced mucositis in patients with head and neck cancer receiving moderate-dose RT
Not recommended	• Sucralfate • Antimicrobial lozenges • Chlorhexidine
Standard-dose CT—prevention	
Recommended	• Oral cryotherapy (30 min) in patients receiving bolus 5-FU • Oral cryotherapy (20–30 min) is suggested to decrease mucositis in patients treated with bolus doses of edatrexate
Not recommended	• Acyclovir and its analogues
Standard-dose CT—treatment	
• Chlorhexidine not to be used to treat established OM	
High-dose CT with or without total body irradiation plus hematopoietic cell transplantation—prevention	
Recommended	Keratinocyte growth factor-1 (palifermin) in a dose of 60 μg/kg/d for 3 d before conditioning treatment and for 3 d posttransplant Cryotherapy Low-level laser therapy (if the technology is available)
Not recommended	Pentoxifylline GM-CSF mouthwashes

Adapted from reference 16.

MASCC/ISOO, Multinational Association of Supportive Care in Cancer and International Society for Oral Oncology; OM, oral mucositis; CT, chemotherapy; RT, radiotherapy; min, minute; 5FU, 5-fluorouracil; d, day; GM-CSF, granulocyte-macrophage colony-stimulating factor.

Meticulous pretreatment assessment and the maintenance of good oral hygiene during and after mucosa toxic therapy will reduce the incidence and duration of OM.

Basic oral care protocols during RT or CT involve brushing in a nontraumatic fashion, two to three times daily with a soft-bristle toothbrush that has to be replaced on a regular basis. The use of daily dental fluoride prophylaxis such as (brushing) gels, rinses, and vacuum-formed vinyl splints loaded with fluoride gel has not been evaluated in clinical trials, but these agents are frequently used to prevent OM in the course of RT or CT because they induce fluoride incorporation into tooth enamel and dentin. They also reduce oral bacterial load.

To maintain oral moistness, patients should frequently rinse with bland solutions, such as normal saline. This saline solution is made by adding half a tablespoon of salt to 1 L of water and can be administered at room or refrigerated temperatures, depending on the patient's preference.[6] The patient should rinse several times as often as necessary to maintain oral comfort. If viscous saliva is present, half a tablespoon of sodium bicarbonate (baking soda) can be added.[6] Saline solution can increase oral lubrication by acting directly as well as by stimulating salivary glands to increase salivary flow.

The daily use of hydrogen peroxide rinses is not recommended, especially if OM is present, because of the potential for damage to fibroblasts and keratinocytes, which can cause delayed wound healing.[17] Using 3% hydrogen peroxide diluted 1:1 with water or normal saline to remove hemorrhagic debris may be helpful; however, this approach should be used for only 1 to 2 days because more extended use may impair timely healing of mucosal lesions associated with bleeding.

Chlorhexidine is an oral broad-spectrum antibiotic rinse known to reduce the colonization of microorganisms in the oral cavity. Pitten et al[18] in his trial concluded that the use of chlorhexidine antiseptic mouthwash was associated with increase in oral mucosal inflammation, general mouth discomfort, taste alteration, and staining of teeth. Based on these trials and updated recommendations of the MASCC/ISOO, the use of chlorhexidine is not recommended.[16]

The "magic mouthwash" or "mouthwash cocktail" is used by different institutions across the world. Such mouthwashes usually have a variety of ingredients, such as lidocaine, diphenhydramine, topical antifungal nystatin, and an antacid containing aluminum/magnesium hydroxide in equal parts.[19] These formulas are popular for OM treatment because of their pain-relieving properties and their coating of the mucosa. However, diphenhydramine is sedating and may carry unpleasant anticholinergic properties. Alternatively, oral ketoconazole and fluconazole are more efficient in controlling oral candidiasis compared with nystatin. Dodd et al[20] evaluated the efficacy and safety of magic mouthwash (lidocaine, diphenhydramine, Maalox [aluminum hydroxide 225 mg, magnesium hydroxide 200 mg; per 5 mL; liq; mint, lemon, or cherry flavor]) versus a salt-and-soda rinse and chlorhexidine. They found no difference in the efficacy between these agents.[20] The MASCC/ISOO guidelines do not recommend the use of such cocktail mouthwashes for the prevention and treatment of OM.[16]

It is also recommended that patients avoid factors that cause irritation such as hot, spicy, and coarse foods, fruits and beverages with a high acid content, and alcohol (including alcohol-containing elixirs) and should abstain from smoking. Although it is accepted that basic oral care is important to maintain dental and mucosal health, there is little direct evidence that it significantly affects the incidence or severity of OM. Nonetheless, basic oral care is considered an essential part of management.

Cryotherapy

Cryotherapy is a procedure of rapid cooling of the oral cavity by chewing ice chips or popsicles, which causes local vasoconstriction and therefore decreases the blood flow to the oral mucosa. Hence, lesser amount of the drug will reach to the oral mucous membrane; consequently, the severity of OM will be greatly reduced. Sucking ice chips for half an hour during intravenous infusion of 5-FU significantly reduces the severity and incidence of OM, successfully studied in randomized trials.[21] The use of cryotherapy is a readily available, cheap, and effective method of minimizing OM induced by bolus 5-FU, but this measure is not effective for continuous infusions. The use of ice chips in patients receiving melphalan- and edatrexate-based CT regimens[22] as a prophylactic measure also indicates reduced incidence of OM.

Current MASCC/ISOO guidelines recommend cryotherapy for the prevention of OM with standard-dose CT.[16]

Pain Management

Pain is the single most important distressing symptom in head and neck RT, and its adequate control affects the treatment outcome favorably. Pain can also lead to decreased oral intake, leading to malnutrition and the need for total parenteral nutrition. Most patients require both systemic and topical analgesics. Many local anesthetic agents, such as diphenhydramine, viscous xylocaine, and lidocaine as oral solutions, are frequently used for the temporary relief of OM-related pain. However, such topical anesthetics interfere with taste perception, thus possibly contributing to hypoalimentation. The most efficacious local anesthetic remains to be determined, as a double-blind randomized trial failed to demonstrate the superiority of any of these local anesthetic agents.[23] Therefore, their frequent and prophylactic use should be discouraged. Few studies suggest the use of combinations of local anesthetics and mouth-coating agents such as sucralfate. However, the use of sucralfate is controversial as most of the randomized trials[24] failed to demonstrate its beneficial effects. The MASCC/ISOO guidelines do not support the use of sucralfate.[16]

The inability to control OM-related pain can be frustrating for both the patient and the treating physician. Such patients should be given narcotic analgesics in the form of morphine or transdermal fentanyl patches along with laxatives to avoid constipation. Irritant laxatives are preferred compared with bulk-forming ones because of compromised oral intake. The dose of narcotic analgesics, their frequency, and duration should be regularly adjusted to meet the level of pain intensity. Despite the recommendations from the MASCC/ISOO,[16] a recent symptom review study shows that very few patients are being given adequate narcotic analgesia.[25]

Targeting Infection

The oral cavity of normal individual harbors a variety of potentially pathogenic microorganisms. However, healthy individuals are not susceptible to infection because of maintained mucosal integrity and normal immunity. However, in patients with cancer, who are already immunocompromised, oral infections can arise from viral, fungal, and bacterial sources.[26] As a rule, the mucous membrane is a barrier to these agents, but the loss of mucosal integrity can permit systemic entry of organisms, which leads to infection. It is important that patients be monitored closely for any acute exacerbation of signs and symptoms of OM, which will suggest oral/pharyngeal infection and may commonly include candidiasis, bacterial, or HSV. Keeping a high index of suspicion, culture and sensitivity assays should be done if infection is anticipated. Several systemic and topical antimicrobial agents have been evaluated for OM.

Many authors have emphasized the necessity of a variety of disinfectant, antibacterial, antiviral, and antifungal agents for the prophylaxis and treatment of OM, but because of variable results there is no uniform consensus; therefore, their routine use is not recommended.[16]

Targeting Inflammation

Antiinflammatory, steroidal, and nonsteroidal agents such as betamethasone, prednisolone, and prostaglandin E1 have been the focus of many preclinical and clinical researches; however, none have shown a positive effect on OM prevention.[27] Studies evaluating the prophylactic use of the prostaglandin E2 derivate, misoprostol, have produced controversial results.[27]

Benzydamine hydrochloride (BZD) is a nonsteroidal agent, frequently used in Canada and the European Union that exhibits antimicrobial, anti-inflammatory, anesthetic, and analgesic effects. Its action may be mediated by the prostaglandin system. It has been evaluated in phase III trials and found to be effective in low doses of radiation up to 50 Gy.[28] Thus, this study provided preliminary evidence that BZD might be beneficial in patients undergoing RT to the oral cavity. A larger, multicenter, randomized, double-blind, placebo-controlled clinical trial evaluating BZD for the prophylaxis of RT-induced OM demonstrated that that this agent was effective, safe, and well tolerated for prophylactic treatment.[29] Patients were instructed to rinse with BZD for 2 minutes, four to eight times daily, before and during RT and for 2 weeks after completion of RT. The use of BZD was associated with significantly reduced erythema and ulceration and delayed the use of systemic analgesics. BZD was not effective for patients receiving AF-RT. MASCC guidelines recommend the use of BZD for the prevention of OM in patients with HNC receiving moderate-dose RT.[16]

Conformal and Intensity-Modulated Radiation Therapy

OM is virtually universal when the head and neck area is irradiated. The severity depends on the type of ionizing radiation, volume of irradiated tissue, daily and cumulative dose, and duration of RT. OM is a dose- and rate-limiting toxicity of RT. In comparison with CT, where OM usually begins 3 to 5 days after the start of therapy and peaks at 7 to 10 days, RT-induced OM typically appears toward the end of the second week of treatment, plateaus during the fourth week of RT, and may persist for 2 to 3 weeks once treatment is over.[30] RT directly damages the basal epithelial cell layer of the oral mucosa, leading to the loss of the renewal capacity of the epithelium. Erythema of the involved mucosa in the second week of therapy will result because of subepithelial edema aggravating to an epithelial breakdown. As treatment continues, the epithelial surface cells shed, but their replacement by cells from the basal level does not occur. The mucosa becomes thin and superficially ulcerated, appearing as white patches,

commonly mistaken for a yeast infection. As RT progresses, the patches coalesce, forming large fields of superficial ulceration, referred to as confluent OM. By the end of treatment, diffuse erythema, ulceration, spontaneous bleeding, and white or yellow pseudomembrane formation may be present.

AF-RT results in increased rates of grade 3 and 4 OM compared with standard fractionation, and this has been demonstrated in a randomized trial of Fu et al.[31] Treatment of locally advanced HNC had undergone paradigm shift over the last decade in terms of definite use of CRT along with the monoclonal antibody cetuximab.[32] Although such aggressive treatment approach has resulted in better locoregional control and survival, it is at the cost of increased toxicity. Trotti et al[3] in their literature review concluded more incidences of grade 3 and greater OM in patients treated by CRT in comparison to RT alone.

OM is seen more in the neighborhood of prosthesis, and if the detachable part of prosthesis is removed, one can prevent the OM. Similarly, midline blocks also help reduce the incidence of OM.[33] Among the various RT techniques available such as intensity-modulated radiation therapy (IMRT) and two- or three-dimensional RT, only IMRT has the advantage of generating the sharp dose fall off near the targets, thus limiting the radiation dose to critical structures.[34] All the RT techniques result in varying grades of OM, but with the help of IMRT, we can spare the mucosa and thus limit the acute and long-term morbidity associated with grade 3 and 4 OM.[35] MASCC guidelines suggest the use of midline radiation blocks and three-dimensional radiation treatments to reduce OM.

Amifostine

Amifostine is a cytoprotective prodrug that is selectively taken up by nonmalignant cells. It is converted to its active free thiol metabolite at the tissue site. This thiol metabolite is responsible for most of the cytoprotective and radioprotective properties of amifostine. It is preferentially taken up by healthy cells, where it binds to and detoxifies reactive metabolites of platinum and alkylating agents as well as scavenges free radicals. It has a unique antioxidant property acting against reactive oxygen species produced by RT and responsible for OM. A meta-analysis[36] of 1451 has demonstrated a statistically significant role of amifostine in reducing the severity of OM in patients receiving RT. However, this reduction was at the cost of increased adverse effects associated with amifostine, such as nausea, vomiting, hypotension, and allergic reactions. Because of inconsistent results, it has not been approved for the treatment of OM. Till now, amifostine has been approved for reducing the incidence of severe xerostomia in patients with HNC being treated with RT.

Palifermin

Palifermin is a human recombinant keratinocyte growth factor produced in *Escherichia coli*. It reduces the OM because of RT and CT by stimulating the growth of the cells that line the surface of the oral cavity. Palifermin selectively binds to the epithelial cell-surface receptors and stimulates epithelial cell proliferation, differentiation, and upregulation of cytoprotective mechanisms. It reduces the incidence and duration of severe OM[37] by protecting those cells and stimulating the growth of new epithelial cells to build up the mucosal barrier. Clinical trials have demonstrated that palifermin can exert a mucoprotective effect in patients who were treated with RT or CT.[37] Palifermin-related adverse effects include skin toxicities (rash, erythema, edema, and pruritus), oral toxicities (dysesthesia, tongue discoloration, tongue thickening, and dysgeusia), and arthralgia. Further studies are ongoing to confirm its role in reducing OM.

Glutamine

Glutamine is a nonessential amino acid that reduces mucosal injury by reducing the production of proinflammatory cytokines and cytokine-related apoptosis. Many malignancies are characterized by decreased glutamine levels, which can be further exacerbated by cell damage caused by cancer therapy. Glutamine supplementation can reverse this effect and may help to protect mucosal tissues from damage by RT or CT and thus accelerate recovery. Glutamine has been used in different trials as oral, systemic, and as mouthwashes. Data suggest that this agent may be useful in preventing or reducing the incidence and severity of OM in patients undergoing cancer therapy.[38] However, because of incoherent results, the MASCC/ISOO do not recommend its routine use in present guidelines.[16] Further studies on this approach are warranted.

Granulocyte Colony-Stimulating Factor and Granulocyte-Macrophage Colony-Stimulating Factor

Granulocyte colony-stimulating factor (G-CSF) and granulocyte-macrophage colony-stimulating factor (GM-CSF) are used extensively with high-dose CT as systemic agents. Such systemic administration of G-CSF and GM-CSF leads to local accumulation of activated neutrophils in the oral mucosa, thus enhancing the defense mechanism. Systemic[39] as well as local (as topical mouthwash)[40] uses of G-CSF and GM-CSF have been evaluated in different trials for the prevention and treatment of OM. Results of these trials suggest a significant effect of GM-CSF and G-CSF on the prevention of OM in the systemic intervention group.[39] No effect was found for the topical administration group.[40] In view of inconsistent results, the MASCC/ISOO guidelines do not recommend their routine use.[16]

Low-Level Laser Therapy

Low-level laser therapy or "soft laser" has analgesic, anti-inflammatory, and wound-healing effects by speeding up the oral reepithelialization. There is no known clinical toxicity or side effects of the application of low-energy helium-neon lasers (soft lasers), and it positively influences the outcome of OM. Still there is no specific guidelines regarding the type of light source, wavelength, and dose schedule that have to be used, and it requires special training and necessary technology. MASCC guidelines suggest low-level laser therapy use in the transplant setting,[16] but do not propose its use during RT for HNC.

References

1. Russo G, Haddad R, Posner M, Machtay M. Radiation treatment breaks and ulcerative mucositis in head and neck cancer. Oncologist 2008;13(8):886–898

2. Bese NS, Hendry J, Jeremic B. Effects of prolongation of overall treatment time due to unplanned interruptions during radiotherapy of different tumor sites and practical methods for compensation. Int J Radiat Oncol Biol Phys 2007;68(3):654–661

3. Trotti A, Bellm LA, Epstein JB, et al. Mucositis incidence, severity and associated outcomes in patients with head and neck cancer receiving radiotherapy with or without chemotherapy: a systematic literature review. Radiother Oncol 2003;66(3):253–262

4. Rapoport AP, Miller Watelet LF, Linder T, et al. Analysis of factors that correlate with mucositis in recipients of autologous and allogeneic stem-cell transplants. J Clin Oncol 1999;17(8):2446–2453

5. Dodd MJ, Miaskowski C, Shiba GH, et al. Risk factors for CT-induced oral: dental appliances, oral hygiene, previous oral lesion, and a history of smoking. Cancer Invest 1999;17(4):278–284

6. Borowski B, Benhamou E, Pico JL, Laplanche A, Margainaud JP, Haya M. Prevention of oral mucositis in patients treated with high-dose chemotherapy and bone marrow transplantation: a randomized controlled trial comparing two protocols of dental care. Eur J Cancer B Oral Oncol 1994;30(2):93–97

7. Sonis ST. The pathobiology of mucositis. Nat Rev Cancer 2004;4(4):277–284

8. Hickok JT, Morrow GR, Roscoe JA, Mustian K, Okunieff P. Occurrence, severity, and longitudinal course of twelve common symptoms in 1129 consecutive patients during radiotherapy for cancer. J Pain Symptom Manage 2005;30(5):433–442

9. World Health Organization. WHO Handbook for Reporting Results of Cancer Treatment. Geneva, Switzerland: World Health Organization; 1979:15–22

10. National Cancer Institute. Common Terminology Criteria for Adverse Events (CTCAE) Version 4.0. Rockville, MD: U.S. Dept of Health and Human Services; May 28, 2009 (v4.03, June 14, 2010) Publication No. 09-5410. Available from: http://evs.nci.nih.gov/ftp1/CTCAE/About.html. Accessed 23-6-2012

11. Trotti A, Colevas AD, Setser A, et al. CTCAE v3.0: development of a comprehensive grading system for the adverse effects of cancer treatment. Semin Radiat Oncol 2003;13(3):176–181

12. Sonis ST, Eilers JP, Epstein JB, et al; Mucositis Study Group. Validation of a new scoring system for the assessment of clinical trial research of oral mucositis induced by radiation or chemotherapy. Cancer 1999;85(10):2103–2113

13. Cox JD, Stetz J, Pajak TF. Toxicity criteria of the Radiation Therapy Oncology Group (RTOG) and the European Organization for Research and Treatment of Cancer (EORTC). Int J Radiat Oncol Biol Phys 1995;31(5):1341–1346

14. Rubenstein EB, Peterson DE, Schubert M, et al; Mucositis Study Section of the Multinational Association for Supportive Care in

Cancer; International Society for Oral Oncology. Clinical practice guidelines for the prevention and treatment of cancer therapy-induced oral and gastrointestinal mucositis. Cancer 2004;100(9, Suppl)2026–2046

15. McGuire DB, Correa ME, Johnson J, Wienandts P. The role of basic oral care and good clinical practice principles in the management of oral mucositis. Support Care Cancer 2006;14(6):541–547

16. Keefe DM, Schubert MM, Elting LS, et al; Mucositis Study Section of the Multinational Association of Supportive Care in Cancer and the International Society for Oral Oncology. Updated clinical practice guidelines for the prevention and treatment of mucositis. Cancer 2007;109(5):820–831

17. Tombes MB, Gallucci B. The effects of hydrogen peroxide rinses on the normal oral mucosa. Nurs Res 1993;42(6):332–337

18. Pitten FA, Kiefer T, Buth C, Doelken G, Kramer A. Do cancer patients with chemotherapy-induced leukopenia benefit from an antiseptic chlorhexidine-based oral rinse? A double-blind, block-randomized, controlled study. J Hosp Infect 2003;53(4):283–291

19. Chan A, Ignoffo RJ. Survey of topical oral solutions for the treatment of chemo-induced oral mucositis. J Oncol Pharm Pract 2005;11(4):139–143

20. Dodd MJ, Dibble SL, Miaskowski C, et al. Randomized clinical trial of the effectiveness of 3 commonly used mouthwashes to treat chemotherapy-induced mucositis. Oral Surg Oral Med Oral Pathol Oral Radiol Endod 2000;90(1):39–47

21. Cascinu S, Fedeli A, Fedeli SL, Catalano G. Oral cooling (cryotherapy), an effective treatment for the prevention of 5-fluorouracil-induced stomatitis. Eur J Cancer B Oral Oncol 1994;30B(4):234–236

22. Gandara DR, Edelman MJ, Crowley JJ, Lau DH, Livingston RB. Phase II trial of edatrexate plus carboplatin in metastatic non-small-cell lung cancer: a Southwest Oncology Group study. Cancer Chemother Pharmacol 1997;41(1):75–78

23. Carnel SB, Blakeslee DB, Oswald SG, Barnes M. Treatment of radiation- and chemotherapy-induced stomatitis. Otolaryngol Head Neck Surg 1990;102(4):326–330

24. Carter DL, Hebert ME, Smink K, Leopold KA, Clough RL, Brizel DM. Double blind randomized trial of sucralfate vs placebo during radical radiotherapy for head and neck cancers. Head Neck 1999;21(8):760–766

25. Epstein JB, Stevenson-Moore P, Jackson S, Mohamed JH, Spinelli JJ. Prevention of oral mucositis in radiation therapy: a controlled study with benzydamine hydrochloride rinse. Int J Radiat Oncol Biol Phys 1989;16(6):1571–1575

26. Pico JL, Avila-Garavito A, Naccache P. Mucositis: its occurence, consequences, and treatment in the oncology setting. Oncologist 1998;3(6):446–451

27. Labar B, Mrsić M, Pavletić Z, et al. Prostaglandin E2 for prophylaxis of oral mucositis following BMT. Bone Marrow Transplant 1993;11(5):379–382

28. Epstein JB, Stevenson-Moore P, Jackson S, Mohamed JH, Spinelli JJ. Prevention of oral mucositis in radiation therapy: a controlled study with benzydamine hydrochloride rinse. Int J Radiat Oncol Biol Phys 1989;16(6):1571–1575

29. Epstein JB, Silverman S Jr, Paggiarino DA, et al. Benzydamine HCl for prophylaxis of radiation-induced oral mucositis: results from a multicenter, randomized, double-blind, placebo-controlled clinical trial. Cancer 2001;92(4):875–885

30. Wong PC, Dodd MJ, Miaskowski C, et al. Mucositis pain induced by radiation therapy: prevalence, severity, and use of self-care behaviors. J Pain Symptom Manage 2006;32(1):27–37

31. Fu KK, Pajak TF, Trotti A, et al. A Radiation Therapy Oncology Group (RTOG) phase III randomized study to compare hyperfractionation and two variants of accelerated fractionation to standard fractionation radiotherapy for head and neck squamous cell carcinomas: first report of RTOG 9003. Int J Radiat Oncol Biol Phys 2000;48(1):7–16

32. Bonner JA, Harari PM, Giralt J, et al. Radiotherapy plus cetuximab for locoregionally advanced head and neck cancer: 5-year survival data from a phase 3 randomised trial, and relation between cetuximab-induced rash and survival. Lancet Oncol 2010;11(1):21–28

33. Perch SJ, Machtay M, Markiewicz DA, Kligerman MM. Decreased acute toxicity by using midline mucosa-sparing blocks during radiation therapy for carcinoma of the oral cavity, oropharynx, and nasopharynx. Radiology 1995;197(3):863–866

34. Intensity Modulated Radiation Therapy Collaborative Working Group. Intensity-modulated radiotherapy: current status and issues of interest. Int J Radiat Oncol Biol Phys 2001;51(4):880–914

35. Sanguineti G, Endres EJ, Gunn BG, Parker B. Is there a "mucosa-sparing" benefit of IMRT for head-and-neck cancer? Int J Radiat Oncol Biol Phys 2006;66(3):931–938

36. Sasse AD, Clark LG, Sasse EC, Clark OA. Amifostine reduces side effects and improves complete response rate during radiotherapy: results of a meta-analysis. Int J Radiat Oncol Biol Phys 2006;64(3):784–791

37. Spielberger R, Stiff P, Bensinger W, et al. Palifermin for oral mucositis after intensive therapy for hematologic cancers. N Engl J Med 2004;351(25):2590–2598

38. Anderson PM, Schroeder G, Skubitz KM. Oral glutamine reduces the duration and severity of stomatitis after cytotoxic cancer chemotherapy. Cancer 1998;83(7):1433–1439

39. Schneider SB, Nishimura RD, Zimmerman RP, et al. Filgrastim (r-metHuG-CSF) and its potential use in the reduction of radiation-induced oropharyngeal mucositis: an interim look at a randomized, double-blind, placebo-controlled trial. Cytokines Cell Mol Ther 1999;5(3):175–180

40. van der Lelie H, Thomas BL, van Oers RH, et al. Effect of locally applied GM-CSF on oral mucositis after stem cell transplantation: a prospective placebo-controlled double-blind study. Ann Hematol 2001;80(3):150–154

29 Surgical Reconstruction

Oleg Militsakh and Jason Jay Miller

Core Messages

- Oncologic surgery is a prominent modality in the treatment of head and neck cancers.

- The majority of the resultant defects will require some type of surgical reconstruction.

- Thus, the reconstructive surgeon becomes a principal figure in safeguarding patients' posttreatment function, cosmesis, and quality of life.

- It is paramount that the reconstructive surgeon is well skilled in various reconstructive methods and chooses carefully an appropriate reconstructive technique.

- This chapter describes a full gamut of reconstructive techniques, including healing by secondary intention, grafting, local and regional flaps, and microvascular tissue transfer.

Excluding laryngeal malignancies, the survival rate for head and neck cancers (HNCs) has been steadily improving since 1975.[1] While enjoying better survival rates, the focus is increasingly being placed on functional aspects and quality of life.[2–4] According to the National Comprehensive Cancer Network guidelines, the surgical extirpation is either a preferred modality or an accepted alternative in the treatment algorithm for all stages of the majority of HNCs.[5] Proper surgical reconstruction is a paramount aspect of rehabilitation of the patient with HNC and ideally should be completed or planned for at the time of the initial oncologic surgery. Furthermore, advanced reconstructive surgery becomes even more significant in either the setting of salvage surgery or the correction of the sequelae of the primary treatment modalities.

The reconstructive surgeon is frequently challenged to restore not just a surface area of the defect but a complex three-dimensional (3D) anatomy to preserve numerous affected physiologic functions. The integrity of an aerodigestive tract is frequently breached during tumor extirpation and requires a repair to prevent a salivary and microbial cross-contamination to deep tissues of the neck and/or the central nervous system. Moreover, in ideal circumstances, the removed tissues must be replaced with similar type of tissues to maintain mastication, deglutition, airway, articulation, oral competence, and other important bodily functions. With most of the human senses concentrated around the head and neck region, hearing, vision, smell, and taste can be unnecessarily affected by a lack of or inadequate reconstruction. In addition, cosmesis must not be overlooked in these patients, as prominent facial features are often affected by head and neck tumors and

their treatment. Functional deficits and cosmetic deformities may negatively affect patients' personality and lifestyle. Consequently, patients with HNCs have a disproportionally high rate of depression and one of the highest rates of suicide as compared with patients with other malignancies.[6,7]

Several defects, such as small defects of oral tongue or small skin defects, can be closed primarily with excellent long-term cosmetic and functional outcome.

Pearl

- One must be careful in evaluating patients with anterior oral cavity defects. Seemingly small defects may result in a significant decrease in tongue volume or tethering of the tongue to the mandible, particularly when the floor of the mouth is involved. Primary closure in these situations is undesirable because of a high potential for future functional dysfunction. The decrease in tongue volume has been shown to affect both swallowing and articulation.[8]

Healing by secondary intention may also be possible and even advisable in some specific situations. It can be used in the setting of previous irradiation, although not as effectively as it is in nonirradiated tissues. Often, secondary healing is suitable as the initial treatment of fistulas. Nonetheless, it should be used only in the areas where contracture is not going to result in disfigurement or functional compromise. More importantly, an exposure of major organs or vessels may preclude the use of this delayed type of therapy altogether. Healing by secondary intention can be further facilitated by providing continuously moist environment.[9] Several commercially available products provide the technology that can wick away an excess of exudate and provide the necessary moist environment as well as antimicrobial properties.[10] Furthermore, the use of hydrocolloid, film, foam, and gel dressings has been shown to be more bacteriostatic and effective than a traditional wet-to-dry dressing.[11]

Negative pressure wound therapy, otherwise known as vacuum-assisted closure, has revolutionized how we manage wounds left to heal by secondary or tertiary intention.

Since its introduction in 1997 by Argenta and Morykwas, the use of the negative pressure therapy has been tested in a variety of head and neck defects.[12] It has been shown to be safe and efficacious. Various foams and dressings can be used in conjunction with a negative pressure device to control exudate evacuation and new granulation tissue formation. It has been used to aid the closure of difficult head and neck wounds either as a primary modality or as a preparation step for future grafting.[13–15] If used appropriately, the negative pressure therapy has been shown to be a useful adjunct in the closure of orocutaneous and pharyngocutaneous fistulas.[15,16]

When surrounding tissues are not sufficient to support primary closure, healing by secondary intention, or nonvascularized grafts fails, a tissue transfer becomes necessary. Commonly, both medical professionals and patients use the term *flap* to describe various types of tissue transfers. This term is derived from a Middle English or Dutch word *flappe*, which originally meant "a partially attached broad flat piece or shingle." Medical terminology redefined it as "a piece of tissue partly severed from its place of origin for use in surgical grafting."[17] Over the last four decades, with the advent of free tissue transfer, this term has become outdated as, unlike other flaps, free flaps are completely detached from its place of origin before transfer. Nonetheless, the definition of the word *flap* still holds water when applied to local and regional transfers. Furthermore, it is one of the most recognized and widely used terms in reconstructive surgery.

Successful reconstruction of posttumor ablative defects of the head and neck region requires thoughtful consideration of many variables. Consideration must first be given to the overall health status of the patient and associated comorbidities. Factors such as metastatic disease, significant systemic disease, or extreme advanced age may influence the choice of reconstruction with possible avoidance of heroic measures or lengthy operations. Other patient factors such as diabetes, smoking, peripheral vascular disease, and radiation must be assessed as they will affect the healing process of the chosen reconstructive maneuver. Once a patient is deemed a candidate for reconstruction, attention is directed toward the thought process of choosing an individualized treatment plan. The basic concepts of restoration of form and function and avoiding donor site deformity must be kept in mind. A thorough and logical approach involves following certain steps to obtain optimal results: (1) accurate defect analysis and definition of specific tissue requirements, (2) understanding the detailed anatomy of the local and distant tissues as they may relate to the reconstruction, and (3) reviewing all surgical options and choosing the intervention that satisfies the tissue requirements with good cosmesis, provides the least morbidity, and allows for a stable and long-lasting result. For the reconstructive surgeon, steps 1 and 2 above are easily followed. Step 3, choosing the right option, comes from advanced training, experience, thoughtfulness, and knowledge of current and previous literature as it relates to the specific reconstruction. A thorough understanding of the reconstructive options is paramount in achieving a successful outcome.

Secondary Intention Healing

This option of reconstruction obviously requires little thought process in its planning and minimal to no intervention by the surgeon. It does require patience by the physician and patient and appropriate follow-up to assure adequate healing. Proper wound care and reassurance are also important aspects of the postoperative course. Fortunately, the excellent vascularity of the head and neck region allows open wounds to heal secondarily in an acceptable time period.

Areas that are good candidates for secondary intention healing include small defects of the nasal tip and also medial canthal region. Minor defects in these areas may actually heal with improved cosmesis as compared with attempts at primary closure, which may actually cause more deformity. The upper forehead is another area that may obtain an improved aesthetic result if allowed to granulate as opposed to attempts at closure of the defect. The paramedian forehead flap donor site is an excellent example of this, where aggressive attempts at closure may result in distortion of the hairline or eyebrows. Defects of 2 to 3 cm or larger oftentimes heal remarkably well.

It must be kept in mind, though as a prerequisite for secondary intention healing to occur, a well-vascularized wound bed must be present. In cases of exposed bone or cartilage, another reconstructive option should be used. Also, wounds that have previously been irradiated will also heal in a much delayed fashion. Other choices should also be considered in this situation.

Primary Closure

Another simple option low on the reconstructive ladder is primary closure. Wounds that can be closed directly without undue tension and that do not distort adjacent structures are best managed by this approach. A meticulous suturing technique that incorporates atraumatic tissue handling, tension-free skin closure, and eversion of skin edges allows for the best cosmetic result.

Delicate handling of tissues is paramount to avoid unnecessary trauma to tissues and allow appropriate healing. Tissue should be grasped gently with forceps and skin hooks used, when applicable, to avoid crushing delicate skin. Sutures should also be placed properly to allow gentle eversion of wound edges to avoid depressed scars.

Incision placement can sometimes be challenging for the beginning surgeon. Ideally, scars should be placed in the lines of minimal tension. This usually allows for the most inconspicuous scar. Other areas that lend to a well-camouflaged scar are incisions placed along the hairline, or along borders of facial subunits, for example, within the nasolabial crease. Before committing to an incision, one must look closely at the surrounding structures to assure that they will not be significantly distorted when the incision is closed.

Skin Grafts

Skin grafts are classified as split-thickness skin graft (STSG) or full-thickness skin graft (FTSG) based on their composition of either epidermis and some portion of dermis or epidermis and entire dermis, respectively. STSG can be classified as very "thin" (approximately 6/1000 in.) to "thick" (more than 20/1000 in.) grafts. Both STSG and FTSG have advantages and disadvantages in terms of their donor and recipient site properties. STSGs have the advantage of ease of harvest and no need to close the donor site. Disadvantages of STSG include the need for specialized equipment, that is, dermatome, and the need for wound care for the donor defect. Other negative aspects include possible prolonged pain for the patient and unsightly scarring. FTSGs have the advantage of improved color and texture match. They can also be harvested from inconspicuous areas such retro- or preauricular skin creases. Disadvantages of FTSGs include the need for the closure of the donor site and possibly slightly less predictable "take."

Defects on the face are often reasonable candidates for FTSG. Areas that are particularly well suited for this are nasal defects and temporal defects. In general, local flaps provide a better option for nasal reconstruction, but in certain circumstances an FTSG is a viable option. An example would be a defect with a well-vascularized wound bed in which multiple previous scars on the nose preclude many typical local flap options. FTSG might also be considered in large defects in the temporal region in which no small local flaps are possible because of the likelihood of distorting the brow or hairline. Again, typically not a first-line option, an FTSG should always be kept in mind as a fairly simple option that provides an acceptable result.

Large defects on the scalp or neck are often amenable to STSG as long as there is a well-vascularized wound bed, that is, no exposed bone, and so forth. Removal of the outer cortex of calvarium and skin grafting onto the diploic cancellous bone can circumvent this situation in select cases.

Tissue Expansion

The process of tissue expansion was introduced in the early 1900s and further refined and popularized in the 1950s.[18] Its main benefit is that it provides an adjacent tissue of similar color and texture to the recipient area. It can also transfer hair-bearing and sensate tissue, if needed, for the reconstruction. Although not typically used in the acute setting for reconstruction of HNC defects, it is quite useful in the management of late post-tumor ablative defects or other nonmalignant settings such as congenital nevi and posttraumatic defects. It should also be noted that the previous radiation somewhat precludes the use of expansion.

The expansion process is performed as a staged procedure. The first stage involves choosing an appropriately sized expander and inserting it into an area adjacent to the defect. There are multiple shapes and sizes of expanders available and the choice depends on the size of the defect, surrounding tissues, and the surgeon's preference. In general, the amount of tissue gained is roughly equal to half of the width of the expander.[19] After insertion, the incision is allowed to heal for 2 to 4 weeks before expansion is started. The patient visits the office on a weekly or biweekly basis for expansion. In the head and neck region, smaller volumes (25 to 50 cm³) are typically injected during each visit. Larger volumes may be injected depending on the site and patient tolerance. The expansion process is typically completed in 2 to 3 months. The second stage involves removal of the expander and rotation of the newly expanded tissue into the defect. In cases of large defects, multiple expanders or multiple expansion procedures may be required.

Unfortunately, tissue expansion has a relatively high complication rate ranging from 25 to nearly 50%.[20,21] The most common complication associated with the expansion process is infection. Other complications include hematoma, seroma, skin breakdown, expander exposure, and expander leakage or deflation. Fortunately, in certain circumstances, some of these complications can still allow for enough tissue expansion to complete the reconstruction. It is best to minimize these possible complications, though with meticulous planning and technique.

Local Flaps

Local flap reconstruction is quite commonly the best option to repair defects that cannot be closed primarily. They provide tissue of similar color, thickness, and texture. Reconstruction of defects of the head and neck with local flaps is oftentimes the most challenging and thought-provoking process for the reconstructive surgeon. Multiple considerations must be kept in mind. First of all, a thorough defect analysis should be performed noting 3D size of the defect. Structural analysis of the defect should also be performed, including the assessment of tissue requirements, that is, skin, cartilage, mucosa, and so on. It should also be noted which subunits of the face are involved and their proximity to anatomic landmarks, which is, eyebrow margin, eyelid margin, lip margin, and so on. One should visualize the placement of tissues into the area in such a way that it minimizes distortion and potential complication. Once a grasp has been obtained on specific details of the wound/recipient bed, one should begin to review different options for local flap reconstruction. This, of course, first requires knowledge of the multiple different local flaps available to the reconstructive surgeon.

There are many ways to classify the various types of local flaps. Flaps may be classified by their composition (e.g., cutaneous, chondrocutaneous, myocutaneous, fasciocutaneous), their blood supply (random or axial pattern), or direction of their movement (e.g., advancement, rotation).

"Random flaps" as the name implies are not vascularized by a named blood vessel. These flaps maintain their blood supply via the subdermal plexus entering the flap from its base. In the face, length-to-width ratios of up to 5:1 may be possible because of the excellent vascularity but clinical judgment should be exercised in design.[22] In certain situations, it may be possible to improve the vascularity of a random flap by performing a "delay" phenomenon.[23] This involves incising the flap margins sometimes with elevation and placing back into the donor bed that allows for opening of "choke" vessels and perhaps vasculogenesis. One to three weeks later, the flap is elevated and transferred to the recipient site. A delay might also be considered intraoperatively if a flap demonstrates signs of vascular compromise after elevation. In contrast to random flaps, "axial pattern flaps" obtain their blood supply via a discrete blood vessel. They are generally more reliable than random flaps and should be considered for specific larger defects, for example, paramedian forehead flap.

Local flaps are also classified based on the direction of their movement. An "advancement flap" is one in which the flap is advanced in a linear fashion. The simplest form of such a transfer is undermining and direct advancement of tissue into a defect. Usually, incisions are made to create a discrete flap, which is then transferred to the recipient area in an advancing fashion. Sometimes, the bipedicled flap can be created by leaving two separate bases to the flap. This provides additional blood supply to the flap but obviously limits its movement. Bipedicled flaps are potentially useful for select eyelid and intraoral defects. Another type of advancement flap that is quite useful is the V-Y advancement flap. This flap is created by making a V incision and releasing the flap from the deeper tissues along the periphery while maintaining the blood supply along the deep surface. The flap is then advanced into the defect and the donor area closed in a straight-line fashion creating a Y. A Y-V advancement can also be performed by making a Y incision and advancing the triangular flap into the Y limb, thereby creating a V. The Y-V flap is used less commonly to close defects but finds its utility in rearranging malpositioned facial structures. Another technique of movement is the "rotation flap." This is a semicircular-shaped flap that rotates along an arc. Pure rotation flaps are relatively uncommon in head and neck reconstruction. A bilobed flap would be an exception as it is a type of rotation flap, although not semicircular in shape. A "transposition flap" is similar to a rotation flap except it typically is more rectangular in shape and does not necessarily rotate along an arc when transposed into

the defect. Numerous types of transposition flaps have been described in the literature, with the more familiar ones being the Z-plasty and rhomboid flaps. Finally, an "interpolation flap" is a flap that is transferred to a nonadjacent defect being brought over some intervening skin or underneath a skin tunnel. The most commonly used interpolation flap is the paramedian forehead flap used in nasal reconstruction.

Once a thorough understanding has been obtained regarding the basic concepts of reconstruction, a more detailed discussion regarding site-specific defects is helpful in understanding the nuances of local flap reconstruction of the head and neck region. Areas to be discussed include the scalp, forehead, ear, eyelids, nose, cheeks, and lips.

Scalp

The scalp is composed of the skin, subcutaneous tissue, galea aponeurotica, loose areolar tissue, and pericranium. The scalp tissue is the thickest and least mobile of tissues in the head and neck area, making small local flaps less useful. Oftentimes, larger and more complex flaps are required to close a defect on the scalp. This sometimes is accompanied by skin grafting of the donor defect given the limited mobility of the calvarial soft tissues.

The blood supply to the scalp is derived mainly from the occipital and superficial temporal arteries. The occipital artery supplies the majority of the posterior scalp. The superficial temporal artery has two branches—frontal and parietal—which branch about 2 cm above the zygomatic arch. The parietal branch supplies the majority of the lateral and superior scalp. Some additional blood supply is provided by the posterior auricular artery laterally and supratrochlear and supraorbital arteries anteriorly.

Sensory innervation to the scalp is obtained by the supratrochlear and supraorbital nerves anteriorly. The lesser occipital nerve supplies the posterior scalp and the auriculotemporal nerve the lateral scalp. No significant motor nerves travel in the scalp tissue proper.

The management of scalp defects begins with a thorough analysis of the defect. Important factors include dimensions of the defect, involvement of periosteum and/or bone, and proximity to the hairline. Small defects less than approximately 2 cm in size can usually be managed by undermining and direct closure or advancement flap. Undermining is typically done in the subgaleal plane as this provides an avascular dissection plane. Scoring of the undersurface of the galea can also provide some mobility of the scalp tissues. Defects larger than 2 cm often require some form of the rotation flap to close.[24] As defects progress in size, additional flaps can be incorporated. Bilateral rotation flaps and the pinwheel (three-flap) techniques are useful for these larger defects. When defects get much larger than 6 cm, large scalp flaps (**Fig. 29.1**) sometimes accompanied by skin grafting of the donor defect is required. The orticochea flap is another three-flap technique, but is reserved for very large defects.[25]

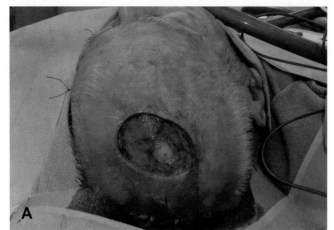

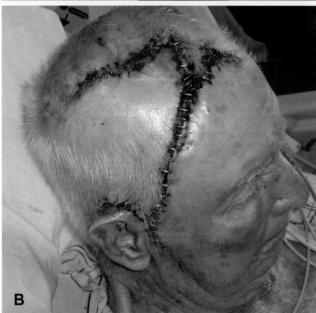

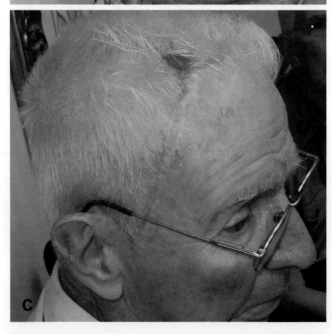

Figure 29.1 Approximately 4 × 6-cm scalp defect closed with multiple large rotation flaps.

Skin grafting scalp defects is less than ideal as it leaves a suboptimal cosmetic result. Unfortunately, this is not avoidable in some situations. In cases of exposed bone with large soft tissue defect, a few options exist. The outer cortex can be removed with a drill, exposing the more vascularized cancellous diploic space. The exposed skull can then be directly grafted onto or an intervening layer of the allogenic or xenogenic material can be placed and secured for a few weeks until it vascularizes.[26] This thicker and possibly more durable tissue can then be skin grafted. Another option involves rotation of a pericranial flap with subsequent skin grafting. Unsightly skin grafted areas can sometimes be removed at a later date, with subsequent tissue expansion and scalp flap rotation.

If defects are present in the calvarium, they can be reconstructed by a variety of means including autologous split calvarial bone grafting, bone grafting from a distant site (e.g., rib), titanium mesh with alloplastic bone paste, or free vascularized bone flap.

Total and near-total scalp defects with exposed bone will require free flap reconstruction usually in the form of a latissimus dorsi free flap (LDFF).[27]

Forehead

Reconstruction of the forehead can be challenging for the reconstructive surgeon. The forehead skin is fairly immobile as is scalp skin, but additional considerations exist. Not only must one consider distortion of the frontal hairline, the brow location must also be kept in mind and maintained as much as possible to avoid significant distortion. Avoidance of motor and sensory nerves is also important.

Blood supply to the forehead is derived from the frontal branch of the superficial temporal artery laterally and the supratrochlear and supraorbital arteries centrally. The robust vascular supply to the area also allows for a variety of random flap options to close multiple defects.

The main sensory nerves of the forehead are the supraorbital and supratrochlear nerves. Motor nerve supply to the frontalis muscle is provided by the frontal branch of the seventh cranial nerve. This nerve travels a path from a point approximately 5 mm below the tragus to within 1.5 cm of the lateral brow. It travels deep to or within the superficial temporal fascia to innervate the muscle on its deep surface. The nerve is at greatest risk of injury in the temporal area as the tissue becomes thinner over and above the zygomatic arch. To prevent injury to the nerve, flaps should be elevated either in the subcutaneous plane or in the subgaleal plane underneath the muscle.

Many flap options for forehead reconstruction exist.[28] Small defects of the central forehead can usually be closed with small tissue advancement, leaving a horizontal or vertical scar. For larger defects, unipedicled or bipedicled flaps can be used. Defects of the upper forehead may be closed by unilateral or bilateral advancement flaps created by incising along the hairline on each side moving the lateral forehead skin toward the midline.

Many flap options exist for lateral brow defects including advancement flaps, rotation flaps, and transposition flaps.

The main consideration in this area is avoidance of the complications of hairline and brow distortion as well as nerve injury. Large defects of the upper lateral forehead may be best reconstructed with a skin graft when flap reconstruction will likely create deformity (**Fig. 29.2**). If portions of the eyebrow have been resected, they can be reconstructed often in a delayed fashion with either hair transplantation or composite grafting.

Ear

The ear is frequently affected by skin cancer and therefore frequently needs reconstructive intervention. Although oftentimes defects are limited to the helical rim, it is important to accurately identify all anatomic elements that are missing. Small defects involving only the skin can sometimes be closed in a simple fashion. More commonly, some amount of cartilage defect also occurs. For defects less than 1 cm in size, a small wedge or star-shaped excision can produce an acceptable result without significant distortion of the helical rim contour.[29] For slightly larger defects (less than 2 cm), chondrocutaneous advancement flaps (Antia-Buch technique) can be used with success (**Fig. 29.3**).[30]

For larger defects, costal cartilage may be required and covered with a retroauricular advancement flap that is divided later. If the defect also includes other anatomic sites of the ear, rib cartilage or an alloplastic framework may be placed and covered with a temporoparietal fascial flap and skin graft.

Defects of the conchal bowl or helical rim are usually closed directly or can be covered with an FTSG if viable perichondrium is present. For larger defects of this area, a trap door flap from the retroauricular crease provides a vascularized flap of similarly colored and textured skin.[31]

Eyelids

Reconstruction of the eyelids must not only restore adequate cosmesis and function but also, most importantly, protect the integrity of the underlying globe. A thorough understanding of the function, anatomy, and physiology of the eyelids and periorbita is a prerequisite to obtain an acceptable result.

The upper eyelid provides approximately 90% of eyelid closure, while the lower eyelid provides the remaining 1 to 2 mm of closure. Although the upper eyelid provides the majority of the function of the eyelids, both are of paramount importance in maintaining adequate protection and lubrication of the globe. Even small malpositions of the lower eyelid can lead to discomfort, epiphora, and eventual exposure keratopathy. From a reconstructive standpoint, the eyelids can be thought of as being composed of lamellae. The anterior lamella of the lids is composed of skin and orbicularis. The middle lamella of the upper lid consists of orbital septum, preaponeurotic fat, and levator complex. The middle lamella of the lower eyelid is composed of orbital septum, orbital fat, and capsulopalpebral fascia. The

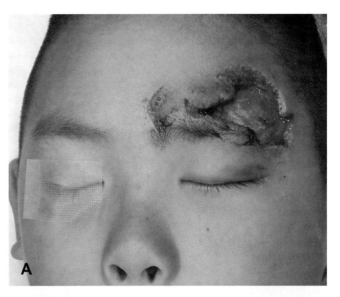

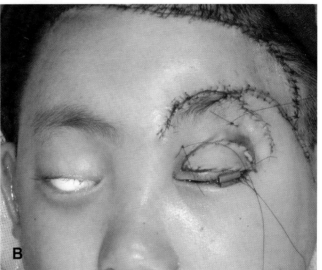

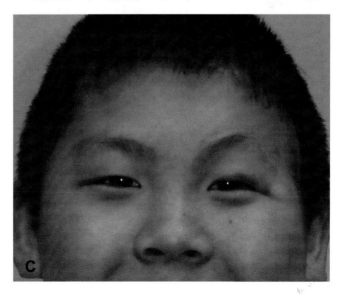

Figure 29.2 Large forehead/brow defect reconstructed with a combination of rotation and advancement flaps and a full-thickness skin graft.

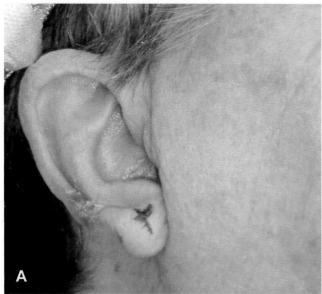

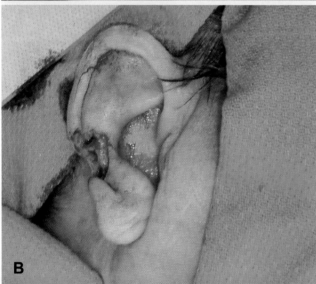

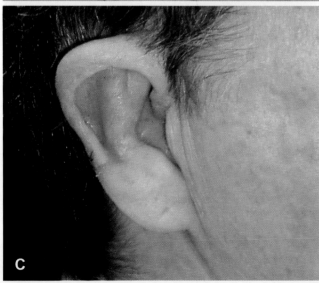

Figure 29.3 Helical rim defect reconstructed with chondrocutaneous advancement flaps.

posterior lamella consists of tarsal plate, Müller muscle, and conjunctiva. The tarsal plate height is approximately 10 mm in the upper lid and 5 mm in the lower lid.

Surgical defects of the anterior lamella are ideally reconstructed with soft tissues from the surrounding area. In older individuals, skin laxity may allow the surgeon to close fairly large defects. Younger patients with less skin laxity may require an FTSG to address large defects of the anterior lamella. The upper eyelid, retroauricular sulcus, and supraclavicular fossa are acceptable donor sites. Unipedicled or bipedicled myocutaneous flaps from the upper eyelid may also be used to reconstruct skin defects of the lower eyelid (**Fig. 29.4**).

Full-thickness defects of the eyelids can be closed primarily if their size is less then 25% of total lid length. Layered closure involves reapproximating anatomic landmarks of the lash line and gray line. The tarsal plate and orbicularis, if needed, can be repaired with resorbable suture. The skin edges can then be closed with a fine permanent suture. Fine fast-absorbing sutures can be used to close the anatomic structures at the lid margin. If the closure is tight, it may be necessary to perform a lateral canthotomy. For larger defects, up to two-thirds of the upper or lower eyelid local tissue must be incorporated to obtain closure. The semicircular flap of Tenzel is useful for defects of either the upper or the lower eyelid.[32] In some cases, it may be helpful to provide reconstruction of the posterior lamella with a cartilage graft or periosteal flap. Defects greater than two-thirds may require a lid sharing type of procedure. The Cutler-Beard flap is useful for reconstruction of the upper eyelid.[33] This is a staged reconstruction that involves the creation of a full-thickness flap of lower eyelid tissue starting just below the tarsal plate to maintain integrity and vascularity to the lower eyelid. The skin-muscle-conjunctival flap is then advanced into the upper eyelid defect and allowed to "take" place for 6 to 8 weeks before division. The Hughes tarsoconjunctival flap is an analogous flap from the upper eyelid used to reconstruct the lower eyelid.[34] This flap leaves 3 to 4 mm of the upper tarsus intact to maintain upper eyelid integrity. The flap is elevated from the inner aspect of the eyelid and involves tarsus and conjunctiva as the name implies. The dissection plane is between the conjunctiva and Müller muscle to avoid the dysfunction of upper eyelid excursion. The flap is mobilized as needed and then advanced inferiorly into the lower eyelid defect. The anterior lamella is then reconstructed with either a skin graft or a local skin flap. Division then takes place 4 to 6 weeks later.

Nose

Somewhat analogous to the eyelids, the nose can be thought of in a layered fashion. The three layers of the nose that are important from a reconstructive standpoint are external covering, supporting structures, and internal lining. Reconstruction of part or all of the necessary layers should result in restoration of function in terms of a patent

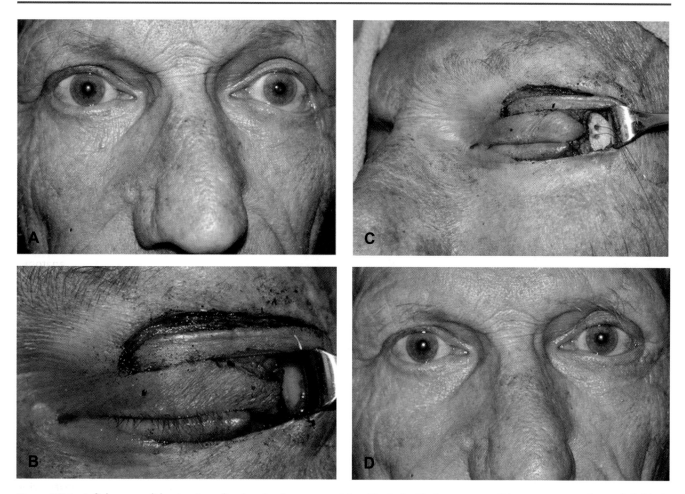

Figure 29.4 Left lower eyelid ectropion after basal cell cancer excision. Treated with the upper eyelid myocutaneous flap and drill-hole canthopexy. (A) Left lower eyelid cicatricial ectropion. (B) Myocutaneous flap elevated and lateral orbital rim exposed. (C) Drill hole canthopexy performed and canthal sutures passed. (D) 12-month postoperative view.

airway as well as a normal appearing nose. Not only is it important to evaluate the nasal defect within the context of the facial subunits, the nose itself is also divided into nine subunits. The regional subunits of the nose are the dorsum, tip, columella, and the paired sidewalls, ala, and soft triangles. The "subunit principle" proposed by Burget and Menick states that if greater than 50% of a subunit is involved in a defect, consideration should be given to discarding the remaining defect and including it in the reconstruction.[35] This also allows for scars to be positioned along the normal contour changes of the nose, thereby improving cosmesis.

Small defects less than 5 mm in size can often be closed by direct closure after undermining of adjacent tissues. Some minor deformity of the nose may result, but this often improves with time as the soft tissues undergo relaxation. An exception to this would be defects near the alar margin where even small defects, if closed, can primarily cause distortion and notching. In these cases, small local flaps, FTSGs, or composite grafts from the ear may give a better result. The nasolabial flap, which is a random flap harvested from the nasolabial fold skin, is also useful for larger alar

defects. It can be used in conjunction with cartilage graft placement, if needed, but has the disadvantage of being a staged flap that typically requires division and contouring to recreate the alarfacial groove. Defects of the alar rim up to 1.5 cm that involve skin and cartilage are also amenable to the composite graft that provides skin and structural support. For defects with intact cartilage and up to 1.5 cm, bilobed flaps are also useful on the nasal and alar areas.[36] These may also be used on the dorsum and sidewalls. A variety of rotation and transposition flaps work well in this area, also given the fact that some increased tension on the closure will not cause distortion of the ala or tip. The dorsal nasal (glabellar) flap is another useful flap for reconstruction of skin defects of the midnasal and central tip defects of up to 2.5 cm. This flap takes advantage of skin laxity in the dorsum and glabellar regions by elevating a large flap and closing the glabellar donor area primarily (**Fig. 29.5**).

For larger nasal defects or full-thickness nasal defects, the paramedian forehead flap is extremely useful (**Fig. 29.6**). In cases of full-thickness defects, nasal lining and structural support must also be added. Internal

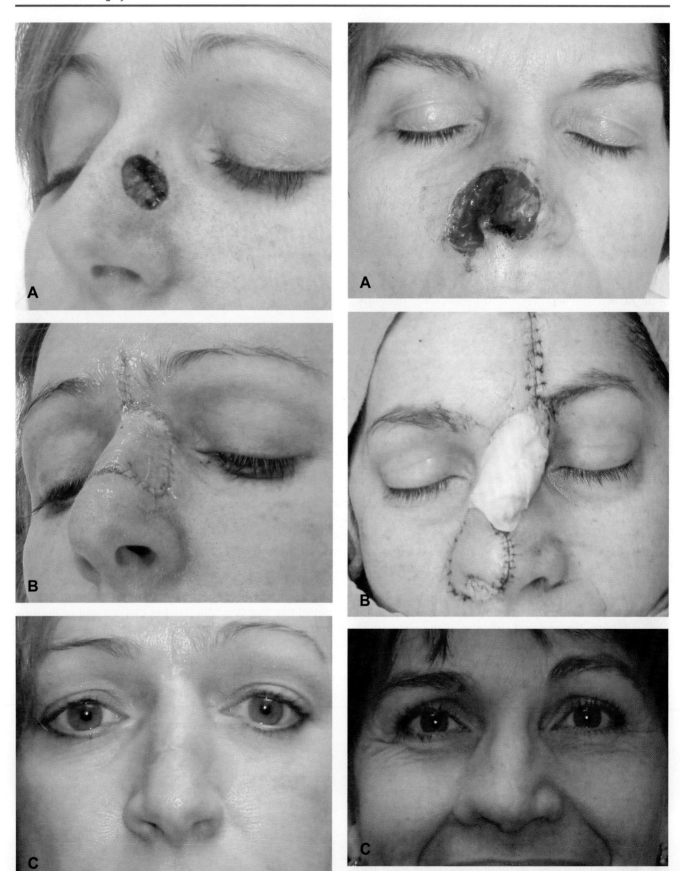

Figure 29.5   Lateral midnasal defect of 1.8 cm repaired with a dorsal nasal flap.

Figure 29.6   Right nasal and cheek defect reconstructed with the paramedian forehead flap, conchal cartilage, and cheek advancement flap.

lining ideally comes from adjacent nasal mucosa. For small lining defects near the nasal tip, bipedicled vestibular advancement flaps are simple and useful. For larger defects, either ipsilateral or contralateral septal mucoperichondrial hinge flaps provide the necessary tissue.[37] In the event that the septum has been partially or totally removed, lining can be provided by a radial forearm free flap (RFFF) or a paramedian forehead turnover flap. Structural support usually comes from harvested septal cartilage or conchal cartilage. If more significant dorsal support is needed, a cantilevered cranial bone graft or rib graft can restore support.

Once the lining and support are restored, a template of the skin defect is usually made through a variety of means. The template is then transferred to the forehead skin and the flap outlined. One must be sure that there is an adequate arc of rotation and the flap will reach the most inferior aspect of the defect. The flap itself is an axial pattern flap based on the supratrochlear vessels. Its base can therefore be fairly narrow (approximately 1.5 cm) that allows for primary closure of the inferior aspect of the donor site. The superior aspect can also be closed primarily in some cases, but wider flap defects are usually left to heal secondarily. After the flap is closed into the defect, it is allowed to heal for 2 to 3 weeks and then divided in a second-stage operation. Oftentimes, cosmesis of the flap can be optimized by subsequent debulking and contouring, which can be performed in the office under local anesthesia. Dermabrasion can also be helpful and is easily done under local anesthesia as well.

Cheeks

The cheeks are composed of the skin, subcutaneous fat, muscles of facial expression, and oral mucosa. Many defects of the cheek can be closed primarily given the significant laxity of the soft tissues in this area. When possible, it is ideal to hide incision lines in the facial subunit borders, that is, nasolabial fold, preauricular skin crease, or lid cheek junction. Multiple rotation, advancement, and transposition flaps have been described and work fairly well in this area for closure of larger defects. Attention must always be given to avoidance of distortion of structures such as the lower eyelid and lips. It is also important to avoid damage to the underlying facial nerve during flap elevation. These flaps are raised in the subcutaneous plane to assure safe flap elevation. Larger defects that cannot be closed by smaller local flaps may be amenable to closure with flaps that incorporate skin from the lax skin of the neck. For defects located more inferiorly on the cheek, simple rotation or transposition flaps from the neck may be used (**Fig. 29.7**).

For large defects of the superior cheek, loose neck skin can be used in the form of a cervicofacial flap. This flap is very useful for large cheek defects and hides donor incisions in the pre- and retroauricular skin creases (**Fig. 29.8**). The cervicofacial flap can also reach defects in the temporal area (**Fig. 29.9**).

Larger defects or full thickness of the cheek and midface region are typically candidates for reconstruction with free tissue transfer.

Lips

Knowledge of the topographic landmarks and the underlying anatomy of the lips are essential in achieving an ideal result in upper and lower lip reconstruction. The upper lip is divided into two lateral and one central elements by the paired philtral columns. The philtral columns end inferiorly

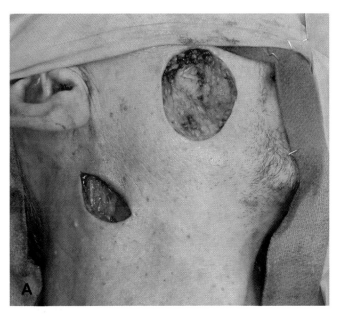 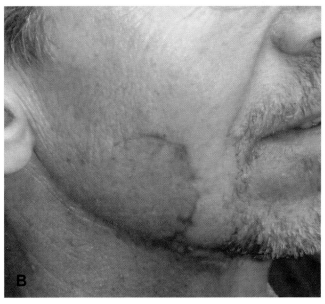

Figure 29.7 Transposition flap used to reconstruct a 4-cm inferior cheek defect. Inferior neck incision for sentinel lymph node biopsy was incorporated into the flap design.

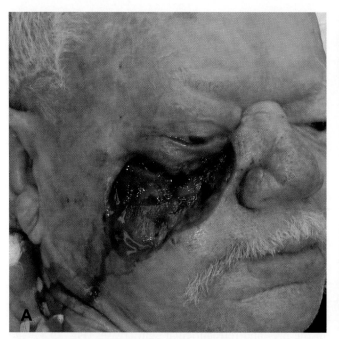
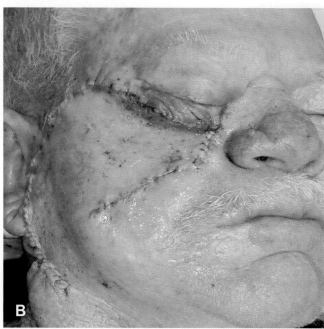

Figure 29.8   Cheek defect of 4 × 6 cm reconstructed with a cervicofacial flap.

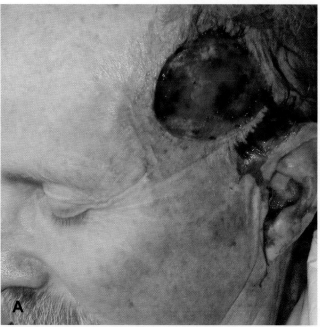
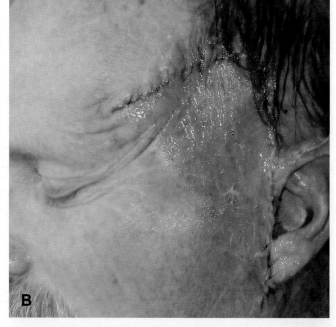

Figure 29.9   Cervicofacial flap used for the 4 × 4-cm temporal defect.

at the high points of the Cupid's bow. The Cupid's bow makes the central aspect of the upper lip white roll, which is the junction of the lip vermilion and skin. The wet-dry line marks the transition of wet and dry mucosa of the lip. Underlying the skin is the orbicularis oris muscle that allows for mouth closure and oral competence. The orbicularis oris muscle is tightly adherent to the overlying skin because of the paucity of subcutaneous fat in the lips. The inner aspect of the lips is composed of oral mucosa. Arterial supply to the lips comes

from the superior and inferior labial arteries via the facial artery.

Defects of the vermilion of the lips can often be reconstructed with local vermilion flaps. This can be accomplished in the form of lateral advancement flaps in cases of small lateral defects or bilateral advancement flaps in the case of central defects (**Fig. 29.10**).

When near or complete defects in the vermilion exist, a mucosal advancement flap (lip shave procedure) can be

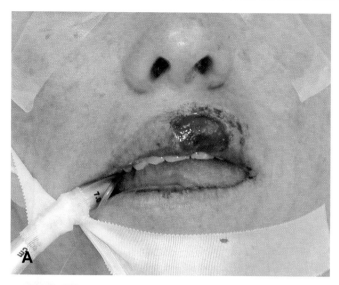

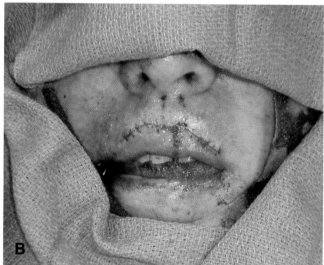

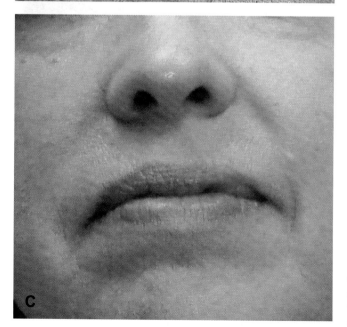

Figure 29.10 Central upper lip defect reconstructed with mucosal advancement flaps.

performed with acceptable cosmetic outcome. In cases where some skin involvement is also present, it is better to convert the defect into a full-thickness defect and reconstruct in a layered fashion (**Fig. 29.11**).

Defects of up to one-third are typically amenable to primary closure. Larger defects that comprise between one-thirds and two-thirds typically require local flap reconstruction. In these situations, cross-lip flaps can be used with success. The Abbe flap can be transferred on a small myomucosal pedicle that includes the labial artery.[38] The flap is inset into the opposite lip defect and then divided approximately 10 to 14 days later. For defects involving the oral commissure, a variation of this flap, the Abbe-Estlander flap is the reconstructive option of choice (**Fig. 29.12**).

For defects greater than two-thirds of the lower lip, the Karapandzic flap provides a pedicled composite flap that can restore oral competence (**Fig. 29.13**). The Gilles fan flap is a similar flap in design but includes a back cut on the back edge of the flap to enhance rotation.[39] The main disadvantage of these flaps is the potential for causing microstomia. A commissuroplasty may be needed after healing has occurred to enhance mouth opening.

Historically, total lower lip defects were repaired with a variety of local and regional flaps with mixed results. However, microsurgical tissue transfer has become the preferred technique to reconstruct total lower lip defects (**Fig. 29.14**).

Regional and Pedicled Flaps

In contrast to local flaps, regional flaps provide an increased tissue quality, larger size, and greater arc of rotation or flexibility of transfer. Most common regional and/or pedicled flaps used for head and neck reconstruction include pectoralis major muscle (PMM) or musculocutaneous flap, temporalis muscle flap, deltopectoral flap (DPF), and paramedian forehead flap. Temporoparietal, trapezius, latissimus, sternocleidomastoid, platysma, submental flaps, and several other regional flaps have been described and successfully used for reconstruction of head and neck defects. For the brevity of the discussion, we will concentrate our efforts on the description of the previously mentioned and more commonly used regional transfers.

Deltopectoral Flap

DPF was first described by Bakamjian in 1965 as a new way to reconstruct a pharyngoesophageal defect.[40] Originally known as a Bakamjian flap, this flap revolutionized the approach to head and neck reconstruction and jolted an investigation of various other donor sites. Over the following decades, the number of flaps used for head and neck reconstruction multiplied exponentially. While very important from a historical standpoint, the use of a DPF is rarely indicated in the current practice.

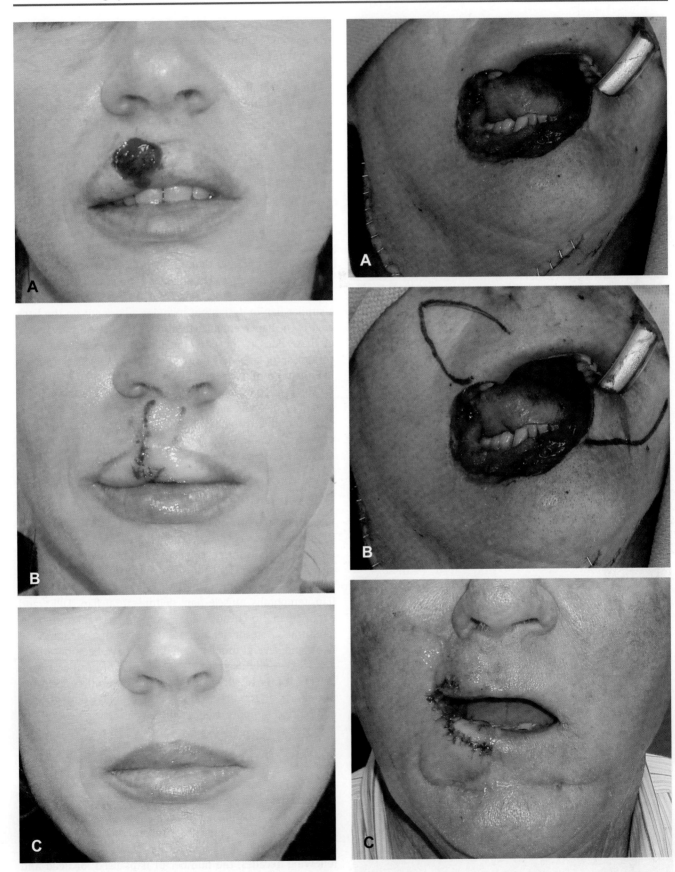

Figure 29.11 Upper lip defect of 1 cm involving the skin reconstructed with wedge excision and layered closure. Z-plasty performed along the vermilion to camouflage the scar.

Figure 29.12 Large lower lip involving right oral commissure reconstructed with the Abbe-Estlander flap and the lower lip advancement flap.

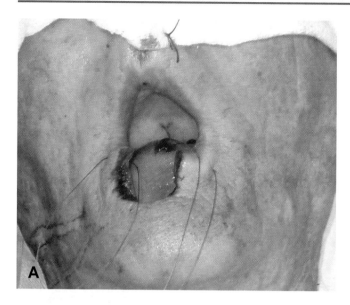

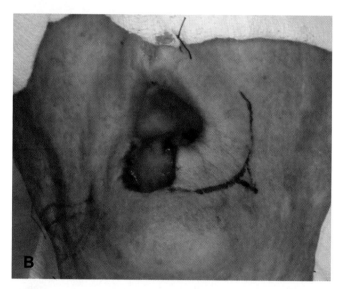

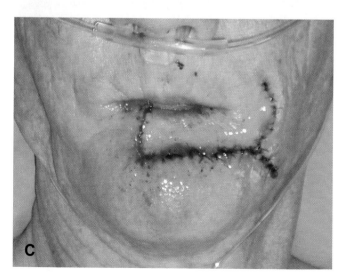

Figure 29.13   Reconstruction of lower lip defect with the Karapandzic flap.

Based on the second and third intercostal branches of the internal mammary artery, this flap is simple to harvest. Normally, the distal extent of the nonrandom vascular supply of the flap terminates at the anterior axillary line. However, formerly described "delay phenomenon" technique will allow for a significantly greater length if desired. The advantages of the DPF include the ease of harvest and an ability to close a secondary defect primarily. One of the few continuing indications of the DPF in the present-day practice is the use in the view of salvage surgery with history of multiple previous surgical interventions. This donor site for DPF is usually spared from radiotherapy or scarring from other head and neck extirpative and/or reconstructive procedures and can be used to reconstruct recalcitrant pharyngocutaneous fistulas or for neck vessel coverage (**Fig. 29.15**).

Pectoralis Major Flap

For over a decade, DPF was the best option available for pharyngoesophageal reconstruction. However, in 1979 another fundamental milestone in head and neck reconstruction was reached when Ariyan described and popularized the pectoralis major myocutaneous flap.[41] The pectoralis flap provided a better flexibility, less complication at the recipient site, and at the same time a one-stage reconstructive procedure.

The anatomy of the pedicle is consistent and reliable. The harvest allows for a large area/volume transfer with a narrow base. Subsequently, a 180° transposition is possible and often used. The flap can be harvested only as a muscle or as a musculocutaneous transfer. The variety of indications includes pharyngoesophageal reconstruction, reconstruction of oral cavity, oropharynx, skull base, and a range of external head and neck defects.

The harvest of the flap is straightforward and starts by outlining the skin paddle (if one is desired) at the inferior aspect of the PMM. An area of 60% or more of the skin paddle should overlie the PMM, while the rest can be positioned distally over the rectus fascia, which in that case is harvested altogether with the flap. A curvilinear incision is placed in the inframammary crease in women. The same type of incision can be used in men. Alternatively, incision can be extended from the skin paddle in the curvilinear fashion toward axilla, parallel and four fingerbreadths below the clavicle.

Pearl

- The incision described by Ariyan in his original description is not generally recommended, as it transects and eliminates the future potential use of deltopectoral flap. For the same reasons, second and third intercostal perforators and underlying fascia are preserved during subcutaneous tunnel elevation superiorly.

A lateral incision is placed before committing to circumferential skin paddle incision. This technique allows

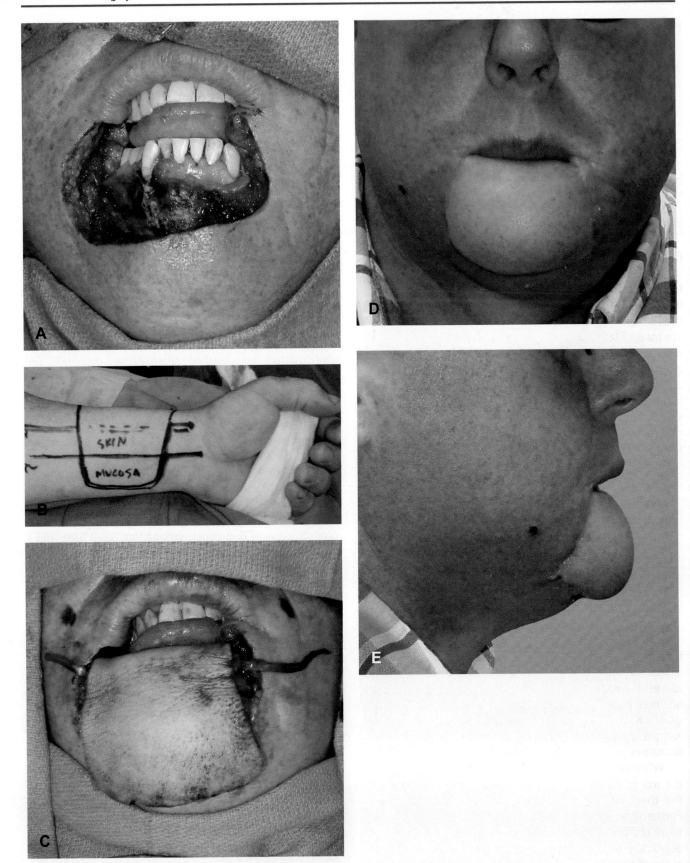

Figure 29.14 (A) Near-total lower lip defect. (B) Radial forearm outlined on donor arm. (C) Flap at inset, (D, E) 12-month postoperative result.

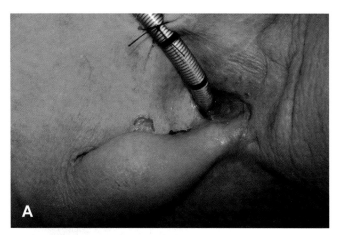

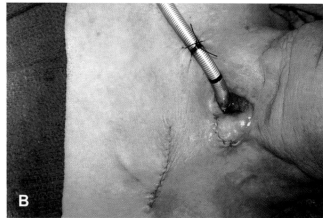

Figure 29.15 Deltopectoral flap fistula repair.

for skin paddle adjustment if PMM happened to terminate in an unusually superior position. Once the lateral border of the PMM is identified, the rest of the skin paddle incisions are made. Many surgeons prefer tacking a skin paddle to a muscle belly with temporary sutures to prevent sheering. Inferiorly, rectus fascia is incised at the level of the inferior extend of the skin paddle and the entire flap is elevated in the plain deep to the PMM. Superior elevation proceeds in the subfascial plane to preserve a potential future DPF. Intercostal perforators should be ligated or cauterized and divided. Once the pectoral vascular pedicle is identified on the deep surface of the PMM, the nerve to the muscle is divided.

> **Pearl**
>
> - Division of the motor nerve to the pectoralis major muscle will allow for muscle atrophy in the future and subsequently will decrease a mass effect on the clavicle. Even more importantly, it will prevent flap jerking with shoulder movement.

Following this, medial sternocostal and lateral humeral muscle attachments can be divided using cautery, harmonic sheers, or other hemostatically dividing device. Once the harvest is complete, the flap can be transposed into the head and neck region for the inset. The donor chest skin defect can usually be closed without difficulty by adjacent tissue transfer. A drain is placed into the donor wound to prevent a seroma formation.

While many head and neck surgeons still rely heavily on the use of this flap, with advancements in microvascular-free tissue transfer, its use and indications have diminished. Furthermore, because free flap reconstructions have become more reliable and facile, a bigger emphasis is placed on the donor site morbidity. For example, Moukarbel et al found a significant effect on the shoulder range of motion as compared with dissected necks without pectoralis major.[42] Moreover, shoulder strength and neck range of motion are also negatively affected by PMM flap harvest.[42]

Temporalis Muscle Flap

Since 1970, temporalis muscle flap has been used for both reconstruction of maxillofacial defects and dynamic rehabilitation of facial nerve paralysis.[43,44] One of the few facial muscles not innervated by a facial nerve, over the years it has offered a valuable option for rehabilitation of facial paralysis in the cases where reinnervation of the facial nerve is not feasible. Furthermore, this dynamic correction can be achieved by using a temporalis tendon without the need for the entire muscle transfer.[45,46] Hemicoronal incision with preauricular extension is placed for the conventional harvest. Minimally invasive approach for a tendon transfer has also been described.[46] Once the temporalis muscle is exposed, the distal aspect of the muscle is elevated from the skull. Care is taken to preserve a vascular supply to the flap that arrives via deep temporal vessels of the internal maxillary artery. Zygomatic arch may need to be removed and subsequently replaced to achieve an adequate reach. Reconstruction of orbitomaxillary defects is easily accomplished with such a transfer.[40] Furthermore, maxillectomy defects can be successfully reconstructed with this technique (**Fig. 29.16**). The donor defect produces temporal hollowing and can be reconstructed with acellular allograft or cranioplastic material in the same stage.

Paramedian Forehead Flap

Arguably, the first description of this flap dates back to 970 BC. Regardless of whether this fact is true, it is clear that the surgical experience in India with this flap predates modern medicine.[47] Forehead flaps were introduced to Western World in the 18th century. Older descriptions of the forehead flaps mostly described a midline forehead flap. More recent advancements in the knowledge of vascular anatomy has allowed for the harvest of a flap based on supratrochlear vasculature.[47] Using newer techniques, the base of the pedicle can be narrowed to as small as 1 cm and extended to below the level of the brow. As a result, the arc of rotation is improved along with decreased tension exerted to the

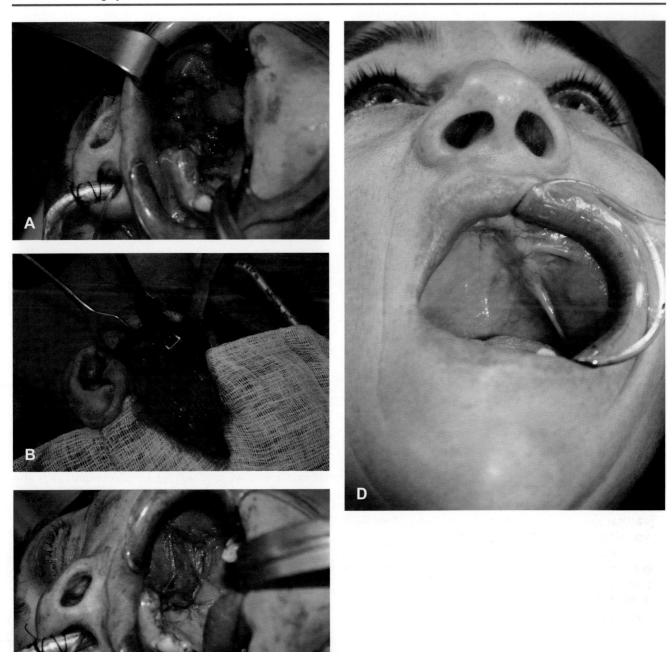

Figure 29.16 Temporalis flap and maxillectomy repair. (A) maxillectomy defect, (B) temporalis flap, (C) flap inset, and (D) appearance at 6-month follow-up.

pedicle and ultimately enhancement of the distal reach. Furthermore, the narrower base facilitates primary closure of the forehead defect.

Cadaveric dissections confirmed that the supratrochlear artery consistently exits the orbit 1.7 to 2.2 cm lateral to the midline.[47] This point frequently corresponds to the medial part of the brow. The same cadaveric study found that the nutrient vessel is also consistently pierced through orbital septum, exiting the orbit and coursed in

between corrugator and orbicularis muscles. It then passes deep to the frontalis muscle but transverses superficially into subcutaneous tissues as it ascends superiorly. This anatomic knowledge can be applied clinically, as the distal portion of the flap can be harvested devoid of the frontalis muscle, resulting in a decrease of the bulk of the flap.

While several adaptations of the forehead flaps exist, the paramedian forehead flap that is based on the supratrochlear pedicle has been a reliable and valuable technique for reconstruction of various nasal and orbital defects.

Free Tissue Transfer

Although the term *free flap* is disliked by some practitioners, it is the most frequently used synonym for a microvascular tissue transfer. Microvascular tissue transfer is defined as an autograft that is transferred from the donor site to another location in the body and is revascularized by using microsurgical techniques. The major advantage of such a transfer is a plethora of the donor sites. Unlike locoregional flaps, free flaps allow for unparalleled freedom of selection of the type and size of tissues transferred. Consequently, bony defects can be reconstructed with vascularized bone grafts, while composite defects that encompass soft tissue and bony defects can have a transfer such as osteocutaneous or musculocutaneous flaps. The wide selection of the donor sites also allows for improved reconstruction of large surface area versus large volume soft tissue defects as well.

In contrast to nonvascular grafts, free flaps are more resilient to the radiation effects. They can withstand salivary and polymicrobial exposure of the aerodigestive tract and also offer an excellent option for reconstruction in the setting of previously irradiated recipient bed.

While there are innumerous flap donor sites that have been described, only a few are used most commonly for head and neck reconstruction.

Some prefer to categorize microvascular flaps by donor body regions (trunk, lower, upper extremity, etc.). However, because of a focused nature of this chapter and also for the practical reasons, we stratify and describe free flaps by the type of transferred tissue (**Table 29.1**).

Numerous other free flap donor sites, such as ulnar forearm, dorsalis pedis, temporoparietal, and free pectoralis, have been described and used effectively for reconstruction of head and heck defects.[48-50] Nonetheless, this chapter covers the descriptions of most frequently used flaps.

Group I: Skin Free Flaps

The first group of flaps includes cutaneous, fascial, and fasciocutaneous flaps. Used for both external and internal lining defects, these are the most commonly performed microsurgical procedures.

Radial Forearm Free Flap

RFFF was described in 1981, although the first report in English literature did not appear until 1982. Since then, it has become a workhorse flap in head and neck reconstruction.[51]

The flap can be harvested as a fasciocutaneous or osteocutaneous transfer. Numerous advantages of the flap include a reliable anatomy, long pedicle with large caliber vessels, ability for reinnervation, and thin, pliable skin paddle.

Preoperative clinical assessment or vascular testing must be performed to assure an adequate hand perfusion after the flap harvest. A modified Allen test is usually performed as part of the clinical assessment. It involves a compression of both radial and ulnar arteries, while the patient clenches his or her fist. Thereafter, the patient relaxes the hand and the ulnar artery is decompressed. The test is considered to be positive if the capillary refill returns within 5 to 15 seconds.

> **Pearl**
>
> - A modified Allen test is positive if palmar arch is complete and there is an adequate collateral hand circulation via the ulnar artery, making the donor extremity suitable for harvest.

The Allen test may suffice for the patients with obvious brisk capillary refill, as we have found a 100% correlation between clinical assessment and digital waveforms in such cases. However, in the cases when clinical examination is

Table 29.1 Classification of Microvascular Flaps by the Type of Transferred Tissue

Group I: Fascial, Cutaneous, Fasciocutaneous	Group II: Muscle, Musculocutaneous	Group III: Bone, Osteocutaneous	Group IV: Internal
RFFF	LDFF	OCFFF	Jejunum
ALTFF	Rectus	OCRFFF[a]	Omentum-x
SFF	Vastus (ALTFF)	OCSFF[a]	Colon-x
Lateral arm-x	Gracilis	OCICFF	Ileocolic-x
DIEP[b]			
Groin-x			

[a]Description included in the fasciocutaneous flap counterpart.
[b]Description included in the musculocutaneous flap counterpart.
RFFF, radial forearm free flap; LDFF, latissimus dorsi free flap; OCFFF, osteocutaneous forearm free flap; ALTFF, anterolateral thigh free flap; OCRFFF, osteocutaneous radial forearm free flap; -x, less frequently used and not described in detail in this chapter; SFF, scapular free flap; OCSFF, osteocutaneous scapular free flap; OCICFF, osteocutaneous iliac crest free flap; DIEP, deep inferior epigastric artery perforator flap.

equivocal, vascular testing proves to be of a great benefit. Most commonly, the vascular testing is performed by recording digital waveforms, paying particular attention to the first and fifth digits (**Fig. 29.17**). Alternatively, digital pulse volume recording/segmental pressures studies can be performed.

The harvest of RFFF is commonly simplified by performing the procedure under the tourniquet. If the tourniquet is used, it is placed over the brachial region of the upper extremity. Commonly, the inflation pressure varies between 150 and 250 mm Hg. It is unnecessary to use the pressures more than 50 to 75 mm Hg above the patient's systolic blood pressure.[52] The skin paddle can be centered over the radial artery. However, if vascularized radius is harvested concomitantly, the ulnar biased positioning of the skin paddle is advised. In addition, in many male and some female patients, the skin paddle with ulnar bias will provide a lesser amount of hair-bearing skin.

The dissection can be started from either the ulnar or radial sites. The initial description and many current descriptions of the RFFF harvest advise for subfascial dissection, harvesting the deep fascia with the flap. Conversely, recent studies have shown that subfascial vascular plexus does not contribute significantly to the perfusion of RFFF.[53] Thus, suprafascial dissection is safe, easy, and provides great wound bed for a skin graft. If the ulnar site is approached initially, then the dissection proceeds in the suprafascial plane until the flexor carpi radialis tendon is encountered. Thereafter, the dissection is transcended into the subfascial plane, and the radial pedicle is identified. Normally, the pedicle consists of a radial artery and two venae comitantes. Once identified distally, the vessels can easily be followed into the antecubital fossa. The superficial venous system is frequently harvested with the flap as well and can provide either additional or sole venous outflow drainage from the flap. The superficial venous anatomy, however, is variable. Most commonly, a cephalic or median antecubital vein will have dominant venous contributories from the flap. The radial side dissection is more tedious as the branches of the superficial radial nerve must be preserved during the skin flap elevation. Furthermore, if vascularized radius is being brought up with the flap, care must be taken to preserve fine osteocutaneous perforators that lie in close relation to the brachioradialis tendon.[54] During the fasciocutaneous flap harvest, however, these perforators are divided. The distal pedicle is ligated, and after release of the tourniquet the flap harvest is complete.

If an osteocutaneous flap is desired, once the brachioradialis tendon and superficial radial nerve are retracted laterally, the flexor digitorum superficialis attachments to the radius are released. Flexor pollicis longus along with radial periosteum is incised longitudinally for the required length of the bone graft. Typically, a bone length of 5 to 8 cm can be harvested. If a longer bone graft is required, the pronator teres tendon can be released to achieve lengths up to 10 to 12 cm. In that case, the released tendon needs to be reattached after the flap harvest is complete. The

longitudinal osteotomy is then placed through the radius harvesting 40 to 50% of the total radius circumference for the length required. The bone harvest is completed by placing keel-shaped proximal and distal osteotomies (**Fig. 29.18**).[55]

Initially, the osteocutaneous radial forearm flap did not gain a widespread popularity, as several reviews reported a 15 to 30% rate of donor radius fracture.[56,57] While some abandoned the use of this flap, others used a technique of prophylactic radius plating during the initial harvest. Using this technique, the risk of postoperative radius fracture has been nearly completely eliminated.[54,58] Locking and nonlocking fixation plates have been successfully used.[59,60] Usually, the plate is placed dorsolaterally with two screws distally and three screws proximally to the bone defect (**Fig. 29.19**). Placing additional screws through the osteotomized portion of the radius will weaken the donor bone, which is detrimental to the desired effect.[61]

After the flap is transferred out to the recipient site, a resultant soft tissue defect is reconstructed by either adjacent tissue transfer or coverage with STSG (**Fig. 29.20**). The skin graft can be bolstered with a nonadhesive gauze or with a negative pressure device. Negative pressure devices are helpful not only in preventing sheering but also in evacuating excess fluids at the donor site and providing additional stabilization of surrounding tissues. Coverage with acellular dermis or healing by secondary intention will prolong the healing of the donor site.[62] While temporary splinting of the donor forearm is used by some, it is not absolutely necessary.

Anterolateral Thigh Free Flap

Anterolateral thigh free flap (ALTFF) was first described in 1984 by Song et al.[63] It has been proclaimed by some as an "ideal flap" for reconstruction of soft tissue defects.[64] Indeed, ALTFF is quite versatile. The size of the skin paddle can be as large as 250 cm². The thickness of the flap can be controlled by either thinning the skin paddle down to subdermal fat (but yet preserving the subdermal vascular plexus) or increasing transferred tissue volume by designing it as a musculocutaneous flap and harvesting vastus lateralis muscle. Furthermore, multiple skin perforators allow for separate independent skin paddles (**Fig. 29.21**). A chimeric flap can be easily designed if vascularized tendon tissue of the fascia lata is required.

Many mention a variable vascular anatomy as a disadvantage. Conversely, while the course of the skin perforators is not consistent, a sizable skin perforator can be located in more than 95% of the cases.[64] Occasionally, the skin paddle may have to be adjusted once the dominant perforator is located. Furthermore, the perforator should be dissected until its entrance onto the pedicle as the course of it is variable and the oblique branch of the lateral femoral circumflex vessels may have to be used instead of the traditionally described descending branch. Several publications have described the variations of vascular anatomy of the anterolateral thigh. However, commonly, there is a sizable perforator within a 5-cm circle that is

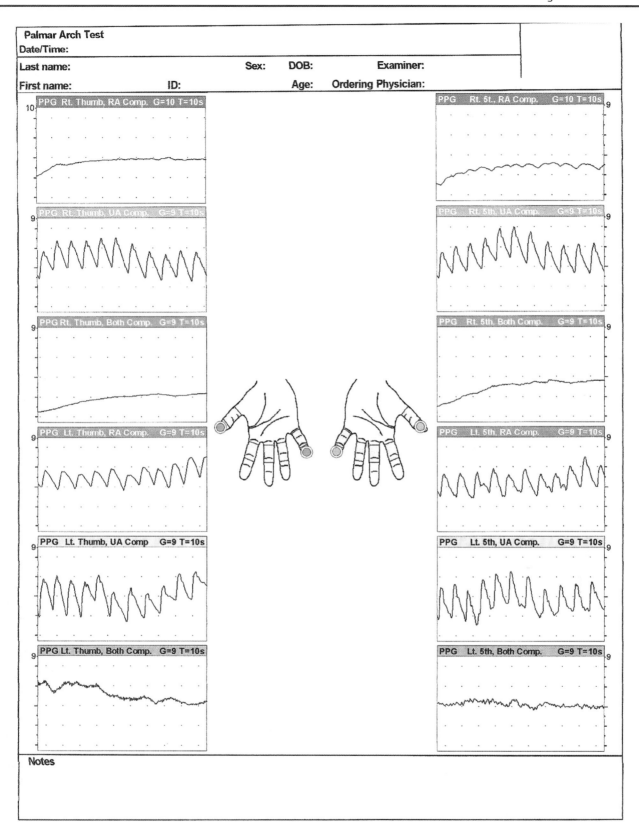

Figure 29.17 An example of vascular studies. Simultaneous compression of the radial artery (RA) and ulnar artery (UA) performed to confirm test reliability. In this example, alternate RA and UA compression reveal RA dominant right arm with incomplete palmar arch. The left arm study confirms a complete palmar arch. On the basis of this study, the left radial forearm flap can be harvested without a significant vascular compromise to the hand. Conversely, while the right forearm donor site could be used for ulnar free flap harvest, it is not acceptable as a donor site for a radial forearm free flap.

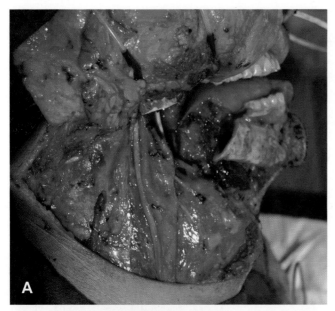

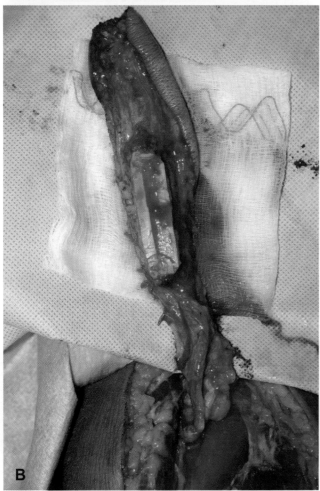

Figure 29.18 Small segmental mandibular defect with a three-dimensional soft tissue defect (base of tongue, floor of mouth, pharynx) can be effectively reconstructed with the osteocutaneous radial forearm free flap. Soft pliable skin that is not tethered to the bone graft will allow for an excellent contouring without tongue tethering.

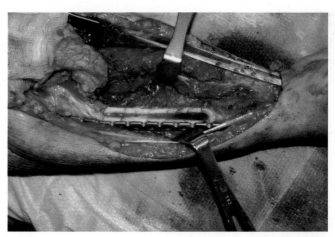

Figure 29.19 Donor radius defect is prophylactically treated with a reconstruction plate.

centered over the middle point of the line drawn from anterior superior iliac spine and superior lateral patella. In a majority of these cases, the perforators are musculocutaneous. Septocutaneous perforators occur 15% of the time and, if encountered, simplify the harvest significantly.

Once the perforator(s) is located, a skin paddle of the desired size is drawn out. The dissection starts from the medial side. The skin paddle elevation can be performed in either the subfascial or the suprafascial plane. Once the skin perforator is identified, it is then traced back to its origin from the pedicle.

Pearl

- Failure to dissect the perforator to the pedicle may compromise the entire cutaneous portion of the flap, as the musculocutaneous perforator course is highly variable in its path through the muscle and may have a variable vascular origin.

A small cuff of fascia and muscle should be preserved around the perforator. Because of the vascular variation, it is important to follow the perforator all the way to the pedicle, as the perforator course may find itself originating from an accessory descending branch or oblique branch of the lateral femoral circumflex vessels. The artery of the pedicle is of a good caliber and of adequate length. It is usually accompanied by two venae comitantes. Once the vascular system is identified during its entire length, the lateral incision is made. The rest of the muscular attachments can be divided around the perforator(s) with the help of bipolar electrocautery. Alternatively, a gastrointestinal anastomosis stapler device or harmonic sheers can be used to quickly divide the muscle, while maintaining hemostasis.

Unless, the defect width exceeds 10 cm, the donor defect can be repaired by primary closure. A closed suction drain and a compression bandage can be used to prevent a donor site seroma formation.

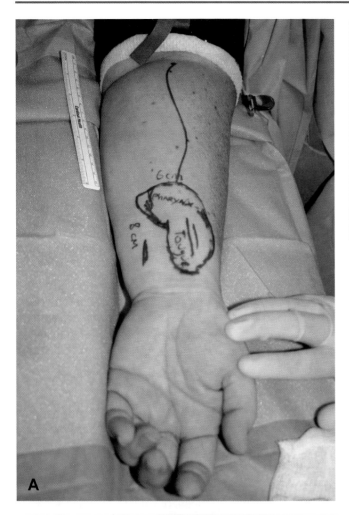

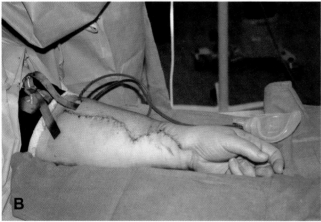

Figure 29.20 Radial forearm defect closed primarily by the advancement of adjacent tissues.

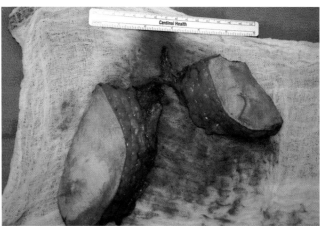

Figure 29.21 Large volume anterolateral thigh free flap with two skin paddles based on two separate perforators.

Scapular/Parascapular Free Flap

The scapular flap vascular anatomy was first described by Saijo in 1978.[65] Early 1980s were then marked by a widespread use of the scapular free flap (SFF) as both scapular and parascapular paddles were used separately and along with a newly described vascularized scapula bone graft.[66–69] Combination of these two skin paddles makes this flap a

unique tool for the reconstructive surgeon, allowing a possibility of a 3D reconstruction. While the skin and a layer of subcutaneous fatty tissue are thicker on the back, the flap can provide a remarkable area of soft tissue for harvest. Furthermore, the soft tissue flap can easily be combined with vascularized bone of the lateral border of the scapula. Further refinements of the vascular anatomy by Coleman gave a better understanding of the blood supply of the scapular tip.[70] Knowing the anatomy of the angular artery has opened the door for a reliable harvest of the tip of the scapula either as one segment contiguous with a lateral border of the scapula or as a separate bipedicle flap. SFF can be harvested as a chimeric flap by an addition of the latissimus dorsi or serratus anterior muscle flaps that are supplied by the same subscapular vascular system.[67]

The subscapular artery arises from the axillary artery and then branches into the circumflex scapular artery (CSA) and the thoracodorsal artery. The descending and transverse branches of the CSA supply the skin of scapular and parascapular flap skin paddles. There are a few minor variations of the arterial system, but none preclude harvest of the SFF. In 5% of the cases, a thoracodorsal artery arises directly from the axillary artery and this would disallow the harvest of the "megaflap."[67] Either one or two venae comitantes are identified along the pedicle.

While both lateral and medial approaches to the flap harvest have been described, the lateral approach is used more frequently. For ease of harvest, the patient is usually seated on the bean bag patient holder in the lateral decubitus position. Because most of the head and neck procedures are performed while supine, this need for an intraoperative position change has been the loudest criticism of the CSA-based flaps. To counter that, the patient can be placed in a 30 degrees lateral decubitus position at the beginning of the procedure. This allows extirpative and reconstructive procedures to be accomplished without turning the patient. Furthermore, a concurrent harvest becomes possible.

> **Pearl**
>
> • Preparing and draping the entire ipsilateral upper extremity along with the axilla into the operative field will facilitate exposure to the surgical site.

Once an adequate scapular and/or parascapular skin paddle has been drawn out and skin incisions are made, the dissection proceeds in a suprafascial plane from lateral to medial. The intermuscular triangle is then identified and dissection of the pedicle proceeds into the axilla. Osteocutaneous perforators to the bone of the lateral scapula can be quite large and need be ligated if no bony transfer is planned.

> **Pearl**
>
> • Teres major muscle is usually divided during the osteocutaneous transfer. Dividing this muscle before the dissection of main pedicle can simplify the procedure by improving the visualization of the vessels into the axilla.

If scapula bone is required for the transfer, the dissection of the osteocutaneous pedicle is avoided and instead osteotomies are placed to harvest the lateral border of the scapula. The blood supply to the tip of the scapula is unreliable, unless the angular artery is dissected out and preserved. Furthermore, this distinct pattern of the blood supply to the tip allows for a harvest of two individual vascularized bone grafts that are depended on the common pedicle of the subscapular vessels and yet have a great degree of separation.[70] This unique configuration can allow for osseous reconstruction of maxillary and mandibular or contralateral mandibular defects during a single-stage procedure by using the same flap.[71]

Once the flap harvest is complete, an abundance of the back skin allows for an easy primary closure of the cutaneous defect. Some advocate reattaching previously divided musculature of the teres major to a new lateral border of the scapular. While this practice makes sense anatomically and may improve postoperative shoulder mobility, clinically it has not shown to make a significant difference.[72]

Group II: Muscle and Musculocutaneous Free Flaps

Group II is composed of muscle and musculocutaneous flaps. These allow for large volume transfers, particularly when combined with overlying skin and adipose tissue. Furthermore, the muscle flaps can be reinnervated and used for facial reanimation. The best suited and most commonly used flap for this purpose is a gracilis muscle flap.

Gracilis Flap

The gracilis flap was first reported in 1976 by Harii et al, who described two cases of reinnervated gracilis muscle free flap.[73] Gracilis muscle provides an adequate length, thin muscle belly, and consistent vascular pedicle and nerve anatomy.

The harvest is accomplished in a supine position with the donor thigh abducted. A two-team approach can easily be accomplished if desired. A 10-cm incision is placed proximally, along the line drawn from pubic attachment of the usually palpable adductor longus tendon down to medial epicondyle of the femur. Dissection is carried down to the muscular fascia. The fascia is divided and the adductor longus muscle can be retracted anterolaterally. This allows for the identification of the vascular bundle and the anterior branch of the obturator nerve.

> **Pearl**
>
> • The point of the location of the vascular bundle can be predicted by placing a mark 10 cm inferior to the pubic tubercle.

If a longer length of the gracilis muscle is desired, a skin incision can be extended distally. Alternatively, if the total muscle harvest is planned, a second, distal incision can be placed separately from a former proximal incision. In that case, the distal muscle tendon can be easily identified by traction technique posterior to the sartorius muscle. The vessels are of an adequate caliber, allowing for easy microvascular anastomosis. The pedicle, however, is only 5 to 6 cm long and recipient vessel geometry must be carefully planned preoperatively. The gracilis flap can be easily harvested as a myocutaneous flap in a similar fashion, if needed. However, it is not used as often for its cutaneous properties, mostly because of a wide availability of other fasciocutaneous or myocutaneous flaps.

> **Pearl**
>
> • Measure the length of the muscle before dividing it. The muscle fibers will contract upon harvest, and if this is not taken into account, understretched graft will not provide an adequate muscle pull when used in cases of facial reanimation.

Latissimus Dorsi Flap

A muscle flap that clearly stands out in our abbreviated list of reconstructive options is the LDFF. While the original report by Maxwell et al described it as a musculocutaneous flap, it is now used more commonly as a muscle-only flap.[74] This flap provides an unparallel area of soft tissue and can easily be used for resurfacing of large head and neck defects. The area of 35 × 20 cm² (700 cm²) muscle can be harvested without difficulty. It is not advisable to harvest the entire area of overlying skin, and it would rarely, if ever, be indicated anyway. Large area with a relatively low volume defects, such as total scalpectomy or large neck soft tissue defects, are ideal for reconstruction with the LDFF along with concurrent skin grafting (**Fig. 29.22**).

The patient positioning, preparation, and draping of the donor site is similar to the harvest of SFF. An incision is placed along the posterior axillary line. A skin paddle overlying the muscle can be incorporated at this time, if desired. Following this, the anterolateral border of the muscle is exposed along with adequate exposure of the muscle posteromedially and inferiorly, depending on the desired flap size. The pedicle passes on the deep surface of the latissimus dorsi. Its dissection starts by identifying, ligating, and dividing the branch to the anterior serratus muscle. This branch can be preserved if a larger area of coverage would dictate a need for a serratus/latissimus combined flap. The vascular pedicle, which consists of the thoracodorsal artery and one or two venae comitantes, can then be easily dissected proximally. If a longer length of the pedicle is required, the CSA and vein can be ligated and then subscapular vessels are included with a flap. Medial and distal muscular attachments are divided either before or after pedicle identification. To prevent an injury to a pedicle, the humeral attachment should be divided only after the vessels are identified. Following harvest completion, one or two closed-circuit suction drains are placed and the wound is closed primarily. The use of the postoperative shoulder immobilizer may reduce the rate of seroma formation.

Rectus Flap

In the past, the rectus musculocutaneous flap had been used extensively for reconstruction of a variety of large volume head and neck soft tissue defects.[75,76] The use of this flap has waned in the recent years, mostly because of an increased use of anterolateral thigh/vastus lateralis flap. The rate of the donor site complications such as seromas, abdominal hernias, and/or mesh problems (if used), while acceptable, is greater than the donor site risks of ALTFF. While the traditional rectus musculocutaneous flap is no longer as common, the use of recently popularized perforator version of this flap has been on an upsurge. This deep inferior epigastric artery–based perforator flap is harvested sparing the rectus muscle, and as a result the complications of the abdominal well, defects have diminished significantly and mesh use is rarely, if ever, indicated.[77,78]

The rectus flap is harvested in a supine position. This facilitates a two-team approach with concomitant harvest and defect closure. The majority of skin perforators are located in the periumbilical area. Whether transverse, vertical, or oblique, the traditional skin paddle design should include the periumbilical area. Alternatively, if the microvascular surgeon is proficient with perforator dissecting techniques, then the flap paddle design can be more flexible and centered over one or two of the other major perforators of the deep inferior epigastric artery. Preoperative localization of the perforators with a handheld Doppler can substantially decrease operative harvest time if a perforator (deep inferior epigastric perforator) flap is considered.

For the traditional rectus myocutaneous flap harvest, the circumferential skin incisions are made and dissection is carried down to the abdominal wall fascia. The incisions are typically beveled outward to incorporate as many perforators as possible. Once the lateral and medial borders of the rectus muscle are identified, the fascia is incised along its length as well as superiorly and inferiorly. The muscle is transected superiorly, and the dissection progresses in a superior to inferior direction, lifting the myocutaneous flap off the posterior rectus sheath. Small perforators and intercostal nerves are ligated as encountered. Care is taken to avoid damage to the posterior sheath. Once the semicircular line is encountered, the vascular pedicle should be monitored. The deep inferior epigastric vessels enter the lateral aspect of the muscle approximately 4 cm superior to the fibers of origin. The artery and paired venae

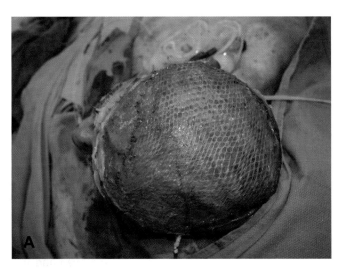 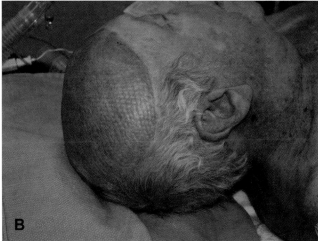

Figure 29.22 Total scalpectomy defect reconstructed with the latissimus dorsi free flap and meshed partial-thickness skin graft. Second photograph was taken 6 months postoperatively when the patient was undergoing unrelated surgical procedure.

comitantes are dissected until their takeoff from the external iliac artery. The vessels are typically 2 to 3 mm in diameter and quite sufficient for microvascular techniques.

Group III: Bone-Containing Flaps

Fibula Free Flap

Since the original description of a vascularized fibula flap for mandibular reconstruction by Hidalgo, the fibula free flap has been a workhorse flap for reconstruction of bony head and neck defects.[79] The flap harvest is straightforward with consistent donor site anatomy. Being the farthest removed from a head and neck site, this site allows for an easy concurrent harvest by a second team. The vascular pedicle consists of a peroneal artery and two venae comitantes. The caliber of the vessels is large and of adequate length; 25 to 30 cm of the bone can be safely harvested, depending on the individual's native skeletal structure. While the pedicle is most often of adequate length, it becomes shorter when a longer segment of bone is used. This consideration becomes important for total or near-total mandibular reconstructions. The stock of the bone is great and allows for either concomitant or postoperative placement of the osseointegrated implants.[7]

Before the harvest, the entire lower extremity is prepared and draped into the field. Including a thigh into a sterile field allows for a sterile placement of the tourniquet and also provides a site for the harvest of a partial-thickness skin graft if it is required for the closure of the donor site.

Traditionally, the pressures of 300 to 350 mm Hg have been used for the tourniquet. However, orthopedic literature has shown that there is no significant improvement in hemostasis when lower extremity tourniquet pressure exceeds more than 90 to 100 mm Hg above systolic blood pressure.[52] Furthermore, there is evidence that higher pressures may induce more local tissue damage, and as a result patients endure higher levels of pain postoperatively, which is significantly more difficult to control.[80,81]

If a skin paddle is desired, it needs to be centered over the posterior intermuscular septum. A Doppler device can help to locate skin perforators and further assist with placement of the skin paddle.

Pearl

- If no dominant perforator is identified, harvesting a longer skin paddle can decrease the risk of a skin paddle failure.

Topography of the perforator distribution has been studied and has shown that there is at least one consistent skin perforator from the peroneal artery located at the junction of middle and distal thirds of the fibula.[82,83]

Once the lower extremity is exsanguinated and the tourniquet inflated, an anterior skin incision is placed and the dissection proceeds in the subfascial plane until the posterior intermuscular septum and cutaneous perforators are identified. At this juncture, if a bone-only flap is desired, these perforators are ligated and the entire septum is divided. If an osteocutaneous flap is being harvested, a posterior skin incision is made around the skin paddle. Dissection proceeds in the subfascial plane anteriorly to identify the posterior septum from the other side.

Pearl

- By making either an anterior or a posterior, but only one at a time, incision allows for adjustment of the skin paddle either superiorly or inferiorly to incorporate a major septocutaneous perforator once it has been identified.

Dissection is then directed over the fibula, dividing the attachments of the peroneus longus and brevis. The anterior septum is identified and sharply incised. The dissection in the anterior compartment is performed with greater care, as, while the muscular attachments to the fibula are released, one must pay attention not to injure an anterior tibial pedicle. The interosseous membrane is the next layer that needs to be divided before making osteotomies through the fibula. The distal osteotomy is placed 5 cm proximal to the lateral malleolus to preserve an ankle mortise. The proximal osteotomy is recommended to be placed 5 cm distal to the fibular head to preserve a common peroneal nerve. However, the common peroneal nerve is easily identified and can be retracted superiorly if a longer segment of the vascularized bone is required for reconstruction. Once osteotomized, the fibula flap can be retracted laterally and the distal peroneal pedicle is visualized, ligated, and divided. Division of the tibialis posterior muscle allows for the visualization of the peroneal pedicle, which can now be traced to its take off from the tibioperoneal trunk. Posterior leg musculature is then divided with a 1-cm cuff of muscle along the fibula to preserve the perforators to complete the flap harvest. At this point, the tourniquet can be released and after a brief reperfusion time the flap is ready for a transfer. In appropriate cases, if the width of the skin paddle is less than 5 cm, a donor site can be closed primarily.[84] However, the increased rate of donor site complications has been observed in patients who were poor candidates for primary closure.[85] Nevertheless, a partial-thickness skin graft is a safe and effective modality. It can be harvested from a previously prepared ipsilateral thigh.

Pearl

- Fibula free flap is a workhorse flap for reconstruction of bony defects in pediatric population as well. One must remember that the distal fibular remnant must be fixated to the tibia to prevent a valgus ankle deformity in pediatric patients.[86]

Controversy

- Preoperative vascular evaluation of the lower extremity is essential before contemplating to use fibula free flap. While everybody agrees that a clinical evaluation of dorsalis pedis and posterior tibial pulses is a standard procedure, there is a controversy on whether and/or what radiologic studies should be used. Some surgeons are comfortable to proceed based on a good clinical examination. However, to avoid disastrous postoperative foot devascularization problems, an additional radiologic evaluation is recommended. While there are several congenital anomalies of lower extremity vessels, such as absences of anterior or posterior tibial arteries or peroneus magna, it is acquired abnormalities such as atherosclerotic disease that are more common. Traditionally, an angiogram has been a gold standard for vascular evaluation of the lower extremity.[87,88] At the present time, however, less invasive studies such as CT angiogram, magnetic resonance angiography, and Doppler ultrasound are used.[89–91] Doppler ultrasound is the most cost-effective option and has been shown to be adequately comparable for preoperative evaluation before the fibula harvest.[91,92]

Scapula Osteocutaneous and Radial Forearm Osteocutaneous Free Flap

Scapular osteocutaneous flap and radial forearm osteocutaneous flap harvests are similar to their kin fasciocutaneous flap harvests and have been described in section "skin free flaps" of this chapter.

Iliac Crest Osteocutaneous Free Flap

Iliac crest osteocutaneous and osseous free flaps are based on the deep circumflex iliac artery (DCIA). Originally, this flap was described as the treatment used to aid a reconstruction of lower extremity.[93] In the following decade, the use of this flap has extended to head and neck reconstruction. Because of the thickness of the available bone, it was found to be particularly useful for reconstruction of the mandible and maxilla.[94,95] Iliac crest was shown to be an excellent recipient for osseointegrated implants.[7] While the main skin paddle is fairly tethered to the harvested bone, the flexibility of the soft tissue can be augmented by incorporating an internal oblique muscle.[96] Nonetheless, despite many advantages and uses of this flap in head and neck reconstruction, because of significant donor site morbidity, it has not become a widely popular choice of reconstruction.

The anatomy and harvest of the flap are consistent and straightforward. If a skin paddle is being used, it is usually centered over the iliac crest and posterior to the anterior superior iliac spine. Dissection proceeds down to the muscular fascia. The external oblique muscular layer is incised. If one chooses to include an internal oblique muscle with the flap, then at this juncture the incision is made through the muscle below the costal margin. The attachments to the rectus sheath are released. The ascending branch of the DCIA is identified on the undersurface of the internal oblique muscle and preserved. Thereafter, transversalis fascia is released and DCIA and venae comitantes are dissected to their takeoff from the external iliac vessels. Gluteus medius attachments are released laterally, and once the iliacus muscle fibers are incised, osteotomies through the ilium will complete the harvest. It is possible, however, and less morbid to harvest a split-thickness vascularized bone graft. While not applicable for mandibular reconstruction, this thinner graft often will suffice for skull base and/or orbital reconstructions. The reconstruction of the donor defect should be meticulous to prevent the herniation of abdominal contents. Two-layer closure is accomplished by approximation of the transversalis abdominis fascia to the iliacus muscle and external oblique to the tensor fascia lata and gluteal musculature. The use of synthetic mesh may be required to achieve an adequate closure.

Pearl

- Lateral femoral cutaneous nerve course is variable and can be either deep or superficial to the vascular pedicle. In the latter case, the nerve is divided during the harvest but can be repaired to diminish anesthesia of the lateral thigh skin.

Group IV: Bowel Flaps

The category of bowel flaps is another helpful adjunct to the reconstructive surgeon's armamentarium. Several bowel flaps have been described and include transverse colon, ileocolic, and jejunum, with the jejunum being the most common.[97–100]

Jejunal Flap

In 1959, Seidenberg et al experimented with dogs by reconstructing a segment of the esophagus with the revascularized jejunum.[101] This breakthrough in reconstructive surgery was the first reported description of a microvascular free tissue transfer.

To the current date, the jejunal flap is still used for reconstruction of laryngopharyngeal and upper esophageal defects. While the harvest is not complex, it requires general surgical expertise and a traditional laparotomy approach.[97,98] With the advancement of laparoscopic techniques, this alternative to a traditional open approach has been used as well.[102,103] The blood supply to a harvested segment of the jejunum comes from the second or third jejunal branch of the superior mesenteric artery. Before a harvest of the flap, proximal and distal ends of the proposed graft are marked to assure an inset in an isoperistaltic direction. A tubular structure of the jejunum allows for a straightforward inset (**Fig. 29.23**).

Pearl

- Oropharyngeal aperture is larger than the lumen of the jejunum; thus, additional care must be taken while advancing mucosa to close proximal anastomosis. This size mismatch has encouraged surgeons to search for other possible sites, such as ileocolic flaps, to mitigate this problem.[99]

Historically, an additional segment of the vascularized jejunum was externalized to allow for easy monitoring. However, the use of arterial and venous implantable Doppler devices abated the necessity of this step. The inset should be done with neck in the flexed position to prevent the redundancy of the flap, as this could contribute to postoperative swallowing difficulties. Native lubricative properties of the jejunum can assist with food propulsion through a reconstructive segment. An innate jejunal peristalsis, however, is uncoordinated with esophageal peristalsis and probably does not help as much as it was previously believed. Furthermore, while there are many reports of successful alaryngeal speech rehabilitation, jejunal secretions can create some difficulties with the quality of produced voice.[104,105] While this flap is time tested and performs quite well, the need for intra-abdominal surgery and potential donor site morbidity should be taken into consideration (**Table 29.2**).

Controversies

Microvascular Anastomosis

The geometry and the type of vascular anastomosis have been studied as well as the choice for the recipient vessel(s).[106,107]

End-to-end anastomosis has been compared with end-to-side anastomosis, and no benefit has been found to either approach.[108,109] The coupler system has revolutionized microsurgery, significantly decreasing the time required for anastomosis as compared with a suturing technique.[110,111] Furthermore, the coupler device allows for easy overcoming of a significant venous size mismatch.[112] While it is quite a bit easier to apply a coupler in the end-to-end fashion, an end-to-side coupler anastomosis is possible and also has shown to have a good efficacy.

Continuous suture technique offers similar patency rate but decreased flap ischemia time as compared with a most commonly used interrupted suture technique.[113]

The advantage of supplementary anastomoses, both venous and arterial, for the same flap has also been studied. Supercharged flaps have an additional arterial anastomosis. While the need for supercharging the flap is exceedingly rare, it could provide a benefit for long jejunal flaps or for perforator flaps in certain populations.[114–116]

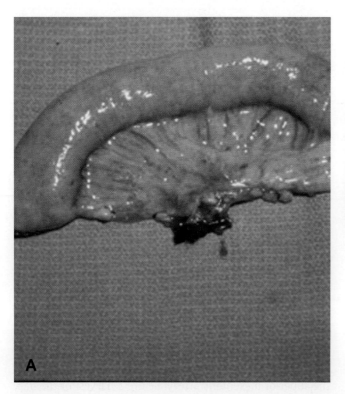
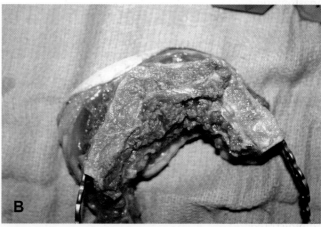

Figure 29.23 Tubular structure of the jejunum has been used extensively for reconstruction of pharyngoesophageal defects.

Table 29.2 Microvascular Head and Neck Reconstruction Reference Table

Tongue reconstruction	
• < 50%	RFFF, UFFF, lateral arm, ALTFF-p
• > 50%	ALTFF (± vastus), rectus, DIEP-p, scapula
Mandible	
• Posterior defect <5 cm	Soft tissue or bone flaps
• Anterior defect(s) > 5 cm, but < 10 cm	FFF, SFF, ICFF, OCRFFF
• Defects >10 cm	FFF, double flaps can be considered
Oral cavity/pharyngeal lining defects	RFFF, ALTFF, UFFF
Total laryngopharyngectomy defects	ALTFF, RFFF, jejunum, ileocolic
Cervical esophageal defects	
Orbital defects	RFFF, OCRFFF
Orbitomaxillary defects	SFFF, OCRFF, ICFF, FFF, rectus, ALTFF
Total scalpectomy defects	LDFF, omentum

RFFF, radial forearm free flap; UFFF, ulnar forearm free flap; ALTFF, anterolateral thigh free flap; DIEA-p; deep inferior epigastric artery perforator flap; FFF, forearm free flap; SFF, scapular free flap; ICFF, iliac crest free flap; OCRFFF, osteocutaneous radial forearm free flap; LDFF, latissimus dorsi free flap.

Double venous outflow has been suggested by some as a "safer" microvascular anastomosis.[117-119] In selected cases, it has been shown that anastomosing deep and superficial venous draining systems may reduce flap venous congestion.[119] The use of a single venous outflow system, however, is safe, as long as the dominant venous vessel is identified intraoperatively.[64,120]

Antithrombogenic Therapy

Several pharmacologic agents have been evaluated in an attempt to reduce the risk of thrombus formation at the anastomotic site. Aspirin (Bayer Aspirin), heparin (Heparin Sodium ADD-Vantage), ketorolac (Toradol), low-molecular-weight dextran, and clopidogrel (Plavix) have been used clinically and studied in the animal models.[121-124] Some of these studies have found marginal benefits, while others found no significant differences. Furthermore, intravenous administration of dextran was shown to have an increased rate of systemic complications without a significant benefit of flap survival.[121] Impeccable surgical techniques are paramount, and the most important factor for the anastomosis-related flap survival. The authors of this chapter prefer and recommend a daily use of aspirin postoperatively. Subcutaneous heparin can be used for prophylaxis of the deep venous thrombosis in this patient population as aspirin administration does not offer a protection in that regard.

Preservation of Preoperative Dimensions during Mandibular Reconstruction

Preserving adequate mandibular dimensions during mandibular reconstruction is of paramount significance for future dental rehabilitation. There are several means available at the disposal of the reconstructive surgeon in that regard. Commonly, a reconstructive plate is prebent before the oncologic extirpation. This straightforward and reliable technique allows for precise mandibular reconstruction but has several disadvantages. Tumors with buccal cortex involvement preclude the preresection placement of the plate. Also, rounded contour of the plate that was bent to abut the mandible is not ideal for osteotomized straight bone grafts. And lastly, this technique fails in the anterior mandibular reconstructions. While the external mandibular contour is preserved, the "new" alveolar ridge of the reconstructed symphysis ends up being overprojected. As a result, this will effectively impair prospective dental rehabilitative efforts and may require orthognathic surgery in the future.

The temporary use of the external fixator intraoperatively has been suggested. It is a reliable technique that preserves preoperative dimensions but allows for relative freedom of placement of the osteotomized bone grafts.[125] Drilling into a native mandible for the device placement is a minor disadvantage. More importantly, it is a bulky piece of equipment that can interfere with other aspects of the extirpative and reconstructive procedures.

Experienced surgeons have found the preoperative use of the 3D models beneficial. The models can be manufactured with the tumor or mandible subtracted. Alternatively, a mirror image from the contralateral mandible can be incorporated if needed. The entire reconstructive procedure can be designed preoperatively with grafts and plates placement. In our experience, this decreases the complexity of the case and the length of time needed for reconstruction. When reconstruction is planned taking into consideration the future dental rehabilitative needs, the need for postreconstruction orthognathic work is also decreased (**Fig. 29.24A, B**).

Conclusions

Surgical reconstruction is an integral part of the rehabilitation of a patient with HNC. Tumors and their treatments result in

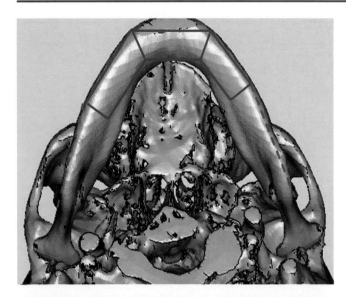

Figure 29.24 Osteotomies and bone grafts are designed preoperatively. Mandibular neosymphsis is placed taking into consideration the position of the neoalveolus to enable an effective future reconstruction with implant-borne denture. Mandibular reconstruction plate is manufactured based on the three-dimensional computed tomography imaging. Preoperative position of the native mandible is preserved.

functional deficits and cosmetic deformities. Reconstruction of these defects is strikingly different from other sites in the body. Consequently, up to 50% of the patients undergoing the treatment for HNCs suffer from major depression.[6] The suicide rate among these patients is one of the highest as compared with patients with other malignancies.[126] With this in mind, the restoration of patients' appearance and functionality becomes of major importance. Over the past three decades, we have enjoyed a marked improvement in reconstructive techniques including the greatest advance seen with the introduction of microvascular tissue transfer. Currently, these reconstructions have become very reliable, and an increasing emphasis is being placed on the refinement of techniques, resulting in improved functionality and decreased donor site morbidity. In addition, prevention and early detection of tumors, along with improvements of treatment modalities, will result in decreased morbidity, requiring less-intensive reconstructive efforts or eliminating the need for it altogether. New advancements in tissue engineering techniques may completely eliminate the need for donor sites in the future and will revolutionize the field of reconstructive surgery.

References

1. Surveillance epidemiology and end results. Available from: http://seer.cancer.gov/faststats. Accessed June 5, 2011
2. Karnell LH, Funk GF, Hoffman HT. Assessing head and neck cancer patient outcome domains. Head Neck 2000;22(1):6–11
3. Weymuller EA Jr, Yueh B, Deleyiannis FW, Kuntz AL, Alsarraf R, Coltrera MD. Quality of life in head and neck cancer. Laryngoscope 2000;110(3 Pt 3):4–7
4. Tschiesner U, Linseisen E, Baumann S, et al. Assessment of functioning in patients with head and neck cancer according to the International Classification of Functioning, Disability, and Health (ICF): a multicenter study. Laryngoscope 2009;119(5):915–923
5. Pfister DG, Ang KK, Brizel DM, et al; National Comprehensive Concer Network. Head and neck cancers. J Natl Compr Canc Netw 2011;9(6):596–650
6. Lydiatt WM, Moran J, Burke WJ. A review of depression in the head and neck cancer patient. Clin Adv Hematol Oncol 2009;7(6):397–403
7. Moscoso JF, Keller J, Genden E, et al. Vascularized bone flaps in oromandibular reconstruction. A comparative anatomic study of bone stock from various donor sites to assess suitability for endosseous dental implants. Arch Otolaryngol Head Neck Surg 1994;120(1):36–43
8. Yun IS, Lee DW, Lee WJ, Lew DH, Choi EC, Rah DK. Correlation of neotongue volume changes with functional outcomes after long-term follow-up of total glossectomy. J Craniofac Surg 2010;21(1):111–116
9. Chang H, Wind S, Kerstein MD. Moist wound healing. Dermatol Nurs 1996;8(3):174–176, 204
10. Barnea Y, Weiss J, Gur E. A review of the applications of the hydrofiber dressing with silver (Aquacel Ag) in wound care. Ther Clin Risk Manag 2010;6:21–27
11. Spear M. Wet-to-dry dressings—evaluating the evidence. Plast Surg Nurs 2008;28(2):92–95
12. Argenta LC, Morykwas MJ. Vacuum-assisted closure: a new method for wound control and treatment: clinical experience. Ann Plast Surg 1997;38(6):563–576, discussion 577
13. Dhir K, Reino AJ, Lipana J. Vacuum-assisted closure therapy in the management of head and neck wounds. Laryngoscope 2009;119(1):54–61
14. Lee DL, Ryu AY, Rhee SC. Negative pressure wound therapy: an adjuvant to surgical reconstruction of large or difficult skin and soft tissue defects. Int Wound J 2011;8(4):406–411
15. Andrews BT, Smith RB, Hoffman HT, Funk GF. Orocutaneous and pharyngocutaneous fistula closure using a vacuum-assisted closure system. Ann Otol Rhinol Laryngol 2008;117(4):298–302
16. Hanasono MM, Lin D, Wax MK, Rosenthal EL. Closure of laryngectomy defects in the age of chemoradiation therapy. Head Neck 2012;34(4):580–588
17. Flap. Available from: http://www.merriam-webster.com. Updated 2011. Accessed June 21, 2011
18. Neumann CG. The expansion of an area of skin by progressive distention of a subcutaneous balloon: use of the method for securing skin for subtotal reconstruction of the ear. Plast Reconstr Surg (1946) 1957;19(2):124–130
19. Sasaki GH. Tissue Expansion in Reconstructive and Aesthetic Surgery. 1st ed. Mosby, MO: Mosby Elsevier Health Science; 1998:373
20. Manders EK, Schenden MJ, Furrey JA, Hetzler PT, Davis TS, Graham WP III. Soft-tissue expansion: concepts and complications. Plast Reconstr Surg 1984;74(4):493–507
21. Antonyshyn O, Gruss JS, Zuker R, Mackinnon SE. Tissue expansion in head and neck reconstruction. Plast Reconstr Surg 1988;82(1):58–68
22. Larrabee WF Jr, Sutton D. The biomechanics of advancement and rotation flaps. Laryngoscope 1981;91(5):726–734
23. Pearl RM. A unifying theory of the delay phenomenon—recovery from the hyperadrenergic state. Ann Plast Surg 1981;7(2):102–112
24. Seline PC, Siegle RJ. Scalp reconstruction. Dermatol Clin 2005;23(1):13–21, v
25. Orticochea M. Four flap scalp reconstruction technique. Br J Plast Surg 1967;20(2):159–171

26. Cordaro ER, Calabrese S, Faini GP, Zanotti B, Verlicchi A, Parodi PC. Method to thicken the scalp in calvarian reconstruction. J Craniofac Surg 2011;22(2):598–601

27. Lutz BS, Wei FC, Chen HC, Lin CH, Wei CY. Reconstruction of scalp defects with free flaps in 30 cases. Br J Plast Surg 1998;51(3):186–190

28. Jackson IT. Forehead reconstruction. In: Jackson IT, ed. Local Flaps in Head and Neck Reconstruction. 2nd ed. St. Louis, MO: Quality Medical Publishing; 2007:43–85

29. Song R, Chen Z, Yang P, Yue J. Reconstruction of the external ear. Clin Plast Surg 1982;9(1):49–52

30. Antia NH, Buch VI. Chondrocutaneous advancement flap for the marginal defect of the ear. Plast Reconstr Surg 1967;39(5):472–477

31. Renard A. Postauricular flap based on a dermal pedicle for ear reconstruction. Plast Reconstr Surg 1981;68(2):159–165

32. Tenzel RR, Stewart WB. Eyelid reconstruction by the semicircle flap technique. Ophthalmology 1978;85(11):1164–1169

33. Cutler NL, Beard C. A method for partial and total upper lid reconstruction. Am J Ophthalmol 1955;39(1):1–7

34. Hughes WL. A new method for rebuilding a lower lid: report of a case. Arch Ophthal 1937;17(6):1008–1017

35. Burget GC, Menick FJ. Nasal support and lining: the marriage of beauty and blood supply. Plast Reconstr Surg 1989;84(2):189–202

36. Zitelli JA. The bilobed flap for nasal reconstruction. Arch Dermatol 1989;125(7):957–959

37. Baker SR. Nasal lining flaps in contemporary reconstructive rhinoplasty. Facial Plast Surg 1998;14(2):133–144

38. Abbe RA. A new plastic operation for the relief of deformity due to double hairlip. Plast Reconstr Surg 1968;42:481–483

39. Renner GJ, Zitsch RP III. Reconstruction of the lip. Otolaryngol Clin North Am 1990;23(5):975–990

40. Bakamjian VY. A two-stage method for pharyngoesophageal reconstruction with a primary pectoral skin flap. Plast Reconstr Surg 1965;36:173–184

41. Ariyan S. The pectoralis major myocutaneous flap. A versatile flap for reconstruction in the head and neck. Plast Reconstr Surg 1979;63(1):73–81

42. Moukarbel RV, Fung K, Franklin JH, et al. Neck and shoulder disability following reconstruction with the pectoralis major pedicled flap. Laryngoscope 2010;120(6):1129–1134

43. Baker DC, Conley J. Regional muscle transposition for rehabilitation of the paralyzed face. Clin Plast Surg 1979;6(3):317–331

44. Bakamjian VY, Souther SG. Use of temporal muscle flap for reconstruction after orbito-maxillary resections for cancer. Plast Reconstr Surg 1975;56(2):171–177

45. Byrne PJ, Kim M, Boahene K, Millar J, Moe K. Temporalis tendon transfer as part of a comprehensive approach to facial reanimation. Arch Facial Plast Surg 2007;9(4):234–241

46. Boahene KD, Farrag TY, Ishii L, Byrne PJ. Minimally invasive temporalis tendon transposition. Arch Facial Plast Surg 2011;13(1):8–13

47. Shumrick KA, Smith TL. The anatomic basis for the design of forehead flaps in nasal reconstruction. Arch Otolaryngol Head Neck Surg 1992;118(4):373–379

48. Wax MK, Rosenthal EL, Winslow CP, Bascom DA, Andersen PE. The ulnar fasciocutaneous free flap in head and neck reconstruction. Laryngoscope 2002;112(12):2155–2160

49. Antunes MB, Chalian AA. Microvascular reconstruction of nasal defects. Facial Plast Surg Clin North Am 2011;19(1):157–162

50. Corten EM, Hage JJ, Schellekens PP, Kreulen M, Kon M. Clinical application and outcome of the segmental pectoralis major free flap in five head and neck patients. Plast Reconstr Surg 2009;123(5):1462–1467

51. Song R, Gao Y, Song Y, Yu Y, Song Y. The forearm flap. Clin Plast Surg 1982;9(1):21–26

52. Tejwani NC, Immerman I, Achan P, Egol KA, McLaurin T. Tourniquet cuff pressure: the gulf between science and practice. J Trauma 2006;61(6):1415–1418

53. Schaverien M, Saint-Cyr M. Suprafascial compared with subfascial harvest of the radial forearm flap: an anatomic study. J Hand Surg Am 2008;33(1):97–101

54. Militsakh ON, Werle A, Mohyuddin N, et al. Comparison of radial forearm with fibula and scapula osteocutaneous free flaps for oromandibular reconstruction. Arch Otolaryngol Head Neck Surg 2005;131(7):571–575

55. Tsue TT, Shnayder Y, Girod DA, Militsakh ON. Free tissue transfer, osteocutaneous radial forearm flap. Available from: http://emedicine.medscape.com.library1.unmc.edu:2048/article/881055-overview. Accessed June 25, 2011

56. Inglefield CJ, Kolhe PS. Fracture of the radial forearm osteocutaneous donor site. Ann Plast Surg 1994;33(6):638–642, discussion 643

57. Thoma A, Khadaroo R, Grigenas O, et al. Oromandibular reconstruction with the radial-forearm osteocutaneous flap: experience with 60 consecutive cases. Plast Reconstr Surg 1999;104(2):368–378, discussion 379–380

58. Villaret DB, Futran NA. The indications and outcomes in the use of osteocutaneous radial forearm free flap. Head Neck 2003;25(6):475–481

59. Militsakh ON, Wallace DI, Kriet JD, Girod DA, Olvera MS, Tsue TT. Use of the 2.0-mm locking reconstruction plate in primary oromandibular reconstruction after composite resection. Otolaryngol Head Neck Surg 2004;131(5):660–665

60. Karamanoukian R, Gupta R, Evans GR. A novel technique for the prophylactic plating of the osteocutaneous radial forearm flap donor site. Ann Plast Surg 2006;56(2):200–204

61. Edmonds JL, Bowers KW, Toby EB, Jayaraman G, Girod DA. Torsional strength of the radius after osteofasciocutaneous free flap harvest with and without primary bone plating. Otolaryngol Head Neck Surg 2000;123(4):400–408

62. Wax MK, Winslow CP, Andersen PE. Use of allogenic dermis for radial forearm free flap donor site coverage. J Otolaryngol 2002;31(6):341–345

63. Song YG, Chen GZ, Song YL. The free thigh flap: a new free flap concept based on the septocutaneous artery. Br J Plast Surg 1984;37(2):149–159

64. Wei FC, Jain V, Celik N, Chen HC, Chuang DC, Lin CH. Have we found an ideal soft-tissue flap? An experience with 672 anterolateral thigh flaps. Plast Reconstr Surg 2002;109(7):2219–2226, discussion 2227–2230

65. Saijo M. The vascular territories of the dorsal trunk: a reappraisal for potential flap donor sites. Br J Plast Surg 1978;31(3):200–204

66. dos Santos LF. The vascular anatomy and dissection of the free scapular flap. Plast Reconstr Surg 1984;73(4):599–604

67. Hamilton SG, Morrison WA. The scapular free flap. Br J Plast Surg 1982;35(1):2–7

68. Gilbert A, Teot L. The free scapular flap. Plast Reconstr Surg 1982;69(4):601–604

69. Baker SR, Sullivan MJ. Osteocutaneous free scapular flap for one-stage mandibular reconstruction. Arch Otolaryngol Head Neck Surg 1988;114(3):267–277

70. Coleman JJ III, Sultan MR. The bipedicled osteocutaneous scapula flap: a new subscapular system free flap. Plast Reconstr Surg 1991;87(4):682–692

71. Urken ML, Bridger AG, Zur KB, Genden EM. The scapular osteofasciocutaneous flap: a 12-year experience. Arch Otolaryngol Head Neck Surg 2001;127(7):862–869

72. Nkenke E, Vairaktaris E, Stelzle F, Neukam FW, Stockmann P, Linke R. Osteocutaneous free flap including medial and lateral scapular crests: technical aspects, viability, and donor site morbidity. J Reconstr Microsurg 2009;25(9):545–553

73. Harii K, Ohmori K, Torii S. Free gracilis muscle transplantation, with microneurovascular anastomoses for the treatment of facial paralysis. A preliminary report. Plast Reconstr Surg 1976;57(2):133–143

74. Maxwell GP, Stueber K, Hoopes JE. A free latissimus dorsi myocutaneous flap: case report. Plast Reconstr Surg 1978;62(3):462–466

75. Urken ML, Turk JB, Weinberg H, Vickery C, Biller HF. The rectus abdominis free flap in head and neck reconstruction. Arch Otolaryngol Head Neck Surg 1991;117(8):857–866

76. Wax MK, Burkey BB, Bascom D, Rosenthal EL. The role of free tissue transfer in the reconstruction of massive neglected skin cancers of the head and neck. Arch Facial Plast Surg 2003;5(6):479–482

77. Koshima I, Soeda S. Inferior epigastric artery skin flaps without rectus abdominis muscle. Br J Plast Surg 1989;42(6):645–648

78. Woodworth BA, Gillespie MB, Day T, Kline RM. Muscle-sparing abdominal free flaps in head and neck reconstruction. Head Neck 2006;28(9):802–807

79. Hidalgo DA. Fibula free flap: a new method of mandible reconstruction. Plast Reconstr Surg 1989;84(1):71–79

80. Kam PC, Kavanagh R, Yoong FF. The arterial tourniquet: pathophysiological consequences and anaesthetic implications. Anaesthesia 2001;56(6):534–545

81. Worland RL, Arredondo J, Angles F, Lopez-Jimenez F, Jessup DE. Thigh pain following tourniquet application in simultaneous bilateral total knee replacement arthroplasty. J Arthroplasty 1997;12(8):848–852

82. Papadimas D, Paraskeuopoulos T, Anagnostopoulou S. Cutaneous perforators of the peroneal artery: cadaveric study with implications in the design of the osteocutaneous free fibular flap. Clin Anat 2009;22(7):826–833

83. Yu P, Chang EI, Hanasono MM. Design of a reliable skin paddle for the fibula osteocutaneous flap: perforator anatomy revisited. Plast Reconstr Surg 2011;128(2):440–446

84. Urken ML, Weinberg H, Buchbinder D, et al. Microvascular free flaps in head and neck reconstruction. Report of 200 cases and review of complications. Arch Otolaryngol Head Neck Surg 1994;120(6):633–640

85. Shindo M, Fong BP, Funk GF, Karnell LH. The fibula osteocutaneous flap in head and neck reconstruction: a critical evaluation of donor site morbidity. Arch Otolaryngol Head Neck Surg 2000;126(12):1467–1472

86. Omokawa S, Tamai S, Takakura Y, Yajima H, Kawanishi K. A long-term study of the donor-site ankle after vascularized fibula grafts in children. Microsurgery 1996;17(3):162–166

87. Young DM, Trabulsy PP, Anthony JP. The need for preoperative leg angiography in fibula free flaps. J Reconstr Microsurg 1994;10(5):283–287, discussion 287–289

88. Disa JJ, Cordeiro PG. The current role of preoperative arteriography in free fibula flaps. Plast Reconstr Surg 1998;102(4):1083–1088

89. Ribuffo D, Atzeni M, Saba L, et al. Clinical study of peroneal artery perforators with computed tomographic angiography: implications for fibular flap harvest. Surg Radiol Anat 2010;32(4):329–334

90. Manaster BJ, Coleman DA, Bell DA. Magnetic resonance imaging of vascular anatomy before vascularized fibular grafting. J Bone Joint Surg Am 1990;72(3):409–414

91. Futran ND, Stack BC Jr, Zaccardi MJ. Preoperative color flow Doppler imaging for fibula free tissue transfers. Ann Vasc Surg 1998;12(5):445–450

92. Smith RB, Thomas RD, Funk GF. Fibula free flaps: the role of angiography in patients with abnormal results on preoperative color flow Doppler studies. Arch Otolaryngol Head Neck Surg 2003;129(7):712–715

93. Sanders R, Mayou BJ. A new vascularized bone graft transferred by microvascular anastomosis as a free flap. Br J Surg 1979;66(11):787–788

94. Brown JS. Deep circumflex iliac artery free flap with internal oblique muscle as a new method of immediate reconstruction of maxillectomy defect. Head Neck 1996;18(5):412–421

95. Urken ML, Vickery C, Weinberg H, Buchbinder D, Lawson W, Biller HF. The internal oblique-iliac crest osseomyocutaneous free flap in oromandibular reconstruction. Report of 20 cases. Arch Otolaryngol Head Neck Surg 1989;115(3):339–349

96. Urken ML, Vickery C, Weinberg H, Buchbinder D, Biller HF. The internal oblique-iliac crest osseomyocutaneous microvascular free flap in head and neck reconstruction. J Reconstr Microsurg 1989;5(3):203–214, discussion 215–216

97. Coleman JJ III, Searles JM Jr, Hester TR, et al. Ten years experience with the free jejunal autograft. Am J Surg 1987;154(4):394–398

98. Disa JJ, Pusic AL, Mehrara BJ. Reconstruction of the hypopharynx with the free jejunum transfer. J Surg Oncol 2006;94(6):466–470

99. Mardini S, Chen HC, Salgado CJ, Ozkan O, Cigna E, Chung TT. Free microvascular transfer of the reverse ileo-colon flap with ileocaecal valve valvuloplasty for reconstruction of a pharyngoesophageal defect: indication and usage of the 'funnel flap'. J Plast Reconstr Aesthet Surg 2006;59(11):1241–1246

100. Wei FC, Carver N, Chen HC, Tsai MH, Wang JY. Free colon transfer for pharyngo-oesophageal reconstruction. Br J Plast Surg 2000;53(1):12–16

101. Seidenberg B, Rosenak SS, Hurwitt ES, Som ML. Immediate reconstruction of the cervical esophagus by a revascularized isolated jejunal segment. Ann Surg 1959;149(2):162–171

102. Rosenberg MH, Sultan MR, Bessler M, Treat MR. Laparoscopic harvesting of jejunal free flaps. Ann Plast Surg 1995;34(3):250–253, discussion 253

103. Wadsworth JT, Futran N, Eubanks TR. Laparoscopic harvest of the jejunal free flap for reconstruction of hypopharyngeal and cervical esophageal defects. Arch Otolaryngol Head Neck Surg 2002;128(12):1384–1387

104. Sharp DA, Theile DR, Cook R, Coman WB. Long-term functional speech and swallowing outcomes following pharyngolaryngectomy with free jejunal flap reconstruction. Ann Plast Surg 2010;64(6):743–746

105. Yu P, Lewin JS, Reece GP, Robb GL. Comparison of clinical and functional outcomes and hospital costs following pharyngoesophageal reconstruction with the anterolateral thigh free flap versus the jejunal flap. Plast Reconstr Surg 2006;117(3):968–974

106. Chalian AA, Anderson TD, Weinstein GS, Weber RS. Internal jugular vein versus external jugular vein anastomosis: implications for successful free tissue transfer. Head Neck 2001;23(6):475–478

107. Egemen O, Ugurlu K, Ozkaya O, Sacak B, Sakiz D, Bas L. Anastomosis with fish-mouth technique using fibrin glue. J Craniofac Surg 2011;22(3):1047–1051

108. Graham BB, Varvares MA. End-to-side venous anastomosis with the internal jugular vein stump: a preliminary report. Head Neck 2004;26(6):537–540

109. Dotson RJ, Bishop AT, Wood MB, Schroeder A. End-to-end versus end-to-side arterial anastomosis patency in microvascular surgery. Microsurgery 1998;18(2):125–128

110. Jandali S, Wu LC, Vega SJ, Kovach SJ, Serletti JM. 1000 consecutive venous anastomoses using the microvascular anastomotic coupler in breast reconstruction. Plast Reconstr Surg 2010;125(3):792–798

111. Rozen WM, Whitaker IS, Acosta R. Venous coupler for free-flap anastomosis: outcomes of 1,000 cases. Anticancer Res 2010;30(4):1293–1294

112. Sullivan SK, Dellacroce F, Allen R. Management of significant venous discrepancy with microvascular venous coupler. J Reconstr Microsurg 2003;19(6):377–380

113. Chen YX, Chen LE, Seaber AV, Urbaniak JR. Comparison of continuous and interrupted suture techniques in microvascular anastomosis. J Hand Surg Am 2001;26(3):530–539

114. Barzin A, Norton JA, Whyte R, Lee GK. Supercharged jejunum flap for total esophageal reconstruction: single-surgeon 3-year experience and outcomes analysis. Plast Reconstr Surg 2011;127(1):173–180

115. Numajiri T, Sowa Y, Nishino K, et al. Double vascular anastomosis in the neck for reliable free jejunal transfer. Br J Oral Maxillofac Surg 2010;48(7):511–514

116. Wu LC, Iteld L, Song DH. Supercharging the transverse rectus abdominis musculocutaneous flap: breast reconstruction for the overweight and obese population. Ann Plast Surg 2008;60(6):609–613

117. Alan Turner MJ, Smith WP. Double venous anastomosis for the radial artery forearm flap. Improving success and minimising morbidity. J Craniomaxillofac Surg 2009;37(5):253–257

118. Mao C, Yu GY, Peng X, Zhang L, Guo CB, Huang MX. [168 cases of free flap transplantation with double vein anastomoses for reconstruction of head and neck defects]. Hua Xi Kou Qiang Yi Xue Za Zhi 2006;24(6):530–532

119. Enajat M, Rozen WM, Whitaker IS, Smit JM, Acosta R. A single center comparison of one versus two venous anastomoses in 564 consecutive DIEP flaps: investigating the effect on venous congestion and flap survival. Microsurgery 2010;30(3):185–191

120. Wei FC, Demirkan F, Chen HC, Chen IH, Liao CT, Hau SP. Management of secondary soft-tissue deficits following microsurgical head and neck reconstruction by means of another free flap. Plast Reconstr Surg 1999;103(4):1158–1166

121. Disa JJ, Polvora VP, Pusic AL, Singh B, Cordeiro PG. Dextran-related complications in head and neck microsurgery: do the benefits outweigh the risks? A prospective randomized analysis. Plast Reconstr Surg 2003;112(6):1534–1539

122. Veravuthipakorn L, Veravuthipakorn A. Microsurgical free flap and replantation without antithrombotic agents. J Med Assoc Thai 2004;87(6):665–669

123. Moore MG, Deschler DG. Clopidogrel (Plavix) reduces the rate of thrombosis in the rat tuck model for microvenous anastomosis. Otolaryngol Head Neck Surg 2007;136(4):573–576

124. Harsha WJ, Kau RL, Kim N, Hayden RE. Effects of antithrombogenic agents on microvenous anastomoses in a rat model. Arch Otolaryngol Head Neck Surg 2011;137(2):170–174

125. Ung F, Rocco JW, Deschler DG. Temporary intraoperative external fixation in mandibular reconstruction. Laryngoscope 2002;112(9):1569–1573

126. Misono S, Weiss NS, Fann JR, Redman M, Yueh B. Incidence of suicide in persons with cancer. J Clin Oncol 2008;26(29):4731–4738

30 Prosthetic Rehabilitation: Intraoral and Extraoral Prostheses

Betsy K. Davis and David J. Reisberg

Core Messages

- Defects of the maxillofacial complex are due to tumor surgery, a congenital condition, or trauma.

- They affect function and esthetics and have a great effect on a patient's quality of life.

- Surgical reconstruction alone may not completely resolve these problems.

- Oral and facial prostheses restore function and esthetics either alone or in conjunction with reconstructive surgery.

- The prosthesis covers and protects sensitive tissues, restores oral and facial anatomy and function, improves psychological well-being and quality of life.

- Successful maxillofacial rehabilitation requires a team approach.

- The prosthesis may serve as an interim measure until reconstructive surgery is performed or as definitive treatment.

Although head and neck cancers make up less than 5% of all cancers,[1] the resulting hard and soft tissue deficits, either intraorally or extraorally, can present a difficult challenge to the reconstructive surgeon and maxillofacial prosthodontist. The successful outcome depends on a team approach to both resection and rehabilitation. The maxillofacial prosthodontist is an integral part of the team approach from diagnosis to treatment to rehabilitation.[2] With advances in microvascular surgery, vascularized free flaps, distraction osteogenesis, and other improvements in hard and soft tissue grafting, surgical reconstruction is a viable option in many cases. However, not all situations are amenable to surgery alone. Surgical reconstruction may be limited by the size or location of the defect, quantity and quality of available tissue, the patient's physical and/or mental health, or their personal wishes regarding reconstructive surgery. Prosthetic rehabilitation instead of, or in conjunction with, reconstructive surgery may be a viable alternative to achieve the goals of functional, esthetic, and psychosocial normalcy.

Intraoral defects include tumors of the tongue, floor of the mouth, mandible, and adjacent structures as well as maxillary defects of the hard and soft palate. There are significant differences between maxillary surgical defects and mandibular surgical deficits with respect to quality, mode, and effectiveness of rehabilitation, the role of surgical reconstruction, and psychosocial profiles.[2] The goal of rehabilitating hard and soft palate defects and mandibular defects is to restore, to some degree of normalcy, functions of speaking, swallowing, and chewing. Rehabilitation of acquired hard and soft palate defects usually can be restored to close to normal function and physical appearance with an obturator prosthesis (**Figs. 30.1** to **30.3**).[2–5] The use of surgical reconstruction of both hard and soft palate defects is gaining acceptance.[6–12] However, surgical reconstruction of hard and soft palate defects still has not been shown to have better functional outcomes (Beumer J, Garrett N. Personal communication, 2010). There are some preliminary reports that show promising results with surgical reconstruction.[8–12] With respect to mandibular defects, the use of free vascularized tissue flaps and dental implants have revolutionized our ability to rehabilitate these patients (**Figs. 30.4** to **30.6**).[13] Although many advances have been made, many patients with surgical resections of the tongue, mandible, and adjacent soft tissues still have functional disabilities of speech, mastication, and deglutition (**Fig. 30.7**). Control of saliva is difficult, and xerostomia, a side effect of radiation, compounds the problems with deglutition. Patients with mandible/tongue deficits generally have a greater alteration in their quality of life than do patients with maxillary deficits of the hard and soft palate.[13]

Extraoral defects involve defects of the auricle, orbit, nasal, or midfacial region. The decision between surgical reconstruction of a facial defect and a prosthetic restoration should be made based on several general guidelines while taking into consideration the specifics of each case. The natural history of the tumor, the size and location of the defect, the quantity and quality of available tissue, the patient's physical and/or mental health, and their personal wishes

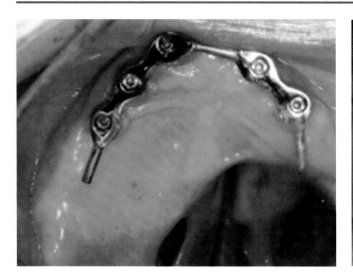

Figure 30.1   Endosseous screw retained (implant) bar.

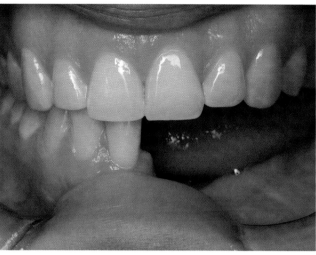

Figure 30.4   Resulting mandibular defect from resection of a benign tumor.

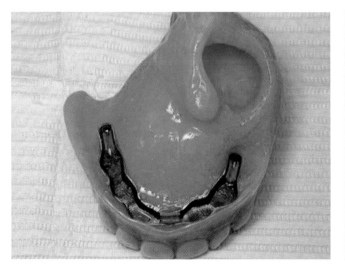

Figure 30.2   Obturator prosthesis.

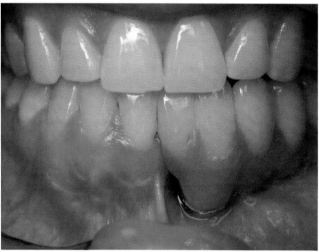

Figure 30.5   Endosseous screw retained (implant) mandibular prosthesis.

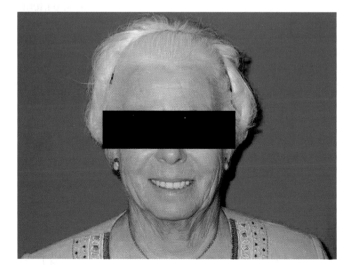

Figure 30.3   Minimum facial disfigurement with obturator prosthesis.

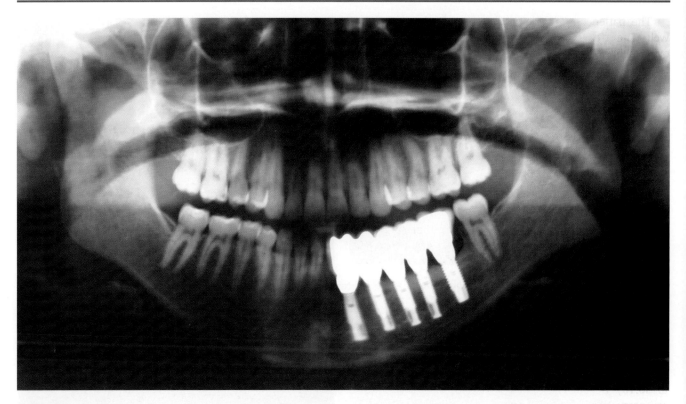

Figure 30.6   Panorex.

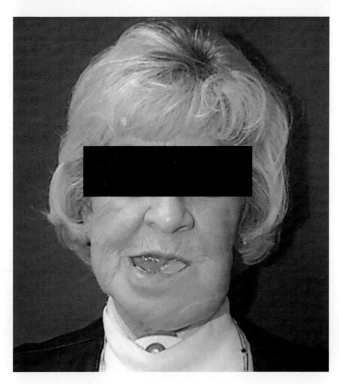

Figure 30.7   Mandibular reconstruction with resulting disabilities of speech, mastication, and deglutition.

regarding reconstructive surgery should be considered. As a rule, it is difficult for the surgeon to reconstruct a facial part that is as cosmetic as a well-made prosthesis (or in as little time), although a surgical reconstruction does result in an autologous, nonartificial outcome that does not require the maintenance of a prosthesis.[14]

There is limited information in the literature to confirm that a facial prosthesis restores lost function. In a pilot study, Reisberg and Lipner[15] demonstrated some limited improvement in hearing with an ear prosthesis. However, an orbital prosthesis does not restore sight and there are no data to indicate improved function with a nasal prosthesis. It should not be overlooked, however, that in addition to restoring normal anatomic contour, a facial prosthesis does cover and protect the sensitive soft tissues of a facial defect. What is even more important is to recognize the benefit of a facial prosthesis in improving the quality of life of a cancer victim.

Team Approach

Whatever be the method of rehabilitation for either intraoral or extraoral defects, a team approach is necessary for a successful outcome. The team should consist of not only medical and dental specialists but allied health professionals as well. A comprehensive oncology team includes an otolaryngologist/head and neck surgeon, plastic and reconstructive surgeon, maxillofacial prosthodontist, medical oncologist, radiation oncologists, dental oncologist, speech and language pathologist, dietician, nurse, social worker, and psychologist. From the outset, rehabilitation becomes part of the overall treatment plan. Communication between team members is a key to success. A weekly team meeting to discuss new patients and monitor the progress of those receiving care is useful.

The patient should be considered a team member as well. The treatment and rehabilitation process may be overwhelming and confusing for the patients and their family. They must be fully informed of treatment options and participate in the decision-making process of the treatment plan. The objective is a well-informed patient with realistic expectations.

Intraoral Defects: Hard Palate Defects

Surgical Reconstruction versus Prosthetic Reconstruction

Several factors influence the decision of either surgical or prosthetic reconstruction. For example, the etiology, size, and location of the defect influence the reconstructive options.[2] As a general rule, defects resulting from trauma are more amenable to surgical reconstruction whereas defects resulting from malignant tumor ablation tend to do better with prosthetic reconstruction. Plank et al,[16] Rieger et al,[4] and Sullivan et al[17] found that speech and swallowing can be restored to normal levels in almost all patients with an obturator prosthesis with adequate retention (**Figs. 30.8** to **30.10**). Defects from benign tumors can have surgical reconstruction if the margins are negative; however, some advocate a waiting period of 2 years before surgical reconstruction with prosthetic obturation used as an interim measure. Patients with either midline granuloma or mucormycosis are not candidates for surgical reconstruction when the disease is in an active state.[2] Defects resulting from adenoid cystic carcinoma are not candidates for surgical reconstruction because of its propensity for recurrence.[2] Small defects of the alveolar ridge and hard palate can be easily closed surgically with local flaps, whereas larger hard palate defects are more amenable to prosthetic obturation or to free vascularized osteocutaneous tissue flaps such as the fibula. The fibula with its bicortical bone provides

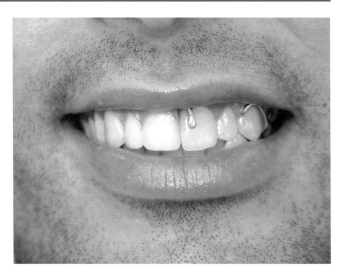

Figure 30.9 Resection of a benign tumor with obturator prosthesis.

an ideal placement for osseointegrated implants and can be easily osteotomized to provide favorable alveolar ridge contours. The use of these flaps is particularly desirable for restoration of total palatectomy defects and for total maxillectomy defects. The success of surgical reconstruction is proper planning with the maxillofacial prosthodontist, so the patient can be rehabilitated with dental implants.[8,9] If the

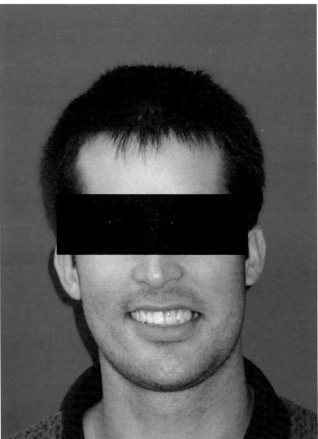

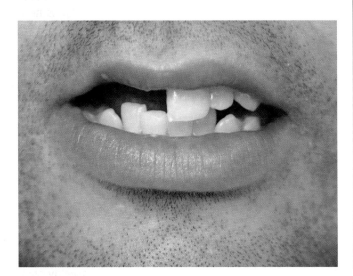

Figure 30.8 Resection of a benign tumor without obturator prosthesis.

Figure 30.10 Facial appearance after rehabilitation with an obturator prosthesis.

surgical reconstruction is not properly planned, prosthetic rehabilitation may not be possible because of poorly contoured bulky tissues, lack of suitable bone volume for dental implant placement, and improper positioning of the bone (**Figs. 30.11** and **30.12**). Generally, younger patients are better suited for surgical reconstruction. Patients who are incapable of wearing an obturator prosthesis, such as a patient with Alzheimer disease, would be more amenable to surgical reconstruction.

Rohner et al[8,9] and Jaquiéry et al[6] have reported on the successful use of computer-aided design and computer-aided manufacturing technologies using a combined surgical and prosthodontic approach. The success of the technique depends on multidisciplinary treatment planning and communication. This technique advocates preplanning the maxillary surgical reconstruction based on the occlusion and the opposing mandible configuration. A free vascularized bony flap, usually the fibula, is used to replace the missing alveolar bone and to retain an implant prosthesis. This technique uses a two-stage procedure by placing implants in the donor bone and creating a new per-implant tissue by placing a split thickness skin graft around the implants. The second stage involves harvesting the bone and osteomized the bone and securing it to the preprepared prosthesis. The bone is then attached to the residual maxilla and skull base to create a new maxilla. Any remaining palatal defect can be closed with either an overlay denture or soft tissue flaps.

As a general rule, soft tissue flaps should not be used to close large palatal defects. Soft tissue flaps such as a radial forearm flap distort palatal contours and the mobility of the soft tissues makes prosthetic rehabilitation with a removable partial denture difficult. It is important that the patient be informed, before surgical resection, that prosthetic rehabilitation may not be possible with the use of soft tissue flaps. The buildup of mucus on the nasal side of the defect creates a strong unpleasant odor for some patients. Also, facial contours, particularly the lip and cheek area, are compromised with soft tissue flaps.[2] Functional outcomes of speech and mastication are also compromised with this flap.[18] The inability to fabricate a removable partial denture prosthesis compromises masticatory efficiency. Matsui et al[18] found that with the loss of anterior dentition and normal palatal contours, normal speech cannot be effectively restored with these flaps, particularly the lingual dental, lingual alveolar, lingual palatal, and velar consonant speech sounds. The exception would be a patient who was not capable of proper hygiene of the defect, nor had the manual dexterity required for an obturator prosthesis.

Prosthetic Rehabilitation

Prosthetic rehabilitation consists of three distinct phases: surgical, interim, and definitive obturation. The surgical phase involves the placement of an immediate surgical obturator at the time of surgical resection. Its purpose is to restore and maintain oral functions of speaking

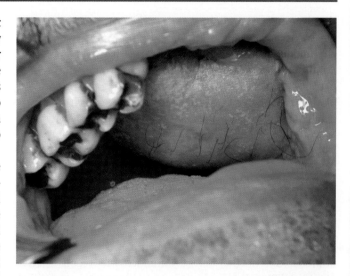

Figure 30.11   Surgical reconstruction with resulting bulky tissues.

and swallowing during the initial postoperative therapy. The interim obturator phase begins at the unpacking visit of the immediate surgical obturator. It still provides speaking and swallowing functions until healing is complete. Usually, this obturator will require multiple relines during the healing phase. The definitive obturation phase usually begins 3 to 6 months after surgical resection.[2]

Initial Treatment Phase

The patient is evaluated with the maxillofacial prosthodontist. During this appointment, a thorough dental examination with recording of the periodontal evaluation and restorative charting is accomplished. Impressions for diagnostic casts, a jaw relationship record, and dental radiographics can be made. Depending on the clinical situation and the timing of the surgical procedure, a dental prophylaxis can be accomplished along with restoration of carious teeth. Dental extractions can be coordinated at the time of surgical resection. Most importantly, a discussion with the patient concerning the advantages and

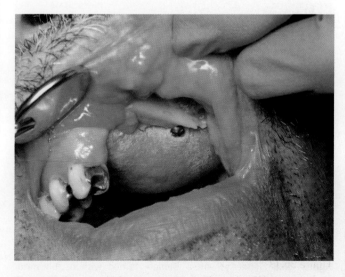

Figure 30.12   Surgical reconstruction with exposed bone.

disadvantages of prosthetic rehabilitation is accomplished. Once a decision is made concerning prosthetic rehabilitation, the maxillofacial prosthodontist and the resection surgeon communicate as to the best method to prepare the defect for the prosthesis. It is critical that the surgeon understand that the success of the prosthesis is in large part related to how well the defect is prepared for the prosthesis. Surgical resection of hard palate defects usually can be rehabilitated quite easily with an obturator prosthesis. As Curtis and Beumer[2] outlined, the goals of an obturator prosthesis are to restore partition between the nasal and oral cavities, restore palatal contours, maintain tongue space, replace the missing dentition, restore midfacial contours, and provide retention, stability, and support for the obturator prosthesis without compromising the health of the residual dentition and supporting structures. With proper communication between the resection surgeon and the maxillofacial prosthodontist, a defect can be optimized to accept a prosthesis without a compromise in the surgical resection of the tumor.

Surgical Modifications

Hard Palate Resection

The more of the hard palate, particularly the premaxillary segment, that can be preserved without compromising tumor control contributes to increased stability and support for the obturator prosthesis (**Fig. 30.13**). The premaxillary segment is the most desirable site for implant placement in the edentulous patient. Preservation of the premaxillary segments allows an increased number of implants to be placed while increasing the anterior-posterior spread of the implants. From a biomechanical standpoint, the greater the anterior-posterior spread of the implants, the greater the retention of the obturator prosthesis and the greater the ability of the obturator prosthesis to withstand the forces of mastication.[2]

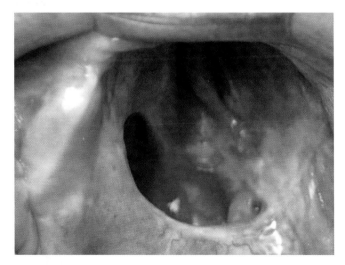

Figure 30.13   Linear arrangement of alveolar arch reduces stability and support of the obturator prosthesis.

Skin Grafting the Defect

Lining the reflected cheek flap with a split thickness skin graft allows the maxillofacial prosthodontist to engage the scar band, resulting in an improvement of the retention and stability of the obturator prosthesis. This skin-lined surface is a more suitable prosthesis-bearing surface. It also increases flexibility of the cheek, allowing the maxillofacial prosthodontist to displace the cheek on the resected side, resulting in a relatively normal midfacial symmetry (**Fig. 30.14**). If this is not done, the reflected cheek flap will granulate and will be surfaced with either respiratory mucosa or poorly keratinized squamous epithelium, resulting in a more irritation of the prosthesis to the reflected cheek surface (**Fig. 30.15**). Skin grafting the raw tissue surfaces of total palatectomy defects is particularly crucial with anterior defects. Skin grafting prevents contraction of the upper lip, resulting in an obturator prosthesis with which the patient can function. For total maxillectomy procedures, the resection surgeon should consider skin grafting the sinus side of the floor of the orbit. If possible, engaging this surface with the obturator prosthesis will improve support; however, for patients with postsurgical trismus, this may not be possible to engage.[2]

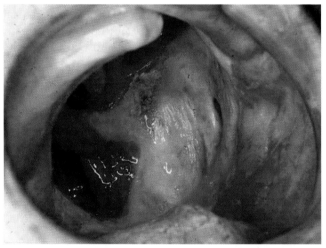

Figure 30.14   Skin grafting the defect increases stability and retention of the prosthesis.

Image Courtesy: Dr. John Beumer.

Retention of Teeth Adjacent to the Defect

Surgical resection through the transeptal bone approximating the tooth of the defect side results in loss of bony support with eventual loss of the tooth (**Fig. 30.16**). Therefore, transalveolar resections should be made as far as possible from the tooth beside the proposed defect. The next distal tooth should be extracted. This allows the surgeon to make transalveolar cuts through the middle or distal of the socket, resulting in more bony support. The abutment tooth adjacent to the defect is one of the many fulcrums that the obturator prosthesis will rotate around. This additional bony support improves the clinical viability of the tooth. If oncologically sound, the cuspid tooth provides greater bony

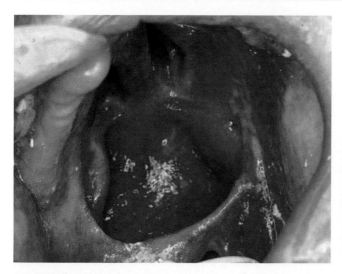

Figure 30.15   Respiratory mucosa is a poor prosthesis-bearing surface. *Image Courtesy*: Dr. John Beumer.

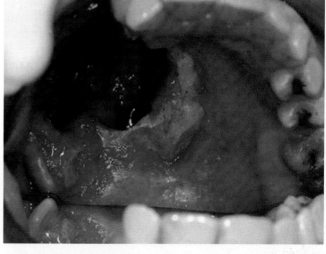

Figure 30.17   Lack of proper use of the palatal mucosa on the medial margin.

support than the lateral incisor and should be preserved if possible.[2]

Palatal Mucosa

The medial bony margin of the palatal bones should be rounded and covered with palatal mucosa or a skin graft. This allows the maxillofacial prosthodontist to engage the surface, enhancing the lateral stability of the obturator prosthesis. The medial bony margin is a fulcrum for the obturator prosthesis to rotate during function for the edentulous patients. If allowed to granulate in, the poorly keratinized squamous epithelium or respiratory mucosa is an inadequate prosthesis-bearing surface (**Fig. 30.17**).[2]

Soft Palate Resection

If the tumor resection involves more than two thirds of the soft palate, then the resection surgeon should remove the remaining one third of the posterior aspect of the soft

palate for dentate patients. The levator veli palatini muscle, located in the middle third of the soft palate, is responsible for elevating the soft palate. Leaving a nonfunctional band of soft palate intact posteriorly interferes with access for proper obturation to achieve velopharyngeal closure during speech and swallowing, resulting in hypernasal speech and leakage of fluids into the nose. The exception to the rule is for edentulous patients who have had a total maxillectomy. The posterior band of soft palate in this situation allows extension onto the nasal side, aiding in retention of the obturator prosthesis.[2]

Access to the Defect

Removal of the turbinates and bands of oral mucosa allows the maxillofacial prosthodontist access to the superior and lateral aspects of the defect (**Fig. 30.18**). Engaging the lateral nasal side of the orbital floor along with extension

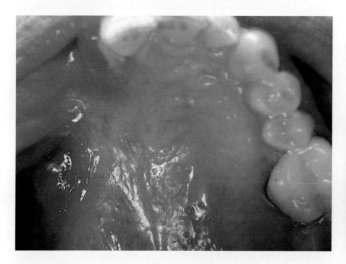

Figure 30.16   Loss of bone around abutment tooth.

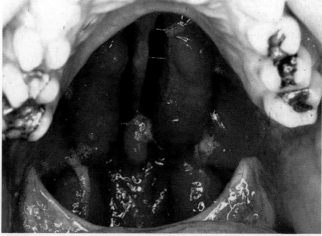

Figure 30.18   Need to remove turbinates to have access to the defect. *Image Courtesy*: Dr. John Beumer.

of the obturator prosthesis up the lateral wall of the defect increases retention and stability of the obturator prosthesis. The exception is midline defects of the hard-soft palate junction. Extension superiorly for these defects is not as critical as in larger defects.[2]

Osseointegrated Implants

Osseointegrated implants have improved the prosthetic prognosis immensely for edentulous patients undergoing a maxillectomy. Garrett[3] has shown that placement of osseointegrated implants will dramatically improve the function of the obturator prosthesis, particularly for edentulous patients. Usually, the implants can be placed after tumor resection in the premaxillary segment and the maxillary tuberosity or placement can be delayed. The alveolar arch below the maxillary sinus, if present, can be used for implant placement. It is not recommended to place implants within the defect itself because of difficulty in adequate hygiene of the implants. For patients receiving postoperative radiation therapy, implant placement should be delayed if the implant site is to receive excess of 60 Gy. Scwartz et al[19] and Mian et al[20] found that the backscatter of radiation from the implant increases the radiation dose to the bone by an additional 11 to 15%, resulting in nonvital bone. If intensity-modulated radiation therapy is used, it is advantageous to reduce the dose to the implant site, if oncologically sound.[2]

Surgical Obturation

The immediate surgical obturator is placed at the time of surgical resection and is made of acrylic resin. The prosthesis may or may not have teeth. Surgical packing is used in the defect and the prosthesis is either wired or screwed into place. This prosthesis is used for either edentulous or dentate patients requiring a partial or total maxillectomy or a partial or total palatectomy. The advantages of an immediate surgical obturator include maintaining the surgical packing in place, ensuring close adaptation of the split thickness skin graft to the raw surfaces of the cheek flap; reducing oral contamination of the wound; reducing the incidence of local infection; enabling the patient to speak more effectively; proper deglutition, eliminating the need for nasogastric tube; lessening the psychological effect of surgery; and reducing the period of hospitalization.

The immediate surgical obturator is placed for 7 to 10 days. At the unpacking visit, either the surgical obturator is relined and used as an interim obturator or a new interim obturator is delivered to the patient.[2]

Interim Obturation

The purpose of the interim obturator is to maintain patient comfort and function during the healing phase. A new prosthesis is fabricated if the surgical resection was different from the presurgical resection plan. Fabrication of a new prosthesis allows the addition of the teeth, which aids the patient psychologically and helps to restore occlusal contact on the defect side, increasing retention and stability. The interim obturator prosthesis will need relines every 4 to 8 weeks to account for tissue changes within the defect.[2]

Definitive Obturation

Three to four months after surgery or after adequate healing of the defect, fabrication of the definitive obturator prosthesis may begin. Soft tissue changes of the defect will continue at least for 1 year. Patient factors such as the prognosis for tumor control and the general health and desire of the patient have to be considered in treatment planning for the definitive obturator prosthesis. If implants have been placed at the time of surgical resection, implants will need to be exposed with adequate healing of the peri-implant tissues. In certain situations, it may be decided to proceed ahead with implant placement at this time. This will delay the fabrication of the definitive obturator. Roumanas et al,[21] Hoshaw et al,[22] Miyata et al,[23] and Miyamoto et al[24] have shown that implants are subjected to overload, resulting in bone loss and subsequent loss of the implants. To prevent implant overload, treatment planning of implant tissue bar designs must be implant assisted and accommodate multiple axis of rotation of the obturator prosthesis. Davis et al[25] found that implant-assisted designs resulted in less stress around the implants and hence less overloading of the implants. Of note, the successful use of zygoma implants has been reported by Schmidt et al[11] for patients with large or total palatectomy defects. They recommend placement of two zygoma implants into each residual zygoma and splinting all four implants together with a tissue bar. Landis et al[26] also reported on the use of zygoma implants in this patient population and found that 8 of the 36 zygoma implants placed were lost because of either implant overload and/or chronic infections or resection of recurrent disease.

Functional Outcomes

Masticatory Performance

Both Matsuyama et al[27] and Koyama et al[28] found that the remaining maxillary dentition is a critical factor in the restoration of masticatory function. Each found that maxillectomy patients with residual dentition to support an obturator prosthesis had masticatory efficiency that was not that significantly different from dentate controls. Garret[3] found significant improvement in masticatory performance on both the defect side and the nondefect side with the use of osseointegrated implants for edentulous patients. Although these improvements reach the level of a conventional edentulous patient restored with an implant-supported prosthesis, their performance levels still remained lower than dentate individuals.

Air and Fluid Leakage

Watson and Gray[29] found air leakage of the obturator prosthesis by using either simple lung function tests or sequential radiographic assessment of a radiopaque liquid during swallowing. The authors theorized that during forced exhalation, the soft tissues peripheral to the obturator contract more, leading to an improved seal and found leakage more likely to occur during sustained exhalation. The use of contrast medium showed most leakage around the obturator, particularly along the posterior-medical and posterior-lateral margins of the defect when the obturator is improperly contoured in those areas. Leakage may also occur most posteriorly during swallowing because of movement of the soft palate. In addition, the functional movement of the coronoid process posterolaterally may contribute to leakage. The authors concluded that complete and total closure may be unobtainable at times, but a sufficient level of obturation exists to permit acceptable speech and swallowing. Minsley et al[30] found the oral opening around the definitive obturator was less than 0.05 mm, which did not significantly affect speech but may lead to the leakage of fluids into the nasal cavity during swallowing.

Speech

The size and location of the defect significantly affect the restoration of speech. There have been several studies that have reported normal speech after the placement of an obturator prosthesis for patients with acquired surgical defects of the maxillae.[31,32] Plank et al[16] found speech intelligibility for both dentate and edentulous patients rehabilitated with an obturator prosthesis after surgical resection to be 98.8% intelligible presurgically, 92.1% intelligible with an immediate surgical obturator, and 97.3% correct with their definitive obturator. A patient with a bilateral maxillectomy defect exhibited a 12% reduction in speech intelligibility with the definitive prosthesis. Sullivan et al[17] found a 30% improvement in the mean speech intelligibility ratings with an obturator prosthesis compared with no prosthesis. Communication effectiveness was restored to 75% of the original level with the obturator prosthesis compared with the level before the cancer resection. Hypernasality was found to have a strong correlation with communication effectiveness. A 95% or greater intelligibility score was obtained with obturation for all defects except for the combined unilateral hard and soft palate. Rieger et al[4] found that average speech with obturation was not significantly different from the preoperative speech.

Quality of Life

In a study of 47 maxillectomy patients who had worn an obturator for at least 5 years, Kornblith et al[33] found that satisfactory functioning of the obturator was significantly related to psychological adjustment and quality of life. They concluded that a well-functioning obturator significantly improves quality of life. They also concluded that the most significant predictor of obturator function was the extent of soft palate resection. In a study evaluating quality of life in patients with obturator maxillectomy compared with similar patients who had surgical reconstruction, Rogers et al[5] found no statistically significant difference in patient perceptions between the 28 patients with obturators and the 18 patients undergoing surgical reconstruction.

Intraoral Prostheses: Soft Palate Defects

Just as with hard palate defects, rehabilitation of soft palate defects requires a multidisciplinary team approach with communication between all members of the team, particularly the surgeon, speech and swallowing pathologist, and the maxillofacial prosthodontist. Soft palate defects usually affect resonance of speech. The major determinant of resonance balance is the degree of velopharyngeal closure.[34] Other factors such as tongue position[35-37] relative to velar elevation and the structural resistance within the nasal cavity[38] also influence the resonance balance.

Several differences exist between hard and soft palate defects.[34] Usually, hard palate defects are of a static nature with very little movement. In contrast, soft palate defects are of a dynamic nature that must function in concert with surrounding moveable tissues. The goal of a hard palate obturation is to separate the oral cavity from the nasal cavity. Superior extension of the obturator for hard palate defects improves retention, support, and stability of the prosthesis. The goals of soft palate obturation are to control nasal emission during speech and to prevent the leakage of material into the nasal passage during swallowing.[39] Soft palate defects are rarely in the soft palate alone. Many of the resections that affect the soft palate originate in the tonsil, retromolar trigone, base of tongue, oropharynx, or nasopharynx.

Surgical Reconstruction versus Prosthetic Obturation

In recent years, prosthetic obturation was considered the treatment of choice for soft palate rehabilitation. When properly prepared for a prosthesis, soft palate obturation was highly predictable and the treatment of choice. Surgical reconstruction often resulted in excessive scarring and impaired movement. The end result was a deficient, nonfunctioning velopharyngeal mechanism. Many times, prosthetic obturation was not possible because of limited access to the residual velopharyngeal mechanism. Rieger et al[40] and Seikaly et al[41] have reported on soft palate reconstruction with excellent function results. Reconstruction of soft palate defects is becoming more popular but requires a multidisciplinary approach.

Surgical Modifications

The success of either surgical or prosthetic rehabilitation depends on communication between the maxillofacial prosthodontist and the surgeon. Prosthetic rehabilitation depends on the mobility of the residual velopharyngeal mechanism and access to the areas of movement and the quality of retention available for the obturator prosthesis. In many clinical situations, the raw surfaces of the defect are lined or closed with a radial forearm free flap and the prosthodontist has to restore a nonfunctional velopharyngeal defect. If the opposite lateral pharyngeal wall exhibits movement and the prosthodontist has access to engage the dynamic areas during velopharyngeal function, then speech and swallowing can be restored to normal limits. If there is limited movement of the soft tissues peripheral to the defect, then speech will not be normal with either prosthetic obturation or surgical reconstruction. Zlotolow[42] reported that the movement of at least one lateral wall is necessary for either method of rehabilitation.

Once a decision is made to proceed with prosthetic obturation, the surgeon needs to prepare the soft palate defect for the prosthesis. If the tumor resection involves more than two-thirds of the soft palate, then the resection surgeon should remove the remaining one-third of the posterior aspect of the soft palate for dentate patients. The levator veli palatini muscle, located in the middle third of the soft palate, is responsible for elevating the soft palate. Leaving a nonfunctional band of soft palate intact posteriorly interferes with access for proper obturation to achieve velopharyngeal closure during speech and swallowing, resulting in hypernasal speech and leakage of fluids into the nose. The exception to the rule is for edentulous patients who have had a total maxillectomy. The posterior band of soft palate in this situation allows extension onto the nasal side, aiding in retention of the obturator prosthesis. If the resection stops short of the midline, then it is possible to reconstruct the unilateral soft palate defect with a vascularized free flap. If more than one half of the soft palate is to be resected, the residual portion of the soft palate should not be connected to the free flap. If the free flap is connected to the residual soft palate, speech is compromised. Also, if more than one half of the soft palate is to be resected, the residual soft palate should not be tethered to the hard palate or the lateral pharyngeal wall. This limits the movement of the levator muscle and limits access to the lateral pharyngeal area on the side opposite the resection. It is better for the residual portion of the soft palate to hang free. Doing this will allow maximum movement of the velopharyngeal mechanism and will allow access for proper obturation.[34]

Prosthesis Evaluation

Fabrication of a soft palate obturator requires close communication with the speech and swallowing pathologist. Working in a large tertiary center provides an environment where specialized equipment such as nasal videoendoscopy and pressure airflow equipment are readily available. The use of this equipment allows better visual inspection and useful information in the fabrication process. It has been shown that better speech outcomes are achieved with the aid of nasal videoendoscopy for prosthetic rehabilitation of soft palate defects.[43] Several reported studies[44-46] have also advocated the use of pressure airflow equipment to determine the velopharyngeal orifice opening and nasal airflow.

Immediate Surgical Obturation

Immediate surgical obturation may or may not be indicated depending on the clinical situation. For example, immediate surgical obturation is useful for dentate patients, in which the whole soft palate is resected. In contrast, for edentulous patients, delayed obturation may be indicated. As it is not possible to obtain an impression of the nasopharynx before surgical resection and of the dynamic movements of the velopharyngeal mechanism before surgical resection, delayed obturation may be preferred. If an immediate surgical obturator is used, it is imperative that the posterior margins of the obturator be short so as not to cause an interference with either the lateral or posterior pharyngeal walls.[34]

Interim Obturation

Because of the frequent relines during the postsurgical treatment phase resulting often in a heavy and uncomfortable prosthesis, an interim obturator may need to be fabricated. The interim obturator may be used as a guide for the initial contours of the definitive prosthesis.[34]

Definitive Obturation

The primary prognostic indicator of either surgical or prosthetic reconstruction is a reasonable movement of the residual velopharyngeal mechanism during function.[47-50] Of particular importance is lateral pharyngeal wall movement to control nasal emission. Curtis and Beumer[34] outlined the guidelines for soft palate obturation as follows: (1) obturation should be located in the nasopharynx at the level of normal velopharyngeal closure; (2) inferior margin of the obturator should not extend below the lower level of muscular activity exhibited by the residual velopharyngeal mechanism; (3) superior margin of the obturator should not extend above the level of muscular activity; (4) inferior extension of the obturator usually is an extension of the palatal plane as extended to the posterior pharyngeal walls; and (5) oral side of the obturator should be concave to accommodate for tongue movement during swallowing. Special consideration should be given for the edentulous patients with soft palate defects. Because of a lack of retention, placement of osseointegrated implants may be advantageous. Two implants in the cuspid region provide adequate anterior-posterior spread, providing adequate retention for the soft palate obturator.[34]

Palatal Lift Prosthesis

A palatal lift prosthesis is fabricated for patients with velopharyngeal incompetence. Palatal incompetence occurs when patients with normal velopharyngeal structures lack movement to affect velopharyngeal closure. This occurs most often in patients who have some type of neurological disorder secondary to a cerebrovascular accident or a neurological disease such as myasthenia gravis or closed head injuries. The palatal lift displaces the soft palate to the level of normal palatal elevation to affect closure by pharyngeal wall action. In contrast, palatal insufficiency refers to patients with inadequate length of the soft palate to affect velopharyngeal closure; however, the remaining structures have normal movement. For palatal insufficiency, an obturator prosthesis is indicated.[34]

Intraoral Prostheses: Mandibular Defects

Rehabilitation of mandibular defects requires a multidisciplinary approach to successful rehabilitation. For many years patients with mandibular defects were known as the "forgotten patients." The use of free tissue transfers along with dental implants has made a dramatic effect on mandibular reconstruction (**Figs. 30.19** and **30.20**). The fibula is an ideal donor site because it has adequate bony support for the placement of dental implants and prosthetic rehabilitation. The goals of mandibular reconstruction—form and function—are met if the reconstructed mandible is positioned close to the original position of the native mandible. In addition, prosthetic rehabilitation is much easier to achieve if the bony support is properly positioned and contoured. This allows adequate intercuspation and occlusion of remaining teeth and a proper jaw relationship of the maxilla and mandible for prosthetic rehabilitation. This aids in proper positioning of the condyles within the temporomandibular joint, thus minimizing dysfunction. Anatomically, the position of the bone along the lower border

of the mandibular body and symphysis region is critical to success. Positioning the reconstructed bone along the lower border of the mandibular body complicates implant placement. The use of dental implants may result in a cantilever effect, particularly if the bony support is not of substantial size. Attention must be given to the peri-implant soft tissues for successful rehabilitation. It is preferred that the oral portion of the reconstructed mandible be surfaced with keratinized attached epithelium. This contributes to successful prosthetic rehabilitation with either a conventional removable partial or complete denture or an implant prosthesis.[13] Rehabilitation, hence, requires the efforts of both the reconstructive surgeon and the maxillofacial prosthodontist working in concert. Of late, the use of computer-aided surgical planning software (SurgiCase, Materialise Helm Court, Plymouth, Michigan, United States) along with the increased use of three-dimensional models has allowed better reconstruction outcomes. The use of this software allows the reconstruction of plates to be preformed before resection. It also allows the osteotomy cuts to be planned either with the three-dimensional model or with surgical planning software. The use of the prefabricated surgical guides and implant drill guides can be planned before resection. It is hoped that the end result is positioning of the reconstructed mandible in the proper maxillomandibular relationship to aid in prosthetic rehabilitation.

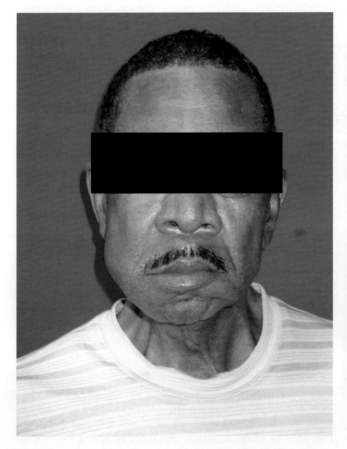

Figure 30.19 Mandibular reconstruction with fibula without prosthesis.

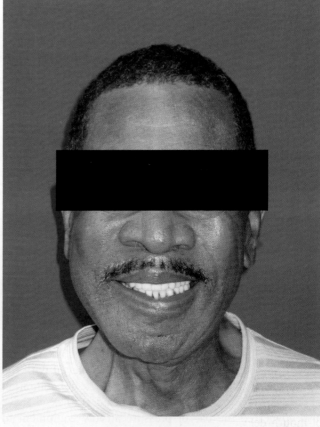

Figure 30.20 Mandibular reconstruction with fibula with prosthesis.

It is also possible to virtually plan not only the surgical reconstruction but also the dental implant placement (Materialise). Both immediate and delayed implant placements have been reported in the literature. Some advocate a delay of implant placement for 6 to 12 months with the use of an interim prosthesis. Their position is such that waiting for 6 to 12 months will allow more accurate positioning of the dental implants. Even with a delay approach, implant placement can be planned virtually, although a new computed tomography (CT) scan will be required. Often times, debulking may be required as well as the removal of a reconstruction plate.[13]

Surgical Modifications

Lateral Tongue-Mandible Defects

If the resection involves both the tongue and the mandible, reconstruction of the tongue is of higher importance. The tongue is the critical oral structure for speech, swallowing, mastication, and saliva control. The goal is to restore bulk and to maximize mobility of the remaining tongue. Even though the mandible may still have continuity, if the tongue is not reconstructed the patient will be severely disabled with respect to function.

If the mandible cannot be reconstructed, it is important that the condyle and remaining ascending ramus be removed for edentulous patients. Keeping this fragment prevents proper extension of the maxillary complete denture into the pterygomaxillary space, thus compromising retention and stability. If the resection includes a lateral portion of the mandible and the planned reconstruction includes a musculocutaneous flap with a reconstruction plate, it is vital that the posterior resection line should be made vertically from sigmoid notice to the angle rather than horizontally across the ramus. This allows relatively normal anatomic position.

Bony cuts should be made intraseptal, not interproximal, for dentulous portions of the mandible. The goal here is to try and maintain as much bone as possible for the tooth adjacent to the surgical defect, which helps it to be more desirable for a removable partial denture abutment. If oncologically sound, bony resections through the body of the mandible should be made as far posteriorly as possible. For edentulous patients, the more of the mandible that can be maintained the better the prosthetic prognosis. If mandibular continuity has been maintained or restored, usually dental implants are not necessary, if the patient's dentition is in a healthy state.

The greater the amount of tongue resected, the greater are the functional disabilities. It is preferable not to close the surgical defect primarily, which compounds the functional disabilities. In many situations, patients lack the ability to control their saliva, speak, and swallow or appear presentable.[13]

Anterior Mandible Floor-of-Mouth Defects

The primary goal for patients with anterior mandible floor-of-mouth defects is to restore mandibular continuity. The fibula is the preferred donor site. The use of dental implants aids in prosthetic rehabilitation. For these defects, the sensory and motor innervation of the tongue are largely not affected.[13]

Tonsil-Tongue-Soft Palate Defects

The radial forearm free flap has been used for these defects. Functional occlusal relationships are maintained and the use of dental implants for the edentulous patient aids in prosthetic rehabilitation with removable overlay dentures. An obturator prosthesis can be used to rehabilitate velopharyngeal defects. Most patients have normal speech, swallowing, and mastication. As outlined previously, the residual soft palate should not be tied to the flap if greater than one half of the soft palate is involved.[13]

Functional Outcomes

As a general rule, the degree to which deglutition, speech, and mastication are adversely affected depends on the extent of surgery, the method of closure, the affect of radiation and/or chemotherapy, and the extent of tongue involvement. If the defect is closed primarily, those patients experience the poorest functional outcomes. Patients whose tongue have been reconstructed with free flaps and have tongue bulks restore or patients who maintained mandibular continuity with little or no tongue involvement experience the least difficulty.

The integrity of the mandible; tooth-to-tooth stops or implant stops; support and retention of the dental prosthesis by tissue, teeth or implants, tongue, cheek, and perioral function; and radiation history influence masticatory efficiency.[13] Maintaining mandibular continuity optimizes function and esthetics. When mandibular continuity is not maintained, joint loading mandibular movement, occlusal contact time, and the angle of occlusal contact are altered.[51] The end result is that the remaining mandible has an altered path of rotation with the residual mandible shifting toward the defect side.[52] Mandibular movement and functional disability are influenced by numerous factors including the patient's level of depressive symptoms before surgery,[52] volume of hard and soft tissue removed,[54,55] whether radiation is used,[54,56] and the type of reconstruction completed.[57] However, Marunick et al[58] and Curtis et al[59] have shown that continuity of the mandible as an independent variable has an effect on masticatory function. The clinical findings of the significance of mandibular continuity are supported by the work of Hannam et al,[60,61] with modeling data of jaw biomechanics. Mandibular continuity should optimize the number of opposing tooth-to-tooth contacts. Helkimo et al[62,63] have shown a high correlation between the number of opposing tooth-to-tooth contacts and masticatory efficiency. Mandibular continuity increases the number of stable posterior occlusal contact, resulting in improved masticatory efficiency.[54,57,59]

Another factor affecting masticatory efficiency is the support and retention of the prosthesis. Schoen et al[64] reported that more than 50% of the patients with oral cancer who were edentulous were dissatisfied with their mandibular prosthesis and wore the prosthesis only a few hours each day. Roumanas et al[65] advocated placement of dental implants to improve retention, support, and stability of the prosthesis, hence an improvement in function. Garret et al[66] and Roumanas et al[65] reported that implant prostheses had an improvement in masticatory efficiency on the defect side. Both Roumanas et al[65] and Hundepool et al[67] found that rehabilitation of this patient population was limited because of patient deaths and complications, with only 25% of the patients benefited from dental implant rehabilitation.

The tongue can aid in the stabilization of mandibular prosthesis. Several reports found that tongue mobility, volume, and sensation were indicators of masticatory efficiency.[57,68,69] It has also been shown that an independent surgical management radiation therapy adversely affects masticatory efficiency.[13,54,56] The direct effects of radiation and the side effects of xerostomia make wearing a prosthesis difficult. The most common patient concerns following radiation alone was oral dryness, pain, lack of taste, and diminished appetite.[54] Following surgery, patient complaints included difficulty in eating, swallowing, and chewing or disfigurement.[70] It has been reported by Garret et al[71] that a patient's perception of chewing ability is influenced by comfort, rather than objective measures of chewing performance. Both radiation and surgery have an additive negative affect on function as reported by Bozec et al.[54]

Extraoral Prostheses

A facial prosthesis restores anatomy, soft tissue contour, appearance, and function after surgical resection of a tumor. It may replace an ear, orbit, nose, or combination of facial components that are missing because of surgery. A prosthesis may serve as an interim measure until reconstructive surgery is performed or as a definitive restoration. In some cases, it may be the only option for rehabilitation.

The ideal facial prosthesis should be undetectable in public. Its color, texture, form, and translucency must duplicate that of the missing structures and adjacent skin. A conspicuous prosthesis will increase patient anxiety and will compromise social readjustment. The final esthetic result is the most important factor relative to clinical success or failure.[72]

Pathology

Malignant neoplasms of the face are often derived from the epithelium, the most common being basal cell and squamous cell carcinomas. Basal cell carcinomas arise from basal keratinocytes and are the most common form of skin cancer, often associated with overexposure to UV light or the sun. While they are regarded as noninvasive, they do have the potential for aggressive behavior characterized by extension into adjacent and underlying soft and hard tissues. They do not typically metastasize but are considered locally aggressive with the potential for persistent growth and recurrence. In most cases, local excision is the preferred treatment. In some instances, the Mohs technique of excision may be used.[73] Squamous cell carcinomas of skin are true

malignancies with significant growth potential and invasion into underlying muscle, bone, and cartilage. These tumors also have a propensity to metastasize to regional lymph nodes. Their treatment is often more aggressive than that of basal cell tumors because of this metastatic factor. Squamous cell lesions may also originate in hard or soft tissues and erode into the overlying facial skin. Because of their invasive and metastatic nature, squamous cell lesions are often treated with a combination of surgery and radiation therapy. In advanced cases, chemotherapy may also be part of the treatment.

Malignant melanoma is a more aggressive type of skin cancer. It originates in melanocytes, the pigment-producing cells of the skin. Melanin pigment shields and protects the skin from the effects of solar irradiation. The benign type of this tumor, a nevus, is self-limiting in its growth. Malignant melanoma proliferates and invades with the potential for hematogenous spread. Although it is a less common type of skin cancer, it causes the majority of skin cancer-related deaths. Because of its aggressive nature, treatment often includes surgical removal in addition to chemotherapy, immunotherapy, and/or radiation therapy.

Surgical Reconstruction versus Prosthetic Rehabilitation

The decision between surgical reconstruction of a facial defect and a prosthetic restoration should be made based on several general guidelines while taking into consideration the specifics of each case. The natural history of the tumor, the size and location of the defect, the quantity and quality of available tissue, the patient's age and physical and mental health, as well as their personal wishes regarding reconstructive surgery should be considered. As a rule, it is difficult for the surgeon to reconstruct a facial part that is as cosmetic as a well-made prosthesis, or in as little time (**Fig. 30.21**). However, a surgical reconstruction does result in a natural, permanent outcome that does not require the maintenance or commitment to care of prosthesis.

Smaller defects are more amenable to surgical reconstruction alone. The larger the defect, the more challenging and unpredictable the surgical outcome may be. Defects of all or a portion of the auricle may be amenable to surgical reconstruction, but quality of the soft tissue at the defect and donor sites must be considered. Autogenous reconstruction of an auricle is much more common for a congenital deformity than a tumor resection, particularly if the area has been irradiated. Nasal reconstruction with a forehead, cheek, or free flap is more common in cases of tumor, but these often require multiple procedures over a period of time.

It is, of course, impossible to surgically reconstruct the entire orbit and eye. In the best-case scenario, an ocular prosthesis may be used after successful surgery to create a brow, socket, lids, and adequate fornices—a considerable challenge for even the most talented reconstructive surgeon. More commonly, surgery may decrease the size of a large orbital defect by augmenting missing soft tissue in the

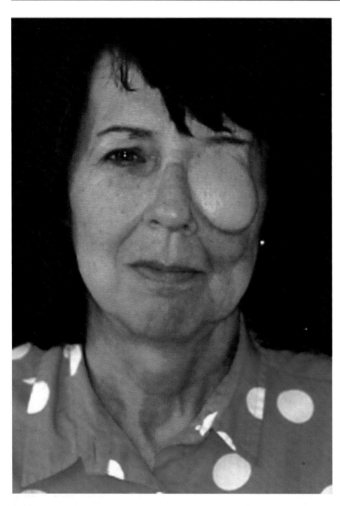

Figure 30.21 Reconstructive flap obliterates orbital defect and prevents prosthesis.

malar/infraorbital area or close off the orbital defect from the nasal cavity to improve hygiene and outcome of an orbital prosthesis. If a flap is used for this purpose, it must not be too bulky or it will interfere with an esthetic prosthetic result.

Whether reconstructive surgery is used alone or to augment a planned prosthesis, not only must the quality of the tissue at the defect site be considered but also the quality of local vascularity. If the reconstructive site was irradiated, this may compromise the blood supply in the area and may result in a poor surgical outcome. Beumer et al[74] cited several conditions that favor prosthetic restoration over surgical reconstruction:

- When a large resection is necessary and recurrence of tumor is likely, it is advantageous to be able to monitor the surgical site closely. A prosthesis permits such observation, whereas primary surgical reconstruction makes this more difficult.
- Surgical restoration of large defects is technically difficult and requires multiple procedures and hospitalizations. Patients confronted with this type of defect may be medically compromised and less able or willing to tolerate the multiple procedures required for surgical reconstruction.

- Even when surgical reconstruction is possible, many surgeons prefer to wait at least 1 year after a large tumor resection before considering surgical reconstruction of a facial defect resulting from a malignant tumor. Therefore, an interim prosthesis may be fabricated during this interval.

A final consideration is that many of the patients who undergo oncologic resections are older and may already be in compromised health. They may not be physically or mentally prepared for the rigors of reconstructive surgery, the lengthy anesthesia, or the time required to recover from these procedures. In these cases, especially if the defect is large, a well-made facial prosthesis is the treatment of choice.

Preoperative Evaluation and Planning

Prosthetic rehabilitation after tumor surgery requires a team approach. It is imperative for members of the surgical and prosthetic teams to work together to ensure an optimal outcome. The maxillofacial prosthodontist should see the patient before surgery. At this visit, the patient and family members have an opportunity to learn more about a facial prosthesis including its purpose, how it is made and attached, timing of treatment, and its limitations as well as to see examples. Most patients are completely unaware of the prosthetic treatment option or have incorrect or incomplete information about a facial prosthesis.

In addition to providing information about the prosthesis to the patient, during this initial visit presurgical records may be made. These may include two-dimensional and/or three-dimensional photographs or a facial moulage, if necessary. These will be useful during the design and fabrication phases of the prosthesis and the planning for placement of osseointegrated implants, if applicable. These records may also be used by the surgeon and the prosthodontist to plan the surgery and the design of the ideal defect with respect to the planned prosthesis.

Tumor Treatment and Idealization of the Defect

Because of the aggressive nature of tumors that affect the face, surgery is most often the treatment of choice. Depending on the histology, size, and extent of the tumor, radiation therapy with or without chemotherapy may also be part of the treatment. The first goal of surgery is to obtain adequate margins around the tumor, but then the surgeon should turn attention to the defect.

Firm, immobile skin at the defect site is ideal. For an auricular prosthesis, it is preferable to save the tragus or a portion of the conchal bowl. Leaving a portion of the helix may be problematic as the remnant tends to move away from the cranial base and project further than the auricle on the opposite side. In most cases, a complete resection of the external ear will yield a preferred site on which to place an auricular prosthesis (**Fig. 30.22**).

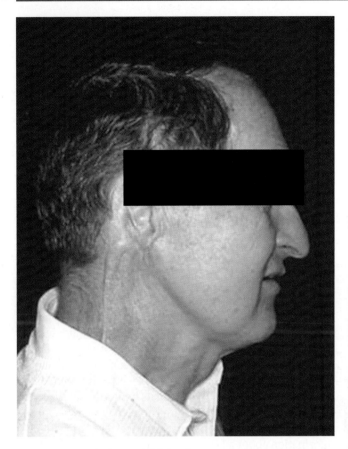

Figure 30.22   Ideal auricular defect.

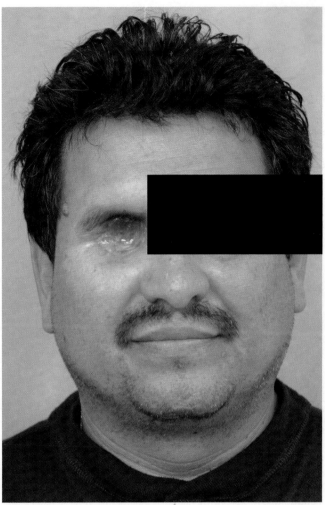

Figure 30.23   Ideal orbital defect.

The ideal orbital defect is one which follows the outline of the bony orbital rim and leaves the brow intact and in position. There must be adequate depth to the defect to allow for an ideal position of the ocular portion of the orbital prosthesis. The ocular piece should be in the same frontal plane as the unaffected eye to allow for balance and symmetry of the orbital prosthesis. A layer of soft tissue separating the nasal and oral cavities from the orbital defect not only makes for a more hygienic condition but also simplifies impression making and fabrication of the orbital prosthesis (**Fig. 30.23**).

As with the resection of the auricle, residual soft tissue remnants may likewise contribute to a less esthetic nasal prosthesis. If soft tissue in the alar region is retained, it must be overlaid by the prosthesis, making it appear excessively wide. Otherwise the margin of the prosthesis may have to be placed in a more prominent and noticeable position at or near the midsagittal line of the nose (**Fig. 30.24**). As with the orbital defect, closing off any communication between the nasal and oral cavities will improve hygiene for the patient as well as assist in eating and speaking.

Osseointegrated Implants

Facial prostheses have, in the past, been retained by skin adhesives. These held relatively well but always had the potential to weaken and come loose while the patient was wearing the prosthesis in public. Aside from this retention issue, adhesive-retained facial prostheses pose several other problems as well.

Adhesives may be messy and time-consuming to apply and remove; they may cause skin irritation (especially if the site has been irradiated); they may make the proper positioning of the prosthesis difficult; and they may compromise the marginal integrity, esthetics, and longevity of the prosthesis because of the need to clean this area of the adhesive on a daily basis. The margins or edges of the prosthesis are more liable to tear during cleaning. This will require repair or remake of the prosthesis and one that has thicker margins for tear resistance that will be less esthetic.

In 1985, Tjellström et al[75] introduced the use of osseointegrated implants to retain facial prostheses. This procedure evolved from the original work of Brånemark et al,[76] who pioneered the use of osseointegrated implants to retain oral prostheses. The use of these titanium implants to retain facial prostheses was approved in the United States by the Food and Drug Administration in 1995.[77] While requiring one or two surgical procedures to place and expose the implants, these may be performed on an outpatient basis under local

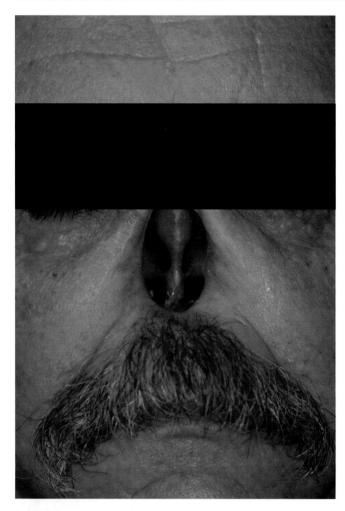

Figure 30.24 Ideal nasal defect.

anesthesia or sedation. There are very few contraindications to performing this procedure; however, consideration should be given to the ability of a patient or caregiver to perform daily skin hygiene procedures around the implants and retention components to which they are attached and to come in for periodic follow-up visits to check the health of the skin, the implants, and the condition of the prosthesis.

By eliminating the use of adhesive, placement and removal of the prosthesis are much easier and faster. There is no need to clean adhesive from the prosthesis, so the edges remain intact with less wear and tear on the prosthesis and thus its longevity is extended. The marginal edges may be made thinner to blend with the surrounding natural skin so the prosthesis is more esthetic. Accurate positioning of the prosthesis each time it is placed is assured by the guiding effect of the retentive elements connected to the implants and those reciprocating ones incorporated within the prosthesis. The implant-retained facial prosthesis is actually more retentive when compared with adhesive retention.[76] The introduction of osseointegrated implants to retain facial prostheses has actually changed patient perceptions about facial prostheses because of the effectiveness of retention and the improved esthetic results.[79,80]

Implants are most often placed after completion of all tumor therapy, but some report placing them at the time as the tumor resection surgery.[81] Another area of controversy exists regarding the placement of implants in irradiated bone. Opinions vary widely from never placing them in a field that has been irradiated to placement in irradiated bone with or without the use of hyperbaric oxygen therapy. Some surgeons believe that a compromised vascular bed and implant survival will be improved with the use of hyperbaric oxygen therapy,[82–85] while others[86,87] disagree with its use because it is costly, time-consuming, and unnecessary. This latter group argues that there are no randomized clinical trials to support its use in these situations.

The implant positions should be preplanned to ensure that at the skin level, they lie within the confines of the prosthesis so as not to compromise the ideal shape and esthetic outcome. There are few things more frustrating than healthy, stable osseointegrated implants that are so poorly positioned as to be unusable. The use of a surgical guide is necessary to this end. This may be accomplished in a variety of ways. Reisberg and Habakuk[88]and Wolfaardt et al[89] have described traditional techniques for the fabrication of such a guide. A more recent technique incorporates digital technology.

A cone-beam CT scan (i-CAT Imaging Sciences International, Hatfield, Philadelphia, United States) of the head and neck is taken along with a three-dimensional digital photograph. The photograph of the facial defect is overlaid onto the radiograph. A photograph of the facial portion that is missing is overlaid onto the 3-day scan. If a presurgical 3-day photograph was taken, this may be used to extract the portion of the face that is now missing. If not, then a postoperative 3-day photograph may be used and the unaffected auricle or orbit may be extracted, reversed, and overlaid onto the scan. In the case of a nasal tumor, either a presurgical photograph is used or a nose from another individual's 3-day photograph may be imported onto the radiograph.

Digital implants are imported and placed into the available bone with the defect, with consideration given to the ideal contour of the imported ear, orbit, or nose so that they will not interfere with the contour of the planned prosthesis. A three-dimensional resin model of the defect along with a fitted resin surgical guide with access holes indicating the desired position of the implants are generated via stereolithography. The surgical guide may be borne on either bone or skin. The stability and intimate fit of the guide on bone versus skin makes it the preferred method. For an auricular prosthesis, two to three implants are placed in the temporal bone (**Fig. 30.25**). For an orbital, usually three to four implants are placed along the superior and lateral orbital rims. Implants may be placed along the inferior rim as well, but this may create a technical problem for prosthesis fabrication and path of insertion (**Fig. 30.26**). For a nasal prosthesis, two to three implants are placed at the inferior aspect of the defect at the base of the nose (**Fig. 30.27**). Rarely, a single implant may also be placed at

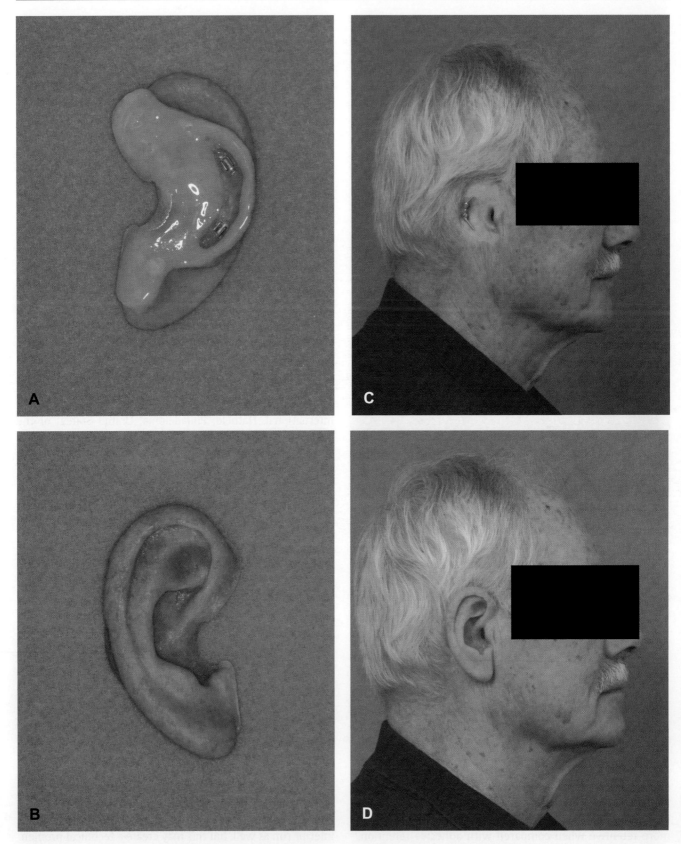

Figure 30.25 (A) Auricular prosthesis, finished surface; note clips for retention to bar. (B) Auricular prosthesis, tissue side. (C) Auricular defect; note retaining bar. (D) Implant-retained auricular prosthesis in position. (*Prosthesis made by Rosemary Seelaus.*)

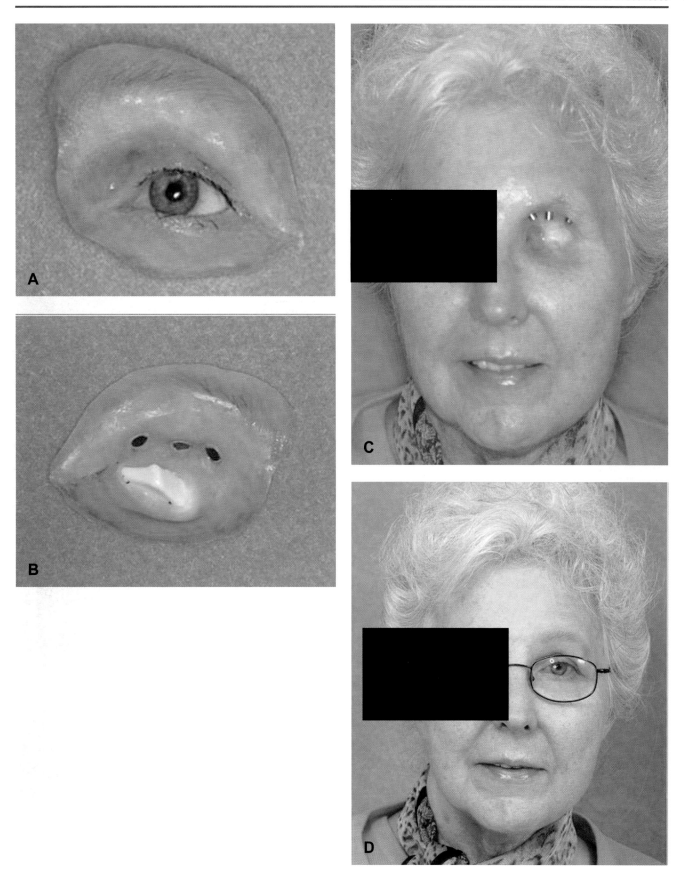

Figure 30.26   (A) Orbital prosthesis, finished surface; note ocular portion, eyebrow, eyelashes. (B) Orbital prosthesis, tissue surface; note magnets for retention. (C) Orbital defect; note magnets attached to implants. (D) Implant-retained orbital prosthesis in position. (*Prosthesis made by Camille Rea.*)

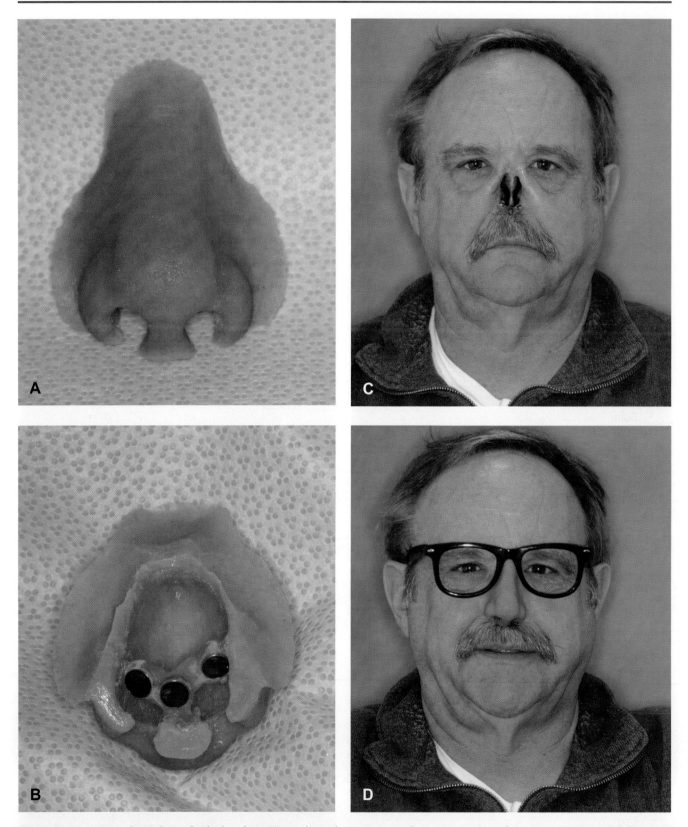

Figure 30.27 (A) Nasal prosthesis, finished surface. (B) Nasal prosthesis, tissue surface; note magnets for retention. (C) Nasal defect; note magnets attached to implants. (D) Implant-retained nasal prosthesis in position. (*Prosthesis made by Camille Rea.*)

the superior aspect of the defect but often the position of the frontal sinus prevents this.

The technique for site preparation and placement of the implants has been well documented.[90] Using the openings on the guide, the positions for the implants are marked on the bone with an electrocautery tip or straight fissure bur. Each site is prepared to proper depth with a round guide drill. Then the site is widened with a drill countersink, and the implant is placed, first with a handpiece set at a slow speed so as not to overheat the bone and then hand tightened to place with a torque driver.

In most cases, cover screws are placed in the threaded access openings on top of the implants and the soft tissue is closed over them. After 3 to 6 months of healing while osseointegration occurs where the bone chemically bonds to the implant surface, the implants are uncovered through the skin and prosthesis fabrication begins. Various systems may be connected to the implants to achieve retention and stability of the prosthesis. These may use a bar-clip, magnetic, or male-female snap connector or some combinations of these.[91] The fabrication of the prosthesis involves several visits. The basic steps include

- Impression making.
- Sculpting a wax prototype and fitting on the patient.
- Color matching to the skin.
- Processing the final wax prototype in medical grade silicone elastomer.
- Fitting the prosthesis on the patient and instructing on skin hygiene and prosthesis maintenance.
- Follow-up visits every 6 to 12 months.

The restoration of a facial defect after tumor resection is a challenge for both the patient and the treatment team.

Tips to Avoid Complications

- The maxillofacial prosthodontist evaluates the patient before surgery.
- Surgical and prosthetic treatment plans are coordinated to ensure that the outcome provides maximum benefit to the patient.

Clinical Pearls

- Oral and facial prostheses restore function, esthetics, and quality of life.
- Prosthetic rehabilitation should be considered as part of the overall treatment plan in the management of patients with head and neck cancer.
- A maxillofacial prosthodontist is part of the head and neck cancer team.

There are physical and psychological issues with which to deal, beginning with the patient's very real concern for survival. Although prosthetic rehabilitation may not be an ideal restoration for all facial defects, it should be considered a reasonable treatment option in this process and an important step in restoring a quality of life to the patient with head and neck cancer.

References

1. Jemal A, Siegel R, Ward E, et al. Cancer statistics, 2008. CA Cancer J Clin 2008;58(2):71–96
2. Curtis TA, Beumer J. Restoration of acquired hard palate defects: etiology, disability, and rehabilitation. In: Beumer J, Curtis Ta, Marunick MT, eds. Maxillofacial Rehabilitation Prosthodontic and Surgical Considerations. St. Louis, MO: Ishiyaku EuroAmerica, Inc; 1996:225–286
3. Garrett N. 2008. Outcomes of maxillectomies with conventional and implant restorations. Paper presented at: International Congress on Maxillofacial Rehabilitation; September 24–27, 2008; Bangkok, Thailand
4. Rieger J, Wolfaardt J, Seikaly H, Jha N. Speech outcomes in patients rehabilitated with maxillary obturator prostheses after maxillectomy: a prospective study. Int J Prosthodont 2002;15(2):139–144
5. Rogers SN, Lowe D, McNally D, Brown JS, Vaughan ED. Health-related quality of life after maxillectomy: a comparison between prosthetic obturation and free flap. J Oral Maxillofac Surg 2003;61(2):174–181
6. Jaquiéry C, Rohner D, Kunz C, et al. Reconstruction of maxillary and mandibular defects using prefabricated microvascular fibular grafts and osseointegrated dental implants—a prospective study. Clin Oral Implants Res 2004;15(5):598–606
7. Okay DJ, Genden E, Buchbinder D, Urken M. Prosthodontic guidelines for surgical reconstruction of the maxilla: a classification system of defects. J Prosthet Dent 2001;86(4):352–363
8. Rohner D, Kunz C, Bucher P, Hammer B, Prein J. [New possibilities for reconstructing extensive jaw defects with prefabricated microvascular fibula transplants and ITI implants]. Mund Kiefer Gesichtschir 2000;4(6):365–372
9. Rohner D, Jaquiéry C, Kunz C, Bucher P, Maas H, Hammer B. Maxillofacial reconstruction with prefabricated osseous free flaps: a 3-year experience with 24 patients. Plast Reconstr Surg 2003;112(3):748–757
10. Santamaria E, Cordeiro PG. Reconstruction of maxillectomy and midfacial defects with free tissue transfer. J Surg Oncol 2006;94(6):522–531
11. Schmidt BL, Pogrel MA, Young CW, Sharma A. Reconstruction of extensive maxillary defects using zygomaticus implants. J Oral Maxillofac Surg 2004;62(9 Suppl 2)82–89
12. Smolka W, Iizuka T. Surgical reconstruction of maxilla and midface: clinical outcome and factors relating to postoperative complications. J Craniomaxillofac Surg 2005;33(1):1–7
13. Beumer J, Marunick MT, Curtis TA, Roumanas E. Acquired defects of the mandible: etiology, treatment, and rehabilitation. In: Beumer J, Curtis TA, Marunick MT, eds. Maxillofacial Rehabilitation Prosthodontic and Surgical Considerations. St. Louis, MO: Ishiyaku EuroAmerica, Inc; 1996:113–224
14. Beumer J, Tsun M, Marunick MT, Roumanas E, Nishimura R. Restoration of facial defects: etiology, disability, and rehabilitation. In: Beumer J, Curtis TA, Marunick MT, eds. Maxillofacial Rehabilitation Prosthodontic and Surgical Considerations. St. Louis, MO: Ishiyaku EuroAmerica, Inc; 1996:377–454

15. Reisberg DJ, Lipner M. Audiometric evaluation of prosthetic ears: a preliminary report. J Prosthet Dent 1993;69(2):196–199

16. Plank DM, Weinberg B, Chalian VA. Evaluation of speech following prosthetic obturation of surgically acquired maxillary defects. J Prosthet Dent 1981;45(6):626–638

17. Sullivan M, Gaebler C, Beukelman D, et al. Impact of palatal prosthodontic intervention on communication performance of patients' maxillectomy defects: a multilevel outcome study. Head Neck 2002;24(6):530–538

18. Matsui Y, Ohno K, Shirota T, Imai S, Yamashita Y, Michi K-I. Speech function following maxillectomy reconstructed by rectus abdominis myocutaneous flap. J Craniomaxillofac Surg 1995;23(3):160–164

19. Schwartz H, Wollinn M, Leak D, et al. Interface radiation dosimetry in mandibular reconstruction. Arch Otolaryngol 1979;105:293

20. Mian TA, Van Putten MC, Kramer DC, et al. Backscatter radiation at bone litanium interface from high energy X and gamma rays. Int J Radiat Oncol Biol Phys 1987;13:1943

21. Roumanas ED, Nishimura RD, Davis BK, Beumer J III. Clinical evaluation of implants retaining edentulous maxillary obturator prostheses. J Prosthet Dent 1997;77(2):184–190

22. Hoshaw SJ, Brunski JB, Cochran GVB. Mechanical loading of Brånemark implants affects interfacial bone modeling and remodeling. Int J Oral Maxillofac Implants 1994;9:345–360

23. Miyata T, Kobayashi Y, Araki H, Ohto T, Shin K. The influence of controlled occlusal overload on peri-implant tissue. Part 3: A histologic study in monkeys. Int J Oral Maxillofac Implants 2000;15(3):425–431

24. Miyamoto Y, Koretake K, Hirata M, Kubo T, Akagawa Y. Influence of static overload on the bony interface around implants in dogs. Int J Prosthodont 2008;21(5):437–444

25. Davis B, Roumanas E, Hong S, Nishimura R. Stress distributions of implants used for retention of maxillary obturators. In: Zlotolow I, Esposit S, Beumer J, eds. Proceedings of the 1st International Congress on Maxillofacial Prosthetics. Seoul, Korea: Shin Jin; 1995:204–208

26. Landes CA, Paffrath C, Koehler C, et al. Zygoma implants for midfacial prosthetic rehabilitation using telescopes: 9-year follow-up. Int J Prosthodont 2009;22(1):20–32

27. Matsuyama M, Tsukiyama Y, Tomioka M, Koyano K. Clinical assessment of chewing function of obturator prosthesis wearers by objective measurement of masticatory performance and maximum occlusal force. Int J Prosthodont 2006;19(3):253–257

28. Koyama M, Inaba S, Yokoyama K. Quest for ideal occlusal patterns for complete dentures. J Prosthet Dent 1976;35(6):620–623

29. Watson RM, Gray BJ. Assessing effective obturation. J Prosthet Dent 1985;54(1):88–93

30. Minsley GE, Warren DW, Hinton V. Physiologic responses to maxillary resection and subsequent obturation. J Prosthet Dent 1987;57(3):338–344

31. Warren DW. Restorative treatment of the dentofacial complex. Proceedings of the Workshop on Speech and the Dentofacial Complex: The State of the Art; 1970:132. ASHA Reports #5

32. Bradley DP. Congenital and acquired palatopharyngeal insufficiency. Speech Hearing Dis 1966;31:362–369

33. Kornblith AB, Zlotolow IM, Gooen J, et al. Quality of life of maxillectomy patients using an obturator prosthesis. Head Neck 1996;18(4):323–334

34. Curtis TA, Beumer J. Speech, velopharyngeal function, and restoration of soft palate defects. In: Beumer J, Curtis TA, Marunick MT, eds. Maxillofacial Rehabilitation Prosthodontic and Surgical Considerations. St. Louis, MO: Ishiyaku EuroAmerica, Inc; 1996:285–330

35. Subtelny JD, Worth JH, Sakuda M. Intraoral pressure and rate of flow during speech. J Speech Hear Res 1966;9:498–518

36. Shelton RL, Lindquist AF, Arndt WB, Elbert MA, Youngstrom KA. Effect of speech bulb reduction on movement of the posterior wall of the pharynx and posture of the tongue. Cleft Palate J 1971;8:10–17

37. Shelton RL, Lindquist AF, Knox AW, et al. The relationship between pharyngeal wall movements and exchangeable speech appliance sections. Cleft Palate J 1971;8:145–158

38. Warren DW, Ryon WE. Oral port constriction, nasal resistance, and respiratory aspects of cleft palate speech: an analog study. Cleft Palate J 1967;4:38–46

39. Rahn AO, Boucher LJ. Maxillofacial Prosthetics. Philadelphia, PA: WB Saunders; 1970

40. Rieger JM, Zalmanowitz JG, Li SY, et al. Speech outcomes after soft palate reconstruction with the soft palate insufficiency repair procedure. Head Neck 2008;30(11):1439–1444

41. Seikaly H, Rieger JM, Zalmanowitz JG, et al. Functional soft palate reconstruction: a comprehensive surgical approach. Head Neck 2008;30(12):1615–1623

42. Zlotolow I. Restoration of the acquired soft palate deformity with surgical resection and reconstruction. In: Zlotolow I, Esposito S, Beumer J, eds. Proceedings of the 1st International Congress on Maxillofacial Prosthetics. Seoul, Korea: Shin Jin; 1995:49–55

43. Rieger JM, Zalmanowitz JG, Wolfaardt JF. Nasopharyngoscopy in palatopharyngeal prosthetic rehabilitation: a preliminary report. Int J Prosthodont 2006;19(4):383–388

44. La Velle WE, Hardy JC. Palatal lift prostheses for treatment of palatopharyngeal incompetence. J Prosthet Dent 1979;42(3):308–315

45. Reisberg DJ, Smith BE. Aerodynamic assessment of prosthetic speech aids. J Prosthet Dent 1985;54(5):686–690

46. Minsley GE, Warren DW, Hairfield WM. The effect of cleft palate speech aid prostheses on the nasopharyngeal airway and breathing. J Prosthet Dent 1991;65(1):122–126

47. Mazaheri M, Millard RT. Changes in nasal resonance related to differences in location and dimension of speech bulbs. Cleft Palate J 1965;31:167–175

48. Rosen MS, Bzoch KR. The prosthetic speech appliance in rehabilitation of patients with cleft palate. J Am Dent Assoc 1958;57(2):203–210

49. Harkins CS, Harkins WR, Harkins JF. Principles of Cleft Palate Prosthesis. New York, NY: Columbia University Press; 1960

50. Terkla LC, Laney WR. Partial Dentures. St. Louis, MO: Mosby; 1963

51. Curtis DA, Plesh O, Hannam AG, Sharma A, Curtis TA. Modeling of jaw biomechanics in the reconstructed mandibulectomy patient. J Prosthet Dent 1999;81(2):167–173

52. Beumer J III, Curtis T, Harrison RE. Radiation therapy of the oral cavity: sequelae and management, part 2. Head Neck Surg 1979;1(5):392–408

53. de Graeff A, de Leeuw JR, Ros WJ, Hordijk GJ, Blijham GH, Winnubst JA. Pretreatment factors predicting quality of life after treatment for head and neck cancer. Head Neck 2000;22(4):398–407

54. Bozec A, Poissonnet G, Chamorey E, et al. Free-flap head and neck reconstruction and quality of life: a 2-year prospective study. Laryngoscope 2008;118(5):874–880

55. Marunick M, Mathes BE, Klein BB, Seyedsadr M. Occlusal force after partial mandibular resection. J Prosthet Dent 1992;67(6):835–838

56. Epstein JB, Emerton S, Kolbinson DA, et al. Quality of life and oral function following radiotherapy for head and neck cancer. Head Neck 1999;21(1):1–11

57. Urken ML, Buchbinder D, Weinberg H, et al. Functional evaluation following microvascular oromandibular reconstruction of the oral cancer patient: a comparative study of reconstructed and nonreconstructed patients. Laryngoscope 1991;101(9):935–950

58. Marunick MT, Mathes BE, Klein BB. Masticatory function in hemimandibulectomy patients. J Oral Rehabil 1992;19(3):289–295

59. Curtis DA, Plesh O, Miller AJ, et al. A comparison of masticatory function in patients with or without reconstruction of the mandible. Head Neck 1997;19(4):287–296

60. Hannam AG, Stavness I, Lloyd JE, Fels S. A dynamic model of jaw and hyoid biomechanics during chewing. J Biomech 2008;41(5):1069–1076

61. Hannam AG, Stavness IK, Lloyd JE, Fels SS, Miller AJ, Curtis DA. A comparison of simulated jaw dynamics in models of segmental mandibular resection versus resection with alloplastic reconstruction. J Prosthet Dent 2010;104(3):191–198

62. Helkimo E, Carlsson GE, Helkimo M. Bite force and state of dentition. Acta Odontol Scand 1977;35(6):297–303

63. Helkimo E, Carlsson GE, Helkimo M. Chewing efficiency and state of dentition. A methodologic study. Acta Odontol Scand 1978;36(1):33–41

64. Schoen PJ, Raghoebar GM, Bouma J, et al. Prosthodontic rehabilitation of oral function in head-neck cancer patients with dental implants placed simultaneously during ablative tumour surgery: an assessment of treatment outcomes and quality of life. Int J Oral Maxillofac Surg 2008;37(1):8–16

65. Roumanas ED, Garrett N, Blackwell KE, et al. Masticatory and swallowing threshold performances with conventional and implant-supported prostheses after mandibular fibula free-flap reconstruction. J Prosthet Dent 2006;96(4):289–297

66. Garrett N, Roumanas ED, Blackwell KE, et al. Efficacy of conventional and implant-supported mandibular resection prostheses: study overview and treatment outcomes. J Prosthet Dent 2006;96(1):13–24

67. Hundepool AC, Dumans AG, Hofer SO, et al. Rehabilitation after mandibular reconstruction with fibula free-flap: clinical outcome and quality of life assessment. Int J Oral Maxillofac Surg 2008;37(11):1009–1013

68. McConnel FM, Teichgraeber JF, Adler RK. A comparison of three methods of oral reconstruction. Arch Otolaryngol Head Neck Surg 1987;113(5):496–500

69. Kapur K, Garrett N, Fischer E. Effects of anaesthesia of human oral structures on masticatory performance and food particle size distribution. Arch Oral Biol 1990;35(5):397–403

70. Langius A, Lind MG. Well-being and coping in oral and pharyngeal cancer patients. Eur J Cancer B Oral Oncol 1995;31B(4):242–249

71. Garrett NR, Kapur KK, Perez P. Effects of improvements of poorly fitting dentures and new dentures on patient satisfaction. J Prosthet Dent 1996;76(4):403–413

72. Anderson JD, Szalai JP. The Toronto outcome measure for craniofacial prosthetics: a condition-specific quality-of-life instrument. Int J Oral Maxillofac Implants 2003;18(4):531–538

73. Mohs FE. Chemosurgery for the microscopically controlled excision of cutaneous cancer. Head Neck Surg 1978;1(2):150–166

74. Beumer J, Curtis TA, Marunick MT, eds. Maxillofacial Rehabilitation, Prosthodontic and Surgical Considerations. St. Louis, MO: Ishiyaku EuroAmerica, Inc ; 1996

75. Tjellström A, Yontchev E, Lindström J, Brånemark P-I. Five years' experience with bone-anchored auricular prostheses. Otolaryngol Head Neck Surg 1985;93(3):366–372

76. Brånemark PI, Hansson BO, Adell R, et al. Osseointegrated implants in the treatment of the edentulous jaw. Experience from a 10-year period. Scand J Plast Reconstr Surg Suppl 1977;16:1–132

77. Tolman DE, Taylor PF. Bone-anchored craniofacial prosthesis study. Int J Oral Maxillofac Implants 1996;11(2):159–168

78. Del Valle V, Faulkner G, Wolfaardt J, Rangert B, Tan HK. Mechanical evaluation of craniofacial osseointegration retention systems. Int J Oral Maxillofac Implants 1995;10(4):491–498

79. Markt JC, Lemon JC. Extraoral maxillofacial prosthetic rehabilitation at the M. D. Anderson Cancer Center: a survey of patient attitudes and opinions. J Prosthet Dent 2001;85(6):608–613

80. Chang TL, Garrett N, Roumanas E, Beumer J III. Treatment satisfaction with facial prostheses. J Prosthet Dent 2005;94(3):275–280

81. Flood TR, Russell K. Reconstruction of nasal defects with implant-retained nasal prostheses. Br J Oral Maxillofac Surg 1998;36(5):341–345

82. Marx RE. A new concept in the treatment of osteoradionecrosis. J Oral Maxillofac Surg 1983;41(6):351–357

83. Marx RE. Osteoradionecrosis: a new concept of its pathophysiology. J Oral Maxillofac Surg 1983;41(5):283–288

84. Granström G. Placement of dental implants in irradiated bone: the case for using hyperbaric oxygen. J Oral Maxillofac Surg 2006;64(5):812–818

85. Granström G. Osseointegration in irradiated cancer patients: an analysis with respect to implant failures. J Oral Maxillofac Surg 2005;63(5):579–585

86. Franzén L, Rosenquist JB, Rosenquist KI, Gustafsson I. Oral implant rehabilitation of patients with oral malignancies treated with radiotherapy and surgery without adjunctive hyperbaric oxygen. Int J Oral Maxillofac Implants 1995;10(2):183–187

87. Keller EE. Placement of dental implants in the irradiated mandible: a protocol without adjunctive hyperbaric oxygen. J Oral Maxillofac Surg 1997;55(9):972–980

88. Reisberg DJ, Habakuk SW. Use of a surgical positioner for bone-anchored facial prostheses. Int J Oral Maxillofac Implants 1997;12(3):376–379

89. Wolfaardt JF, Troppmann R, Wilkes GH, Coss P. Surgical templates for auricular reconstruction. J Facial Somato Prosthet 1996;2:131–136

90. Tjellström A. Osseointegrated implants for replacement of absent or defective ears. Clin Plast Surg 1990;17(2):355–366

91. Rubenstein JE. Attachments used for implant-supported facial prostheses: a survey of United States, Canadian, and Swedish centers. J Prosthet Dent 1995;73(3):262–266

SECTION II: Emerging Technologies and Therapeutics in Head and Neck Oncology

31 Computer Planning and Intraoperative Navigation for Head and Neck Cancer

Michael R. Markiewicz and R. Bryan Bell

Core Messages

- Virtual surgical planning is useful as an educational and teaching instrument by allowing three-dimensional analysis of the clinical problem and visualization of idealized digital manipulations. Without the ability to transfer the virtual plan into reality, however, it remains just that: an educational tool.

- The incorporation of computer-aided design and computer-aided modeling technology into the head and neck workflow process facilitates transfer of the virtual plan into reality and theoretically has a positive effect on functional and esthetic treatment outcomes, reduced operating times, and improved quality.

- Computer planning and intraoperative navigation (computer-aided surgical simulation) may add safety and predictability during extirpative and reconstructive surgery of the head and neck.

The age of virtual surgery made its clinical debut in the early 1990s with the use of frameless stereotaxy, or intraoperative navigation. Intraoperative navigation was initially developed for medical purposes as an aid to performing safe neurosurgical and endoscopic sinus surgical procedures.[1-5] Recently, its use has been expanded to a variety of anatomic regions and it is now used to improve accuracy and predictability in reconstructive head and neck/craniomaxillofacial surgery, including complex orbital repair,[6] head and neck oncologic surgery,[7-9] and craniofacial surgery.[10] Intraoperative navigation offers the advantage of three dimensional (3D) visualization of the patient's anatomy and access to areas of the facial skeleton that once required larger incisions and increased hard tissue exposure. Modern navigation systems allow precise location of anatomic landmarks or implants with a margin of error of 1 to 2 mm when compared with the projected computer tomography (CT) in the operating room.[11,12]

Computer-aided design (CAD) and computer-aided modeling (CAM) software and the easy acquisition and transfer of Digital Imaging and Communications in Medicine (DICOM) data have facilitated the development of various proprietary software programs for use in planning and implementing surgical procedures in the head and neck region/craniomaxillofacial skeleton. These software systems have been incorporated into previously developed navigation systems to create a computer-aided surgical simulation (CASS) system that may be applied in head and neck ablative and reconstructive surgery. Contemporary software allows the surgeon to analyze the patient with head and neck cancer by performing three-dimensional (3D) measurements of tumor volume and skeletal relationships and to manipulate deformed or missing anatomy by mirror imaging, segmentation, or insertion of unaltered or ideal skeletal constructs (**Fig. 31.1**). The virtual reconstruction may be transferred to reality (the patient) by using custom stereolithographic models (SLMs), implants, and/or cutting jigs that are constructed by using a CAD/CAM process or through image-guided surgery in the form of intraoperative navigation performed to the idealized virtual image (**Fig. 31.2**).

The accuracy of the surgical procedure may then be confirmed by using modern portable intraoperative CT scanners (**Fig. 31.3**). Third-party service providers have made this software and rapid prototyping technology available and accessible to most surgeons.

Site-Specific Applications for Computer Planning and Intraoperative Navigation

Skull Base

Surgery of the anterior and lateral skull base has traditionally been characterized by lengthy and extensive transcranial operations, often performed with suboptimal visualization and with a modest degree of unpredictability in terms of obtaining negative resection margins and minimizing complications. Frameless stereotaxy has been advocated as a method to facilitate subcranial approaches to the anterior skull base, to improve the surgeon's ability to achieve safe, clear resection margins, and to minimize complications.[13-16] Virtual approaches using intraoperative navigation can be incorporated into existing anterior skull base protocols, such

Virtual surgery

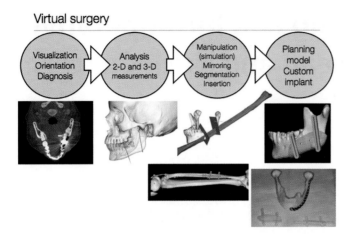

Transfer of the virtual reconstruction to the patient

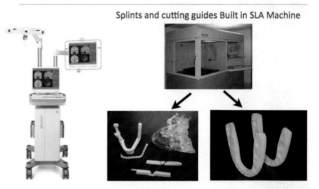

Figure 31.1 Workflow diagram of the initial clinical and radiographic analysis. Virtual two-dimensional and three-dimensional measurements of surgical resection are made. Fibula is virtually osteotomized and adapted to native mandibular margins. Virtual splints are made and then fabricated to replicate virtual cuts during surgery. A reconstruction plate is then adapted to a stereolithographic model.

Figure 31.2 Splints and cutting guides for ablative and donor sites are fabricated in the SLA machine to replicate osteotomies made during virtual surgery. SLM, stereolithographic model.

as that defined by Dubin et al, to facilitate both subcranial ablation and reconstructive surgery when indicated.[17]

Intraoperative navigation has also been advocated as a method to increase safety in mandibular ankylosis release or resection of lateral skull base tumors or other lesions involving the temporomandibular joint (TMJ), pterygomaxillary fossa, and/or infratemporal fossa.[14,18] The senior author has combined these techniques into a protocol for skull base tumors that uses navigation-assisted tumor resection to aid in safely achieving negative en block resection margins, followed by custom CAM as a guide for accurate fibular reconstruction of the mandible.

Schmelzeisen et al first described the use of navigation for improved safety in lateral skull base surgery in general and ankylosis release in particular.[14] Malis et al later described a single-stage approach for ankylosis release combined with total TMJ replacement by using navigation as a guide to accurately place osteotomies and inset custom prostheses.[19]

Zhang et al recently reported the outcome of a case series by using digital preoperative segmentation, osteotomies, and preoperative shaping of a reconstruction plate on an SLM derived from patients undergoing costochondral graft reconstruction of the TMJ.[20] Compared with a control group, computer-assisted TMJ reconstruction was found to have significantly shorter operating time; however, it was found to have no significant difference in accuracy when compared with those subjects who underwent conventional TMJ reconstruction. Similar methodology in a patient with TMJ bony ankylosis was used by Chandran et al,[21] who built on the previous application of navigation protocols.[22,23] Preoperative digital resection of the TMJ fossa and condylar head was performed; cutting guides to duplicate the resection were fabricated; and an appropriate alloplastic stock prosthesis was adapted to an SLM model, rendering successful total joint reconstruction.

Mandibular Reconstruction

Perhaps the most significant advancement in reconstruction of the midface and mandible during the past 30 years has been the development of microvascular osteocutaneous flaps, particularly the free fibular osteocutaneous free flap (FFOF) and its ability to achieve dental implant-supported prosthetic rehabilitation.[24–30] SLMs developed from 3D preoperative imaging have been used to assist in overcoming some of the limitations of the FFOF as it relates to ideal positioning of the neomandibular constructs and to allow the surgeon to assess the contour of the maxillomandibular complex by removal of the external deformation left by the tumor, creating "ideal" anatomic surfaces.[31] In addition to transverse assessment of the jaws, sagittal relationships of the jaws may be assessed for proper anteroposterior positioning to create ideal orthogonal relationships. Inaccurate insertion of the neomandibular (fibular)

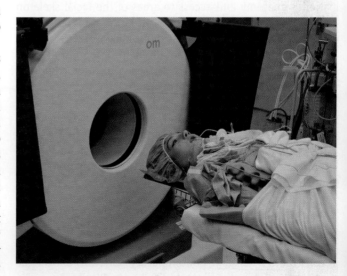

Figure 31.3 Intraoperative computed tomography can be used before the patient leaves the operating room to confirm surgical resection and implant and graft placement.

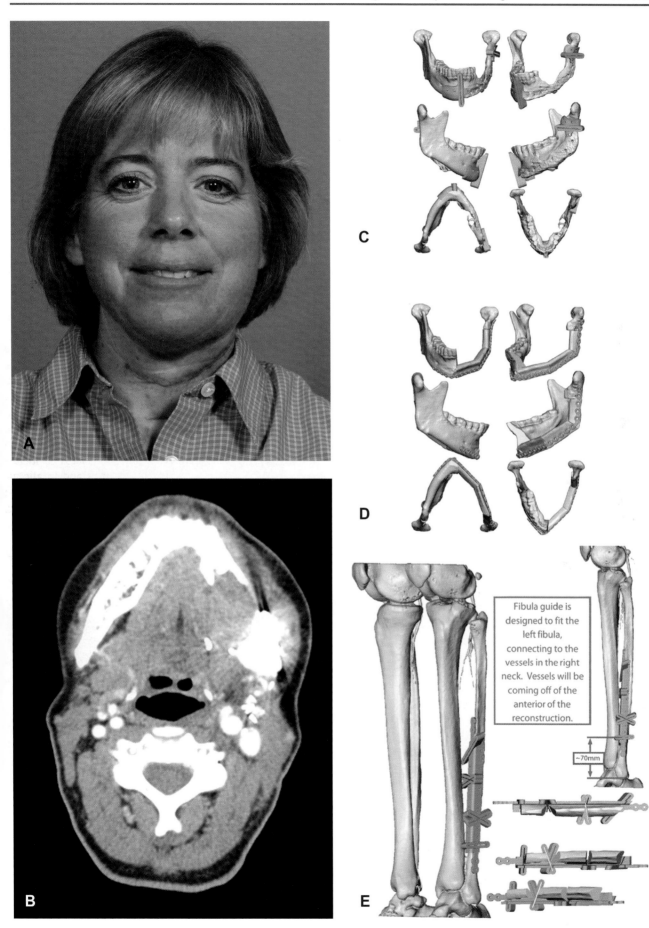

Fibula guide is designed to fit the left fibula, connecting to the vessels in the right neck. Vessels will be coming off of the anterior of the reconstruction.

~70mm

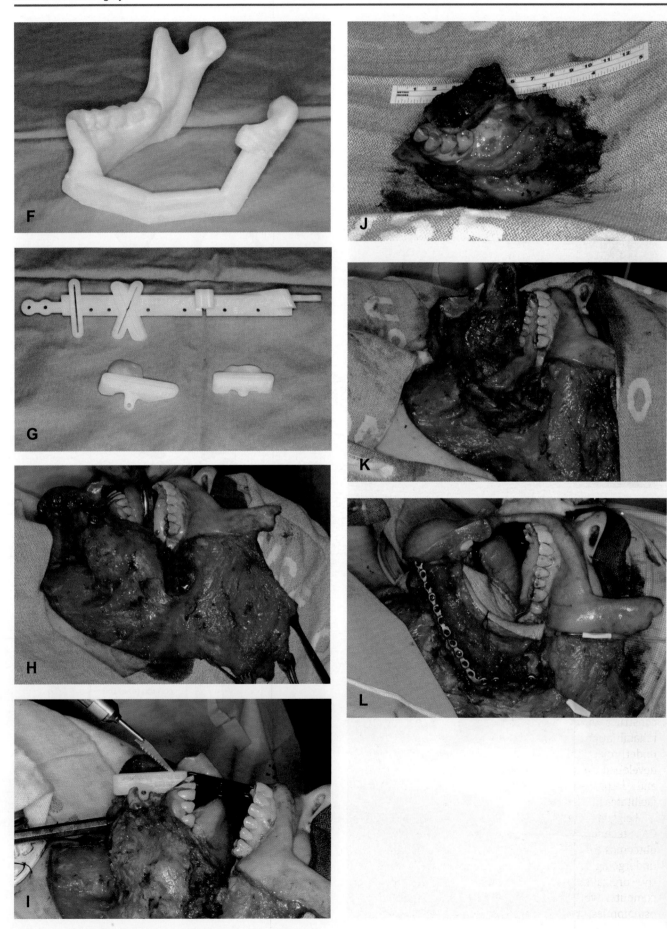

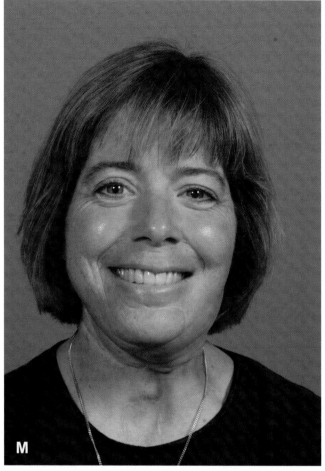

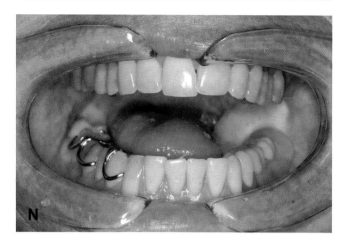

Figure 31.4 A 37-year-old woman with recurrent, previously resected squamous cell carcinoma of the tongue, invading the mandible and previous fibular reconstruction. (A) Preoperative appearance. (B) Preoperative computed tomography (CT) image demonstrating recurrent tumor with the erosion of the mandible. (C) CT images in the Digital Imaging and Communications in Medicine format imported into Surgicase CMF software (Materialise, Ann Arbor, Michigan, United States) for segmentation and insertion. The resection is planned, and the defect is analyzed for fibular reconstruction. Cutting paths are created and virtual cutting guides are planned. (D) By using custom CT fibular data, the virtual fibula is imported into the mandible to create ideal position of the neomanidbular construct. (E) Virtual fibular cutting guides are constructed based on the planned fibular reconstruction to provide cutting guides for the closing wedge osteotomies at the time of surgery. (F) Virtually altered stereolithographic model demonstrating the neomandible. The model is used to prebend a stock locking reconstruction plate. (G) Neomandible, mandibular cutting guides, and fibular cutting guides. (H) Surgical approach. (I) Mandibular resection using cutting guide. (J) Resection specimen. (K) Composite tissue defect following composite resection of the tongue, floor of mouth, and mandible. (L) Fibular construct inset into defect with prebent reconstruction plate. (M) Postoperative appearance following adjuvant chemoradiation therapy. (N) Postoperative intraoral appearance of patient prosthesis in place.

construct will render dental implant-supported prosthetic rehabilitation difficult or impossible because of over- or underprojection of the reconstructed mandible. SLMs developed from 3D imaging allow for precise plate bending and improved maxillomandibular relationship, which facilitates ideal dental implant placement.

Leiggener et al[32] and Hirsch et al[33] described the use of CAD/CAM technology to produce orthognathically ideal surgical outcomes for patients with segmental mandibular defects undergoing reconstruction with fibular free flaps. Using the surgical simulation software, surgery is simulated on a computer workstation. The virtual fibular and mandibular osteotomies are transferred to a rapid prototyping instrument and a guide stent is constructed to allow for accurate placement of osteotomies (Medical Modeling, Inc., Golden, Colorado, United States). The guide stent is sterilized and used intraoperatively for mandibular osteotomies at the time of resection and fibular closing-wedge osteotomies. In this fashion, the vascularized composite tissue is transferred to the appropriate anteroposterior, vertical, and transverse position (**Fig. 31.4**). Custom guide stents may also be used to aid the accurate dental implant placement to facilitate prosthetic rehabilitation.[34]

Roser et al, in 2010, compared their ability to reproduce the computer plan in a series of 11 patients who underwent segmental mandibulectomy with FFOF.[35] 3D computer models of the final reconstruction were obtained for comparison with the preoperative virtual plan. To make the desired comparisons, the 3D objects representing the postoperative surgical outcome were superimposed onto the preoperative virtual plan by using manual alignment techniques. These objects were then compared by 1-to-1 magnification for measurements of fibular bone volume, location of mandibular osteotomies, location of fibular osteotomies, plate contour, plate position on the fibula, and plate position on the mandible. Comparison was made between the virtual and final plates with regard to contour and position through superimposition overlays of the 3D models that are registered in the same coordinate system. The authors noted that the mean distance of the actual mandibular osteotomy compared with the virtual mandibular osteotomy was 2.00 ± 1.12 mm. The mean volume determined by the software program of the 11 virtual fibulas was 13,669.45 ± 3874.15 mm^3 (range 9568 to 22,860 mm^3), and the mean volume of the 11 actual postoperative fibulas was 12,361.09 ± 4161.80 mm^3 (range 7142 to 22,294 mm^3). The mean percentage volumes of the actual postoperative fibula compared with the planned fibula were 90.93% ± 18.03%.

Katikaneni et al[36] performed a study similar to that of Roser et al. In 16 patients and 104 osteotomies, the average linear variance from the preoperative plan in all tested locations was 1.49 to 4.91 mm, with the transverse dimension being the most unpredictable location (mean 4.91 mm difference) compared with the accuracy of the mandibular osteotomies (1.49 mm difference from planned) and length of fibular segments (2.27 mm difference). Additional studies that will evaluate the cost relative to a similar group of patients treated without computer planning are underway.

Palatomaxillary Reconstruction

Bell et al described the use of intraoperative navigation combined with custom cutting guides and guide stents to implement the virtual plan for patients undergoing maxillectomy or midface resection reconstruction using fibular free flaps.[7–9] The planned reconstruction data from patients undergoing maxillary ablation were "back converted" from their proprietary language to the standard DICOM format, so that digital reconstruction may then be imported into a surgical navigation system (Intellect Cranial Navigation System, Stryker, Freiburg, Germany). The resection is performed under navigation guidance so that the ablative defect matches the planned fibular reconstruction. Custom guide stents are then used to recreate the fibular closing wedge osteotomies, so that the neomaxillary construct fits the ablative defect. The entire neomaxillary construct is then inserted under navigation guidance (**Fig. 31.5**).

Hanasono et al also described favorable results in a single patient who underwent reconstruction of a total maxillectomy defect.[37] Besides providing a chance for preoperative planning, the authors noted that computer-assisted preoperative planning also limits the number of incisions that has to be made on the face. Lethaus et al reported a similar method of reconstruction of midface defects by using computer-assisted free-fibula graft reconstruction and found favorable results.[38]

Orbital Reconstruction

Despite the use of traditional reconstructive principles, lasting functional and esthetic complications, such as enophthalmos, may persist following orbital reconstruction of postablative defects.[39] This is especially true following tumor resection with margins spanning multiple orbital walls. In these defects it is especially difficult to obtain premorbid orbital dimensions because of the lack of reliable bony landmarks to guide the placement of bony plates and implants. Specific areas of difficulty are reestablishing proper orbital volume, considering the need to reestablish the critical ethmoidal and antral bulges of the medial and inferior floors, respectively, as well as plate adaptation around the orbital apex. 3D virtual planning combined with intraoperative navigation has been shown to assist the surgeon in achieving ideal orbital volume and globe projection when compared to unoperated controls.[39–41]

Gellrich et al used 3D imaging in a study on subjects with increased enophthalmos and decreased globe projection secondary to posttraumatic orbital deformities.[39] In their landmark study, the investigators mirrored the unaffected orbit to the affected, traumatized orbit by using 3D preoperative image software. They used this as their "goal" orbital dimensions, and the subjects then underwent orbital reconstruction by using intraoperative navigation. Navigation guidance was used to confirm plate placement of grafts at the "goal" dimensions set preoperatively. The investigators found a significant decrease in orbital volume and increase in globe projection in their study cohort. Markiewicz et al performed a similar study, using the imaging software Analyze (Mayo Clinic Biomedical Imaging Resource, Rochester, Minnesota, United States) to assess the change in orbital volume and globe projection in a cohort of subjects with defects secondary not only to trauma but to tumor ablation as well.[42,43] In addition, they used SLMs for preoperative graft contouring as well as confirming graft placement by using intraoperative navigation. They found results similar those of the study by Gellrich et al, with a significant decrease in orbital volume, an increase in globe projection, a linear correlation between goal and actual orbital volume, and globe projection measurements following orbital reconstruction.

Computer-Aided Surgical Simulation

CASS can be divided into four phases: (1) data acquisition phase, in which all clinical information, anthropometric

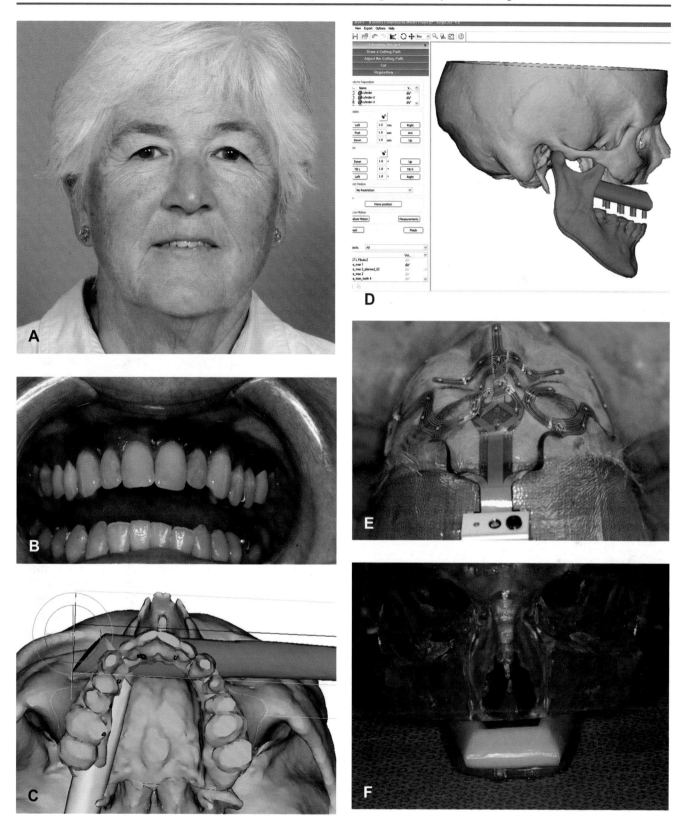

Figure 31.5 A 67-year-old woman with invasive mucosal melanoma involving the maxillary gingiva extending from second molar to contralateral second molar. (A) Preoperative appearance. (B) Preoperative appearance of lesion. (C) Virtual image based on computed tomography (CT) data set of the patient illustrating planned resection osteotomies and virtual reconstruction using a fibula (average female dimensions) illustrating inset with care to position fibular construct into a favorable position relative to the dental arch and into the pterygoid plates. (D) Virtual implants are placed into the virtual neomaxilla in a prosthetically favorable position relative to the opposing dental arches. (E) Stereolithographic model with the neomaxilla template and dental implant stent milled based on the virtual reconstruction. (F) Fiducial mask for intraoperative navigation.

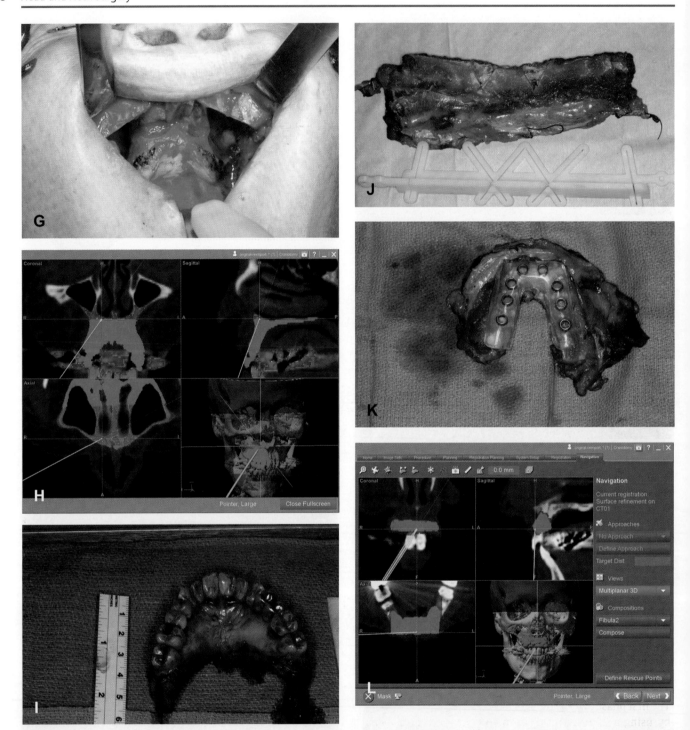

Figure 31.5 (*contd.*) (G) Navigated resection defect. (H) The virtual reconstruction is "back converted" into the navigation system generating intraoperative navigation images that are used to transfer the virtual reconstruction into reality. (I) Resection specimen. (J) Closing-wedge fibular osteotomies are performed by using cutting guides and templates from the virtual reconstruction. (K) Neomaxilla is formed from the fibula and implants are then placed by using a stent constructed from the virtual images. (L) Accurate inset of the fibular construct is confirmed by using intraoperative navigation.

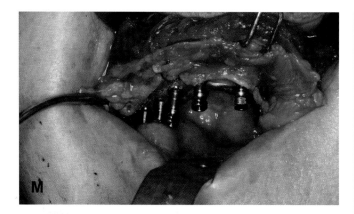

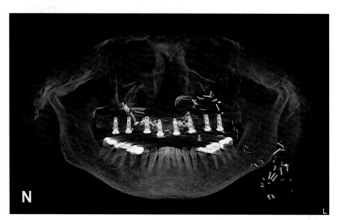

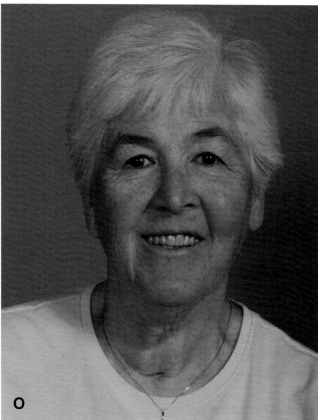

Figure 31.5 (*contd.*) (M) Planned anteroposterior and vertical position of the anterior neomaxilla is confirmed. (N) Postoperative cone-beam CT images. (O) Postoperative appearance.

measurements, and bite registrations are obtained; (2) planning phase, in which CT data are imported into a proprietary software program for the purposes of virtual planning before surgery; (3) surgical phase, which is performed by using CAD/CAM-derived SLMs, guide stents, occlusal splints, and/or intraoperative navigation; and (4) assessment phase, in which the accuracy of the treatment plan transfer is evaluated using intraoperative (or postoperative CT imaging).

Data Acquisition

The first phase of treatment for patients considered for surgery by using a CASS protocol is data acquisition. This includes quantifying the clinical deformity or problem through clinical examination, obtaining all necessary anatomicl "bite registrations" and/or dental or anaplastic models, and acquiring a CT scan of the patient, with the DICOM data to be imported into the appropriate planning software.

The patient data necessary for computer planning depend on the clinical application. Specific information necessary for use in head and neck surgery includes pathologic diagnosis (benign vs. malignant), tumor volume, existing deformity, hard and soft tissue involvement, the extent of the planned surgical resection, and the type of reconstruction planned for the patient (**Fig. 31.6**). CASS for craniofacial/orthognathic

surgery requires additional data, including registration of centric relation before CT imaging, registration of natural head position, laser scanning of plaster dental models, and high-quality facial photography, in addition to accurate anthropometric data.

Once the clinical evaluation is completed and presurgical records have been obtained, the CT scan is completed by using the standard scanning algorithm, matrix of 512×512 degree at 0.625-mm slice thickness, 25 cm or lesser field of view, 0-degree gantry tilt, and 1:1 pitch. The CT images are then transferred to the appropriate surgical planning software in the DICOM format.

Surface imaging, or scanning, is an adjunctive technique in which a laser of other capturing device is used to replicate the 3D surface of soft tissue, bone, or a dental cast. These data can then be imported digitally into a computer software program and integrated with the existing 3D CT data, thus creating a composite image that can be manipulated based on the clinical indications.

Planning Phase

The ablative or reconstructive operation is virtually planned by using the CT data set in the following manner: (1) tumor volume is outlined, and planned resection margins are delineated; (2) the virtual surgical "defect" is quantified and manipulated to optimize position, proportion, or contour of the patient's anatomy (segmentation, mirroring, or insertion of specific anatomic regions from other data sets), (3) a custom SLM is constructed for analysis, preoperative plate bending, and/or intraoperative assessment; (4) custom SLM cutting guides, jigs, or splints are constructed to transfer the virtual plan to reality; and (5) the virtual reconstruction is imported into a navigation system via a process called "back conversion," which can then be used intraoperatively to guide placement of hardware, bone grafts, movement of bone segments, resection of tumor, and/or osteotomy design (midface and skull base applications).

Surgical Phase

The preoperative virtual plan is transferred to the patient undergoing head and neck extirpative surgery in one of two ways, depending on the clinical problem. Reconstruction of the mandible and the inset of microvascular bone flaps may be facilitated by using virtually reconstructed or idealized SLMs, guide stents, and cutting guides. In the maxilla and midface, the cutting guides are augmented by intraoperative navigation, which is also used to aid in orbital reconstruction (restoration of normal orbital volume and malar projection) and by adding safety and predictability to skull base surgery.

Surgeon & Patient Information

Surgeon Name (Head & Neck):_____

   Email Address:_____

   Phone Number:_____

Surgeon Name (Microvascular):_____

   Email Address:_____

   Phone Number:_____

Hospital Affiliation:_____

Patient Name:_____

Surgery Date:_____

Diagnosis:_____

Rigid Fixation Vendor:_____

Vendor Contact:_____

Additional Surgeon Contact:_____

_____

Head & Neck Surgical Plan

The recipient vessels will connect to: ☐ Left Neck   ☐ Right Neck

Surgical Access: ☐ Open   ☐ Limited

The predicted resecting tissue is: ☐ Malignant   ☐ Benign

Notes

Condyle position: ☐ Left side will change
(If mandible is malposed)

☐ Right side will change

☐ No change

Lower Extremity Surgical Plan

Fibula used for reconstruction: ☐ Left   ☐ Right

Lower extremity data: ☐ Patient Specific   ☐ Generic

Notes

Predicted fibula segments in reconstruction: 1 2 3 4 5 6

Fibula positioned on: ☐ Inferior mandible border

☐ ___ mm from inferior mandible border

Predicted Resection & Reconstruction

Please draw the predicted resection on the images below.

A

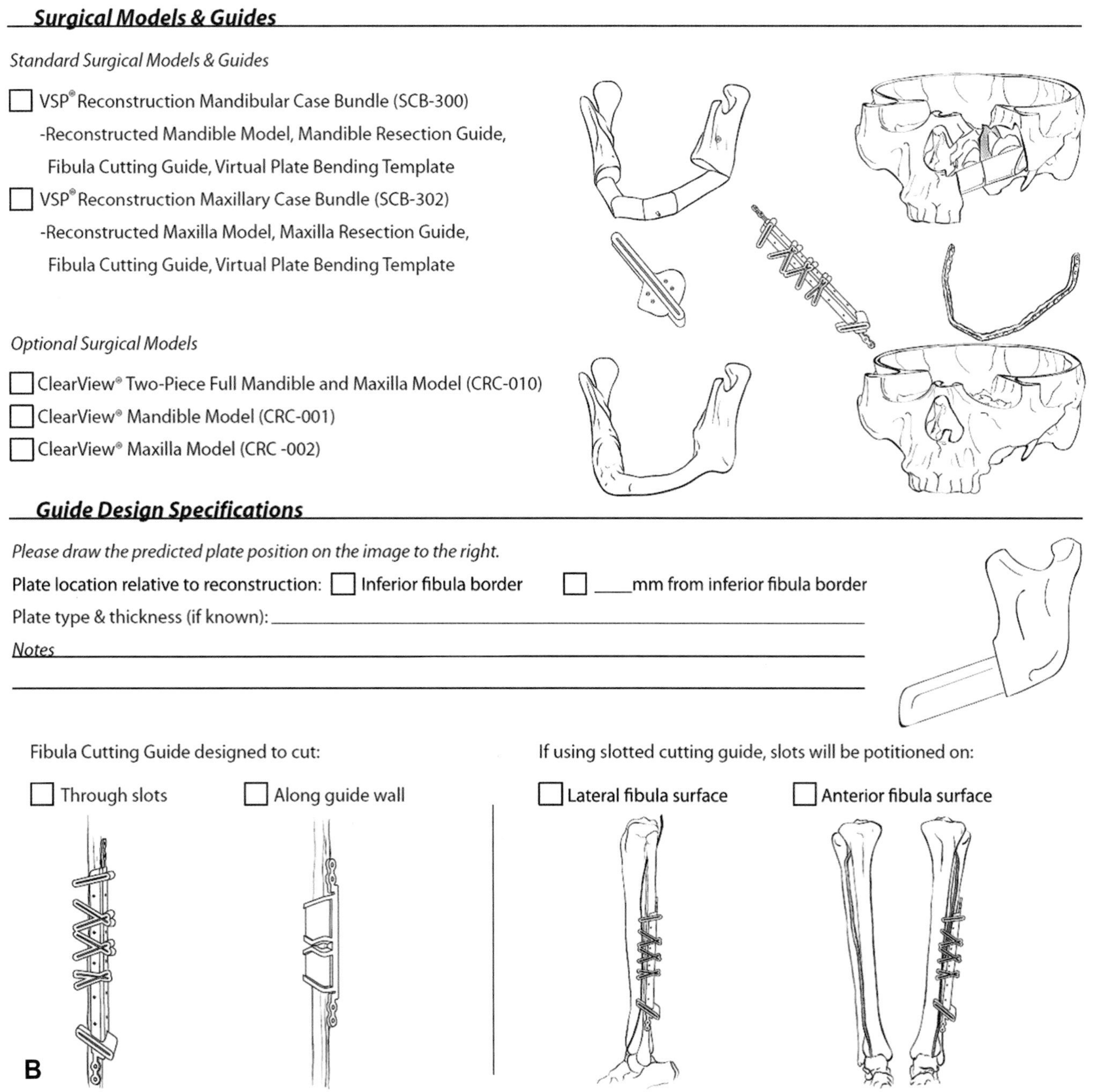

Surgical Models & Guides

Standard Surgical Models & Guides

☐ VSP® Reconstruction Mandibular Case Bundle (SCB-300)
   -Reconstructed Mandible Model, Mandible Resection Guide,
   Fibula Cutting Guide, Virtual Plate Bending Template

☐ VSP® Reconstruction Maxillary Case Bundle (SCB-302)
   -Reconstructed Maxilla Model, Maxilla Resection Guide,
   Fibula Cutting Guide, Virtual Plate Bending Template

Optional Surgical Models

☐ ClearView® Two-Piece Full Mandible and Maxilla Model (CRC-010)
☐ ClearView® Mandible Model (CRC-001)
☐ ClearView® Maxilla Model (CRC -002)

Guide Design Specifications

Please draw the predicted plate position on the image to the right.

Plate location relative to reconstruction: ☐ Inferior fibula border ☐ ____mm from inferior fibula border

Plate type & thickness (if known): _____

Notes _____

_____

Fibula Cutting Guide designed to cut:

☐ Through slots   ☐ Along guide wall

If using slotted cutting guide, slots will be potitioned on:

☐ Lateral fibula surface   ☐ Anterior fibula surface

B

Figure 31.6 (A) Sample worksheet to guide the surgeon in the preoperative work-up, including specific details about the ablative and donor sites. (B) The figure specifically addresses surgical models and cutting guides. (Samples provided by Medical Modeling Inc., Golden, Colorado, Unites States.)

Navigation-assisted surgery in the mandible deserves special mention because of the complexities of navigating a mobile structure. Accurate synchronization of the acquired CT data is made difficult because of the problems associated with determining a stable and reproducible mandibular position. There are three possible solutions to the problem. The first approach is to place the patient in intermaxillary fixation before the CT scan. This method, however, is not feasible for transoral surgery. The second method is to position the mandible in centric relation or centric occlusion, either manually or by using a dental splint. The strategy is sensitive to relative movements of the mandible, which, in turn, undermines the accuracy of the intraoperative navigation. A third approach has been described that uses a special sensor frame that is mounted onto the mandible, thereby allowing surgeons to optically track the jaw's position and to compensate for its continuous movement during surgery. Although time-consuming, this method has the theoretical advantage of improved accuracy by monitoring the position of the mandible directly, rather than by its relative position to other fixed cranial structures. Intraoperative navigation improves visualization of patient's anatomy and increases chances of a successful reconstructive outcome, by making radical tumor surgery more reliable by showing the determined safety margins, preserving vital structures, and guiding reconstruction to preplanned objectives.

Evaluation Phase

Once the virtual plan has been transferred to the patient by performing osteotomies or insetting grafts, flaps, or implants, the accuracy of the surgery is assessed (when appropriate) by using a portable CT scanner. Available at many tertiary care facilities with an active neurosurgical presence, intraoperative CT assessment allows for any revision to occur before the patient leaves the operating room. This is particularly useful in orbital reconstruction, where the surgical access is limited and the relationship of the orbital implant relative to the orbital apex and critical medial and inferior "bulges" is unclear. Outcomes can then be assessed by comparing actual postoperative flap/graft position to that of the virtual plan and to that of the preoperative situation. The accuracy of computer-assisted reconstruction was assessed by comparing preoperative virtual plan to a CT image of the actual postoperative reconstruction, and was found to be reliable (**Fig. 31.7**).[36]

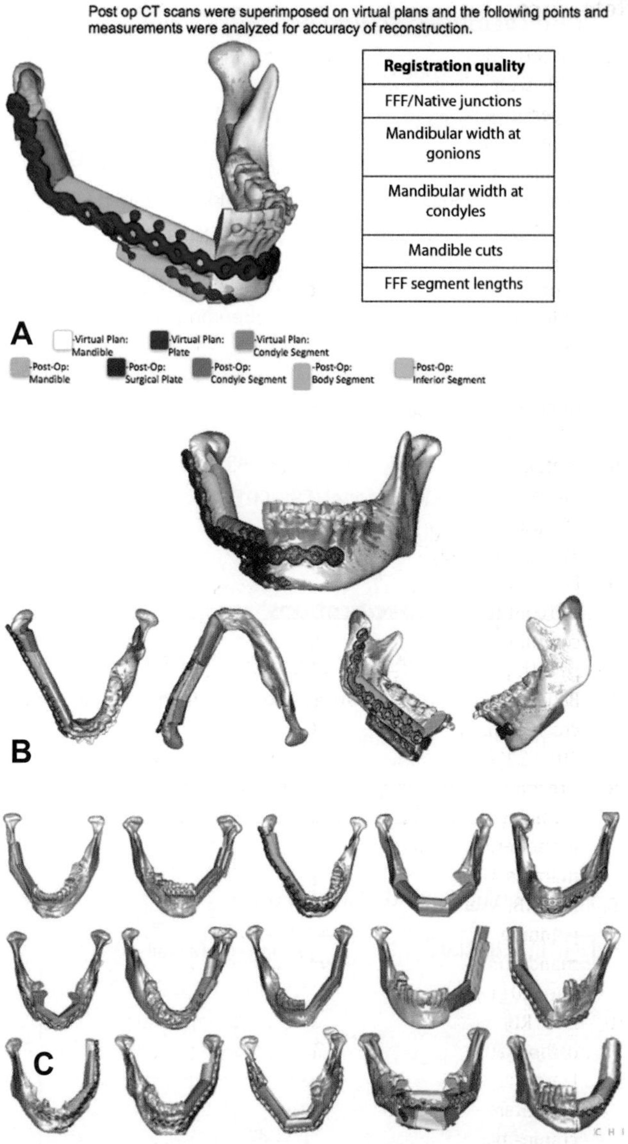

Conclusions

CASS and intraoperative navigation for head and neck oncologic surgery is a recent advancement toward refining surgical technique and improving functional outcomes. It aids the surgeon in the planning and execution of tumor ablation and subsequent reconstruction and has a significant value as an educational tool. Although it is mainly used in maxillomandibular reconstruction, and paranasal sinus, skull base, and orbital surgery, its other potential uses are being investigated. The question of whether intraoperative navigation reduces operating time still remains; however, when taking into account the clinician's work time, it may prove to reduce cost when compared with traditional head and neck oncologic surgery.

Dilemmas/Controversies

- Although several authors advocate that computer-aided surgical simulation (CASS) system and intraoperative navigation reduce operating time, this has yet to be objectively evaluated.
- The accuracy of stereolithographic models in mandibular and craniofacial reconstruction has been validated in several studies; however, they provide a more limited anatomic representation of thin bones of the midface and orbit, making their accuracy in

Figure 31.7 Evaluation of the accuracy of computer-aided surgical simulation system transfer to the patient. (A) Points analyzed for accuracy in the study by Katikaneni et al.[36] (B, C) Series of mandibular reconstructions by using preoperative planning and intraoperative surgical navigation. The pink shaded areas represent the planned postoperative position of the mandible. The green shaded areas represent the actual postoperative position of the mandible.

those areas less than that of the mandible. Newer fabrication techniques, however, are overcoming these inaccuracies.
- CASS and intraoperative navigation can add additional cost and the clinician's work time to the head and neck oncologic procedures. It has been demonstrated that when accounting for the clinician's work time, CASS and intraoperative navigation cost less than traditional surgical procedure.[44]

References

1. Barnett GH, Miller DW, Weisenberger J. Frameless stereotaxy with scalp-applied fiducial markers for brain biopsy procedures: experience in 218 cases. J Neurosurg 1999;91(4):569–576
2. Brinker T, Arango G, Kaminsky J, et al. An experimental approach to image guided skull base surgery employing a microscope-based neuronavigation system. Acta Neurochir (Wien) 1998;140(9):883–889
3. Freysinger W, Gunkel AR, Bale R, et al. Three-dimensional navigation in otorhinolaryngological surgery with the viewing wand. Ann Otol Rhinol Laryngol 1998;107(11 Pt 1):953–958
4. Roberts DW, Strohbehn JW, Hatch JF, Murray W, Kettenberger H. A frameless stereotaxic integration of computerized tomographic imaging and the operating microscope. J Neurosurg 1986;65(4):545–549
5. Watanabe E, Watanabe T, Manaka S, Mayanagi Y, Takakura K. Three-dimensional digitizer (neuronavigator): new equipment for computed tomography-guided stereotaxic surgery. Surg Neurol 1987;27(6):543–547
6. Bell RB, Markiewicz MR. Computer-assisted planning, stereolithographic modeling, and intraoperative navigation for complex orbital reconstruction: a descriptive study in a preliminary cohort. J Oral Maxillofac Surg 2009;67(12):2559–2570
7. Bell RB. Computer planning and intraoperative navigation in cranio-maxillofacial surgery. Oral Maxillofac Surg Clin North Am 2010;22(1):135–156
8. Gregoire C, Adler D, Madey S, Bell RB. Basosquamous carcinoma involving the anterior skull base: a neglected tumor treated using intraoperative navigation as a guide to achieve safe resection margins. J Oral Maxillofac Surg 2011;69(1):230–236
9. Bell RB, Weimer KA, Dierks EJ, Buehler M, Lubek JE. Computer planning and intraoperative navigation for palatomaxillary and mandibular reconstruction with fibular free flaps. J Oral Maxillofac Surg 2011;69(3):724–732
10. Bell RB. Computer planning and intraoperative navigation in orthognathic surgery. J Oral Maxillofac Surg 2011;69(3):592–605
11. Luebbers HT, Messmer P, Obwegeser JA, et al. Comparison of different registration methods for surgical navigation in cranio-maxillofacial surgery. J Craniomaxillofac Surg 2008;36(2):109–116
12. Marmulla R, Niederdellmann H. Computer-assisted bone segment navigation. J Craniomaxillofac Surg 1998;26(6):347–359
13. Batra PS, Kanowitz SJ, Citardi MJ. Clinical utility of intraoperative volume computed tomography scanner for endoscopic sinonasal and skull base procedures. Am J Rhinol 2008;22(5):511–515
14. Schmelzeisen R, Gellrich NC, Schramm A, Schön R, Otten JE. Navigation-guided resection of temporomandibular joint ankylosis promotes safety in skull base surgery. J Oral Maxillofac Surg 2002;60(11):1275–1283
15. Schramm A, Gellrich NC, Gutwald R, et al. Indications for computer-assisted treatment of cranio-maxillofacial tumors. Comput Aided Surg 2000;5(5):343–352
16. To EW, Yuen EH, Tsang WM, et al. The use of stereotactic navigation guidance in minimally invasive transnasal nasopharyngectomy: a comparison with the conventional open transfacial approach. Br J Radiol 2002;75(892):345–350
17. Dubin MG, Sonnenburg RE, Melroy CT, Ebert CS, Coffey CS, Senior BA. Staged endoscopic and combined open/endoscopic approach in the management of inverted papilloma of the frontal sinus. Am J Rhinol 2005;19(5):442–445
18. Lübbers HT, Jacobsen C, Könü D, Matthews F, Grätz KW, Obwegeser JA. Surgical navigation in cranio-maxillofacial surgery: an evaluation on a child with a cranio-facio-orbital tumour. Br J Oral Maxillofac Surg 2011;49(7):532–537
19. Malis DD, Xia JJ, Gateno J, Donovan DT, Teichgraeber JF. New protocol for 1-stage treatment of temporomandibular joint ankylosis using surgical navigation. J Oral Maxillofac Surg 2007;65(9):1843–1848
20. Zhang S, Liu X, Xu Y, et al. Application of rapid prototyping for temporomandibular joint reconstruction. J Oral Maxillofac Surg 2011;69(2):432–438
21. Chandran R, Keeler GD, Christensen AM, Weimer KA, Caloss R. Application of virtual surgical planning for total joint reconstruction with a stock alloplast system. J Oral Maxillofac Surg 2011;69(1):285–294
22. Yeung RW, Xia JJ, Samman N. Image-guided minimally invasive surgical access to the temporomandibular joint: a preliminary report. J Oral Maxillofac Surg 2006;64(10):1546–1552
23. Yu HB, Shen GF, Zhang SL, Wang XD, Wang CT, Lin YP. Navigation-guided gap arthroplasty in the treatment of temporomandibular joint ankylosis. Int J Oral Maxillofac Surg 2009;38(10):1030–1035
24. Chiapasco M, Biglioli F, Autelitano L, Romeo E, Brusati R. Clinical outcome of dental implants placed in fibula-free flaps used for the reconstruction of maxillo-mandibular defects following ablation for tumors or osteoradionecrosis. Clin Oral Implants Res 2006;17(2):220–228
25. Garrett N, Roumanas ED, Blackwell KE, et al. Efficacy of conventional and implant-supported mandibular resection prostheses: study overview and treatment outcomes. J Prosthet Dent 2006;96(1):13–24
26. Hidalgo DA, Pusic AL. Free-flap mandibular reconstruction: a 10-year follow-up study. Plast Reconstr Surg 2002;110(2):438–449, discussion 450–451
27. Odin G, Balaguer T, Savoldelli C, Scortecci G. Immediate functional loading of an implant-supported fixed prosthesis at the time of ablative surgery and mandibular reconstruction for squamous cell carcinoma. J Oral Implantol 2010;36(3):225–230
28. Papadopulos NA, Schaff J, Sader R, et al. Mandibular reconstruction with free osteofasciocutaneous fibula flap: a 10 years experience. Injury 2008;39(Suppl 3):S75–S82
29. Wei FC, Santamaria E, Chang YM, Chen HC. Mandibular reconstruction with fibular osteoseptocutaneous free flap and simultaneous placement of osseointegrated dental implants. J Craniofac Surg 1997;8(6):512–521
30. Sclaroff A, Haughey B, Gay WD, Paniello R. Immediate mandibular reconstruction and placement of dental implants. At the time of ablative surgery. Oral Surg Oral Med Oral Pathol 1994;78(6):711–717
31. Hannen EJ. Recreating the original contour in tumor deformed mandibles for plate adapting. Int J Oral Maxillofac Surg 2006;35(2):183–185
32. Leiggener C, Messo E, Thor A, Zeilhofer HF, Hirsch JM. A selective laser sintering guide for transferring a virtual plan to real time surgery in composite mandibular reconstruction with free fibula osseous flaps. Int J Oral Maxillofac Surg 2009;38(2):187–192
33. Hirsch DL, Garfein ES, Christensen AM, Weimer KA, Saddeh PB, Levine JP. Use of computer-aided design and computer-aided manufacturing to produce orthognathically ideal surgical outcomes: a paradigm shift in head and neck reconstruction. J Oral Maxillofac Surg 2009;67(10):2115–2122
34. Wagner A, Wanschitz F, Birkfellner W, et al. Computer-aided placement of endosseous oral implants in patients after ablative tumour surgery: assessment of accuracy. Clin Oral Implants Res 2003;14(3):340–348

35. Roser SM, Ramachandra S, Blair H, et al. The accuracy of virtual surgical planning in free fibula mandibular reconstruction: comparison of planned and final results. J Oral Maxillofac Surg 2010;68(11):2824–2832

36. Katikaneni R, Hirsch D, Markiewicz M, Bell R. Computer assisted virtual planning in maxillofacial reconstruction using microvascular free fibula flaps. J Oral Maxillofac Surg 2010;68(Suppl 9):e26–e27

37. Hanasono MM, Jacob RF, Bidaut L, Robb GL, Skoracki RJ. Midfacial reconstruction using virtual planning, rapid prototype modeling, and stereotactic navigation. Plast Reconstr Surg 2010;126(6):2002–2006

38. Lethaus B, Kessler P, Boeckman R, Poort LJ, Tolba R. Reconstruction of a maxillary defect with a fibula graft and titanium mesh using CAD/CAM techniques. Head Face Med 2010;6:16

39. Gellrich NC, Schramm A, Hammer B, et al. Computer-assisted secondary reconstruction of unilateral posttraumatic orbital deformity. Plast Reconstr Surg 2002;110(6):1417–1429

40. Hammer B, Kunz C, Schramm A, deRoche R, Prein J. Repair of complex orbital fractures: technical problems, state-of-the-art solutions and future perspectives. Ann Acad Med Singapore 1999;28(5):687–691

41. Yu H, Shen G, Wang X, Zhang S. Navigation-guided reduction and orbital floor reconstruction in the treatment of zygomatic-orbital-maxillary complex fractures. J Oral Maxillofac Surg 2010;68(1):28–34

42. Markiewicz MR, Dierks EJ, Bell RB. Does intraoperative navigation restore orbital dimensions in traumatic and post-ablative defects? J Craniomaxillofac Surg 2012;40(2):142–148

43. Markiewicz MR, Dierks EJ, Potter BE, Bell RB. Reliability of intraoperative navigation in restoring normal orbital dimensions. J Oral Maxillofac Surg 2011;69(11):2833–2840

44. Xia JJ, Phillips CV, Gateno J, et al. Cost-effectiveness analysis for computer-aided surgical simulation in complex cranio-maxillofacial surgery. J Oral Maxillofac Surg 2006;64(12):1780–1784

32 Robotic Surgery for Head and Neck Neoplasms

William R. Carroll, J. Scott Magnuson, Trinitia Y. Cannon, Robert J. Yawn, and Terry A. Day

Core Messages

- The surgical robot is an important tool for expanding the scope of minimally invasive surgery in the head and neck.

- The principles for the proper oncologic management of head and neck tumors are unchanged. The goals of resection are to obtain clear surgical margins and maintain normal function whenever possible.

- Exposure of the tumor remains the most challenging aspect of robot-assisted surgery of the head and neck. The surgeon should determine before proceeding whether there is a reasonable chance of achieving clear margins. The patient rarely benefits, and, in some circumstances, is harmed by partial tumor resection.

- Close collaboration with pathology is mandatory.

Minimally invasive tumor resection is not a new concept for head and neck surgeons. In 1893, U.S. President Grover Cleveland had an oral cavity cancer secretly resected transorally by surgeons on his yacht off the coast of New York. He survived and lived another 16 years. For tumors beyond direct transoral view, the operating microscope has been used for decades with cold instruments and subsequently with laser for tumor resection.

Adaptation of robotic surgery for the head and neck now promises a significant opportunity to expand our minimally invasive capabilities.

History of Robotic Surgery in the Head and Neck

In 2003, investigators at Stanford University first documented the use of a robot in head and neck surgery in porcine models. Procedures performed included submandibular resections, selective neck dissections, a unilateral parotidectomy, and thymectomy. The only complication was one incidence of subcutaneous emphysema.[1] Work began at the University of Pennsylvania in 2005 on transoral approaches as surgeons investigated proper robotic cart and instrument positioning to allow access to the larynx using mannequin models. Cadaver studies followed, demonstrating safe access to the larynx without significant damage to the teeth, mandible, or pharyngeal integrity. Canine studies then confirmed feasibility, safety, and adequate hemostasis during supraglottic laryngectomy. Finally, the procedure was tried in humans as part of a clinical trial under institutional review board supervision. Elsewhere in 2005, 11 endorobotic

submandibular gland resections were successfully performed at the Medical College of Georgia, with an average operating time of 48 minutes.[2] Canine and porcine models were also successfully operated on by using transoral approaches at the Walter Reed Army Medical Center in Washington, DC, in 2005.[3] The acronym TORS (transoral robotic surgery) was coined in 2006 after Weinstein and O'Malley reported the first three human patients with tongue base cancers treated with this innovative technique.[4] In early 2007, other medical centers began to adopt the transoral robot-assisted procedure. At each site, work was originally performed under institutional review board supervision in a clinical trial setting. Reports documenting feasibility, efficacy, and safety began to emerge, indicating that the procedures were reproducible in other settings. In early 2010, the Food and Drug Administration granted approval to use the da Vinci surgical robot for the resection of benign and malignant lesions of the oral cavity, oropharynx, hypopharynx, and larynx, stages T1 and T2.

Surgical Technique

Preoperative Evaluation

The preoperative work-up for a patient undergoing TORS is similar to that for any patient with head and neck cancer (HNC) and includes physical examination, direct laryngoscopy and biopsy, imaging, metastatic work-up, and appropriate laboratory analysis. Many surgeons also insist that they personally perform a diagnostic examination under anesthesia to assess the feasibility of TORS. The rationale is that the robot is an extremely limited resource and the additional examination under anesthesia helps ensure that only those patients whose tumor is accessible by TORS will be scheduled for the procedure. Exclusion criteria specific for TORS management of an oropharyngeal neoplasm are similar to the exclusion criteria for other transoral procedures.[5,6]

These include the following:

- Anatomic characteristics that make exposure and visualization of the tumor impossible via the transoral approach (e.g., trismus and ill-defined margins).
- Lesions fixed to the lateral or posterior pharyngeal wall, indicating deep neck invasion into the parapharyngeal space.
- Lesions intimately associated with the carotid artery, internal jugular vein, or prevertebral fascia as evidenced by physical examination or imaging.
- Skull base invasion.
- Mandibular invasion.
- Stage IVC disease, except for curable distant metastasis.
- Having a retropharyngeal internal carotid artery in which the artery is located directly behind the tonsillar fossa (a contraindication for TORS radical tonsillectomy but not for the resection of other oropharyngeal sites).
- Medical contraindications for either general anesthesia or transoral surgery in which an open wound heals by secondary intention (e.g., the need for chronic anticoagulation).
- Bilateral deep tongue base invasion.

Instruments and Set Up

The da Vinci surgical system is used. The manipulator unit has three laterally placed instrument arms and a centrally located endoscopic arm. For base of tongue (BOT) and supraglottic laryngeal resections, a binocular endoscope angled at 30 degree is positioned in the central arm. For a radical tonsillectomy, a 0-degree binocular endoscope is preferred. Operating instruments commonly include a 5-mm monopolar electrocautery, 5-mm Maryland dissector forceps, 8-mm bipolar scissors, 5-mm needle driver, and 5-mm Debakey forceps. The laryngoscopic clip applier is typically used by the assistant instead of the robotic clip applier to avoid an instrument change on the robotic arms (**Fig. 32.1**).

The surgeon should be prepared that the setup for robotic cases will take extra time initially. As familiarity grows for the surgeon and operating room personnel setup times decrease rapidly. The operation is performed under general anesthesia with nasotracheal intubation. The patient is positioned with the head 180 degrees away from the anesthesia team. Exposure of the tumor is accomplished before moving the robotic cart to the bedside. The teeth are protected with a gauze or molded thermoplastic sheeting. The tumor is exposed with an oral retractor; either the Crow-Davis mouth retractor or the Feyh-Kastenbauer laryngeal

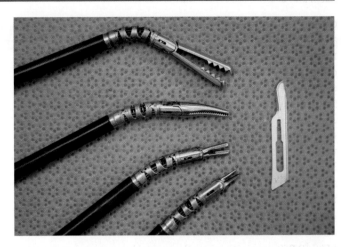

Figure 32.1 Robotic instruments (5 mm): (from top) Schertel forceps, Maryland dissector, Debakey forceps, and needle driver.

retractor is used (**Fig. 32.2**). Distraction of the tongue outward is accomplished with a heavy silk suture. Exposure of the operative site is often the most challenging portion of the TORS procedure. The surgeon should be willing to try different retractors, different blades, and different tongue positions as required to obtain optimal exposure. The retractor is suspended from the surgical bed by using a heavy endoscope holder to facilitate hands-free exposure.

The scrub nurse is positioned to the patient's side, and the surgical assistant is seated at the patient's head. An active and attentive surgical assistant is essential for TORS. The assistant's job is to suction smoke and blood, to apply

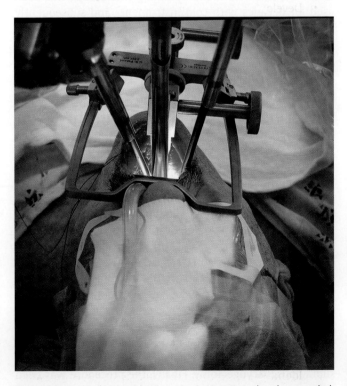

Figure 32.2 Feyh-Kastenbauer retractor postioned and suspended. Note instrument position: camera midline with working arms on sides in triangular configuration.

countertraction at the surgical site, to help with exposure, and to place ligaclips on prominent vessels. The robotic cart for the da Vinci surgical system is positioned on the side opposite the scrub nurse at a 20- to 30-degree angle from the operating room table. The operating console is positioned at some distance away from the patient. The patient is prepped and draped as indicated. Once the robotic cart is positioned, the robotic arms are moved to the oral cavity with the video endoscope centrally and the surgical arms coming in on either side of the endoscope in a roughly triangular arrangement. Because of space limitations, only two of the three robotic operating arms are typically deployed. We prefer the 5-mm monopolar cautery and Maryland dissector as the instruments of choice. Occasionally, the third arm is used to provide static traction at the surgical site.

Operative Procedures

Transoral Robotic Surgery for Radical Tonsillectomy

- Make an incision through the buccal mucosa at the level of the pterygomandibular raphe between the upper and lower molars by using a 5-mm spatula cautery. This landmark is used to guide the surgeon to a dissection plane between the pharyngeal constrictor muscle, which becomes the lateral margin of tumor resection, and the buccopharyngeal fascia.
- Use the 5-mm Maryland forceps to grasp and medially retract the incised buccal mucosa.
- Develop a plane along the lateral aspect of the pharyngeal constrictor muscles and identify the pterygoid musculature laterally.
- Dissect to the level of the styloglossus and stylopharyngeus muscles.
- Transect the soft palate as indicated by the degree of cancer involvement. Dissect through the soft palate musculature to the level of the prevertebral fascia.
- Elevate the constrictor muscles off the prevertebral fascia by using blunt dissection with the 5-mm spatula cautery.
- Identify and divide as necessary the styloglossus and stylopharyngeus muscles.
- Reconfirm the position of the carotid artery via imaging and by assessing for carotid pulsations. Clip any transversing veins and arteries. Attempt to protect the thin layer of fat in the parapharynx around the carotid artery and to prevent communication into the neck.
- At the level of the BOT, incise across the posterior floor of the mouth to the lateral tongue mucosa. The extent of the BOT resection is based on the extent of the tumor, with the goal of achieving negative margins. Identify and preserve the lingual artery unless there is gross tumor involvement.
- Resect the posterior pharyngeal wall from the inferior margin to the level of the soft palate.

- Following resection, the tumor is oriented for pathologic evaluation and margins are taken.
- Remove robotic instruments and assess hemostasis.
- Relax and then reopen retractors to assess for occult bleeding.

Transoral Robotic Surgery for Base of Tongue Resection

- Expose the vallecula inferior to the tumor (**Fig. 32.3**).
- Make an initial inferior horizontal cut at the level of the vallecula. This allows determination of the inferior extent of the tumor and aids in determining the appropriate depth of the resection.
- Next, adjust the retractor to allow the superior and lateral cuts. The end of the retractor blade should be placed anteriorly with just enough room to visualize the anterior extent of the gross tumor and to expose as much of the inferior extent of the tumor as possible.
- Make a mucosal cut at the anterior margin and allow the tumor to fall posteriorly into the field of view. Grasp the normal soft tissue at the edge of the specimen and place it under tension for the remainder of the dissection.
- Make the medial and lateral cuts as defined by the extent of the gross tumor. Identify and preserve, as appropriate, the dorsal lingual artery, the lingual artery trunk, and the hypoglossal nerve.
- Connect the superior cuts to the inferior cuts at the depth defined by the initial tissue incisions to perform an en bloc resection with clear surgical margins.
- Orient the tumor for pathologic evaluation.
- Irrigate the wound bed and control for hemostasis with cautery or hemoclip application.
- Remove all robotic instrumentation and retractors and assess for inadvertent trauma.

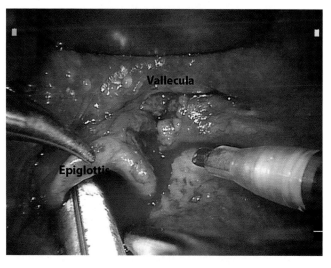

Figure 32.3 T1 vallecular carcinoma with Maryland dissector and monopolar cautery in position.

Transoral Robotic Surgery for Supraglottic Laryngectomy

- Place the laryngeal blade of the Feyh-Kastenbauer retractor within the larynx to expose the inferior portion of the dissection.
- Incise the aryepiglottic fold posteriorly and ventricular mucosa inferiorly.
- Reposition the retractor to expose the vallecula. Change retractor blades if needed.
- Incise the vallecula maintaining an adequate superior tumor margin.
- Laterally, ligate branches of the superior laryngeal artery coursing within the pharyngoepiglottic fold. Be aware of the position of the lingual artery and hypoglossal nerves in the lateral tongue base.
- Dissect deeply into the preepiglottic space and identify the hyoid bone and the inner surface of the thyroid lamina.
- Continue the dissection inferiorly, removing the preepiglottic contents as dictated by tumor extent.
- Communicate the preepiglottic space dissection with the initial aryepiglottic fold and ventricular cuts and remove the specimen.
- Orient the tumor for pathologic evaluation.
- Ensure hemostasis and remove robotic instruments.
- Relax retractors and then briefly reopen to assess for occult bleeding.

Transoral Robotic Surgery for Piriform Sinus Resection

- Repeat direct laryngoscopy to confirm that the inferior tumor margin may be visualized.
- Insert the Feyh-Kastenbauer retractor to visualize the piriform sinus and ipsilateral supraglottic larynx.
- Make inferior cuts initially if possible.
- Incise the vallecula and bivalve the epiglottis as required to establish superior and medial margins.
- Ligate branches of the superior laryngeal artery and the lingual artery.
- Preserve branches of the hypoglossal nerve where feasible. From an internal approach, these will be encountered deep to the lingual artery branches.
- Dissect deeply into the ipsilateral preepiglottic space.
- If tumor involves the anterior or lateral wall of the piriform, the adjacent thyroid ala may be included in the specimen to control the deep margin and to allow the lateral pharynx to collapse inward and obliterate the nonmucosalized dead space.
- Inferior cuts within the larynx are determined by tumor position. Recall that medial wall piriform sinus tumors easily spread up and down in the paraglottic space. The patient will be at a higher risk of aspiration if the ipsilateral vocal cord requires resection.

- Orient the tumor for pathologic evaluation.
- Ensure hemostasis and remove robotic instruments.
- Relax retractors and then briefly reopen to assess for occult bleeding.

Closure

Primary closure is not required for most defects. Palatal reconstruction may be necessary when significant soft palate resection has been performed during a radical tonsillectomy. This is most simply done by suturing the posterior palatal mucosa to the posterior pharyngeal wall with an absorbable suture. In more extensive cases, a rotation flap from the posterior lateral pharyngeal wall may be used to close the palatal defect. In cases with even more extensive soft tissue resection and communication with the neck, flap reconstruction may be indicated. This has been very rare in the authors' experience and is best avoided by proper patient selection. In cases of carotid exposure, the mucosal defect is typically too large for primary reapproximation of the tonsillar pillars. The posterior pharyngeal mucosa may be tacked medially to the fascia adjacent to pterygoid muscles and facilitated by relaxing incisions in the posterior wall to create a rotating pharyngeal flap. If the parapharyngeal fat still protects the anterior surface of the carotid artery, this area is typically allowed to heal by secondary intention.

Postoperative Care

The primary postoperative concerns and most common sources of complications are airway compromise, swallowing dysfunction, and postoperative bleeding. Bleeding is most common in the first 48 hours postoperation, but it has been seen as late as 4 weeks later. Decisions regarding safe times for discharge are similar to those for any patient with HNC. Considerations should include the nature of the surgical defect, ease of patient access to return to the hospital, and social support. Average postoperative length of stay in our institutions is 2 to 3 nights.

Airway management following TORS is evolving in our institutions. Early in our series, most patients remained intubated for 48 hours in the intensive care unit and a few required tracheotomy. Today, radical tonsillectomy patients are rarely left intubated, while tongue base and supraglottic larynx patients are managed on a case-by-case basis. Review of our data has shown that more than two-thirds have been safely extubated.[7] Those patients with bulky or recurrent disease who have a compromised airway preoperatively continue to be intubated or have a tracheotomy tube placed.

Nutritional support postoperatively is also evolving in our institutions, and in contrast to airway management is becoming more aggressive. Early in our experience, Iseli et al[7] reported that 69% of the patients having TORS returned to oral intake before discharge while 83% achieved an oral diet by the first postoperative visit. In his study, requiring a feeding tube before surgery was associated with the need for one after TORS ($p = 0.017$). Today, management is somewhat surgical site specific. Most radical tonsillectomy patients will swallow safely immediately or require nasogastric tube feedings for only a few days. Larger tongue base and supraglottic laryngeal cancer resections, in contrast, usually cause significant temporary swallowing dysfunction. All receive at least nasogastric tube placement, and many are now receiving gastrostomy tubes temporarily. It is important to note that patients who have very poor swallowing function preoperatively will likely require feeding tube support postoperation. These are the only patients we have encountered requiring long-term feeding tubes.

Outcomes of Transoral Robotic Surgery

Safety, Feasibility, Operative Time, and Hospital Stay

Following early studies at the University of Pennsylvania, robot-assisted resection of head and neck tumors has been evaluated in studies from multiple institutions. Early reports focused mainly on safety and efficacy. Boudreaux reported operative times of 99 minutes, mean hospital stay of 3 days, and blood loss ranging from 10 to 90 cm^3 in 29 patients undergoing TORS for upper aerodigestive tract tumors. Eleven of the 29 patients had concomitant neck dissections as well.[8] All patients had negative surgical margins, and there were no adverse events or significant complications. Moore et al reported 49 consecutive patients with oropharyngeal carcinoma resected with robot assistance. All margins were negative, and no patient required a permanent tracheotomy tube or feeding tube. Mean hospital stay was 3.8 days, and there were no significant complications.[6] Genden et al reported similar findings in an early series from Mt Sinai Medical Center.[9] O'Malley et al and Weinstein et al reported results for tongue base resection radical tonsillectomy and supraglottic laryngectomy, finding low rates of complications, early return to oral intake, and negative surgical margins in all but one patient.[4,10,11] Early surgeons commonly reported a learning curve involving setup and procedure times, patient selection, and methods of tumor exposure.

Timing of neck dissection is controversial for patients undergoing transoral resection of pharyngeal and laryngeal tumors. Many surgeons performing robot-assisted resections delay the neck dissection to decrease the risk of pharyngocutaneous fistula. Moore et al reported on 148 patients who had robot-assisted resection and concomitant neck dissection. Forty-two patients (29%) had demonstrated pharyngocervical communication noted at the time of resection. Six patients (4%) developed a leak; all were managed conservatively, and none had delayed adjuvant treatment.[12]

Functional Outcomes: Swallowing and Airway

Once reproducibility and patient safety were demonstrated, attention switched to reporting functional outcomes. Leonhardt et al described patient-reported outcomes following TORS ± chemoradiation and found that swallowing function, as measured by the Performance Status Scale, declined at 6 months but recovered by 12 months. Speech function remained depressed at 6 and 12 months posttreatment. Those patients requiring adjuvant chemoradiation had significantly delayed return of swallowing and speech function.[13] Iseli et al evaluated airway and swallowing function following transoral tumor resection. Twenty-two percent of the patients were intubated for 48 hours, 9% had a tracheotomy tube placed initially, and all were decannulated by day 14. With regard to swallowing, 69% were taking all diet by mouth at discharge, increasing to 83% by 2 weeks postoperation. Predictors of poor swallowing and prolonged feeding tube dependence included surgery for recurrent disease (earlier radiation therapy), higher tumor stage, and poor preoperative swallowing function as measured by the MD Anderson Dysphagia Inventory.[14] In a following publication, Sinclair et al reported patient-perceived outcomes for patients with early stage oropharyngeal tumors undergoing robot-assisted resection. She found that all objective scores fell below baseline measures immediately postoperation but were trending back to baseline by month 3 postoperation. Predictors of delayed swallowing recovery included advanced nodal disease, the need for adjuvant chemotherapy, and poor preoperative physical condition.[15] Proponents suggest that TORS will result in improved functional outcomes over existing treatment options, but there are currently no controlled clinical trials supporting this assertion. A growing fund of data derived from prospective series, however, provides optimistic findings. Alexander et al compared a matched series of oropharyngeal cancers treated with TORS and primary radiation ± chemotherapy. Groups were well matched by patient demographics, tumor site, and stage. There was a significant difference in exposure to chemotherapy between the two groups as would be anticipated. Most significantly, the mean radiation dose was 60 Gy for the TORS group compared with 73 Gy for the primary radiation group ($p = 0.0001$).[16] Dean et al reported similar results in comparing robot-assisted primary surgery, robot-assisted salvage surgery, and open salvage surgery.[17] The robot-assisted groups had less gastrostomy and tracheotomy tube dependence, fewer days of length of stay, and fewer complications than did patients in the open salvage group. Genden et al compared quality-of-life outcomes in 30 patients who underwent TORS with similar patients treated with chemoradiotherapy and found improved swallowing and normalcy of diet in the patients who underwent TORS.[18]

Oncologic Outcomes

Weinstein et al reported oncologic outcomes in 49 patients with previously untreated oropharyngeal scca and detected local recurrence in one patient (2%) and regional recurrence in two (4%).[5] Similar to the Alexander et al study, radiation doses were deescalated and 38% of the patients avoided chemotherapy.[5] In a report of TORS for oropharyngeal cancer, Cohen et al stratified patients by human papillomavirus (HPV) status. While one would expect the disease-free and overall survival to be superior in the HPV(+) group, these investigators found similar overall survival, with a nonsignificant trend toward improved disease-free survival in the HPV(+) group. In most chemoradiation series, the overall and disease-free survival differences are dramatic for HPV(+) versus HPV(–) individuals. These findings may ultimately suggest a role for preferentially including surgery in HPV(–) disease of the oropharynx.[19] Elsewhere, data from two academic centers (Mayo Clinic and University of Alabama, Birmingham) were combined to evaluate early oncologic outcomes of patients with early stage oropharyngeal cancer treated with TORS. The series includes 89 patients with a minimum 2-year follow-up. Recurrence-free survival rates at 1 and 2 years were 89.5% and 86.3%, respectively. Only 3 patients (3.4%) recurred locally in this series.[20]

Complications

Early surgical complications (within 30 days) following TORS include trismus (7%), mucosal bleeding (4%), hypernasality of speech (4%), and unplanned tracheostomy for airway compromise (4%).[10] The orocutaneous fistula rate is as low as 2% and as high as 6.7% and usually occurs in patients with known communication into the neck from the oral cavity at the time of the neck dissection.[6,21] Most agree that the salivary fistula rate can be reduced by delaying neck dissection if a through-and-through defect is anticipated. Review of our own data reveals the following complication rates:

- Bleeding 7.2%
- Aspiration 4.0%
- Pneumonia 1.6%
- Reintubation 2.4%
- Death 3.2%

Emerging Techniques

The ability to work in tight spaces with improved visualization and angles not achievable with nonrobotic instruments is prompting new applications for robotic surgery in the head and neck.

O'Malley et al has described preclinical work and an early series of 10 patients with parapharyngeal space tumors resected with robot assistance. Selected lesions were benign, medial, and anterior to the carotid artery and well circumscribed. Complete tumor excision was possible in nine, but capsular compromise was noted in two patients. No early recurrences have been detected.[22] Hanna et al has

reported preclinical work in four cadavers, demonstrating successful transmaxillary access to the anterior skull base.[23] O'Malley and Weinstein reported transoral cadaver dissection, live canine dissection, and ultimately, clinical application for a patient with a parapharyngeal space mass extending to the infratemporal fossa.[24] In 2008, Kupferman et al demonstrated robotic access to the pituitary gland.[25] In this cadaveric study on four fresh heads, the camera was positioned through the nose, and bilateral Caldwell-luc provided access for the working arms. The authors concluded that this approach provided superior three-dimensional visualization of the sella. A similar approach was used to gain access to the anterior and central skull base.[26]

The nasopharynx is difficult to access for tumor removal. Open surgical approaches to the region require external excisions and translocation of normal structures and are associated with significant morbidity. Transnasal endoscopic techniques address these concerns, but line of sight and intrumentation limitations remain. Wei and Ho recently reported on the use of the robot to resect a small and favorably located residual tumor of the nasopharynx.[27] Access to the lateral nasopharynx was facilitated by a palatal split approach and resulted in excellent tumor visualization and minimal morbidity.

Several investigators have demonstrated robot-assisted free-flap inset following tumor resection. In preclinical investigation, Selber et al created large defects in the oropharynx of cadavers and used the robot to reconstruct the defect by using a radial forearm flap.[28] Genden et al has used this technique clinically as has Mukhija et al.[18,29]

Pearls and Pitfalls

- Select patients carefully. If possible, schedule a separate examination under anesthesia to assess suitability for robot-assisted resection.

- There is a learning curve. Begin with easily accessed and easily visualized cases.

- Be patient and willing to work to obtain optimal exposure at the start of the procedure.

- Do not resect a lesion unless the chance of obtaining clear margins is good.

- Study the anatomy from the "inside-out." Structures are encountered differently than during transcervical approaches.

- Watch for bleeding, aspiration, and airway compromise in the early postoperation period. Use speech pathology liberally to assist with swallowing evaluation and rehabilitation.

References

1. Haus BM, Kambham N, Le D, Moll FM, Gourin C, Terris DJ. Surgical robotic applications in otolaryngology. Laryngoscope 2003;113(7):1139–1144
2. Terris DJ, Haus BM, Gourin CG, Lilagan PE. Endo-robotic resection of the submandibular gland in a cadaver model. Head Neck 2005;27(11):946–951
3. McLeod IK, Mair EA, Melder PC. Potential applications of the da Vinci minimally invasive surgical robotic system in otolaryngology. Ear Nose Throat J 2005;84(8):483–487
4. O'Malley BW Jr, Weinstein GS, Snyder W, Hockstein NG. Transoral robotic surgery (TORS) for base of tongue neoplasms. Laryngoscope 2006;116(8):1465–1472
5. Weinstein GS, O'Malley BW Jr, Cohen MA, Quon H. Transoral robotic surgery for advanced oropharyngeal carcinoma. Arch Otolaryngol Head Neck Surg 2010;136(11):1079–1085
6. Moore EJ, Olsen KD, Kasperbauer JL. Transoral robotic surgery for oropharyngeal squamous cell carcinoma: a prospective study of feasibility and functional outcomes. Laryngoscope 2009;119(11):2156–2164
7. Iseli TA, Kulbersh BD, Iseli CE, Carroll WR, Rosenthal EL, Magnuson JS. Functional outcomes after transoral robotic surgery for head and neck cancer. Otolaryngol Head Neck Surg 2009;141(2):166–171
8. Boudreaux BA, Rosenthal EL, Magnuson JS, et al. Robot-assisted surgery for upper aerodigestive tract neoplasms. Arch Otolaryngol Head Neck Surg 2009;135(4):397–401
9. Genden EM, Desai S, Sung CK. Transoral robotic surgery for the management of head and neck cancer: a preliminary experience. Head Neck 2009;31(3):283–289
10. Weinstein GS, O'Malley BW Jr, Snyder W, Sherman E, Quon H. Transoral robotic surgery: radical tonsillectomy. Arch Otolaryngol Head Neck Surg 2007;133(12):1220–1226
11. Weinstein GS, O'Malley BW Jr, Snyder W, Hockstein NG. Transoral robotic surgery: supraglottic partial laryngectomy. Ann Otol Rhinol Laryngol 2007;116(1):19–23
12. Moore EJ, Olsen KD, Martin EJ. Concurrent neck dissection and transoral robotic surgery. Laryngoscope 2011;121(3):541–544
13. Leonhardt FD, Quon H, Abrahão M, O'Malley BW Jr, Weinstein GS. Transoral robotic surgery for oropharyngeal carcinoma and its impact on patient-reported quality of life and function. Head Neck 2012;34(2):146–154
14. Iseli TA, Kulbersh BD, Iseli CE, Carroll WR, Rosenthal EL, Magnuson JS. Functional outcomes after transoral robotic surgery for head and neck cancer. Otolaryngol Head Neck Surg 2009;141(2):166–171
15. Sinclair CF, McColloch NL, Carroll WR, Rosenthal EL, Desmond RA, Magnuson JS. Patient-perceived and objective functional outcomes following transoral robotic surgery for early oropharyngeal

carcinoma. Arch Otolaryngol Head Neck Surg 2011;137(11):1112–1116
16. Alexander NS, Sullivan BP, Rosenthal EL, Carroll WR, Desmond RA, Magnuson JS. Treatment differences between TORS and primary chemoradiotherapy for T1 and T2 oropharyngeal squamous cell carcinoma. Paper presented at Triology Society Meeting; Orlando, Florida; 2010
17. Dean NR, Rosenthal EL, Carroll WR, et al. Robotic-assisted surgery for primary or recurrent oropharyngeal carcinoma. Arch Otolaryngol Head Neck Surg 2010;136(4):380–384
18. Genden EM, Park R, Smith C, Kotz T. The role of reconstruction for transoral robotic pharyngectomy and concomitant neck dissection. Arch Otolaryngol Head Neck Surg 2011;137(2):151–156
19. Cohen MA, Weinstein GS, O'Malley BW Jr, Feldman M, Quon H. Transoral robotic surgery and human papillomavirus status: oncologic results. Head Neck 2011;33(4):573–580
20. White HN, Moore EJ, Rosenthal EL, et al. Transoral robotic-assisted surgery for head and neck squamous cell carcinoma: one- and 2-year survival analysis. Arch Otolaryngol Head Neck Surg 2010;136(12):1248–1252
21. Moore EJ, Olsen KD, Kasperbauer JL. Transoral robotic surgery for oropharyngeal squamous cell carcinoma: a prospective study of feasibility and functional outcomes. Laryngoscope2009;119(11):2156–2164
22. O'Malley BW Jr, Quon H, Leonhardt FD, Chalian AA, Weinstein GS. Transoral robotic surgery for parapharyngeal space tumors. ORL J Otorhinolaryngol Relat Spec 2010;72(6):332–336
23. Hanna EY, Holsinger C, DeMonte F, Kupferman M. Robotic endoscopic surgery of the skull base: a novel surgical approach. Arch Otolaryngol Head Neck Surg 2007;133(12):1209–1214
24. O'Malley BW Jr, Weinstein GS. Robotic anterior and midline skull base surgery: preclinical investigations. Int J Radiat Oncol Biol Phys 2007;69(Suppl 2):S125–S128
25. Kupferman M, Demonte F, Holsinger FC, Hanna E. Transantral robotic access to the pituitary gland. Otolaryngol Head Neck Surg 2009;141(3):413–415
26. Hanna EY, Holsinger C, DeMonte F, Kupferman M. Robotic endoscopic surgery of the skull base: a novel surgical approach. Arch Otolaryngol Head Neck Surg 2007;133(12):1209–1214
27. Wei WI, Ho WK. Transoral robotic resection of recurrent nasopharyngeal carcinoma. Laryngoscope 2010;120(10):2011–2014
28. Mukhija VK, Sung CK, Desai SC, Wanna G, Genden EM. Transoral robotic assisted free flap reconstruction. Otolaryngol Head Neck Surg 2009;140(1):124–125
29. Selber JC, Robb C, Serlatti JM, Weinstein G, Weber G, Holsinger FC. Transoral robotic free flap reconstruction of oropharyngeal defects: a preclinical investigation. Plast Reconstr Surg 2010;125(3):896–900

33 Endoscopic Approaches to the Anterior Skull Base

Edward D. McCoul, Theodore H. Schwartz, and Vijay Anand

Core Messages

- Endoscopic endonasal approaches offer a minimal-access but maximally invasive alternative to traditional transfacial, transsphenoidal, and transcranial approaches to the anterior skull base.

- The endoscope enables both a panoramic and a microscopic view of the anatomy during dissection, which may be further enhanced by the use of angular optics.

- Because the skull base lies at the anatomic boundary between the fields of head and neck surgery and neurosurgery, the management of tumors in this region can benefit from the collaboration of both disciplines.

- Reconstruction of the skull base is tailored to the individual case. If the dissection entails opening of the dura mater, a multilayered reconstruction using vascularized and nonvascularized components is appropriate.

- Postoperative quality of life may be maintained or improved by the application of endoscopic approaches to tumor resection.

The field of skull base surgery has undergone a rapid evolution over the past 15 years as endoscopic technology has gained increasing prominence.[1] The wide acceptance of endoscopic sinus surgery by otolaryngologists, made possible by the availability of specialized fiberoptic equipment, has expanded the role of the rhinologic surgeon in the management of a variety of disease entities. Sequential developments of technique and ambition have led to endoscopic repair of cerebrospinal fluid (CSF) leaks, resection of sinonasal tumors, intracranial endoscopy, and neurosurgical applications. Other advances that have facilitated progress include digital video systems, specialized endoscopic instrumentation, new biological materials, and intraoperative navigation. Equally important is the spirit of collaboration that has been fostered between rhinologic surgeons and neurosurgeons, who have realized the benefits of a team approach for the treatment of skull base lesions. Refinements of surgical technique now permit completely endoscopic extirpation of tumors at the anterior skull base and enable reconstruction with a low rate of long-term sequellae. This chapter is intended to provide an overview of recent advances in endoscopic skull base surgery, which promise to enhance the field of head and neck oncologic surgery in exciting new ways.

Patient Selection

Tumor Pathology

Success with endoscopic approaches to the skull base begins with appropriate patient selection. A wide variety of skull base tumors are amenable to endoscopic resection, which can be divided into extracranial and intracranial lesions (**Fig. 33.1**). Extracranial tumors are most commonly sinonasal in origin and include squamous cell carcinoma, adenocarcinoma, esthesioneuroblastoma, adenoid cystic carcinoma, and sinonasal mucosal melanoma. Nonsinonasal tumors that arise at the anterior skull base include chondrosarcoma, osteosarcoma, schwannoma, and juvenile nasopharyngioma. Intracranial tumors are predominantly benign lesions such as meningioma and craniopharyngioma, although low-grade malignancy such as chordoma and hemangiopericytoma are not uncommon. Pituitary adenoma, although benign, can be locally aggressive and produce substantial symptoms due to mass effect. Intracranial skull base malignancies are rare and include pituitary carcinoma and anaplastic meningioma.

Surgical Goals

The primary goal of most skull base surgery is complete tumor resection, regardless of whether an open or endoscopic approach is used. The secondary goal is restoration of the anatomic barrier between extracranial and intracranial contents after tumor extirpation. In selected instances where clinical examination and imaging studies result in diagnostic uncertainty, an endoscopic approach may be chosen for biopsy. Debulking of a tumor in anticipation of postoperative radiotherapy, particularly for intracranial tumors, may also be a legitimate surgical goal. Finally, a role may exist for endoscopic surgery in the palliative care of patients with advanced skull base malignancy who suffer

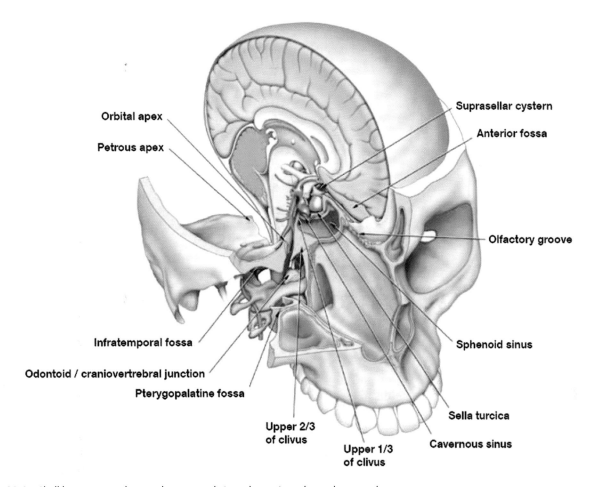

Figure 33.1 Skull base targets that can be accessed via endoscopic endonasal approaches.

from nasal obstruction, sinusitis, visual loss, and other compressive symptoms.[2]

Surgical Outcomes

Systematic review of the literature suggests that endoscopic approaches are equivalent or superior to traditional transcranial or microscope-assisted approaches for the resection of certain anterior skull base tumors.[3] Meningiomas of the tuberculum sellae and planum sphenoidale have equivalent rates of gross total resection by endoscopic or open approaches (73.1 vs. 71.8%). In contrast, meningiomas of the olfactory groove present a greater challenge for endoscopic resection, reflected by a gross total resection rate of 63.2% compared with 92.9% by craniotomy. Endoscopic resection of clival chordoma is more likely to achieve gross total resection (61.0%) compared with transcranial approaches (48.0%), and also produces significantly fewer new cranial nerve deficits. Craniopharyngiomas have significantly higher rates of gross total resection by the endoscopic and microscope-assisted transsphenoidal approaches than by the transcranial route (66.9 vs. 69.1 vs. 48.3%). In addition, improved visual outcome is more likely by endoscopic resection than by transcranial resection (56 vs. 33%). A meta-analysis comparing

endoscopic versus microscope-assisted transsphenoidal pituitary resection found that the endoscopic approach was associated with high rates of gross total resection, normalization of endocrine function, and improved vision.[4]

Direct comparison of endoscopic resection versus craniofacial resection for skull base malignancy has shown no differences in postoperative complication rate or survival, while operative time and length of hospital stay were reduced in the endoscopic resection group.[5,6]

Principles of Endoscopic Skull Base Surgery

General Principles

Adherence to the principles of sound surgical technique is of central importance to endoscopic skull base surgery. The first principle is mastery of the pertinent anatomy, which begins with cadaveric study and continues with a stepwise progression of clinical experience. The second principle is obtaining excellent visualization of the surgical target and surrounding structures, which is facilitated by modern fiberoptic endoscopes that provide a view that is both panoramic and microscopic. The third principle is the maintenance of thorough hemostasis throughout the operation. The fourth principle is minimization of trauma to normal tissue, which can impair postoperative function and counters attempts at maintaining intraoperative hemostasis.

Site-Specific Principles

The essential challenges of skull base surgery are complete tumor extirpation, reliable reconstruction of the skull base, and maintenance of patient's quality of life. The high density of vascular and neurologic structures, as well as the potential for devastating sensory and functional deficits, demands that a highly developed surgical technique be used in the management of skull base lesions.[7] A team-oriented approach between the rhinologic surgeon and the neurosurgeon is advantageous, beginning with preoperative evaluation of surgical goals and continuing throughout the operative procedure and postoperative period.

Complete Tumor Resection

In contrast to the dogma of most oncologic surgery, resection with wide local margins is not mandatory to achieve cure provided that all margins are microscopically free of tumor.[5,8] Similarly, en bloc resection is less important than total tumor removal. Tumor extirpation with negative margins, rather than en bloc resection, has been shown to be an independent predictor of outcome in anterior skull base surgery.[9] The endoscopic approach has not been shown to affect the ability to obtain negative margins.[10] Regardless, the primary goal of tumor resection should never be compromised by the intention to perform endoscopic surgery, and the option to convert to an open approach to ensure clear margins should always be available. In selected cases, endoscopic and open transcranial approaches may be combined to enable complete tumor removal and reliable reconstruction.[5,11]

Watertight Reconstruction

Early attempts at endoscopic skull base tumor resection met with limited acceptance due to a rate of postoperative CSF leak that exceeded 20% in some series.[12,13] With the development of effective reconstructive strategies, postoperative leak rates have been significantly reduced to an overall rate below 5%, which is comparable to the leak rate for open transcranial approaches.[14,15] Multilayered closure of the skull base defect remains the key aspect of complex skull base reconstruction. Creation of a watertight and airtight separation of extracranial and intracranial contents should not be compromised by the use of endoscopic techniques. The potential consequences of inadequate closure include CSF leak, meningitis, pneumocephalus, and death.

Quality-of-Life Preservation

An important consideration for all skull base approaches is the preservation of normal nasal anatomy and nasal function.

Site-specific assessments after open skull base surgery have shown little detrimental effect on patient-reported quality of life.[16,17] Similar assessments after endoscopic skull base surgery suggest that long-term improvements in quality of life are possible.[18] Sinonasal-related quality of life carries particular interest, as the use of an endonasal approach has the potential to disrupt normal mucociliary function and sinus physiology.[19] On the other hand, the use of endoscopic techniques during the approach may have a secondary benefit of correcting preexisting septal deviation, turbinate hypertrophy, or sinus ostium obstruction, which could translate to improved quality of life.[20] The choice of reconstructive option may have an effect on sinonasal-related quality of life, which may be partly dependent on technique.[18,20] Postoperative nasal crusting, which typically results from excessive mucosal trauma, has an influence on sinonasal-related quality of life and may persist for several months postoperatively.[21] Another potentially significant source of reduced quality of life is olfactory dysfunction produced by injury to the olfactory neuroepithelium during the endonasal approach.[22] In general, the destruction of normal sinonasal structures should be avoided with the intention of preserving postoperative function and patient's quality of life. An exception to this principle is the case of sinonasal malignancy, in which the creation of a wide postoperative cavity is desirable to permit surveillance for tumor recurrence on routine examination.

Limits of Resection

The limits of resectability have been defined for open cranial base approaches and are similar for endoscopic approaches. The intracranial portion of the carotid artery cannot be readily sacrificed, and manipulation carries the risk of dissection or hemorrhage with possibly catastrophic results. Involvement of the optic chiasm or bilateral optic nerves is an absolute contraindication to surgical resection. Relative contraindications include the involvement of brain parenchyma and orbital contents, as resection by endoscopic techniques is currently not practicable. Involvement of the bilateral cavernous sinus has been previously considered a contraindication, although the improved anatomic detail and microscopic control afforded by modern endoscopes have made possible the resection of such tumors.

The anatomic limits of the endoscopic approaches continue to be defined. Currently, angled endoscopes can be used to visualize surgical resection as far anteriorly as the frontal sinus, and from lamina papyracea to lamina papyracea.[23] Posteriorly, tumors involving the posterior clinoid processes and the intracranial third ventricle can be accessed by endoscopic techniques.[24] The inferior extent is the craniocervical junction in a plane parallel to the hard palate, while the lateral limit is currently perceived as the parapharyngeal space and jugular foramen.[25,26]

Endoscopic versus Nonendoscopic Approaches

Despite the narrow corridors used to provide the minimal-access approaches, the ultimate goal of endoscopic surgery is to perform resection as aggressively as with traditional approaches. There are several potential benefits of endoscopic surgery compared with traditional microscope-assisted transsphenoidal surgery.[27] Trauma to the nasal mucosa can be minimized with the endoscopic approach, as there is no need for a retractor to create a visual corridor.[28,29] The endoscopic field of view is panoramic, and angled telescopes can be applied to enable the surgeon to see around corners.[29,30] Minimal violation of normal structures is required for access to the target, which has the potential to decrease operative time, obviate the need for nasal packing, and shorten hospital stays.[28,29] With regard to traditional transfacial approaches, the endoscopic approaches avoid large skin incisions and eliminate excessive bony destruction that can contribute to significant pain and deformity. In addition, transfacial approaches can predispose to vestibular stenosis, facial hypoesthesia, and functional impairments. Risks carried by all endonasal approaches include crusting, synechiae, sinusitis, and vestibular abrasions. Excessive turbinate resection may result in excessive turbulent flow and paradoxical nasal obstruction, a disabling condition known as ozena.

Classification of Endoscopic Approaches

A systematic approach is beneficial when considering the endoscopic endonasal approaches to the skull base. The system described by Kassam et al divides the anterior skull base into anatomic planes and modules.[23–25] Under that system, structures from the crista galli to the odontoid process are described in relation to the saggital plane, while the lateral parasphenoidal structures are considered in relation to a coronal plane and the course of the carotid artery. An alternative system described by Schwartz et al considers each approach in relation to the endonasal corridor that is traversed to reach the intended target.[31] Other systems have been described by de Divitiis et al and Cavallo et al.[32–34] Because of the practical division of approaches and the ready adaptability to the skills of the rhinologic surgeon, we have chosen to consider the endoscopic approaches to the skull base using the corridor-approach-target system.

Endoscopic Corridors and Approaches

The practical application of endoscopic skull base surgery can be understood as a combination of three factors: the anatomic target, the skull base approach, and the endonasal corridor (**Table 33.1**).[31] At least 15 targets of the anterior skull base that are amenable to endoscopic approaches have been identified.

Some targets have one possible approach, whereas other targets have multiple approaches. The second component of classification is the endonasal passage that is traversed by the surgeon's instruments. Four passages have been defined, which are referred to as corridors: transnasal, transsphenoidal, transethmoidal, and transmaxillary. These corridors correspond to the paranasal sinuses and can be combined to reach a variety of targets. The link between the nasal corridor and the surgical target is referred to as the approach.

Specific Corridors

Transnasal Corridor

The most basic endoscopic corridor is the transnasal corridor, which can be used to approach skull base targets without traversing any paranasal sinuses (**Fig. 33.2**). The boundaries of the transnasal corridor are the cribriform plate superiorly, the septum medially, the vertical attachment of the middle turbinate laterally, and the hard palate inferiorly. This approach may be unilateral or bilateral if the posterior and superior segments of the nasal septum are removed.

Table 33.1 Endoscopic Endonasal Cranial Base Corridors, Approaches, and Targets

Corridor	Approach	Target
Transnasal	Transcribriform	Olfactory groove
	Transclival	Lower two-thirds of clivus
	Transodontoid	Odontoid/cervicomedullary junction
Transethmoidal	Transfovea ethmoidalis	Anterior cranial fossa
	Transorbital	Orbital apex
	Transsphenoidal	Cavernous sinus
Transsphenoidal	Transsellar	Sella
	Transtuberculum transplanum	Suprasellar cistern
	Transclival	Upper third of clivus
	Transcavernous	Medial cavernous sinus
Transmaxillary	Transpterygoidal	Pterygopalatine fossa
	Transpterygoidal	Infratemporal fossa
	Transpterygoidal	Lateral sphenoid sinus
	Transpterygoidal	Lateral cavernous sinus
	Transpterygoidal	Meckel cave
	Transpterygoidal	Petrous apex
	Transpterygoidal	Jugular foramen

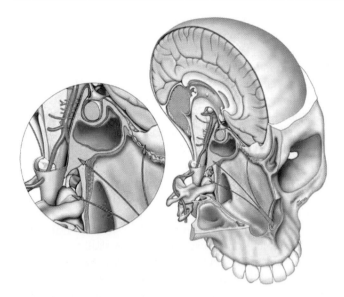

Figure 33.2 The endoscopic transnasal corridor to the anterior skull base.

Printed with permission from: Schwartz TH, Fraser JF, Brown S, Tabaee A, Kacker A, Anand VK. Endoscopic cranial base surgery: classification of operative approaches. *Neurosurgery* 2008;62:994. © Wolters Kluwer Health. All rights reserved. Used with permission.

The transnasal approach may be used to approach targets superiorly at the cribiform plate and olfactory groove, as well as inferiorly at the lower two thirds of the clivus. This can also provide access to the odontoid process and cervicomedullary junction.

Transethmoidal Corridor

The transethmoidal corridor extends the transnasal corridor to address targets lateral to the vertical attachment of the middle turbinate (**Fig. 33.3**). This corridor requires the completion of a total anterior and posterior ethmoidectomy. The boundaries of the transethmoidal corridor are the fovea ethmoidalis superiorly, the lamina papyracea and orbital apex laterally, the sphenoid sinus posteriorly, and the frontal sinus anteriorly. Tumors arising primarily from the ethmoid sinus lie within the transethmoidal corridor. Intracranial targets amenable to the transethmoidal corridor include the anterior cranial fossa and the cavernous sinus.

Transsphenoidal Corridor

The transsphenoidal corridor is the most versatile of the corridors and provides access to primary pathology within the sphenoid sinus as well as a variety of intracranial targets (**Fig. 33.4**). This corridor entails sphenoidotomy and enlargement of one or both sphenoid sinus ostia, which may be facilitated by limited resection of the posterior nasal septum (**Fig. 33.5**). The boundaries of the transsphenoidal corridor are the planum sphenoidale superiorly, the sella and cavernous sinus posteriorly, the middle cranial fossa laterally, and the sphenoid sinus floor inferiorly. Targets accessible by the transsphenoidal corridor include the sella, suprasellar cistern, upper third of the clivus, and the medial cavernous sinus.

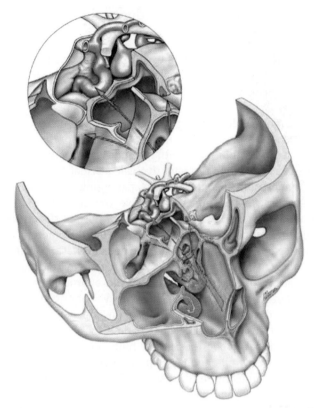

Figure 33.3 The endoscopic transethmoidal corridor to the anterior skull base.

Printed with permission from: Schwartz TH, Fraser JF, Brown S, Tabaee A, Kacker A, Anand VK. Endoscopic cranial base surgery: classification of operative approaches. *Neurosurgery* 2008;62:995. © Wolters Kluwer Health. All rights reserved. Used with permission.

Transmaxillary Corridor

The transmaxillary corridor permits access to targets that lie far laterally from the midline (**Fig. 33.6**). Creation of this corridor begins with uncinectomy, maxillary antrostomy, and ethmoidectomy and passes through the pterygopalatine fossa. The boundaries are the orbital floor superiorly, the maxillary sinus wall anteriorly and laterally, and the plane of the hard palate inferiorly. Targets that are approached by the transmaxillary corridor include the pterygopalatine fossa, infratemporal fossa, lateral sphenoid sinus, lateral cavernous sinus, Meckel's cave, and the petrous apex.

Specific Approaches

Transcribriform Approach

The transcribriform approach uses the transnasal corridor to access the medial anterior cranial fossa and olfactory groove.[35] This approach is best applied to the resection of small esthesioneuroblastomas and olfactory groove meningiomas. Removal of the superior nasal septum facilitates a bilateral approach. The transcribriform approach may be combined with the transfovea approach to improve exposure and

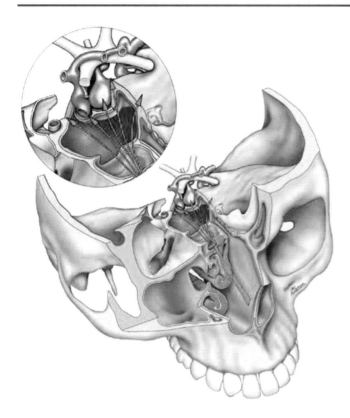

Figure 33.4 The endoscopic transsphenoidal corridor to the anterior skull base.

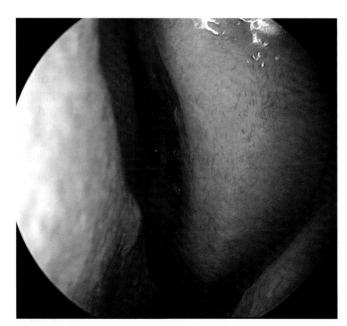

Figure 33.5 Endoscopic view of an unoperated left nasal cavity. The natural sphenoid ostium is visible at the center of the figure, medial to the middle and superior turbinates. The choana is visible at the bottom of the image.

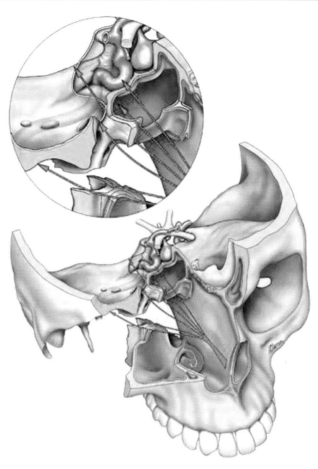

Figure 33.6 The endoscopic transmaxillary corridor to the anterior skull base.

permit the resection of larger tumors. Because the olfactory mucosa lies within this approach, postoperative anosmia is often unavoidable.

Transfovea Ethmoidalis Approach

The transfovea ethmoidalis approach uses the transethmoidal corridor to access the anterior fossa lateral to the cribiform plate.[35] The anterior and posterior ethmoidal arteries are encountered through this approach and must be addressed to ensure vascular control. This approach may be combined with the transcribriform approach to achieve broad exposure of the anterior fossa for the resection of larger tumors. Sacrifice of the superior attachment of the middle turbinate may be necessary. Tumors amenable to this approach include larger olfactory groove meningiomas, esthesioneuroblastomas, juvenile angiofibromas, and sinonasal carcinomas.

Transorbital Approach

The transorbital approach is an extension of the transethmoidal corridor to provide access to the contents of the medial orbit. The orbital apex can be accessed as part of this approach, which is an important consideration when the presence of tumor at the apex poses a threat to normal vision.[36,37] The orbital apex may lie within a posterior ethmoid cell, called an Onodi cell, in up to 25% of the cases.[38] Pathology in this region ranges from benign pseudotumor and hemangioma to malignancies such as lymphoma, sinonasal carcinoma, and esthesioneuroblastoma.

Transsellar Approach

The transsellar approach provides access to the sella turcica via a transsphenoidal corridor. The application of this approach for the management of pituitary adenomas makes this the most commonly used approach by neurosurgeons. Because the sella contents are intradural but extraarachnoidal, tumor resection can typically be accomplished without a significant intraoperative CSF leak (**Fig. 33.7**). Microadenomas as well as macroadenomas can be addressed via the transsellar approach, which can be enhanced by the use of angled scopes and instruments to access tumor that extends into the medial cavernous sinus or the inferior suprasellar cistern (**Fig. 33.8**).[11,39] Less common indications include intrasellar craniopharyngiomas, Rathke cleft cysts, and pituitary carcinoma.

Transplanum Transtuberculum Approach

The transplanum transtuberculum approach expands the transsellar approach to provide exposure to the suprasellar cistern.[40] The tuberculum sellae and planum sphenoidale can be removed in continuation with the superior portion of the anterior sellar wall. Craniopharyngiomas that extend into the third ventricle and interpeduncular cistern can be completely removed via this approach (**Fig. 33.9**).[41] Meningiomas of the tuberculum and planum can be

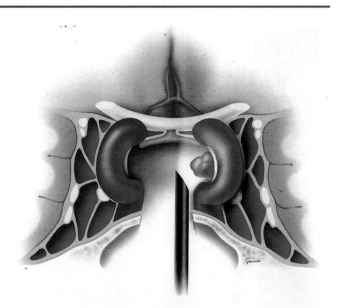

Figure 33.8 Schematic showing the value of using angled endoscopes to visualize residual tumor in obscure locations, which is a major potential benefit of the endoscopic approaches to the skull base. In this instance, residual tumor is present posterior to the carotid artery within the cavernous sinus.

Printed with permission from: Schwartz TH, Anand VK. The endoscopic, endonasal transsphenoidal approach to the sella. In: Anand VK, Schwartz TH, eds., *Practical Endoscopic Skull Base Surgery* 90. Copyright © 2007 Plural Publishing, Inc. All rights reserved. Used with permission.

readily exposed with this approach as well (**Fig. 33.10**). Giant pituitary macroadenomas often extend well into the suprasellar cistern and may require a transplanum transtuberculum approach for adequate tumor extirpation.

Transpterygoidal Approach

The transpterygoidal approach is a versatile technique that uses a transmaxillary corridor to access various

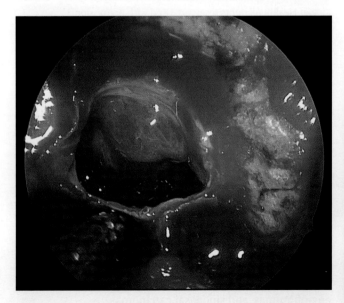

Figure 33.7 Endoscopic view of the defect of the anterior sellar wall after resection of a large pituitary adenoma. The intact arachnoid mater is seen descending into the sella. Preoperative injection of intrathecal fluorescein provides the cerebrospinal fluid with a slight green hue.

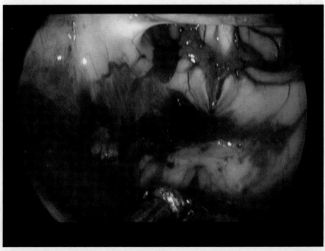

Figure 33.9 Endoscopic intracranial view of the third ventricle after resection of a large craniopharyngioma. The tumor was resected via a transsphenoidal transtuberculum transplanum suprachiasmatic approach.

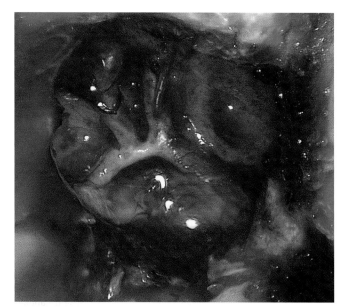

Figure 33.10 Endoscopic view of a surgical defect in the planum sphenoidale after gross total resection of a meningioma. The anterior cerebral arteries and anterior communicating artery are visible, with the optic chiasm visible inferiorly.

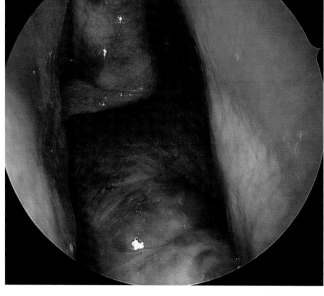

Figure 33.11 Endoscopic view of a large juvenile angiofibroma filling the right nasal cavity. The middle turbinate is at the top of the figure.

anatomic targets situated far laterally from the midline. This approach usually is combined with a transethmoidal and transsphenoidal corridor to achieve the widest possible corridor for surgical access. Drilling of the posterior wall of the maxillary sinus exposes the pterygopalatine fossa, which contains the primary neural and vascular supply to the sinonasal tract. Dissection lateral to the pterygopalatine fossa leads to the infratemporal fossa, parapharyngeal space, and jugular foramen (**Fig. 33.11**).[25,42] Representative lesions of these regions include lymphomas, schwannomas, juvenile angiofibromas, and neoplasms of the deep lobe of the parotid gland. Drilling medially through the pterygoid bone can be used to access the lateral sphenoid sinus, cavernous sinus, Meckel cave, and the petrous apex.[43–45] Pathology in these areas is varied and includes hemangiomas, schwannomas, gliomas, cholesterol granulomas, and chondrosarcomas.

Transclival Approach
The transclival approach provides access to the midline skull base posterior and inferior to the sella. A variable corridor may be used depending on the location of the intended target. For lesions of the upper third of the clivus, a transsphenoidal corridor is appropriate, while lesions of the lower two thirds of the clivus require a transnasal corridor situated parallel to the plane of the hard palate.[46] The two corridors may be combined by removal of the floor of the sphenoid sinus. The pathology that is typically addressed by the transclival approach includes chordomas, chondrosarcomas, keratinaceous cysts, and petroclival meningiomas.[47]

Transcavernous Approach
The transcavernous approach is a heterogeneous designation for three possible approaches to the cavernous sinus.[48,49] The

transsphenoidal transsellar approach to the cavernous sinus has substantial overlap with the approach for the resection of pituitary tumors as described above and is usually selected for the management of pituitary adenoma with invasion of the medial cavernous sinus. The transethmoidal transsphenoidal parasellar approach to the cavernous sinus provides direct access to the medial cavernous sinus without opening the anterior sella wall. This approach may be desirable for pathology that arises primarily within the cavernous sinus or to tumors that extend from other anatomic sites, such as clival chordoma. The transmaxillary transpterygoid approach to the cavernous sinus traverses the lateral sphenoid to address tumors that involve the lateral compartment of the cavernous sinus, which are often associated with cranial neuropathy (**Fig. 33.12**). Tumors arising primarily within the cavernous sinus are rare and include hemangioma, hemangiopericytoma, and chondrosarcoma.[50–52]

Special Considerations

Nasal Cavity Preparation
Preparation of the nasal cavity is of utmost importance to ensure an optimal surgical field. Topical decongestion with 4% cocaine or another sympathomimetic is applied to reduce vascularity and mucosal reactivity. Subsequently, lidocaine with epinephrine is injected into the mucosa at the surgical site. Injection at the sphenopalatine foramen provides a local block of the posterior vascularity, and the mucoperichondrial and mucoperiostial septal flaps can be injected in anticipation of reconstructive needs. Topical

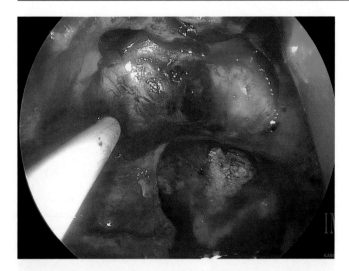

Figure 33.12 Endoscopic view of a tumor of the right cavernous sinus after removal of the posterior sphenoid sinus wall via a transmaxillary transpterygoid approach. A Doppler ultrasound probe has been used to localize the internal carotid artery. The sella is present at the one o'clock position. The final pathology was chondrosarcoma.

application of epinephrine mixed with thrombin facilitates hemostasis and mucosal stability throughout the case.

Nasal Septectomy

The inclusion of nasal septectomy to provide access for endoscopic skull base approaches has not been well studied. We believe that limited resection of the posterior septum, including the vomer and portions of the perpendicular ethmoid plate, has great value in permitting a two-nostril approach to lesions of the skull base. Meanwhile, a detrimental effect on postoperative nasal function has not been demonstrated, likely because nasal resistance is determined by the valve region in the anterior nasal cavity.[53]

Preservation of Nasal Turbinates

Preservation of normal middle turbinates during endoscopic skull base surgery is a plausible prospect in most circumstances, although some authors have described the routine sacrifice of these structures during endoscopic approaches.[23,33] In one series of 163 endoscopic endonasal skull base resections that did not involve the anterior cranial fossa, the rate of middle turbinate preservation was 98%.[54] Given that the middle turbinates participate in the regulation of nasal airflow, contain variable olfactory fibers, and provide a surgical landmark to the skull base and orbit, it is reasonable to advocate for their preservation whenever feasible.

Endoscopic Skull Base Reconstruction

Reconstruction of surgically created defects of the skull base presents a challenge to the endoscopic surgeon.

Separation of intracranial contents from the sinonasal tract is critical to ensuring successful healing and avoiding complications. Failure to achieve this goal can lead to CSF rhinorrhea, chronic headache, pneumocephalus, ascending meningitis, and death. Therefore, a considerable amount of clinical research has been aimed at identifying and refining techniques to reconstruct skull base defects using minimal-access techniques.

An algorithmic approach can be applied to skull base repair depending on the size and location of the skull base defect, the pathology of the lesion, and the volume of the CSF leak.[55] Small defects and low-flow CSF leaks may be repaired with an autologous fat graft, a rigid buttress such as vomer or Medpor (Stryker, Newnan, Georgia, United States), and tissue glue such as DuraSeal (Covidien, Mansfield, Massachusetts, United States). Larger defects with high-volume CSF leak require a more sophisticated reconstruction (**Fig. 33.13**).

Nonvascularized Techniques

Reconstruction can be divided into nonvascularized and vascularized techniques. Autologous bone, fascia, and adipose tissue are well-known nonvascularized materials that have been applied with success in numerous areas of head and neck surgery. The ideal graft tissue has several properties, including ready availability, biocompatibility, minimal resorption, low cost, and the ability to be harvested without cosmetic deformity or functional deficit. The standard locations for fat harvest include the abdomen and the lateral thigh. Fascia lata may be simultaneously harvested from the lateral thigh, which may be required for cases of large defects that require dural closure (**Fig. 33.14**).

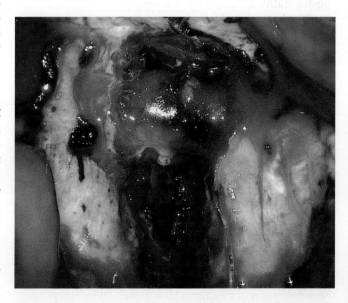

Figure 33.13 Endoscopic view of a complex midline defect involving the clivus, sella, and tuberculum sella after gross total resection of a large epidermoid cyst that extended from the prepontine cistern to the anterior clinoid processes. The cavernous sinuses and carotid arteries remain unexposed on either side.

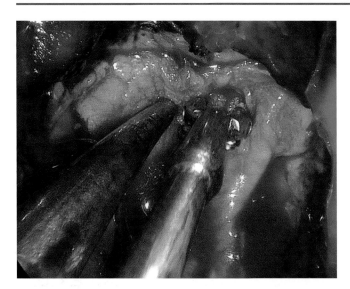

Figure 33.14 Endoscopic view of a fascia lata onlay graft being positioned using microinstruments.

Cartilage and bone may be harvested from the nasal septum, conchal bowl of the ear, and rib.

A simple, single-layer closure has been shown to be sufficient for sellar defects without a CSF intraoperative leak.[56,57] Small CSF leaks may be addressed by a "bath-plug" reconstruction, consisting of an autologous fat inlay held in place with tissue sealant without a rigid buttress.[58] However, because of the unique requirement of creating a watertight seal at the skull base, these simple grafting techniques may not be successful when used in isolation when a significant intraoperative CSF leak is present. The use of multiple layers provides a stronger reconstruction and a lower risk of postoperative CSF leak (**Fig. 33.15A** to **D**).[55]

The choice of graft material is an important consideration. Autologous fat is a reliable choice as it is readily available, has excellent compatibility, and limited resorption. Gelfoam is also useful for obliterating a surgical cavity in which an intraoperative CSF leak is not present. When the dura mater has been widely opened or resected, a pliable dural substitute is needed. Autologous fascia lata is an excellent choice and can be used as an overlay or underlay graft and shares the advantages previously stated for autologous fat. Alternatively, acellular dermis (AlloDerm, LifeCell Corporation, Woodlands, Texas, United States) has been used as primary graft material in large skull base defects.[59] The choice of a rigid buttress may include refined vomer, synthetic Medpor implants, or absorbable or nonabsorbable miniplates. One potential limitation of miniplates is the tendency to spontaneously extrude with long-term healing.

Innovations in reconstructive techniques continue to be developed. The so-called gasket seal closure, described by Leng et al, incorporates an onlay graft of autologous fascia with a rigid buttress of vomer or Medpor that is countersunk into the surgical defect to provide a watertight seal as a single unit (**Fig. 33.16**).[60] The application of this technique includes large defects of the suprasellar region with high-volume CSF

leak or those in which dural resection has been required. A bilayer graft of fascia lata sutured together, described by Luginbuhl et al and termed the button graft, may be useful for dural reconstruction in cases of high-flow, open-cistern CSF leak.[61]

Vascularized Techniques

The introduction of vascularized reconstruction to minimal-access endoscopic surgery has greatly improved the complication rate.[14,15] The workhorse of endoscopic vascularized reconstruction is the nasoseptal flap, which is a regional flap with an axial blood supply pedicled on the posterior septal branches of the spenopalatine artery (**Fig. 33.17A** to **D**).[62] Use of the nasoseptal flap has been associated with improved postoperative CSF leak rates in published series.[14,15] The successful closure of high-flow CSF leaks using the nasoseptal flap has been reported in up to 94% of the cases.[63] Defects with a large surface area that requires coverage can be reconstructed with a bilateral nasoseptal flap, also called the Janus flap.[64] Several other variations on the use of the nasoseptal flap have been proposed for use in a variety of circumstances.[65,66]

The nasoseptal flap is an effective technique with few postoperative complications. Inadequate flap design or compromise of the vascular pedicle may predispose to flap failure and postoperative CSF leak. Insufficient stripping of the sphenoid sinus mucous membrane may result in the long-term development of a mucocele, in which the secretory surface of the mucosa has become trapped on the undersurface of the nasoseptal flap.[15] Management of this condition involves simple surgical revision.

Other forms of vascularized reconstruction are available to the endoscopic surgeon, which may be of interest in cases in which the native nasal septum is not available or is not viable for harvest, or when the course of the sphenopalatine artery has been interrupted by a wide sphenoidotomy. The pedicled inferior turbinate flap, based on the posterior lateral nasal artery, may be applied to the closure of clival or parasellar defects.[67] The temporoparietal fascia transposition flap, which can be tunneled endoscopically through a transpterygoid approach, is another alternative when a nasoseptal flap is not available and coverage of a large endoscopic defect is required.[68]

Reconstruction Outcomes

A systematic review of the literature shows that the success of closure is dependent on tumor pathology, surgical site, and other variables (some analyses unpublished).[69] The rate of postoperative CSF leak after endoscopic closure is 4.9% for pituitary adenomas (43 studies, 2810 patients), 12.3% for clival chordomas (9 studies, 76 patients), 33.3% for meningiomas (12 studies, 75 patients), and 26.0% for craniopharyngiomas (9 studies, 73 patients). Meningiomas

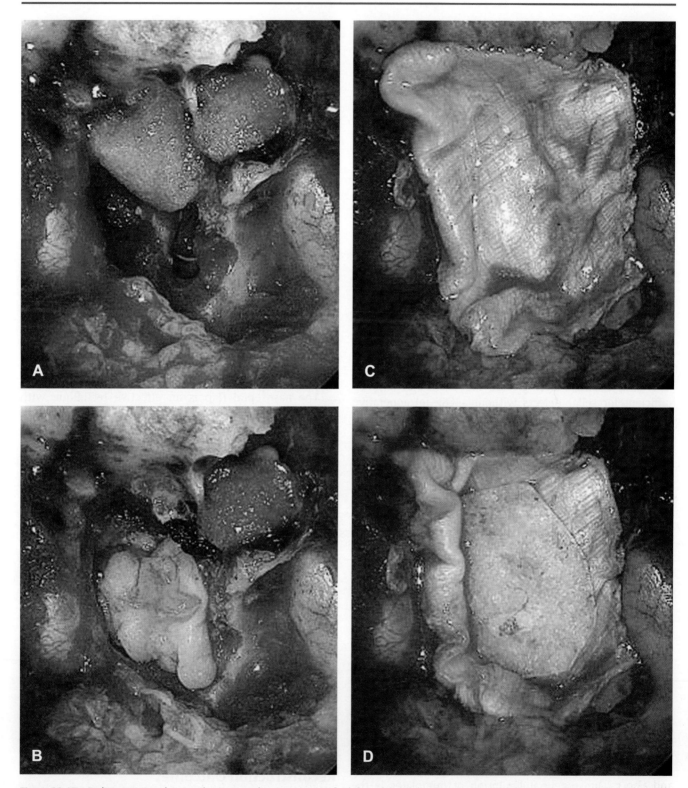

Figure 33.15 Endoscopic view showing the sequential reconstruction of a defect of the clivus after resection of a chordoma. The tumor had significant dural invasion, resulting in an intraoperative cerebrospinal fluid leak after tumor resection. (A) The midline defect communicating with the prepontine cistern and temporary placement of gelfoam. (B) Insertion of an autologous fat graft in the resection cavity. (C) Placement of autologous fascia lata over the reconstruction site. (D) A rigid Medpor prosthesis has been partially countersunk against the fascia to create a watertight "gasket seal" closure.

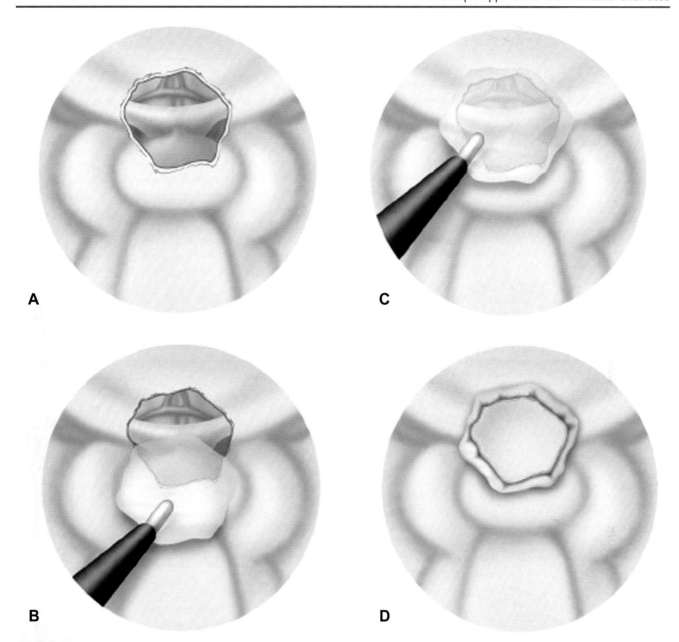

Figure 33.16   The "gasket seal" reconstruction. (A) Surgical defect after a transplanum transtuberculum approach. (B) A piece of fascia lata is fashioned larger than the bone defect. (C) The onlay graft is centered over the defect. (D) A buttress of bone or Medpor is countersunk beneath the bony edges to create a watertight seal.

Printed with permission from: Leng LZ, Brown S, Anand VK, Schwartz TH. "Gasket-seal" watertight closure in minimal-access endoscopic cranial base surgery. *Neurosurgery* 2008;62(ONS Suppl 2):ONSE342–ONSE343. © Wolters Kluwer Health. All rights reserved. Used with permission.

and craniopharyngiomas have a significantly higher rate of leak compared with chordomas and adenomas and also carry a significantly higher rate of reoperation. Intraoperative CSF leak and lumbar drain placement occurs more frequently with tumors involving resection of the anterior cranial fossa compared with hypophyseal, suprasellar, and clival lesions. Closure method also has significance after endoscopic skull base surgery. The rate of postoperative CSF leak was 6.5% with autologous fat alone (23 studies, 1440 patients), 5.6% with gasket seal closure (2 studies, 18 patients), 19.2% with nasoseptal flap alone (5 studies, 78 patients), and 7.5% for multilayer closure without vascularized reconstruction (17 studies, 762 patients). Given that larger defects typically require more complex techniques such as multilayered reconstruction, the postoperative leak rate of large defects is comparable to that achieved with simpler defects. Moreover, these findings indirectly suggest that the success of closure in complex defects can be further improved by the addition of a nasoseptal flap as a final layer of coverage.[14,15]

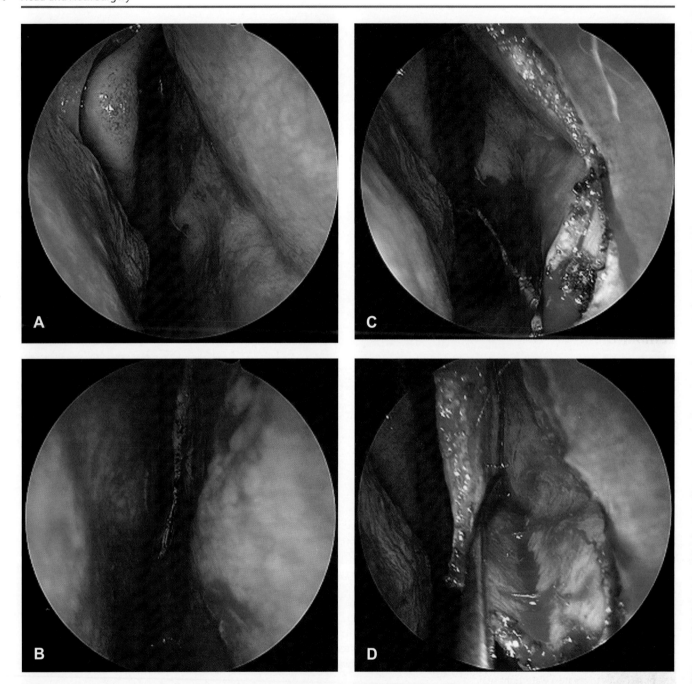

Figure 33.17 Endoscopic view showing the harvest of a pedicled nasoseptal flap from the right nasal cavity. (A) The unoperated nasal cavity, showing the lateralized middle turbinate and the natural sphenoid ostium. (B) The superior cut near the nasal cavity roof. (C) The outline of the nasoseptal flap after completing all incisions. (D) Elevation of the flap from the septum in a submucoperichondrial plane.

Surgical Adjuncts

Intraoperative Navigation

Stereotactic neuronavigation, often referred to as image guidance, provides additional anatomic information that complements the endoscopic view and may increase surgeon understanding of the operative field. During the approach and resection portions of the procedure, the navigation enhances the surgical orientation of the sinonasal structures that are being transgressed, the delineation of

the boundaries of the tumor, and the identification of the surrounding neurovascular structures or orbital structures. One area of particular importance is the relationship of the septations within the sphenoid sinus to the carotid artery, which may precipitate carotid canal fracture and hemorrhage if forcibly fractured. Notable benefit may be observed with use in patients with complex anatomy, revision surgery, or extended procedures.[70,71] Several systems are commercially available, and surgical tracking is performed differently depending on the manufacturer. These systems typically provide a triplanar view that is reconstructed from preoperative imaging that has been coregistered with a navigation protocol. Tracking is typically based on infrared technology or electromagnetic technology, and reproducible accuracy to within 2 mm has been demonstrated.[72]

Intrathecal Fluorescein

Fluorescein is an orange dye that appears bright green when mixed with CSF. When injected intrathecally at the start of the case, fluorescein can improve the detection of a CSF leak that may be otherwise unrecognized in a field of blood and secretions. The resolution of subtle leaks is further increased by the intraoperative application of a blue-light filter (**Fig. 33.18**). Intrathecal injection of fluorescein is currently an off-label use of the product in North America and requires an informed consent discussion with the patient. Although there have been sporadic reports of toxicity, the efficacy and safety of intrathecal fluorescein have been demonstrated.[73]

Lumbar Drainage

Lumbar drainage is an important adjunct for selected cases. The primary goal of lumbar drainage is to decrease the pressure gradient of CSF across the reconstruction site during the postoperative period. However, lumbar drainage may theoretically produce retraction of the brain away from the anterior cranial fossa, which may lead to CSF pooling and intracranial graft displacement. Furthermore, the use of lumbar drainage is associated with complications including meningeal headaches, back pain, local wound infection, pneumocephalus, transtentorial herniation, and retained catheter tip. In addition, lumbar drainage often necessitates

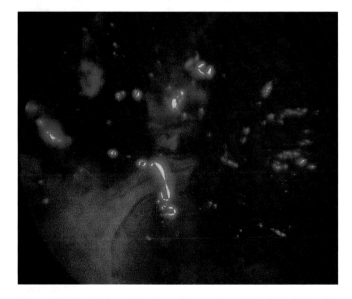

Figure 33.18 Endoscopic view of a cerebrospinal fluid leak after intrathecal injection of fluorescein when viewed by using a blue-light filter.

Printed with permission from: Tabaee A, Placantonakis D, Schwartz TH, Anand VK. Reconstruction after endoscopic skull base surgery. In: Anand VK, Schwartz TH, eds. *Practical Endoscopic Skull Base Surgery* 196. Copyright © 2007 Plural Publishing, Inc. All rights reserved. Used with permission.

prolonged immobility that can predispose to deep vein thrombosis. Given these risks, the routine use of lumbar drainage should be discouraged. The rate of successful endoscopic closure of CSF leaks without lumbar drainage has been reported as 83% to 97%.[74,75] Lumbar drainage may be reserved for cases with a high-volume preoperative CSF leak, evidence of increased intracranial pressure, and those where dural resection or a large intraoperative leak are anticipated. Lumbar drainage is the cornerstone of conservative management for postoperative CSF leaks, which resolve without reoperation in the majority of the cases.[15,35,40,41]

Future Directions

The continual evolution of technology will no doubt promote continued interest in minimal-access surgery of the skull base. Improvements in optics and high-definition video systems allow the surgeon to resolve detail previously unappreciated and enable more precise dissection to remove tumor and preserve normal anatomy. The application of three-dimensional visualization is an area of particular interest that has the potential to overcome the monocular vision of the endoscope. Improvements in intraoperative image-guidance systems, including three-dimensional modeling and fusion with a real-time endoscopic view, also hold promise. The study of surgical outcomes, which has been traditionally measured in terms of survival, operative time, blood loss, and duration of hospitalization, may acquire new measures of success when applied to minimal-access surgery in which quality-of-life concerns become a part of the patient's perception of success. Continued advances in both technology and technique, coupled with thoughtful assessment of surgical outcomes, are likely to promote the integration of endoscopic approaches into the routine management of anterior skull base tumors.

Pearls and Pitfalls

- A team approach between the rhinologic surgeon and the neurosurgeon is critical to the development and execution of endoscopic skull base approaches.

- Complete tumor extirpation with negative margins is a legitimate goal regardless of whether en bloc resection is feasible.

- The use of intraoperative image guidance confirms intraoperative dissection and helps avoid inadvertent injury.

- A mucosa-sparing surgical technique that respects normal anatomy, including the preservation of the middle turbinate, aids in the preservation of postoperative sinonasal function.

- The course of the internal carotid artery and its associations with adjacent structures must be understood, which may be assisted by the use of intraoperative Doppler ultrasonography.

- Intrathecal fluorescein can assist with identification and localization of an intraoperative cerebrospinal fluid (CSF) leak.

- A multilayered watertight closure of the skull base is mandatory whenever the dura mater is disrupted.

- The selection of appropriate grafting material and vascularized reconstruction are important considerations.

- Judicious use of a lumbar drain can help regulate intracranial pressure during the early postoperative period.

- Postoperative CSF leaks should be conservatively managed.

- Conscientious postoperative care with frequent debridement and nasal toilet are beneficial until the surgical defect has fully mucosalized.

References

1. Gandhi CD, Christiano LD, Eloy JA, Prestigiacomo CJ, Post KD. The historical evolution of transsphenoidal surgery: facilitation by technological advances. Neurosurg Focus 2009;27(3):E8

2. Tabaee A, Nyquist G, Anand VK, Singh A, Kacker A, Schwartz TH. Palliative endoscopic surgery in advanced sinonasal and anterior skull base neoplasms. Otolaryngol Head Neck Surg 2010;142(1):126–128

3. Raper DMS, Komotar RJ, Starke RM, Anand VK, Schwartz TH. Endoscopic versus open approaches to the skull base: a comprehensive literature review. Oper Tech Otolaryngol---Head Neck Surg 2011;22(4):302–307

4. Tabaee A, Anand VK, Barrón Y, et al. Endoscopic pituitary surgery: a systematic review and meta-analysis. J Neurosurg 2009;111(3):545–554

5. Eloy JA, Vivero RJ, Hoang K, et al. Comparison of transnasal endoscopic and open craniofacial resection for malignant tumors of the anterior skull base. Laryngoscope 2009;119(5):834–840

6. Hanna E, DeMonte F, Ibrahim S, Roberts D, Levine N, Kupferman M. Endoscopic resection of sinonasal cancers with and without craniotomy: oncologic results. Arch Otolaryngol Head Neck Surg 2009;135(12):1219–1224

7. Schaberg MR, Anand VK, Schwartz TH. 10 pearls for safe endoscopic skull base surgery. Otolaryngol Clin North Am 2010;43(4):945–954

8. Dave SP, Bared A, Casiano RR. Surgical outcomes and safety of transnasal endoscopic resection for anterior skull tumors. Otolaryngol Head Neck Surg 2007;136(6):920–927

9. Ganly I, Patel SG, Singh B, et al. Craniofacial resection for malignant paranasal sinus tumors: report of an International Collaborative Study. Head Neck 2005;27(7):575–584

10. Cohen MA, Liang J, Cohen IJ, Grady MS, O'Malley BW Jr, Newman JG. Endoscopic resection of advanced anterior skull base lesions: oncologically safe? ORL J Otorhinolaryngol Relat Spec 2009;71(3):123–128

11. Greenfield JP, Leng LZ, Chaudhry U, et al. Combined simultaneous endoscopic transsphenoidal and endoscopic transventricular resection of a giant pituitary macroadenoma. Minim Invasive Neurosurg 2008;51(5):306–309

12. Gardner PA, Kassam AB, Thomas A, et al. Endoscopic endonasal resection of anterior cranial base meningiomas. Neurosurgery 2008;63(1):36–52, discussion 52–54

13. Stippler M, Gardner PA, Snyderman CH, Carrau RL, Prevedello DM, Kassam AB. Endoscopic endonasal approach for clival chordomas. Neurosurgery 2009;64(2):268–277, discussion 277–278

14. Kassam AB, Thomas A, Carrau RL, et al. Endoscopic reconstruction of the cranial base using a pedicled nasoseptal flap. Neurosurgery 2008; 63(1 Suppl 1):ONS44–ONS52, discussion ONS52–ONS53

15. McCoul ED, Anand VK, Singh A, Nyquist GG, Schaberg MR, Schwartz TH. Long-term outcomes after endoscopic skull base reconstruction with the nasoseptal flap. World Neurosurg Epub 2012 Sept 25.DOI: 10.1016/j.wnev. 2012.08.011

16. Gil Z, Abergel A, Spektor S, et al. Quality of life following surgery for anterior skull base tumors. Arch Otolaryngol Head Neck Surg 2003;129(12):1303–1309

17. Abergel A, Fliss DM, Margalit N, Gil Z. A prospective evaluation of short-term health-related quality of life in patients undergoing anterior skull base surgery. Skull Base 2010;20(1):27–33

18. McCoul ED, Anand VK, Schwartz TH. Improvements in site-specific quality of life 6 months endoscopic anterior skull base surgery: a prospective study. J Neurosurg 2012;117(3): 498–506

19. Suberman TA, Zanation AM, Ewend MG, Senior BA, Ebert CS Jr. Sinonasal quality-of-life before and after endoscopic, endonasal, minimally invasive pituitary surgery. Int Forum Allergy Rhinol 2011;1(3):161–166

20. McCoul ED, Anand VK, Bedrosian JC, Schwartz TH. Endoscopic skull base surgery and its impact on sinonasal-related quality of life. Int Forum Allergy Rhinol 2012;2(2):174–181

21. de Almeida JR, Snyderman CH, Gardner PA, Carrau RL, Vescan AD. Nasal morbidity following endoscopic skull base surgery: a prospective cohort study. Head Neck 2011;33(4):547–551

22. Rotenberg BW, Saunders S, Duggal N. Olfactory outcomes after endoscopic transsphenoidal pituitary surgery. Laryngoscope 2011;121(8):1611–1613

23. Kassam A, Snyderman CH, Mintz A, Gardner P, Carrau RL. Expanded endonasal approach: the rostrocaudal axis, part I: crista galli to the sella turcica. Neurosurg Focus 2005;19(1):E3

24. Kassam A, Snyderman CH, Mintz A, Gardner P, Carrau RL. Expanded endonasal approach: the rostrocaudal axis, part II: posterior clinoids to the foramen magnum. Neurosurg Focus 2005; 19(1):E4

25. Kassam AB, Gardner P, Snyderman C, Mintz A, Carrau R. Expanded endonasal approach: fully endoscopic, completely transnasal approach to the middle third of the clivus, petrous bone, middle cranial fossa, and infratemporal fossa. Neurosurg Focus 2005; 19(1):E6

26. Falcon RT, Rivera-Serrano CM, Miranda JF, et al. Endoscopic endonasal dissection of the infratemporal fossa: anatomic relationships and importance of eustachian tube in the endoscopic skull base surgery. Laryngoscope 2011;121(1):31–41

27. Schaberg MR, Anand VK, Schwartz TH, Cobb W. Microscopic versus endoscopic transnasal pituitary surgery. Curr Opin Otolaryngol Head Neck Surg 2010;18(1):8–14

28. Jho HD, Alfieri A. Endoscopic endonasal pituitary surgery: evolution of surgical technique and equipment in 150 operations. Minim Invasive Neurosurg 2001;44(1):1–12

29. Cappabianca P, Cavallo LM, de Divitiis E. Endoscopic endonasal transsphenoidal surgery. Neurosurgery 2004;55(4):933–940, discussion 940–941

30. Spencer WR, Das K, Nwagu C, et al. Approaches to the sellar and parasellar region: anatomic comparison of the microscope versus endoscope. Laryngoscope 1999;109(5):791–794

31. Schwartz TH, Fraser JF, Brown S, Tabaee A, Kacker A, Anand VK. Endoscopic cranial base surgery: classification of operative approaches. Neurosurgery 2008;62(5):991–1002, discussion 1002–1005

32. de Divitiis E, Cappabianca P, Cavallo LM. Endoscopic transsphenoidal approach: adaptability of the procedure to different sellar lesions. Neurosurgery 2002;51(3):699–705, discussion 705–707

33. de Divitiis E, Cavallo LM, Cappabianca P, Esposito F. Extended endoscopic endonasal transsphenoidal approach for the removal of suprasellar tumors: part 2. Neurosurgery 2007;60(1):46–58, discussion 58–59

34. Cavallo LM, Messina A, Cappabianca P, et al. Endoscopic endonasal surgery of the midline skull base: anatomical study and clinical considerations. Neurosurg Focus 2005;19(1):E2

35. Greenfield JP, Anand VK, Kacker A, et al. Endoscopic endonasal transethmoidal transcribriform transfovea ethmoidalis approach to the anterior cranial fossa and skull base. Neurosurgery 2010;66(5):883–892, discussion 892

36. Roth J, Fraser JF, Singh A, Bernardo A, Anand VK, Schwartz TH. Surgical approaches to the orbital apex: comparison of endoscopic endonasal and transcranial approaches using a novel 3D endoscope. Orbit 2011;30(1):43–48

37. Murchison AP, Rosen MR, Evans JJ, Bilyk JR. Endoscopic approach to the orbital apex and periorbital skull base. Laryngoscope 2011;121(3):463–467

38. Weinberger DG, Anand VK, Al-Rawi M, Cheng HJ, Messina AV. Surgical anatomy and variations of the Onodi cell. Am J Rhinol 1996;10:365–370

39. Hofstetter CP, Shin BJ, Mubita L, et al. Endoscopic endonasal transsphenoidal surgery for functional pituitary adenomas. Neurosurg Focus 2011;30(4):E10

40. Laufer I, Anand VK, Schwartz TH. Endoscopic, endonasal extended transsphenoidal, transplanum transtuberculum approach for resection of suprasellar lesions. J Neurosurg 2007;106(3):400–406

41. Schwartz TH, Anand VK. The endoscopic endonasal transsphenoidal approach to the suprasellar cistern. Clin Neurosurg 2007;54:226–235

42. McCoul ED, Schwartz TH, Anand VK. Endoscopic approaches to the infratemporal fossa. Oper Tech Otolaryngol---Head Neck Surg 2011;22(4):285–290

43. Hofstetter CP, Singh A, Anand VK, Kacker A, Schwartz TH. The endoscopic, endonasal, transmaxillary transpterygoid approach to the pterygopalatine fossa, infratemporal fossa, petrous apex, and the Meckel cave. J Neurosurg 2010;113(5):967–974

44. Zanation AM, Snyderman CH, Carrau RL, Gardner PA, Prevedello DM, Kassam AB. Endoscopic endonasal surgery for petrous apex lesions. Laryngoscope 2009;119(1):19–25

45. Kassam AB, Prevedello DM, Carrau RL, et al. The front door to Meckel's cave: an anteromedial corridor via expanded endoscopic endonasal approach—technical considerations and clinical series. Neurosurgery 2009; 64(3 Suppl):ons71–ons82, discussion ons82–ons83

46. Fraser JF, Nyquist GG, Moore N, Anand VK, Schwartz TH. Endoscopic endonasal minimal access approach to the clivus: case series and technical nuances. Neurosurgery 2010;67(3 Suppl Operative):ons 150-158; discussion ons 158

47. Fraser JF, Nyquist GG, Moore N, Anand VK, Schwartz TH. Endoscopic endonasal transclival resection of chordomas: operative technique, clinical outcome, and review of the literature. J Neurosurg 2010;112(5):1061–1069

48. Raithatha R, McCoul ED, Woodworth GF, Schwartz TH, Anand VK. Endoscopic endonasal approaches to the cavernous sinus. Int Forum Allergy Rhinol 2012;2(1):9–15

49. McCoul ED, Schwartz TH, Anand VK. Endoscopic approaches to the cavernous sinus. Oper Tech Otolaryngol---Head Neck Surg 2011;22(4):263–268

50. Fraser JF, Mass AY, Brown S, Anand VK, Schwartz TH. Transnasal endoscopic resection of a cavernous sinus hemangioma: technical note and review of the literature. Skull Base 2008;18(5):309–315

51. Alfieri A, Jho HD. Endoscopic endonasal approaches to the cavernous sinus: surgical approaches. Neurosurgery 2001;49(2):354–360, discussion 360–362

52. Frank G, Pasquini E. Endoscopic endonasal cavernous sinus surgery, with special reference to pituitary adenomas. Front Horm Res 2006;34:64–82

53. Eduardo Nigro C, Faria Aguar Nigro J, Mion O, Ferreira Mello J Jr, Louis Voegels R, Roithmann R. A systematic review to assess the anatomical correlates of the notches in acoustic rhinometry. Clin Otolaryngol 2009;34(5):431–437

54. Nyquist GG, Anand VK, Brown S, Singh A, Tabaee A, Schwartz TH. Middle turbinate preservation in endoscopic transsphenoidal surgery of the anterior skull base. Skull Base 2010;20(5):343–347

55. Tabaee A, Anand VK, Brown SM, Lin JW, Schwartz TH. Algorithm for reconstruction after endoscopic pituitary and skull base surgery. Laryngoscope 2007;117(7):1133–1137

56. Couldwell WT, Kan P, Weiss MH. Simple closure following transsphenoidal surgery. Technical note. Neurosurg Focus 2006;20(3):E11

57. Esposito F, Dusick JR, Fatemi N, Kelly DF. Graded repair of cranial base defects and cerebrospinal fluid leaks in transsphenoidal surgery. Neurosurgery 2007; 60(4 Suppl 2):295–303, discussion 303–304

58. Wormald PJ, McDonogh M. The bath-plug closure of anterior skull base cerebrospinal fluid leaks. Am J Rhinol 2003;17(5):299–305

59. Germani RM, Vivero R, Herzallah IR, Casiano RR. Endoscopic reconstruction of large anterior skull base defects using acellular dermal allograft. Am J Rhinol 2007;21(5):615–618

60. Leng LZ, Brown S, Anand VK, Schwartz TH. "Gasket-seal" watertight closure in minimal-access endoscopic cranial base surgery. Neurosurgery 2008; 62(5 Suppl 2):E342–E343, discussion E343

61. Luginbuhl AJ, Campbell PG, Evans J, Rosen M. Endoscopic repair of high-flow cranial base defects using a bilayer button. Laryngoscope 2010;120(5):876–880

62. Hadad G, Bassagasteguy L, Carrau RL, et al. A novel reconstructive technique after endoscopic expanded endonasal approaches: vascular pedicle nasoseptal flap. Laryngoscope 2006;116(10):1882–1886

63. Zanation AM, Carrau RL, Snyderman CH, et al. Nasoseptal flap reconstruction of high flow intraoperative cerebral spinal fluid leaks during endoscopic skull base surgery. Am J Rhinol Allergy 2009;23(5):518–521

64. Nyquist GG, Anand VK, Singh A, Schwartz TH. Janus flap: bilateral nasoseptal flaps for anterior skull base reconstruction. Otolaryngol Head Neck Surg 2010;142(3):327–331

65. Caicedo-Granados E, Carrau R, Snyderman CH, et al. Reverse rotation flap for reconstruction of donor site after vascular pedicled nasoseptal flap in skull base surgery. Laryngoscope 2010;120(8):1550–1552

66. Pinheiro-Neto CD, Prevedello DM, Carrau RL, et al. Improving the design of the pedicled nasoseptal flap for skull base reconstruction: a radioanatomic study. Laryngoscope 2007;117(9):1560–1569

67. Fortes FS, Carrau RL, Snyderman CH, et al. The posterior pedicle inferior turbinate flap: a new vascularized flap for skull base reconstruction. Laryngoscope 2007;117(8):1329–1332

68. Fortes FS, Carrau RL, Snyderman CH, et al. Transpterygoid transposition of a temporoparietal fascia flap: a new method for skull base reconstruction after endoscopic expanded endonasal approaches. Laryngoscope 2007;117(6):970–976

69. Komotar RJ, Starke RM, Raper DM, Anand VK, Schwartz TH. Endoscopic skull base surgery: a comprehensive comparison with open transcranial approaches. Br J Neurosurg 2012;26(5):637-648

70. Lasio G, Ferroli P, Felisati G, Broggi G. Image-guided endoscopic transnasal removal of recurrent pituitary adenomas. Neurosurgery 2002;51(1):132–136, discussion 136–137

71. Jagannathan J, Prevedello DM, Ayer VS, Dumont AS, Jane JA Jr, Laws ER. Computer-assisted frameless stereotaxy in transsphenoidal surgery at a single institution: review of 176 cases. Neurosurg Focus 2006;20(2):E9

72. Kaus M, Steinmeier R, Sporer T, Ganslandt O, Fahlbusch R. Technical accuracy of a neuronavigation system measured with a high-precision mechanical micromanipulator. Neurosurgery 1997;41(6):1431–1436, discussion 1436–1437

73. Tabaee A, Placantonakis DG, Schwartz TH, Anand VK. Intrathecal fluorescein in endoscopic skull base surgery. Otolaryngol Head Neck Surg 2007;137(2):316–320

74. Burns JA, Dodson EE, Gross CW. Transnasal endoscopic repair of cranionasal fistulae: a refined technique with long-term follow-up. Laryngoscope 1996;106(9 Pt 1):1080–1083

75. Casiano RR, Jassir D. Endoscopic cerebrospinal fluid rhinorrhea repair: is a lumbar drain necessary? Otolaryngol Head Neck Surg 1999;121(6):745–750

34 Image Guidance for Sinus Tumors

Benjamin S. Bleier and Rodney J. Schlosser

Core Messages

- Image guidance is helpful in both planning and execution of endoscopic tumor resection. It should never replace a thorough understanding of anatomy and the patient's disease.

- Tracking of surgical instruments may be achieved either through optical or electromagnetic systems although there is no specific advantage of either with respect to surgical accuracy.

- Optimal accuracy requires high resolution preoperative imaging coupled with careful intraoperative registration.

Advances in imaging within the past two decades have led to the widespread use of image-guided surgery (IGS) in the management of sinonasal neoplasms. While the basic tenets of stereotactic surgery were introduced a century ago, current systems allow for detailed triplanar preoperative planning with multiple imaging modalities imaging as well as highly accurate intraoperative surgical navigation. Despite these advances, all systems may be associated with several types of errors and thus should be used only to augment sound clinical judgment and surgical expertise.

Historical Context

While the first stereotactic devices were developed in the early 20th century, the coupling of radiography to surgical navigation did not occur until the 1940s.[1] The introduction of computed tomography (CT) heralded significant improvements in image quality, eventually leading to a CT-guided frame-based system in 1976.[2] With this improved surgical accuracy, the bulky and intrusive stereotactic frame provided an impetus to the development of early frameless systems in the 1980s.[3] Since that time, the use of IGS has become widely accepted for both inflammatory and neoplastic sinonasal diseases and is currently endorsed by the American Academy of Otolaryngology-Head and Neck Surgery (**Table 34.1**).[4]

Operating Principles

While all commercially available IGS systems use a unique method of tracking, they all function to monitor the position of an intraoperative localization device (ILD) within the surgical volume. Each system uses a proprietary software platform designed to construct a virtual data set from preoperative imaging. These data are subsequently correlated to the surgical volume through a process of registration.[1] The ILD may be either fabricated as a surgical implement or directly attached to a preexisting instrument. Current systems use either optical or electromagnetic (EM) technology to track the ILD (**Fig. 34.1**).[3]

EM systems use a radiofrequency field to gather positional information through a receiver in the ILD. Drawbacks of this system include the potential for field distortion by ferromagnetic objects and the reliance on wires to communicate with the system.[3] Some systems also require the patient to use the same headset from the preoperative imaging to the surgery, although some studies suggest that this has little effect on accuracy.[5,6]

In optical systems, the ILD is composed of an array of light-emitting diodes (active tracking) or reflective spheres (passive tracking), which are captured by an overhead camera and referenced to a set of markers on the headset worn by the patient. The principal drawback of this technology is that it requires an uninterrupted line of sight to the overhead camera.[3]

System Setup

Before use, all IGS systems must be registered and calibrated. Registration involves the process of defining the relationship between fiducial position and the corresponding point in the data set volume. Calibration refers only to the confirmation of the relationship between the instrument tip and the ILD.[3] Various registration paradigms include automatic, paired-point, and contour-based registration.

Automatic registration uses a headset that incorporates the fiducial points in a fixed position, allowing the software platform to perform the registration automatically. In this system, changes in the headframe position result in diminished accuracy.[3]

In contrast, paired-point and contour-based registrations require manual mapping of the fiducial points that have

Table 34.1 AAO-HNS Indications for Intraoperative Use of Computer-Aided Surgery

---

Revision sinus surgery

Distorted sinus anatomy of development, postoperative, or traumatic origin

Extensive sinonasal polyposis

Pathology involving the frontal, posterior ethmoid, and sphenoid sinuses

Disease abutting the skull base, orbit, optic nerve, or carotid artery

Cerebrospinal fluid rhinorrhea or conditions where there is a skull base defect

Benign and malignant sinonasal neoplasms

AAO-HNS, American Academy of Otolaryngology-Head and Neck Surgery.

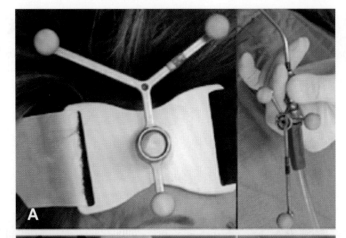

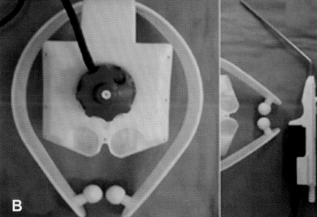

Figure 34.1 Components of optical and electromagnetic tracking systems. (A) The optical system uses reflective spheres in both the headset and the instrument to monitor the intraoperative localization device. (B) In the electromagnetic systems, the headpiece transmits a radiofrequency signal that is detected by a receiver in the handpiece.

been predefined in the virtual data set. In contour-based registration, this is followed by the acquisition of up to 500 points over fixed facial contours. The computer then calculates the registration by aligning these points with the virtual data set.

Preoperative Planning

One of the benefits of the IGS system is the ability to perform detailed preoperative planning with rapid scrolling through sequential high-resolution images in multiple axes. This allows the surgeon to map the location and extent of the neoplasm as well as the degree of involvement of adjacent anatomic structures.[7]

If the lesion involves the skull base, preoperative review aids in the selection of the optimal surgical corridor as well as in the estimation of the size of the expected defect (**Fig. 34.2**).[1] The ability to perform three-dimensional (3D) reconstruction is particularly useful in characterizing morphologically complex lesions at the skull base. Rosahl et al[8] reported that in a series of 110 patients, virtual 3D reconstruction enhanced surgical planning and assisted in targeting structures that would otherwise be hidden or obscured in the surgical field.

Advances in neuroimaging have also allowed for the incorporation of soft tissue data into the preoperative planning stage. CT alone does not allow for accurate delineation of soft tissue and neurovascular structures. This has been addressed by the advent of image-to-image registration software that allows magnetic resonance imaging (MRI) data to be coupled to CT images by using anatomic landmarks, thereby enabling the creation of a fusion image.[9]

The proximity of sinonasal lesions to major sinonasal or intracranial vasculature structures may also be visualized by using 3D CT angiography (3D-CTA). By using this protocol, images are captured as the contrast bolus fills the internal carotid system, thereby allowing for the simultaneous acquisition of the vascular and bony anatomy of the skull base.[9] Leong et al[10] performed 3D-CTA in 18 cases and found an accuracy of 2 mm or more and concluded that 3D-CTA provided an accurate assessment of the location of the internal carotid artery and its relationship to the surgical field. The incorporation of diffusion-weighted MRI and positron emission tomography scanning may also prove to aid in planning approaches to metabolically active tumors.[1]

Intraoperative Image Guidance

One of the significant challenges in the endoscopic management of both benign and malignant sinonasal neoplasms is the distortion of normal anatomy resulting from the presence and growth of the tumor (**Fig. 34.3**). IGS has been shown to decrease surgical disorientation,[6] improve surgical completeness, and decrease overall complication rates[9] in inflammatory disease and may be equally efficacious in the setting of neoplasm.

IGS is also valuable in lesions involving the frontal sinus, where the border between the frontal recess and the adjacent orbit and skull base may be difficult to distinguish. Reardon[11] noted a significant increase in the successful

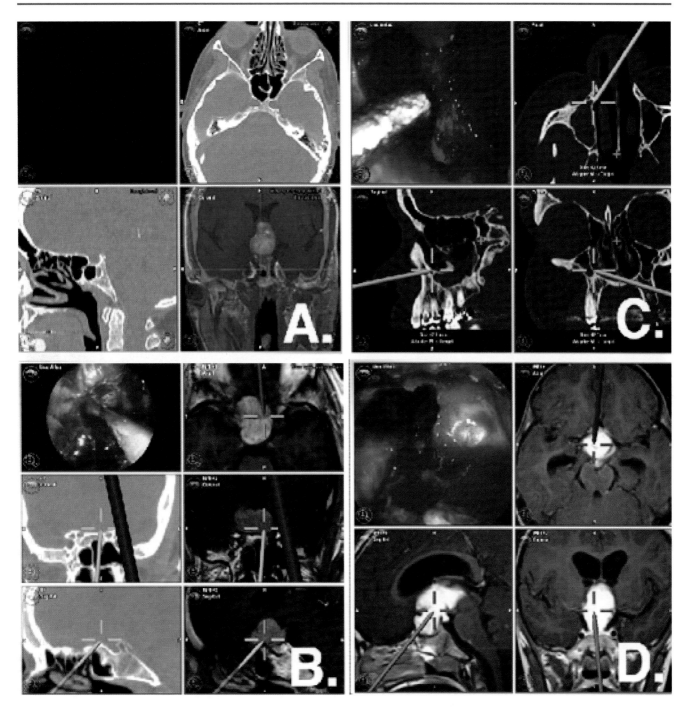

Figure 34.2 The use of image-guided surgery (IGS) in sinonasal and skull base neoplasm. (A) An example of computed tomography/magnetic resonance imaging (MRI) fusion imaging in the setting of a suprasellar pituitary macroadenoma that clarifies the relationship between the lesion and the internal carotid system. (B) IGS is used to map the corridor and the degree of bone removal required in an approach to a tubercular meningioma. (C) The use of IGS to localize the anterior extent of a maxillary sinus inverting papilloma. The angle of approach is achieved by using a transeptal window technique. (D) MRI is used in the setting of a pediatric astrocytoma to assess the extent of resection in the setting of an underpneumatized sphenoid and large cranial base to midface ratio.

frontal sinusotomy for chronic sinusitis following the introduction of IGS in a review of 800 procedures. Success rates in frontal sinus drillout have also been shown to trend toward improvement when using IGS.[12]

External approaches for frontal or anterior cranial fossa lesions may also benefit from the use of IGS by increasing the accuracy of the osteotomy during osteoplastic flap or subfrontal craniotomy.[9] The use of IGS for frontal sinus obliteration was first reported by Carrau et al,[13] who suggested that IGS was more accurate than 6-ft Caldwell radiography, transillumination, and sinus trephination with probing. This finding has been supported by other authors as well.[14]

Finally, the incorporation of CT/MRI fusion and 3D-CTA imaging into the virtual data set provides valuable information with regards to the extent of tumor resection and clarification of boundaries between the lesion and normal adjacent soft tissue and neurovascular structures.[1]

Dilemmas and Controversies

Navigational Accuracy

During the course of endoscopic sinonasal and skull base tumor resection, vital neurovascular structures are

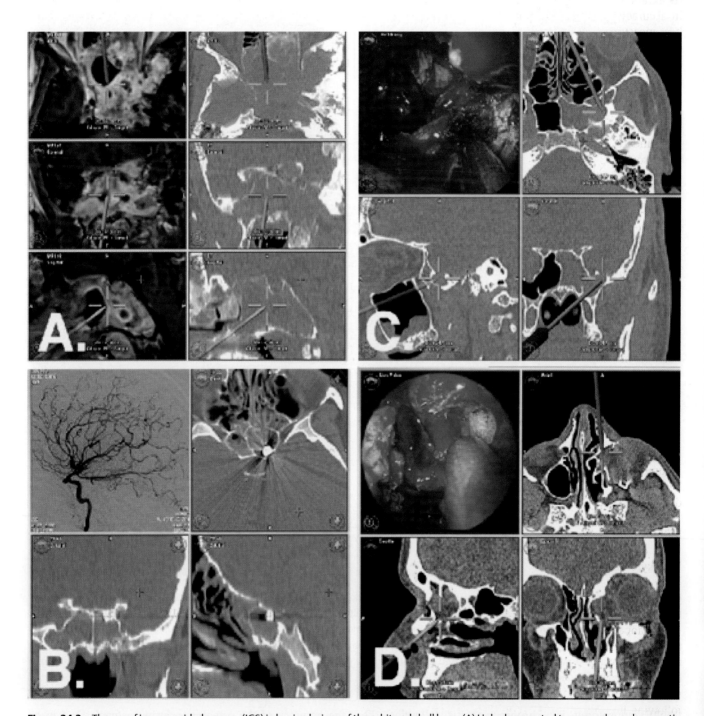

Figure 34.3   The use of image-guided surgery (IGS) in benign lesions of the orbit and skull base. (A) Linked computed tomography and magnetic resonance imaging to aid in optic nerve decompression in the setting of advanced fibrous dysplasia. (B) The use of triplanar imaging to localize and provide mucosal coverage for an internal carotid pseudoaneurysm. The angiographic data were obtained subsequent to surgery. (C) The use of IGS in a transpterygoid approach to a lateral recess sphenoid encephalocele. (D) The use of image guidance to locate and remove an infected medial orbital reconstruction plate following maxillofacial trauma.

commonly encountered; thus, the navigational accuracy of the IGS system is of paramount concern. The degree of baseline accuracy is multifactorial and is derived from the quality of the imaging data set as well as the stability, number, and position of the fiducial points relative to the entire surgical volume. Additional error may then be introduced during the registration process, leading to further subtle degradations in accuracy. Target registration error (TRE) represents the best measure of navigational accuracy and can be assessed clinically by visually comparing known landmarks to their coordinate position in the virtual data set. TRE tends to be lowest proximal to the fiducial points and may increase over time because of fiducial motion, instrument deformation, and tracking errors. As such, the TRE should be assessed intraoperatively in all three axes, as the endoscopic image may underestimate the degree of TRE in any single axis. Other sources of error include fiducial localization error and fiducial registration error.[1]

The reported accuracy of current systems typically falls within 1.5 to 2.4 mm.[3] Of note, Metson et al[15] reported an accuracy within 2 mm by using the InstaTrak and Stealth Station systems with a mean degradation of 0.89 mm during the case, supporting the recommendation that TRE should be assessed throughout the course of the procedure.

Intraoperative Image Updating

Current modeling of registration error presumes that sinonasal anatomy remains static from the preoperative image acquisition through the completion of the procedure. However, during tumor resection both bone and soft tissue structures are subject to displacement secondary to gravitational, physiologic, and hydrodynamic forces. Spring-based and finite element models that attempt to predict volumetric changes based on surface deformation have been developed, although their clinical utility has yet to be determined.[16]

Several reports have investigated the use of intraoperative MRI for skull base lesions and suggest that its use allows for more complete tumor resection. In a retrospective study, Nimsky et al[17] reported a 27% rate of surgical modification in 200 patients based on intraoperative MRI data. However, given the cost of these systems, their practical utility has yet to be determined.

Intraoperative CT systems are more commonly used and represent a significant improvement over earlier attempts at intraoperative fluoroscopic CT.[9] While large series are lacking, preliminary reports are favorable, and one study noted a transition to additional surgery in 30% of the cases following intraoperative CT acquisition.[18] While the use of intraoperative CT and MRI has aided in the ability to update the navigational data set, surgical judgment remains the cornerstone of anticipating discrepancies between the IGS data and the surgical field.

Conclusions

While prospective studies in IGS use are impractical, a wealth of retrospective data supports the use of IGS for sinonasal and skull base tumor resection. Inherent registration and accuracy errors may be compounded by anatomic distortion in the setting of neoplasm, and thus IGS data can be interpreted only in the setting of the entire clinical picture. While IGS allows for improved preoperative planning and enhanced surgical performance, it is not a substitute for sound surgical judgment.

Pearls and Pitfalls

- Image-guided surgery (IGS) systems rely on either optical or electromagnetic tracking systems to monitor an intraoperative localization device. Both formats provide comparable surgical accuracy.

- Surgical accuracy is a product of the quality of the preoperative imaging and inherent registration errors.

- Accuracy should be tested throughout the procedure and can be interpreted only in the context of the entire clinical picture.

- IGS provides for enhanced preoperative planning and intraoperative navigation for sinonasal and skull base tumor resection.

References

1. Tabaee A, Schwartz TH, Anand VK. Image guidance in endoscopic skull base surgery. In: Anand VK, Schwartz TH, eds. Practical Endoscopic Skull Base Surgery. San Diego, CA: Plural Publishing; 2007:57–69

2. Bergström M, Greitz T. Stereotaxic computed tomography. AJR Am J Roentgenol 1976;127(1):167–170

3. Citardi MJ, Batra PS. Image-guided sinus surgery. In: Kountakis SE, ed. Rhinologic and Sleep Apnea Surgical Techniques. Heidelberg: Springer; 2007:189–198

4. American Academy of Otolaryngology Head and Neck Surgery. AAO-HNS Policy on Intra-Operative Use of Computer Aided Surgery. Available from: http://www.entnet.org/ Practice/ policyIntraOperativeSurgery.cfm. Accessed 5/25/10

5. Javer AR, Kuhn FA, Smith D. Stereotactic computer-assisted navigational sinus surgery: accuracy of an electromagnetic tracking system with the tissue debrider and when utilizing different headsets for the same patient. Am J Rhinol 2000;14(6):361–365

6. Metson R, Ung F. Image-guidance in frontal sinus surgery. In: Kountakis SE, ed. The Frontal Sinus. Heidelberg: Springer; 2005:201–209

7. Lee WT, Kuhn FA, Citardi MJ. 3D computed tomographic analysis of frontal recess anatomy in patients without frontal sinusitis. Otolaryngol Head Neck Surg 2004;131(3):164–173

8. Rosahl SK, Gharabaghi A, Hubbe U, Shahidi R, Samii M. Virtual reality augmentation in skull base surgery. Skull Base 2006;16(2):59–66

9. Citardi MJ, Batra PS. Revision functional endoscopic sinus surgery. In: Kountakis SE, ed. Revision Sinus Surgery. Heidelberg: Springer; 2008:251–267

10. Leong JL, Batra PS, Citardi MJ. Three-dimensional computed tomography angiography of the internal carotid artery for preoperative evaluation of sinonasal lesions and intraoperative surgical navigation. Laryngoscope 2005;115(9):1618–1623

11. Reardon EJ. Navigational risks associated with sinus surgery and the clinical effects of implementing a navigational system for sinus surgery. Laryngoscope 2002;112(7 Pt 2, Suppl 99):1–19

12. Samaha M, Cosenza MJ, Metson R. Endoscopic frontal sinus drillout in 100 patients. Arch Otolaryngol Head Neck Surg 2003;129(8):854–858

13. Carrau RL, Snyderman CH, Curtin HB, Weissman JL. Computer-assisted frontal sinusotomy. Otolaryngol Head Neck Surg 1994;111(6):727–732

14. Melroy CT, Dubin MG, Hardy SM, Senior BA. Analysis of methods to assess frontal sinus extent in osteoplastic flap surgery: transillumination versus 6-ft Caldwell versus image guidance. Am J Rhinol 2006;20(1):77–83

15. Metson R, Gliklich RE, Cosenza M. A comparison of image guidance systems for sinus surgery. Laryngoscope 1998;108(8 Pt 1):1164–1170

16. Carter TJ, Sermesant M, Cash DM, Barratt DC, Tanner C, Hawkes DJ. Application of soft tissue modelling to image-guided surgery. Med Eng Phys 2005;27(10):893–909

17. Nimsky C, Ganslandt O, Von Keller B, Romstöck J, Fahlbusch R. Intraoperative high-field-strength MR imaging: implementation and experience in 200 patients. Radiology 2004;233(1):67–78

18. Jackman AH, Palmer JN, Chiu AG, Kennedy DW. Use of intraoperative CT scanning in endoscopic sinus surgery: a preliminary report. Am J Rhinol 2008;22(2):170–174

SECTION III: Miscellaneous

35 Head and Neck Fascial Spaces

Moran Amit and Dan M. Fliss

Core Messages

- Understanding the anatomy and the relationships between the fasciae of the head and neck and their spaces is mandatory for comprehending the manner of spread of most infections and some tumors.

- The cervical fascia is divided into superficial and deep layers, with the deep one further subdivided into superficial, middle, and deep layers.

- The superficial fascia and the superficial layer of the deep fascia surround the entire neck. The middle layer of the deep cervical fascia encircles the center of the anterior neck to contain the viscera of the neck. The deep layer of the deep cervical fascia encircles the spine and the paraspinal muscles.

- The cervical fascia divides the neck into several distinct spaces. The submandibular space corresponds to the submental and submandibular triangles.

- There are four distinct spaces between the pharynx and the vertebral bodies. From anterior to posterior, they are (1) the visceral space, (2) the retropharyngeal space, (3) the danger space, and the (4) prevertebral space.

Understanding the anatomy and the relationships between the fasciae of the head and neck and their spaces is mandatory for comprehending the manner of spread of most infections and some tumors. Proximity of the fascial spaces to various vital structures may cause devastating complications, such as airway obstruction, jugular septic thrombophlebitis, lung abscess, upper airway abscess rupture with asphyxiation, mediastinitis, pericarditis, and septic shock. As such, familiarity with the anatomy and interconnections of the fasciae and spaces of the head and neck is crucial for planning a surgical approach.[1,2]

Fascia does not have well-defined content and texture and varies in thickness and composition. Similarly, its origin and edges are arbitrary in most cases because fasciae may split to surround muscles, vessels, and nerves that have their own surrounding fascia and then merge with other fascial layers. As a result, the compartments they create (i.e., the fascial spaces) are mostly ill-defined areas of relatively loose connective tissues that vary in their content. Computed tomography (CT) and magnetic resonance imaging (MRI) revealed that certain fasciae restricted the growth of some tumors, whereupon knowledge of the anatomy of these fasciae opens the way to understand a disease process and predict its growth patterns. This chapter reviews the major anatomic descriptions of the fasciae and spaces of the head and neck.[3]

Fasciae

The fasciae of the head and neck are divided into superficial and deep layers (**Figs. 35.1** to **35.3**). The superficial cervical fascia (SCF) is a subcutaneous thick, well-defined layer of relatively loose connective tissue. SCF covers the head, face, and neck and contains the platysma, the muscles of facial expression, and portions of the anterior and external jugular veins. The deep cervical fascia (DCF) is thinner and contains denser, more discrete layers. The DCF travels along the neck below the skull base and encloses the muscles of the neck, as well as the mandible and the muscles of mastication and deglutition. The DCF is subdivided into three layers: (1.) the superficial layer of the deep cervical fascia (SLDCF), (2.) the middle layer of the deep cervical fascia (MLDCF), and (3.) the deep layer of the deep cervical fascia (DLDCF).[4-6]

Superficial Fascia

The SCF consists of a loose connective tissue that underlies the skin of the head and neck. It contains sensory nerves, superficial vessels, and lymphatics. It extends from the superior aspect of the head down to the face where its fat content is dense, except around the eyelids. Between it and the periosteum of the calvarium, there is loose areolar tissue that permits motion of the muscles of facial expression and can hold large accumulations of fluid. Within the neck, it contains loose fatty tissue and the platysma muscle. The skin with SCF and the platysma muscle creates a unit that is interconnected by a system of fine connective tissue fibers and less well-defined muscular elements called the superficial musculoaponeurotic system (SMAS).[7] The SMAS interlinks facial muscles with the dermis. It extends from the temporalis and frontalis muscles superiorly down to the platysma.

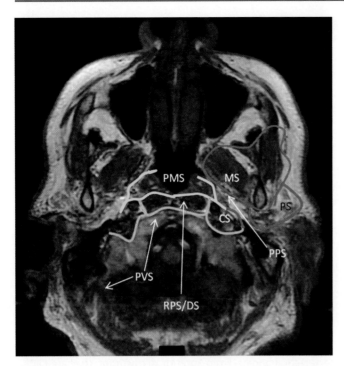

Figure 35.1 Axial T1-magnetic resonance shows fascial spaces at the level of the nasopharynx. Three layers of the deep cervical fascia: superficial (red), middle (yellow), and deep (blue). Notice the relationship between spaces. From anterior to posterior: MS, masticatory space; PS, parotid space; PMS, pharyngeal mucosal space; CS, carotid space; PPS, parapharyngeal space; RPS, retropharyngeal space; DS, danger space; PVS, prevertebral space.

Deep Cervical Fascia

The three layers of the DCF envelop the contents of the head and neck and form the deep neck spaces.[8]

Superficial Layer of the Deep Cervical Fascia

The SLDCF is a well-defined sheet of fibrous tissue that completely envelops the neck. It arises from the ligamentum nuchae of the cervical vertebra and extends laterally and splits to enclose each trapezius muscle. It then crosses the posterior triangle of the neck and splits again to enclose each sternocleidomastoid (SCM) muscle. Anteriorly, it fuses and crosses the midline of the neck in front of the strap muscles as a single fascia. Just deep to the SCM, it contributes to the lateral aspect of the carotid sheath. Inferiorly in the midline, the SLDCF splits to attach the anterior and posterior aspects of the manubrium. Lateral to the sternum, the SLDCF attaches to the superior margin of the clavicle and extends to the spine of the scapula. The SLDCF contains most portions of the anterior and external jugular veins. Above the hyoid bone, the SLDCF extends superiorly to the lower border of the mandible. As it forms the floor of the submandibular space, it fuses and covers the anterior belly of the digastric and mylohyoid muscles.

When the SLDCF reaches the mandible, the fascia divides into superficial and deep leaflets. These leaflets extend superiorly, enclosing the muscles of mastication and forming the masticator spaces. The superficial leaflet

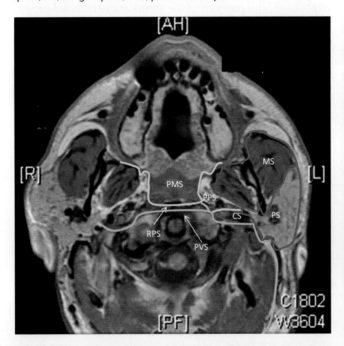

Figure 35.2 Axial T1-magnetic resonance shows fascial spaces at the level of the nasopharynx. Three layers of deep cervical fascia: superficial—red; middle—yellow ; and deep—blue. Notice the relation between spaces. CS, carotid space; DS, danger space; MS, masticatory space; PMS, pharyngeal mucosal space; PPS, parapharyngeal space; PS, parotid space; PVS, prevertebral space; RPS, retropharyngeal space.

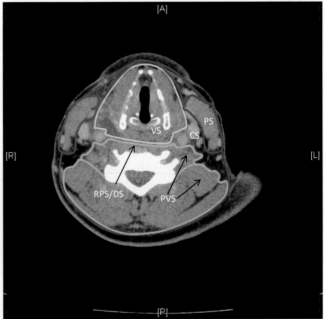

Figure 35.3 Axial computed tomography shows infrahyoid fascial spaces. Three layers of the deep cervical fascia (DCF): superficial (red), middle (yellow), and deep (blue). Notice the relationship between spaces. Superficial and deep layers of the DCF merge at the ligamentum nuchae. CS, carotid space; DS, danger space; PS, parotid space; PVS, prevertebral space; RPS, retropharyngeal space; VS, visceral space.

overlies the masseter muscle and attaches to the zygomatic arch. The fascia at this point splits once again to enclose the zygomatic arch, creating a small space over the superior surface of the arch that is filled with fat. The superficial leaflet then continues superiorly to overlie the temporalis muscle, attaching along the temporal ridge cranially and dorsally and along the lateral orbital margin ventrally. Anteriorly, the fascia covering the masseter muscle curves medially to attach to the mandible. The fascia covering the masseter muscle attaches to the buccinator fascia and to the maxilla, creating the masticator fat pad. This fat pad is intimately associated with the masticator space, and the fat has small projections into the pterygopalatine fossa along the lateral pterygoid muscle. The deep leaflet of the SLDCF extends cranially to form the medial or inner boundary of the masticator space.

The superficial and deep leaflets of the SLDCF fuse along the dorsal border of the mandibular ramus. The space thus enclosed by these leaflets contains the muscles of mastication (the temporalis, masseter, and pterygoid). On each side of the neck, between the angle of the mandible and the anterior border of the SCM muscle, the SLDCF splits again to form the capsule of the parotid gland. The external carotid artery and the retromandibular vein perforate the parotid gland capsule and pass through it. The SLDCF then attaches to the mastoid process and extends posteriorly to attach to the external occipital protuberance.

Middle Layer of the Deep Cervical Fascia

The MLDCF encloses the anterior neck. It has two parts, a muscular one, which encases the infrahyoid strap muscles (sternothyroid, sternohyoid, and thyrohyoid), and a visceral one, which envelops the trachea, larynx, pharynx, esophagus, and the thyroid gland. The muscular division extends inferiorly behind the sternum and then fuses with the pericardium and the great vessels in the superior mediastinum. Superiorly, it fuses with the thyroid cartilage and the hyoid bone. Laterally, the fascia extends to the sternum, clavicle, and scapulae. The visceral division lies posterior to the strap muscles and extends from the pharyngeal constrictor muscles and hyoid bone down into the anterior mediastinum to attach the fibrous pericardium and great vessels. The posterior-superior part of the MLDCF, also known as the buccopharyngeal fascia (BPF), extends from the skull base and follows the pharyngeal constrictors. This fascia is adherent to the muscular wall of the pharynx and the esophagus, and there is no real space between it and the viscera. The BPF encircles the posterior pharynx and forms the anterior wall of the retropharyngeal space. It splits to enclose the more cranial portion of the levator muscle, and a lateral leaflet of the BPF lies in close association with the lateral margin of the tensor veli palatini muscle. A thick fascial sheet extends inferiorly and posterolaterally to the styloid process from the posteroinferior edge of the tensor veli palatini muscle, fusing inferiorly with the fascia covering the styloglossus muscle. This fascial sheet thus

closes the gap between the tensor veli palatini, the skull base, and the styloid process. Anteriorly, this fascia reaches the pterygomandibular raphe where it fuses with both the interpterygoid fascia and the BPF. This fascia contains the ascending palatine artery and vein.

Deep Layer of the Deep Cervical Fascia

The DLDCF encloses the posterior contents of the neck. It originates posteriorly from the vertebral spinous processes and extends anterolaterally under the trapezius muscle enveloping the muscles of the posterior triangle of the neck floor. Laterally, the DLDCF extends between the middle and anterior scalene muscles after which it invaginates outward around the brachial plexus and subclavian artery. More laterally, it continues parallel to the axillary sheath. Medially, as the DLDCF reaches the anterior aspect of the vertebral bodies, it divides into the prevertebral fascia and the alar fascia. The alar fascia lies anteriorly to the prevertebral fascia and forms the posterior wall of the retropharyngeal space. It extends from the skull base down to the level of the C6–T4 vertebrae. The alar fascia is also the anterior wall of the danger space, which extends downward to the level of the diaphragm in the posterior mediastinum. The prevertebral fascia adheres directly to the vertebral bodies and cervical muscles and serves as the posterior wall of the danger space. The potential prevertebral space lies between the vertebral bodies and prevertebral fascia. It extends from the skull base down to the coccyx. Laterally, the DLDCF separates the lower neck and the thorax by extending from the transverse process of C7 to attach to the medial surface of the first rib, covering the dome of the pleura.

Carotid Sheath

The carotid sheath consists of contributions from all three layers of the DCF (**Figs. 35.1** and **35.2**). It contains the carotid artery, internal jugular vein, cervical sympathetic chain, and cranial nerves IX, X, XI, and XII. The inferior and middle portions of the carotid sheath originate from the SLDCF (from the fascia covering the SCM) and from the DLDCF. The upper portion is complex and formed by the SLDCF (from adjacent muscular fasciae), which forms the lateral wall; the DLDCF (alar and prevertebral fasciae), which forms the posterior wall; the cloison sagittale (either part of the DLDCF or the MLDCF), which forms the medial wall; and the stylopharyngeal aponeurosis (MLDCF), which forms the anterior wall. Some areas have overlapping that gives added strength, while there may be focal dehiscences, especially along the medial wall, in other areas.

Fascial Spaces

The fascial spaces are compartments between the fascial layers that are filled with loose connective tissue (**Figs. 35.4** and **35.5**). In some cases, these compartments represent potential spaces. Communication between spaces is variable and considered as normal anatomic variation.[9,10]

Suprasternal Space

The suprasternal space is formed superior to the sternum when the enveloping fascia of the sternal heads of the SCM splits into two layers attached to the anterior and posterior surfaces of the manubrium. It extends from the sternum to halfway up the neck. The primary content of this space is fat and a communicating vein between the left and right anterior jugular veins.

Visceral Space

The visceral space contains the pharynx, cervical esophagus, trachea, thyroid gland, parathyroid glands, larynx, recurrent laryngeal nerves, and portions of the sympathetic trunk (**Fig. 35.5**). This region extends from the skull base down to the upper mediastinum. Its upper part is limited anteriorly by the BPF, posteriorly by the alar fascia, and laterally by the cloison sagittale fasciae. Its inferior portion is divided into two components. The anterior component is covered anteriorly by the strap muscles, laterally by the carotid sheaths, and posteriorly by the alar fascia. The posterior component is considered to have two subdivisions: an anterior pretracheal space and a more posterior retrovisceral space. These spaces communicate freely at the levels of the thyroid cartilage and the inferior thyroid artery. This connection explains why a retropharyngeal abscess can

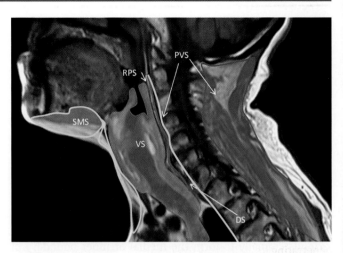

Figure 35.5 Sagittal T1-magnetic resonance image shows infrahyoid neck spaces. Notice that while the RPS ends at the level of T3, the DS continues down to the mediastinum. From anterior to posterior: VS, visceral space; RPS, retropharyngeal space; DS, danger space; PVS, prevertebral space. SMS, submandibular space.

extend down into the pretracheal space and affect the thyroid gland and anterior mediastinum, and why a large thyroid goiter can extend behind the esophagus and grow either upward as a retropharyngeal mass or downward as a retroesophageal mass.

Pretracheal Space

The pretracheal space extends from the hyoid bone toward the upper border of the aortic arch and fibrous pericardium.[9] It is limited superiorly by the attachments of the infrahyoid muscles and their fascia to the thyroid cartilage and to the hyoid bone. It contains the trachea, thyroid gland, parathyroid glands, larynx, cervical esophagus, recurrent laryngeal nerves, and portions of the sympathetic trunk. Lateral attachments of the esophagus to the prevertebral fascia separate the pretracheal and retrovisceral spaces. As a result, the pretracheal space lies anterior to the esophagus and the retropharyngeal space lies posterior to it.

Retrovisceral Space

The retrovisceral space exists posterior to the pharynx and esophagus (**Fig. 35.5**). It is bounded anteriorly by the BPF (covering the posterior pharynx and esophagus) and posteriorly by the alar fascia. It is the largest interfascial space in the neck, and it permits movement of the pharynx, esophagus, larynx, and trachea during swallowing. It extends from the skull base down to the level of the C6-T4 where the alar fascia fuses with the BPF. The retropharyngeal and retroesophageal spaces are the upper and lower aspects of the retrovisceral space, respectively.[6] Laterally, it is bounded by the carotid sheaths. The cloison sagittale separates the retropharyngeal space from the more laterally positioned parapharyngeal space on each side. The retropharyngeal

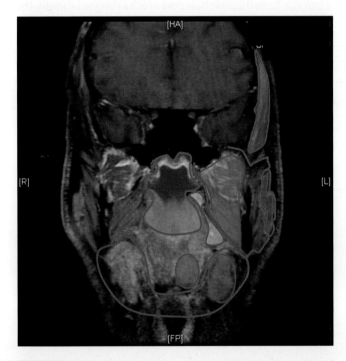

Figure 35.4 Coronal T1-magnetic resonance image shows suprahyoid fascial spaces. MS (masticatory space) (green), has supra- and infrazygomatic compartments. The PPS parapharyngeal space (yellow) and the SLS sublingual space (medial purple) communicate at the posterior border of mylohyoid muscle. PS, parotid space (red); PMS, pharyngeal mucosal space (blue); SMS, submandibular space (lateral purple).

space is fused down the midline and contains two chains of lymph nodes that drain the adenoids, nasal cavities, nasopharynx, and posterior ethmoid sinuses extending down each side.

Danger Space

The danger space (also known as space 4) is bounded anteriorly by the alar fascia and posteriorly by the prevertebral fascia. The space extends from the skull base down to the diaphragm within the posterior mediastinum. It ends where the fused alar and the visceral fascia fuse with the prevertebral fascia. Because this space is sealed superiorly, inferiorly, and laterally, infections must enter the space by penetrating its walls or by direct spread from adjacent spaces. The "danger" lies in the tendency for infections to spread inferiorly through the space and into the thorax because the loose areolar contents offer little resistance.

Prevertebral Space

This is a potential space that exists between the prevertebral fascia and the vertebrae itself. It extends from the skull base down to the coccyx. The prevertebral muscles lie within this space. Pathologies arising within this space originate from hematogenous spread, local instrumentation of the trachea or esophagus, or contiguous spread from vertebral osteomyelitis or discitis. However, dense fibrous attachments between the prevertebral fascia and deep cervical muscles tend to contain and limit prevertebral infections.

Carotid Space

The carotid space is a tubular space lying within the carotid sheath extending from the skull base to the root of the neck. The carotid sheath is a true space only below the level of the carotid bifurcation. The portion of the carotid sheath at the level of the internal carotid artery is embedded within the parapharyngeal space. This space contains the carotid artery, internal jugular vein, cervical sympathetic chain, and cranial nerves IX to XII. Although it is resistant to the longitudinal spread of infection because of the low content of areolar tissue, it nevertheless allows the spread of infections from the upper neck down into the lower neck and mediastinum.

Space of the Body of the Mandible

The SLDCF splits at the inferior border of the mandible. The outer (buccal) layer attaches along the lower outer cortex of the mandible, and the deep (lingual) layer attaches to the inner cortex of the mandible along the line of origin of the mylohyoid muscle. There is a potential space between the deep fascia and the lingual cortex of the bone. This potential space is limited anteriorly by the attachment of the anterior belly of the digastric muscle and posteriorly by the attachment of the internal pterygoid muscle.

Buccal Space

The buccal space contains the buccal fat pad, the parotid duct, and the facial artery. It lies between the fascia overlying the buccinator muscle medially and the skin of the cheek laterally. It is limited by the mandible inferiorly and by the pterygomandibular raphe posteriorly.

Submandibular Space

The submandibular space is limited superiorly by the oral mucosa and inferiorly by the SLDCF sheet extending from the hyoid bone to the mandible (**Fig. 35.4**). The mylohyoid muscle traverses the space horizontally and divides it into a supramylohyoid compartment, also known as the sublingual space, and an inframylohyoid compartment, also known as either the submandibular or submaxillary space. These two compartments communicate freely along the posterior aspect of the mylohyoid muscle. The submandibular gland is folded around the back of the mylohyoid muscle so that the gland lies above and below its posterior edge. The sublingual space contains loose connective tissue, the sublingual glands, the submandibular duct (Wharton's), geniohyoid muscles, and the lingual and hypoglossal nerves. The submaxillary space contains the anterior bellies of the digastric muscles, submandibular glands, and lymph nodes. The "mental space" refers to the portion of the inframylohyoid compartment confined between the anterior bellies of the digastric muscles.

Space of the Parotid Gland

The SLDCF splits around the parotid gland. The fascia is attached by septae to the gland and is inseparable from it (**Fig. 35.4**). Hence, the parotid gland cannot be shelled out leaving behind a real compartment with clear fascial boundaries. The fascia along the deep portions of the gland is thin or deficient in most people. The parotid gland capsule contains the parotid gland, the parotid lymph nodes, the facial nerve, portions of the external carotid artery, the auriculotemporal nerve, the superficial temporal artery, and the posterior facial or retromandibular vein.

Masticator Space

The masticator space lies between the medial pterygoid muscle and the masseter muscle. The SLDCF splits at the lower edge of the mandible, and the superficial layer encloses the masseter muscle, extends over the zygomatic arch, and attaches to the calvarium at the posterosuperior margin of the temporalis muscle and the lateral orbital wall (**Figs. 35.2** and **35.4**). The split layers of the SLDCF fuse again along the anterior and posterior borders of the ramus of the mandible. The fasciae of the masseter, temporalis, and internal pterygoid muscles contribute to the boundaries of this space.[11] Its contents include the lateral pterygoid muscle, temporalis muscle, the ramus of the mandible, the mandibular nerve, and the internal maxillary artery.

Parapharyngeal Space

The parapharyngeal space, also known as the lateral pharyngeal or pharyngomaxillary space, takes the form of an inverted tetrahedral space extending from the base of the skull down to the hyoid bone. It lies between the BPF of the MLDCF covering the lateral surface of the superior constrictor muscle medially and the SLDCF covering the medial aspect of the masticator space and the fascia over the deep surface of the parotid gland laterally. The posterior boundary of the parapharyngeal space is the carotid sheath. The anterior border is the pterygomandibular raphe, which is formed by the junction of the buccinator and the superior constrictor muscles.[7] At its most posterior aspect, the lateral pharyngeal space communicates with the retropharyngeal space, and they are both limited by the prevertebral fascia. The styloglossus muscle forms the inferior boundary of the parapharyngeal space. The styloid process and the stylohyoid, stylopharyngeus, and styloglossus muscles create the three fascial planes of the tensor-vascular-styloid fascia, the stylopharyngeal aponeurosis (aileron), and the sagittal partition (cloison sagittale). These planes divide the parapharyngeal space into two compartments.[11,12] The prestyloid compartment lies anteriorly and just lateral to the pharynx and deep to the masticator space and the ramus of the mandible. It contains the internal maxillary artery, the maxillary nerve, and adipose tissue, and the deep portion of the parotid gland protrudes into it. The poststyloid compartment lies posteriorly and contains the carotid sheath contents. The poststyloid compartment is separated from the retropharyngeal space by the fascia extending from the tensor-vascular-styloid fascia to the prevertebral fascia (the cloison sagittale). The importance of this division into prestyloid and poststyloid compartments comes from the fact that the plane of the tensor-vascular-styloid fascia acts as an important landmark, with the great vessels and cranial nerves lying deep to the plane. One of the main reasons for the interest in the parapharyngeal space is its critical location and anatomic relationships that allow it to act as a route for the spread of tumors and infections to any of the surrounding spaces.[12]

Peritonsillar Space

The peritonsillar potential space lies between the palatine tonsil capsule and the laterally positioned superior pharyngeal constrictor muscle. It is limited anteriorly by the palatoglossus muscle and its fascia (the anterior tonsillar pillar) and posteriorly by the palatopharyngeus muscle and its fascia (the posterior tonsillar pillar) (**Fig. 35.4**). This space mainly contains loose connective tissue. It is medial to the constrictor muscles and the BPF. It lies in proximity to several deeper spaces, and peritonsillar infections can potentially involve both the parapharyngeal and retropharyngeal spaces. A tonsillar infection can also break through the tonsillar capsule into the peritonsillar space. Such an infection (quinsy) can produce bulging of the tissues toward the tonsillar pillars, spreading cranially to the level of the hard palate and caudally to the pyriform sinus.

Paravertebral Space

The DLDCF extends from the spinous processes of the cervical vertebrae bilaterally to attach the transverse processes. The paravertebral space is the one deep to the DLDCF. It contains the muscles of the upper back and the muscles of the floor of the posterior triangle. The DLDCF firmly attaches to the transverse processes of the cervical vertebrae, effectively separating the paravertebral spaces from the adjacent prevertebral space, the danger space, and the carotid sheath.

Posterior Triangle (Cervical) Space

Also known as space 4A, the posterior triangle (cervical) space lies between the SLDCF and the DLDCF, behind the carotid sheath and anterior to the cervical vertebral spinous processes and the ligamentum nuchae. Its deep boundary is the DLDCF lying over the paravertebral space, and its superficial boundary is the SLDCF as it defines the posterior triangle of the neck. This compartment mostly contains fat. It also contains the spinal accessory nerve and its associated lymph node chain, which makes it surgically and radiologically significant.

Clinical Pearls

- Proximity to various vital structures may cause devastating complications, such as airway obstruction, jugular septic thrombophlebitis, lung abscess, upper airway abscess rupture with asphyxiation, mediastinitis, pericarditis, and septic shock.

- The parapharyngeal space is further divided into prestyloid and poststyloid compartments, with the great vessels and cranial nerves lying deep to the tensor-vascular-styloid fascial plane.

- Familiarity with the anatomy and interconnections of the fasciae and spaces of the head and neck allows prediction of tumor growth patterns and is crucial for planning a surgical approach.

- Computed tomography and magnetic resonance imaging are crucial in delineation of disease extension within neck spaces.

References

1. Weed HGFL. Deep neck infection. In: Cummings CW, Harker LA, Haughey BH, et al, eds. Otolaryngology: Head and Neck Surgery. 4th ed. Philadelphia, PA: Elsevier Mosby; 2005:2515–2524

2. Vieira F, Allen SM, Stocks RM, Thompson JW. Deep neck infection. Otolaryngol Clin North Am 2008;41(3):459–483, vii

3. Gray H, Williams PL, Bannister LH. Gray's Anatomy: The Anatomical Basis of Medicine and Surgery. New York, NY: Churchill Livingstone; 1995: xx, 2092

4. Carlson GW. Surgical anatomy of the neck. Surg Clin North Am 1993;73(4):837–852

5. Hiatt JL, Gartner LP. Textbook of Head and Neck Anatomy. Baltimore, MD: Lippincott Williams & Wilkins; 1987

6. Som PM. Fasciae and spaces. In: Som M, ed. Head and Neck Imaging. 3rd ed. St. Louis: Mosby; 1996:738–746

7. Salasche SBG. Superficial musculoaponeurotic system. In: Salasche J, ed. Surgical Anatomy of the Skin. Norwalk, Conn: Appleton & Lange; 1988:89–97

8. Grodinsky MHE. The fasciae and fascial spaces of the head, neck and adjacent regions. Am J Anat 1938;63:367–408

9. Bielamowicz SA, Storper IS, Jabour BA, Lufkin RB, Hanafee WN. Spaces and triangles of the head and neck. Head Neck 1994;16(4):383–388

10. Mukherji SK, Castillo M. A simplified approach to the spaces of the suprahyoid neck. Radiol Clin North Am 1998;36(5):761–780, v

11. Curtin HD. Separation of the masticator space from the parapharyngeal space. Radiology 1987;163(1):195–204

12. Olsen KD. Tumors and surgery of the parapharyngeal space. Laryngoscope 1994;104(5 Pt 2, Suppl 63)1–28

36 Foreign Bodies of the Aerodigestive Tract

Robert J. Yawn and David R. White

Core Messages

- Aspirated foreign bodies are a potentially fatal hazard to children.

- Delayed diagnosis is common, and it increases the rate of complications.

- Rigid bronchoscopy and removal is the treatment of choice in foreign-body aspiration, but role of flexible bronchoscopy is growing.

- Many ingested foreign bodies can be managed expectantly. After 24 hours, it is often necessary to remove the object endoscopically.

- Ingested batteries can be life-threatening and should always be removed expediently.

Foreign body of the aerodigestive tract is a clinical problem that the otolaryngologist must be well equipped to handle. The clinician should have a high index of suspicion in patients with identifiable risk factors to make a prompt diagnosis. Delay in treatment can lead to considerable mortality and morbidity that can often be minimized with the prompt initiation of therapy. The clinical pathway and treatment strategy will vary somewhat with management, depending on the age of the patient and the location of the foreign body in either the airway or the esophagus. Foreign-body aspiration (FBA) should be suspected in all cases of witnessed or reported choking as well as in patients with respiratory or gastrointestinal symptoms that do not appropriately respond to conventional treatment.

Epidemiology

Airway Foreign Bodies

In 2001, FBA accounted for 17,547 emergency room visits for children younger than 14 years.[1] The most common items aspirated in this series were candy/gum and coins. One hundred sixty children died from inhalation or aspiration of foreign body in 2001. Almost three quarters of pediatric FBAs occur in children younger than 3 years, and men appear to have a slightly increased prevalence.[2] Children below 3 years of age have increasing development of fine motor skills and a proclivity for placing things into their mouths but have underdeveloped molars and smaller airways that are prone to obstruction.[3] As the diameter of the airway continues to decrease, airway resistance increases exponentially.

Furthermore, children have lower tidal volumes and decrease cough response, making it more difficult to expel aspirated foreign bodies. The most common objects aspirated by children younger than 3 years are food products, and the most common vary based on regional custom (e.g., peanuts in the Western society and watermelon seeds in the Middle East) (**Fig. 36.1**).[4,5] Children over 5 years of age most commonly aspirate nonfood items, most frequently coins and school supplies.[6] The most frequently involved object in fatal aspirations is the balloon.[7] The ring of the balloon can form a tight seal in the airway, and any pressure within the airway serves to inflate the balloon rather than dislodge it. Other objects commonly involved in fatal aspiration are those that are round, compressible, and smooth and do not break apart easily.

Most aspirated foreign bodies are found within the bronchi, with the right main bronchus accounting for approximately half of all locations.[4] The left main bronchus accounts for approximately 20%, and the larynx and trachea account for portions between 3 and 13%. While laryngeal or tracheal foreign bodies are less common, they are associated with increased morbidity and mortality.[8,9] Obstruction in these areas is typically associated with either large food products or patients with tracheal stenosis.

FBA is much less common in adults than in children; however, adults older than 75 years have increased risk of mortality after FBA.[10] While children are susceptible to FBA owing to a tendency to place objects in their mouths, older adults are more likely to suffer from a decrease in the ability to protect the airway. The most likely type of foreign body is variable and depends on the age and activity level of the patient. Middle-aged adults

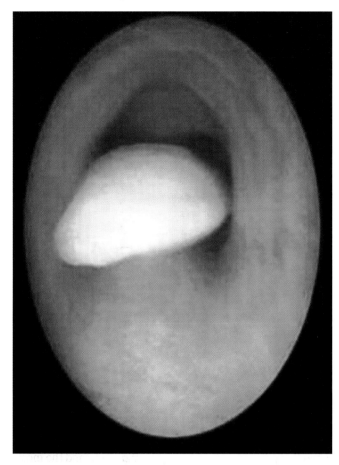

Figure 36.1 A peanut trapped within the airway. It is important to survey the entire airway after extraction for additional or residual foreign body.

may aspirate nails or pins while holding them in their mouth during home maintenance activities. Dental appliances can be aspirated by patients with prostheses, and all patients with a history of neurologic disorder or alcohol and sedative abuse should be considered at increased risk for FBA.[11]

Foreign Body of the Esophagus

Foreign-body ingestion (FBI), like FBA, occurs much more commonly in children than in adults, with incidence being highest in children younger than 3 years.[12] Death from FBI is extremely rare but is possible depending on the object ingested. Sharp objects such as bones and nails can cause esophageal hemorrhage, and button batteries can cause esophageal necrosis and perforation.[13,14] Children have been reported to ingest all kinds of small objects, the most common of which are coins.[15] Repeated FBI, however, is a problem typically associated with developmental delay.[16] In adults, patients at highest risk are those with underlying esophageal pathology (e.g., carcinoma or stricture).[17] In addition, patients with neurologic disability are at higher risk and prison inmates have a high incidence of intentional ingestion.[18]

Presentation

Airway

The presentation of FBA is highly variable and depends on the age of the child, the location of the foreign body within the airway, the degree of obstruction, the type of object aspirated, and whether the event was witnessed. Children who present with cyanosis and respiratory distress require immediate airway management, rigid bronchoscopy for diagnosis and treatment, and supportive care. Patients with FBA with urgent clinical presentations will most often have a laryngotracheal foreign body with near-complete or complete airway obstruction.[8,9]

Patients that present with subacute symptoms or have had an unwitnessed aspiration require a higher index of suspicion. Reports may indicate generalized wheezing. It is important, however, for the clinician to meticulously repeat the physical examination, focusing on localized wheezing and decreased airflow confined to anatomic regions of the lung. The classic triad of FBA includes cough, wheeze, and diminished breath sounds. However, the clinician should be aware that this triad is present only in approximately two thirds of the patients.[19] While the absence of the triad is not sensitive enough to rule out FBA, series data from 370 patients showed this triad to be 96 to 98% specific in children with FBA.[20] Additional symptoms may vary in patients based on their location within the airway. Tracheal foreign bodies may result in stridor and dyspnea. Bronchial foreign bodies may cause shortness of breath, hemoptysis, and coughing in addition to the classic triad.

A witnessed episode of choking has between 75 and 90% sensitivity in FBA.[21,22] The episode may last anywhere from seconds to minutes and often resolves. The clinician should counsel caregivers that even though the acute event may appear to have resolved, FBA is still quite possible. The assumption that the episode is over can lead to delay in diagnosis, which may ultimately lead to pneumonia, lung compromise, or bronchiectasis, which may ultimately require surgical resection such as lobectomy or even pneumonectomy. Should a delay in diagnosis occur, patients often present with signs of airway inflammation and infection. They may have any combination of fever, recurrent pneumonia, wheezing, or chronic cough.[23] FBA in adults is much less common than in pediatric populations, but adults may show atypical symptoms. Diagnosis is much more likely to be delayed in adults than in children, and less than half of adults will have shortness of breath or wheezing. Chronic cough was almost universally present in these patients, with other symptoms (hemoptysis, fever, and chest pain) being less common.[24]

Esophagus

Presentation of patients after FBI is often much less acute than with aspiration. Up to half of pediatric patients may show no signs or symptoms at all. If present, symptoms are often transient and may include chest pain, dysphagia, or indigestion.[25] Patients may also complain of the feeling of something being stuck in their throat. Patients often present for medical care because parents or caretakers witnessed the ingestion.[26] The paucity of symptoms often leads to a delay in diagnosis. Long-term consequences of FBI may include weight loss secondary to malnutrition or aspiration pneumonia owing to the inability to handle excess secretions.[27] Acute presentations are related to sharp or caustic objects that cause esophageal perforation or erosion. This is a potentially life-threatening event that can present with fever, mediastinitis, and crepitus around the neck or upper chest. Adults with FBI most often complain of dysphagia, inability to handle secretions, and neck pain.[28]

Evaluation

The clinical history is the most important aspect in deciding whether to perform bronchoscopy in patients with suspected FBA. Bronchoscopy is the gold standard for diagnosis. Radiographs may be helpful but only when some degree of airway obstruction is present and when patients have aspirated or ingested radiopaque objects. In patients with foreign bodies of the larynx or trachea, posteroanterior and lateral neck films should be obtained, which may show swelling or density in the subglottis.[8] Posteroanterior and lateral chest films should also be obtained, which may show mediastinal shift, obstructive emphysema, or atelectasis (**Fig. 36.2**).[29] In cases of delayed diagnosis, infiltration and regional consolidation may be observed secondary to pneumonia. In addition, bronchiectasis may be observed when the foreign body has been present for a prolonged period of time. Added diagnostic yield may be obtained by obtaining inspiratory and expiratory films, which will indicate hyperinflation of affected lung segments. In uncooperative patients, lateral decubitus films can also be used, which will show hyperinflation on the affected side. Fluoroscopic evaluation has also been shown to have some benefit in the diagnosis, as it can be performed rapidly and does not require precise positioning of the patient for proper evaluation.[30] The most important aspect to remember in using radiographic evaluation for suspected FBA is that imaging should not be obtained if clinical presentation of the patient is severe or has potential to quickly deteriorate.

In patients with suspected FBI, posteroanterior and lateral neck, chest, and abdominal films should be obtained. Traditionally, objects located in the trachea will be oriented in the sagittal plane while objects in the esophagus will be oriented in the coronal plane. If films appear negative, the clinician should consider computed tomography imaging to locate the foreign body within the gastrointestinal tract. Barium studies can be dangerous in suspected perforation and can decrease the utility of endoscopic evaluation.[31] In addition, the clinician should be aware that eosinophilic esophagitis can predispose patients to food impactions in the esophagus, and

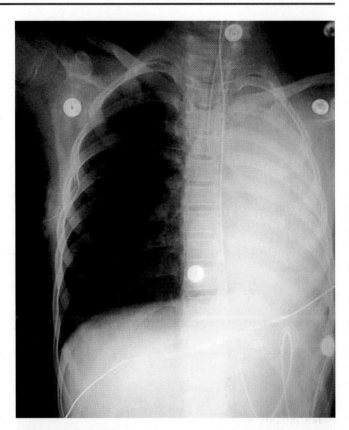

Figure 36.2 Radiograph after foreign-body aspiration. A negative chest X-ray does not exclude the diagnosis of foreign-body aspiration. In cases where the clinical history is unclear but immediate airway compromise is not present, radiographs can be diagnostically helpful.

biopsies should be obtained at the time of removal, especially if the patient has normal neurological development.[32]

Intervention

Trachea

Patients with the inability to cough or speak likely have a complete airway obstruction, and rigid bronchoscopy with direct visualization of the object and removal is the treatment of choice and has been reported to be up to 99% successful (**Fig. 36.3**).[33] In patients with suspected FBA and less than critical clinical presentation, rigid bronchoscopy may still be pursued; however, radiographic evaluation may be warranted as a first step in the work-up. Another valuable tool in the diagnosis is flexible bronchoscopy.[34] This is a reasonable approach to patients with recurrent pneumonia and symptoms of prolonged aspiration. It is also useful in patients who do have less emergent clinical symptoms and do not have the clinical history of a choking event. Rigid or flexible bronchoscopy should always be performed by an experienced physician with surgical capability and airway support available, as there is a chance that bronchoscopy may cause dislodgement or fragmentation of the object and cause migration of the object into other lung segments, which can be potentially lethal.[35] Because of the potential need to convert to rigid bronchoscopy, general anesthesia

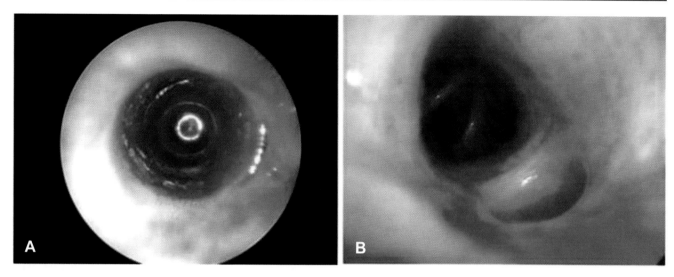

Figure 36.3 Bronchoscopic view of an aspirated pen top (A) before and (B) after removal. Older children have a higher incidence of aspirating school supplies and nonfood objects. After the foreign body has been removed, visualization of the entire airway is necessary to ensure that the object has not fragmented or been displaced into new locations within the bronchial tree.

is recommended for flexible bronchoscopy in foreign-body evaluation. Removal with flexible bronchoscopy is possible through the use of snare devices but should be used cautiously, as the use of simultaneous instrumentation is not possible with flexible scopes. Should bleeding occur, it will not be possible to use suction and the snare to extract the object. If repeated attempts at bronchoscopy are unsuccessful, thoracotomy will be necessary to remove the object.

After the extraction is complete, patients should be placed on corticosteroids to prevent inflammation in the respiratory tract.[36] Also, antibiotics have utility in preventing resultant pneumonia.[37] A repeat bronchoscopic examination of the entire airway should be performed after the extraction is complete to ensure that there are no additional objects or that the object has not fragmented and landed in other lung segments.

Esophagus

FBI is typically less dangerous than FBA, but emergent intervention is indicated in several situations. Ingestion of multiple magnets, especially at differing time frames, can cause necrosis of the bowel or intestinal hemorrhage as loops of bowel or mesenteric vessels can be trapped between the magnets as they travel through the intestinal tract.[38] Ingestion of button batteries requires immediate removal because they can cause esophageal perforation, necrosis, fistula, and erosion into major blood vessels, with damage being significant only for 2 hours after ingestion.[39] If the object is long or sharp, the object should be removed because long objects have a high likelihood of retention in the stomach and sharp objects carry an increased risk of esophageal perforation.[12]

Many patients that have a history of FBI can be managed expectantly if the object ingested is benign and there are no

symptoms of airway compromise or complete esophageal obstruction. Patients should be observed for 24 hours to evaluate for spontaneous passage. If the object does not show signs of passage into the gastrointestinal tract after this time, it should be removed to minimize complications.[27] Should intervention be necessary, several techniques for successful removal have been described.

Flexible endoscopy is the technique of choice in most situations. The benefit of the technique is that it allows direct visualization of the object and manipulation with various instruments, including rat-tooth or alligator forceps, polyp snare, and helical baskets.[40] Foreign-body protector overtubes can be used to safely remove sharp objects, and magnetic extraction devices have been developed for the removal of ingested magnets.[41] Rigid endoscopy can also be used for affected objects in the proximal esophagus or hypopharynx but should only be performed by an experienced operator to prevent damage and perforation to the esophagus.[42] Magill forceps have also been reported to be successful in removing foreign bodies from the oropharynx and upper esophagus with the reported benefit of minimal instrumentation of the aerodigestive tract.[43] For objects that appear stuck in the esophagus but have a high likelihood of passing through the gastrointestinal tract once entering the stomach, using bougienage has been described to push the foreign body into the stomach. Caution should be exercised with this technique, as it does not allow direct visualization of the object, but it has been shown to have significantly less cost than does endoscopic removal.[44] Foley catheters have also been used to extract foreign bodies from the esophagus by passing a catheter beyond the object with fluoroscopic guidance, inflating the balloon, and dragging the object back out through the mouth. This should be performed with caution, as the object can be displaced into the airway.[45] The "penny-pincher" technique has also had success at removing coins. The operator passes grasping forceps through a nasogastric tube and extracts the coin under fluoroscopic guidance.[46] It should always be kept in mind that the optimal technique for extraction is one that allows direct visualization of the object and subsequent evaluation for damage to surrounding structures after extraction.

Prevention

In recent years, much emphasis has been placed on the issue of prevention in FBA and FBI. Unfortunately, regulation of size of toy parts and increased effort to educate the public has had questionable effect. The rate of toy part aspiration appears to be increasing compared with that of past generations.[47]

The Heimlich maneuver, first described by Dr. Henry Heimlich in 1974, has been shown to decrease deaths due to asphyxiation in children over time.[48] Parents and caregivers should be cautioned that if a patient is able to cough or talk, the maneuver should not be performed because the airway is not completely obstructed. In this situation, attempts to remove the object may result in shifting the object into complete obstruction.

Conclusions

In summary, foreign bodies of the aerodigestive tract represent a potentially life-threatening event that the otolaryngologist must be prepared to quickly diagnose and treat. The clinical history and physical examination are the most important aspects in diagnosis, and the safest strategy for removal always involves direct visualization of the object.

Dilemmas and Controversies

- Despite increased legislation and public education, aspiration of nonfood objects appears to be on the rise.

- Endoscopic evaluation of the airway is strongly recommended when there is clinical suspicion for foreign-body aspiration.

Pearls and Pitfalls

- Direct visualization is always preferred in the diagnosis and treatment.

- Flexible bronchoscopy may be a cost-effective way to evaluate the airway, but it should only be used therapeutically by experienced individuals with resuscitative measures and rigid bronchoscopy readily available.

- Parents and caregivers should be instructed that the Heimlich maneuver should not be performed unless total obstruction is evident because complete obstruction may result.

References

1. Centers for Disease Control and Prevention. Nonfatal choking-related episodes among children—United States, 2001. JAMA 2002;288(19):2400–2402
2. Tan HK, Brown K, McGill T, Kenna MA, Lund DP, Healy GB. Airway foreign bodies (FB): a 10-year review. Int J Pediatr Otorhinolaryngol 2000;56(2):91–99
3. Committee on Injury, Violence, and Poison Prevention. Prevention of choking among children. Pediatrics 2010;125(3):601–607
4. Eren S, Balci AE, Dikici B, Doblan M, Eren MN. Foreign body aspiration in children: experience of 1160 cases. Ann Trop Paediatr 2003;23(1):31–37
5. Rothmann BF, Boeckman CR. Foreign bodies in the larynx and tracheobronchial tree in children. A review of 225 cases. Ann Otol Rhinol Laryngol 1980;89(5 Pt 1):434–436
6. Lemberg PS, Darrow DH, Holinger LD. Aerodigestive tract foreign bodies in the older child and adolescent. Ann Otol Rhinol Laryngol 1996;105(4):267–271
7. Lifschultz BD, Donoghue ER. Deaths due to foreign body aspiration in children: the continuing hazard of toy balloons. J Forensic Sci 1996;41(2):247–251
8. Esclamado RM, Richardson MA. Laryngotracheal foreign bodies in children. A comparison with bronchial foreign bodies. Am J Dis Child 1987;141(3):259–262
9. Lima JA. Laryngeal foreign bodies in children: a persistent, life-threatening problem. Laryngoscope 1989;99(4):415–420
10. Rafanan AL, Mehta AC. Adult airway foreign body removal. What's new? Clin Chest Med 2001;22(2):319–330
11. Limper AH, Prakash UB. Tracheobronchial foreign bodies in adults. Ann Intern Med 1990;112(8):604–609
12. Wyllie R. Foreign bodies in the gastrointestinal tract. Curr Opin Pediatr 2006;18(5):563–564
13. Simic MA, Budakov BM. Fatal upper esophageal hemorrhage caused by a previously ingested chicken bone: case report. Am J Forensic Med Pathol 1998;19(2):166–168
14. Yardeni D, Yardeni H, Coran AG, Golladay ES. Severe esophageal damage due to button battery ingestion: can it be prevented? Pediatr Surg Int 2004;20(7):496–501
15. Schunk JE, Harrison AM, Corneli HM, Nixon GW. Fluoroscopic Foley catheter removal of esophageal foreign bodies in children: experience with 415 episodes. Pediatrics 1994;94(5):709–714
16. Reilly S, Carr L. Foreign body ingestion in children with severe developmental disabilities: a case study. Dysphagia 2001;16(1):68–73
17. Li ZS, Sun ZX, Zou DW, Xu GM, Wu RP, Liao Z. Endoscopic management of foreign bodies in the upper-GI tract: experience with 1088 cases in China. Gastrointest Endosc 2006;64(4):485–492
18. Bisharat M, O'Donnell ME, Gibson N, et al. Foreign body ingestion in prisoners—the Belfast experience. Ulster Med J 2008;77(2):110–114
19. Wiseman NE. The diagnosis of foreign body aspiration in childhood. J Pediatr Surg 1984;19(5):531–535
20. Tomaske M, Gerber AC, Stocker S, Weiss M. Tracheobronchial foreign body aspiration in children—diagnostic value of symptoms and signs. Swiss Med Wkly 2006;136(33-34):533–538
21. Ciftci AO, Bingöl-Koloğlu M, Senocak ME, Tanyel FC, Büyükpamukçu N. Bronchoscopy for evaluation of foreign body aspiration in children. J Pediatr Surg 2003;38(8):1170–1176
22. Even L, Heno N, Talmon Y, Samet E, Zonis Z, Kugelman A. Diagnostic evaluation of foreign body aspiration in children: a prospective study. J Pediatr Surg 2005;40(7):1122–1127

23. Blazer S, Naveh Y, Friedman A. Foreign body in the airway. A review of 200 cases. Am J Dis Child 1980;134(1):68–71

24. Lan RS. Non-asphyxiating tracheobronchial foreign bodies in adults. Eur Respir J 1994;7(3):510–514

25. Arana A, Hauser B, Hachimi-Idrissi S, Vandenplas Y. Management of ingested foreign bodies in childhood and review of the literature. Eur J Pediatr 2001;160(8):468–472

26. Louie JP, Alpern ER, Windreich RM. Witnessed and unwitnessed esophageal foreign bodies in children. Pediatr Emerg Care 2005;21(9):582–585

27. Uyemura MC. Foreign body ingestion in children. Am Fam Physician 2005;72(2):287–291

28. Khan MA, Hameed A, Choudhry AJ. Management of foreign bodies in the esophagus. J Coll Physicians Surg Pak 2004;14(4):218–220

29. Mu LC, Sun DQ, He P. Radiological diagnosis of aspirated foreign bodies in children: review of 343 cases. J Laryngol Otol 1990;104(10):778–782

30. Rudman DT, Elmaraghy CA, Shiels WE, Wiet GJ. The role of airway fluoroscopy in the evaluation of stridor in children. Arch Otolaryngol Head Neck Surg 2003;129(3):305–309

31. American Society for Gastrointestinal Endoscopy. Guideline for the management of ingested foreign bodies. Gastrointest Endosc 1995;42(6):622–625

32. Sperry SL, Crockett SD, Miller CB, Shaheen NJ, Dellon ES. Esophageal foreign-body impactions: epidemiology, time trends, and the impact of the increasing prevalence of eosinophilic esophagitis. Gastrointest Endosc 2011;74(5):985–991

33. Black RE, Johnson DG, Matlak ME. Bronchoscopic removal of aspirated foreign bodies in children. J Pediatr Surg 1994;29(5):682–684

34. Martinot A, Closset M, Marquette CH, et al. Indications for flexible versus rigid bronchoscopy in children with suspected foreign-body aspiration. Am J Respir Crit Care Med 1997;155(5):1676–1679

35. Hughes CA, Baroody FM, Marsh BR. Pediatric tracheobronchial foreign bodies: historical review from the Johns Hopkins Hospital. Ann Otol Rhinol Laryngol 1996;105(7):555–561

36. McGuirt WF, Holmes KD, Feehs R, Browne JD. Tracheobronchial foreign bodies. Laryngoscope 1988;98(6 Pt 1):615–618

37. Steen KH, Zimmermann T. Tracheobronchial aspiration of foreign bodies in children: a study of 94 cases. Laryngoscope 1990;100(5):525–530

38. Lee BK, Ryu HH, Moon JM, Jeung KW. Bowel perforations induced by multiple magnet ingestion. Emerg Med Australas 2010;22(2):189–191

39. Litovitz T, Whitaker N, Clark L. Preventing battery ingestions: an analysis of 8648 cases. Pediatrics 2010;125(6):1178–1183

40. Zhang S, Cui Y, Gong X, Gu F, Chen M, Zhong B. Endoscopic management of foreign bodies in the upper gastrointestinal tract in South China: a retrospective study of 561 cases. Dig Dis Sci 2010;55(5):1305–1312

41. Nelson DB, Bosco JJ, Curtis WD, et al; American Society for Gastrointestinal Endoscopy. ASGE technology status evaluation report. Endoscopic retrieval devices. Gastrointest Endosc 1999;50(6):932–934

42. Gilyoma JM, Chalya PL. Endoscopic procedures for removal of foreign bodies of the aerodigestive tract: the Bugando Medical Centre experience. BMC Ear Nose Throat Disord 2011;11:2

43. Janik JE, Janik JS. Magill forceps extraction of upper esophageal coins. J Pediatr Surg 2003;38(2):227–229

44. Arms JL, Mackenberg-Mohn MD, Bowen MV, et al. Safety and efficacy of a protocol using bougienage or endoscopy for the management of coins acutely lodged in the esophagus: a large case series. Ann Emerg Med 2008;51(4):367–372

45. Harned RK II, Strain JD, Hay TC, Douglas MR. Esophageal foreign bodies: safety and efficacy of Foley catheter extraction of coins. AJR Am J Roentgenol 1997;168(2):443–446

46. Gauderer MW, DeCou JM, Abrams RS, Thomason MA. The 'penny pincher': a new technique for fast and safe removal of esophageal coins. J Pediatr Surg 2000;35(2):276–278

47. White DR, Zdanski CJ, Drake AF. Comparison of pediatric airway foreign bodies over fifty years. South Med J 2004;97(5):434–436

48. Ross GL, Steventon NB, Pinder DK, Bridger MW. Living on the edge of the post-nasal space: the inhaled foreign body. J Laryngol Otol 2000;114(1):56–57

37 Sleep-Related Breathing Disorders

Valerie A. Fritsch, Mustafa Gerek, and M. Boyd Gillespie

Core Messages

- Obstructive sleep apnea (OSA) is a prevalent sleep disorder associated with a high risk of morbidity and mortality owing to its correlation with several secondary medical conditions.

- Overnight laboratory polysomnography (PSG) is the current gold standard for establishing the diagnosis of OSA and determining its severity. Portable devices allowing for home PSGs may be used to diagnose otherwise-healthy patients with a high clinical suspicion of moderate to severe OSA.

- Continuous positive airway pressure (CPAP) is the preferred treatment modality in OSA; however, additional options may include any combination of CPAP or other positive airway pressure modalities, oral appliances (OAs), behavioral therapy, surgery, and adjunctive treatments. Effective treatment of OSA significantly reduces morbidity and mortality and improves quality of life.

- Surgical treatment is recommended for a significant number of patients who fail therapy with CPAP and OAs. Several procedures are available to address various sites of obstruction along the upper airway. As most patients with OSA have multiple segments of upper airway collapse, multilevel surgical approaches are often advocated.

Obstructive sleep apnea (OSA) is a disorder that involves frequent episodes of breathing reduction (hypopnea) or cessation (apnea) owing to upper airways obstruction caused by excessive soft tissue compliance, redundant upper airway mucosa, and inadequate motor tone of the tongue and/or pharyngeal dilator muscles. Hypopnea is defined as a decrease in airflow by 50% or more, and apnea is defined as a complete cessation of breathing for at least 10 seconds.[1] Hypopneas and apneas are usually terminated by a brief transient awakening or arousal, followed by resumed sleep. The repetitive cycle of sleep interruption can cause marked daytime sleepiness and cognitive impairment, as well as mood disturbances, social withdrawal, and decreased sexual desire.

An estimated 3 to 7% of men and 2 to 5% of women in the United States are affected by OSA; among patients with a body mass index (BMI) greater than 28 kg/m², the prevalence is estimated to be nearly 50%.[2,3] However, OSA is likely significantly underdiagnosed owing to its often indolent and chronic nature. Patients are not always aware of snoring or apneic episodes, and not all patients present with daytime sleepiness.[4–6]

Regardless of the presence or severity of subjective symptoms, OSA is independently associated with a significant number of adverse health-related outcomes, including systemic and pulmonary hypertension, cardiac arrhythmias, coronary artery disease, heart failure, and cerebrovascular disease, as well as an increased risk of motor vehicle accidents and perioperative complications.[6–10] Successful treatment of OSA attenuates each of these conditions and risks, effectively reducing the risk of morbidity and mortality in addition to improving quality of life[8–13]; hence, early recognition and management of OSA is essential.

Definitions

- **Central sleep apnea:** respiratory distress index ≥ 5 events/h and clinical symptoms related to disrupted sleep. The majority of respiratory events occur without any respiratory effort.

- **Obesity hypoventilation (Pickwickian) syndrome:** daytime hypoventilation that is associated with severe obesity (body mass index > 40 kg/m²) and not secondary to a respiratory or neuromuscular disorder.

- **Obstructive sleep apnea:** respiratory distress index > 5 events/h and clinical symptoms of obstructive sleep apnea, or respiratory distress index > 15 events/h. The majority of respiratory events occur with an increase in respiratory effort.

- **Primary snorer:** snoring that occurs without respiratory-related arousals or disturbances.

- **Upper airway resistance syndrome:** a mild form of obstructive sleep apnea in which there are several respiratory effort-related arousals, but few discrete respiratory disturbances (apnea-hypopnea index < 5).

Anatomy

During normal breathing, negative pressure inspiration stimulates reflexive activation of pharyngeal muscles that dilate and stiffen the upper airway to maintain its patency (i.e., genioglossus, tensor palatine, geniohyoid, and stylohyoid). Pharyngeal dilator activity is usually diminished during sleep in individuals with and without OSA; however, it is more substantially diminished in patients with OSA. In addition, an anatomically smaller upper airway in these patients further limits airflow, predisposing them to apneas and hypopneas during nocturnal inspiration. Upper airway obstruction in OSA frequently occurs along multiple sites. A combination of macroglossia, craniofacial abnormalities, and overly compliant, redundant pharyngeal soft tissues is commonly implicated.

Several anatomic classification systems may be used in the assessment of airway patency among patients with OSA. The Fujita system describes the location airway collapse as retropalatal (type I), retropalatal and retrolingual (type II), and retrolingual (type III).[14] Type I collapse is most commonly encountered in primary snorers and patients with mild OSA and type II in the majority of patients with OSA. Mallampati and Friedman scores describe the completeness of oropharyngeal visualization and suggest the extent of tongue base obstruction. The Mallampati score is determined with the tongue protruded, and the Friedman score is determined with the tongue retained in the oral cavity.[15,16]

Anatomic Classifications

Fujita classification

- Type I: retropalatal collapse
- Type II: retropalatal and retrolingual collapse
- Type III: retrolingual collapse

Mallampati score (measured with tongue extruded)

Friedman score (tongue not extruded while measuring)

- Class I: normal
- Class II: uvula at the base of the tongue
- Class III: uvula not visible
- Class IV: soft palate not visible

Signs and Symptoms

Snoring and excessive daytime sleepiness are the most common presenting symptoms in patients with OSA. Other frequently reported symptoms include fatigue, poor concentration, short-term memory loss, irritability, morning headaches, decreased libido, restless and unrefreshing sleep, gasping or choking while sleeping, repeated awakenings, and excessive nocturia. Bed partners may also report witnessing apneas.

Patients suspected of having OSA should also be assessed for secondary conditions that may occur as a result of OSA, including hypertension, coronary artery disease, heart failure, and stroke. A detailed sleep history is also important to identify other sleep disorders, including poor sleep hygiene, insomnia, and movement disorders, that may occur simultaneously with OSA.

OSA is often suspected in symptomatic patients who are obese or those with a large neck circumference (> 42 cm in men and > 37 cm in women). Additional physical examination findings that are suggestive of OSA include retro- or micrognathia, nasal deformities (turbinate hypertrophy, polyps, valve abnormalities, and septal deviations), a high-arched or narrow hard palate, an enlarged or elongated uvula, macroglossia, tonsillar hypertrophy, and a Mallampati score of 3 or 4.

Diagnostic Testing

OSA's variable and nonspecific clinical features make it nearly impossible to diagnose or exclude without objective testing. Because our ability to clinically predict which patients will meet OSA diagnostic criteria is poor and the consequences of untreated OSA are significant, diagnostic testing is currently recommended for any patient who presents with snoring and excessive daytime sleepiness.[17] In the absence of excessive daytime sleepiness, testing is recommended for snorers with other comorbidities or suggestive clinical symptoms, and those working in mission-critical professions (i.e., truck and bus drivers and pilots).[17]

Polysomnography (PSG) is used to establish the diagnosis of OSA and determine its severity. PSG involves monitoring sleep state (electroencephalography and electrooculography), airflow, oxygen saturation, heart rate (electrocardiography), muscle activity (electromyography), and arousals during sleep. PSG allows for the determination of the apnea-hypopnea index (AHI; calculated by the number of apneas and hypopneas per hour of sleep) and the respiratory distress index (RDI; calculated by the number of apneas, hypopneas, and respiratory effort-related arousals per hour of sleep), which are the most widely used objective assessments of sleep-disordered breathing. The RDI is used to classify OSA severity as mild (5 to 15), moderate (16 to 30), or severe (> 30).

PSG can be performed at home or in a sleep laboratory, which requires an overnight hospital stay. Laboratory PSG offers the most comprehensive evaluation in a monitored, controlled setting and is the current gold standard for OSA diagnosis. However, despite its acceptance as the gold standard, laboratory PSG is associated with a high diagnostic variability, likely owing to various interpretations of nonuniform rules that are used to score events. Furthermore, laboratory PSG is expensive and not always accessible. Patients in rural communities often lack access to centers that perform PSG; and even when access is available, wait times may be exceedingly long.

A simplified version of the laboratory assessment that is performed at home by using a portable monitoring device may be offered as an alternative in select patients. Advantages to home PSG monitoring include the ability to record information in a natural sleep environment; increased access and availability and therefore shorter waiting time; considerably lower cost; and a centralized center for data analysis, which allows for decreased diagnostic variability.[18] However, home PSGs have a higher false-negative rate and likely underestimate disease severity, because home PSG RDI is defined differently (as the number of apneas, hypopneas, and RERAs per hour of recording instead of hours of sleep).[18] Consequently, home PSGs are most effectively used to include the diagnosis of OSA in otherwise-healthy patients with a high pretest probability of moderate to severe OSA.[17] Home PSGs are not appropriate for the diagnosis of OSA in patients with significant comorbid medical conditions (severe pulmonary disease, neuromuscular disease, or congestive heart failure) or in those suspected of having other comorbid sleep disorders (central sleep apnea, periodic limb movement disorder, narcolepsy, insomnia, and circadian rhythm disorder).[17] A repeated laboratory PSG is warranted if clinical suspicion for OSA is high in a patient with a negative home PSG.

Respiratory Scoring Data

- **Apnea:** airflow cessation for ≥10 seconds (represents approximately 2.5 cycles of normal respiration).

- **Hypopnea:** airflow reduction meeting at least one of the following criteria: (1) substantial reduction in airflow (> 50%) lasting at least 10 seconds, (2) a moderate reduction in airflow (< 50%) with desaturation (> 3%), or (3) a moderate reduction in airflow (< 50%) with electroencephalographic evidence of arousal (Chicago criteria).

- **Respiratory effort-related arousal (RERA):** an arousal that is preceded by a brief respiratory effort (< 10 seconds) without significant desaturation.

- **Apnea-hypopnea index (AHI):** an index that measures the number of apneas and hypopneas per hour of sleep.

- **Respiratory distress index (RDI):** an index that measures the number of apneas, hypopneas, and RERAs per hour of sleep.

- **The Epworth Sleepiness Scale:** a validated questionnaire measuring daytime sleepiness severity that is used in the diagnosis of obstructive sleep apnea and in the assessment of symptomatic outcomes following treatment.

Treatment

Treatment of OSA varies according to disease severity and usually involves a combination of behavioral modifications, such as weight loss, alcohol avoidance, and alteration of sleeping position; positive airway pressure (continuous positive airway pressure [CPAP], bilevel positive airway pressure, or automatic positive airway pressure); oral appliances (OAs); and a variety of upper airway surgical procedures.

In mild OSA, CPAP or OAs may be initiated as primary therapy in patients without other medical comorbidities; however, CPAP is preferred in the presence of cardiovascular disease or risk factors (obesity, smoking, hypercholesterolemia, and strong family history). Primary surgical treatment may be considered when patients have severe obstructing anatomy that is surgically amenable (turbinate, tonsillar, or uvula hypertrophy).

In moderate and severe OSA, CPAP is considered first-line therapy because it is the most reliable modality for improving quality-of-life and sleep-disordered-breathing indices.[17] Patients with severe OSA who fail CPAP therapy should be evaluated for surgical treatment, and those with moderate OSA who fail CPAP therapy may consider surgical options or a trial of OAs.[17]

All patients treated for OSA require ongoing, long-term management. OA and CPAP users should be monitored for adherence, continued resolution of symptoms, side effects, and development of secondary medical conditions associated with OSA.[17] Surgical patients and those with resolved OSA owing to weight loss should also be managed long-term for continued risk factor modification and to monitor for returning symptoms.[17]

Continuous Positive Airway Pressure

CPAP decreases snoring and nocturnal respiratory events, improves subjective symptoms, and significantly decreases morbidity and mortality.[19] Accordingly, it is considered first-line therapy in moderate to severe OSA.[17] CPAP prevents airway collapse by delivering fixed inspiratory and expiratory positive pneumatic pressure that reinforces the upper airway. Unfortunately, patient compliance is often imperfect for a variety of reasons, including interface-related claustrophobia, inconvenience, social concerns, and a lack of education by health care professionals. Intensive patient education about the function, care, and maintenance of their equipment as well as continued reinforcement of the benefits of CPAP therapy are essential for maximizing patient adherence and CPAP efficacy.

Close follow-up to assess CPAP compliance and remediate potential problems is especially important during the initial weeks of therapy so that effective CPAP utilization patterns may be established early. Poor compliance may be an effect of discomfort related to the CPAP mask. The standard plastic mask is strapped in place over the nose and mouth and may be the most cumbersome aspect of treatment for some patients. However, a large variety of additional mask options have been developed in a variety of styles, sizes, and materials that may be preferred to the standard device. Advances have also been made to the CPAP machine itself. Some systems have integrated a heated wire into the tubing to maximize inspired humidity, which may improve nasal discomfort; and devices that automatically increase or decrease pressure on the basis of respiratory events (autotitration positive airway pressure) have been developed for patients who cannot tolerate CPAP-generated pressure, usually those who require higher pressures when lying supine. Similarly, bilevel positive airway pressure devices allow for separate inspiratory and expiratory pressure settings and may be more comfortable for patients who require high CPAP or those who have a prolonged poor initial tolerance to CPAP. Treatment of nasal obstruction with decongestants or adjunctive surgery, as appropriate, may improve CPAP adherence as well. When symptoms persist despite CPAP adherence, further evaluation and additional therapy are indicated.

Oral Appliances

Custom-made OAs may be offered as a first-line therapy to otherwise-healthy patients with mild symptomatic OSA or as an alternative therapy to select patients with mild to moderate OSA who are unable to tolerate CPAP.[17] Although slightly less efficacious than CPAP, OAs successfully improve subjective symptoms and indices of sleep-disordered breathing[20]; and the majority of patients who respond to both CPAP and OAs prefer OAs.[20]

Success rates vary by patient selection and appliance. Patients who are most likely to benefit from OAs are those with a lower BMI and less severe, predominantly, supine OSA.[21] Available options include mandibular repositioning appliances, tongue-retaining devices, and appliances that elevate the soft palate. Poor dentition, missing teeth, restricted mouth opening, and temporomandibular joint dysfunction are contraindications to initiating some OAs. Reported side effects of OAs include tooth pain, facial muscle or temporomandibular joint discomfort, bite change, sialorrhea, or xerostomia.[22]

Surgical Treatment

Up to 50% of the CPAP users fail to meet the minimal weekly usage recommendations of at least 5 hours a night for 5 nights a week and require CPAP salvage surgery.[23] The goal of surgical treatment in OSA is to enhance airflow by removing, reconstructing, or bypassing the cause of upper airway obstruction. Surgical treatment may also be considered for patients with mild OSA when there is significant anatomic airway obstruction that is surgically amenable. Adjunctive surgical therapies to improve tolerance of other OSA treatment options are also available.

Identifying the area of airway collapse in OSA surgical candidates is essential to appropriately select which procedure(s) are most likely to be successful. Dynamic magnetic resonance imaging, fluoroscopy, computed tomography imaging, cephalometry, pressure catheters, fiberoptic endoscopy, awake endoscopy with the Müeller maneuver,[a] and sleep endoscopy are commonly employed;

however, a gold standard method of identifying the level of obstruction has not yet been determined.

Drug-Induced Sleep Endoscopy

This procedure is most valuable in patients who are candidates for surgery, and in whom the obstruction sites and the type of surgical procedure that will be applied is unclear. This procedure is performed in a silent, dark surgical room or procedure room under the control of a surgeon and an anesthesiologist. Anticholinergic drugs are used to decrease the secretions and for better visualization. Topical decongestants and anesthetic are applied to the nostril that will undergo endoscopy. Multiple pharmacologic agents such as midazolam, diazepam, propofol, or a combination of propofol and midazolam can be used for sleep endoscopy. Drug-induced sleep endoscopy simulates natural sleep, and ideally, the aim is to see the obstruction that occurs during in natural sleep. The drug dosages should be such that they allow the obstruction to be seen and the patient to remain arousable to verbal stimuli.[24] After enough sedation and sleep are established, fiberoptic examination is performed through the nose to the level of hypopharynx to determine the probable obstruction site. This helps the surgeon in deciding which part of the upper airway should be considered for surgery.

Palatal Implants

Soft palate implants represent a cost-effective, minimally invasive, and reversible procedure that reduces airway collapse by minimizing palatal flutter. Three 18-mm polyester fibers are surgically inserted into the muscular layer of the soft palate at the hard palate junction. The implants induce a chronic inflammatory response that results in a surrounding fibrous capsule that helps maintain palatal rigidity.[25]

Ideal candidates are nonobese patients with milder forms of sleep-disordered breathing. Inserts can be placed in the office as a single procedure or in the operating room when palatal implants are inserted in conjunction with other operations that address additional sites of obstruction as part of a multilevel procedure. Palatal implantation requires minimal recovery time and carries an exceedingly low risk of complications. Partial extrusion of the implant is the most common complication, and extruded implants can be easily removed and replaced.[25]

Uvulopalatopharyngoplasty

Uvulopalatopharyngoplasty (UPPP) involves excision of redundant uvula and posterior palatal soft tissue, tonsillectomy, and closure of the tonsillar pillars to widen the oropharyngeal airway. It is a highly effective procedure for treating snoring and has been the mainstay of upper airway surgery in OSA for years.

UPPP has been shown to significantly reduce AHI; however, postoperative residual AHIs commonly remain elevated.[26]

---

[a]A technique that increases negative intrathoracic pressure by inspiring with closed mouth and nose after a forced expiration.

Although its cure rate is less than 50% in unselected patients, the success rate of UPPP is improved by the addition of a procedure that addresses an additional airway site.[27,28] For this reason, UPPP is now commonly performed as a component of a multilevel procedure. Multilevel operations that use UPPP in combination with other procedures are particularly more successful compared with UPPP alone in obese patients with a crowded oropharynx and tonsillar hypertrophy.[15] UPPP may also be used as an adjunctive procedure to improve CPAP compliance by reducing the pressure requirement. Potential procedure-related adverse effects are uncommon but may include velopharyngeal deficiency, dysphagia, taste disturbances, and voice changes.[29]

Because of the adverse effects of traditional UPPP, several modifications and reconstructive palatal surgical techniques have been described, including uvulopalatal flap, anterior palatoplasty, sphincter pharyngoplasty, and transpalatal advancement procedures. The uvulopalatal flap procedure involves retracting and advancing the uvula superiorly under the soft palate without removal.[30] It reduces the risk of velopharyngeal incompetence and is associated with less postoperative pain, but it is contraindicated in patients with excessively long or bulky soft palates.[30]

Transpalatal advancement pharyngoplasty involves the excision of the posterior hard palate and subsequent advancement of the remaining mucoperiosteal flap and soft palate.[31] It increases the size of the postpalatal airway and decreases retropalatal collapsibility, and it is likely more effective than traditional UPPP.[31]

Anterior palatoplasty includes the resection of the mucosa on the soft palate and moving the distal soft palate superiorly and anteriorly.[32] This technique has been shown to be effective in the management of patients with snoring and mild to moderate OSA.

In the expansion sphincter pharyngoplasty technique,[33] a bilateral tonsillectomy is performed. If the patient has had previous tonsillectomy, a midline anterior pillar incision is made to expose the palatopharyngeus muscle. Once the palatopharyngeus muscle is identified, the next goal is to create a muscle pedicle that will be rotated in a superior lateral direction, which will have the effect of pulling the palate anteriorly and the lateral walls outward. After the muscle is dissected and rotated, a submucosal tunnel is established between the anchoring point just next to the tip of hamulus and tonsillar fossa. The muscle is pulled to this anchoring point and sutured at the apex. Mucosa is closed and the tonsillar pillars are sutured.[33]

Radiofrequency Ablation

Radiofrequency ablation (RFA) is a safe, cost-effective procedure that may be used to reduce the base of tongue, soft palate, and/or turbinates. Radiofrequency (RF) is a form of electrical energy that can penetrate and be absorbed in deep body organs at relatively low temperatures. RF medical devices transmit low-frequency radio waves that cause ionic agitation and friction that increases tissue temperature, causing inflammation, coagulation necrosis, and fibrosis. RF creates a well-demarcated boundary around the affected tissue, allowing for a high degree of precision and minimal damage to surrounding tissues.[34] RFA can be repeated over time with minimal morbidity to titrate the effect for the patient.

RFA can be performed either in the office or as an outpatient procedure. It is often performed in conjunction with other surgeries targeting additional upper airway sites, but it may be used as a primary therapy for selected nonobese patients with mild to moderate OSA. Alternatively, it may be offered as an adjunctive measure for patients who wear the CPAP device for less than the recommended minimum (5 hours a night for at least 5 days a week) or those who require an uncomfortably high CPAP owing to excessive soft tissue collapse.[34] Discomfort and recovery time are usually minimal; complications are rare but may include mucosal ulcerations, palatal perforations, floor of mouth and tongue edema, postoperative bleeding, and infections or abscesses.[29,34]

Submucosal Minimally Invasive Lingual Excision

Similar to RFA, submucosal minimally invasive lingual excision (SMILE) is a technique that involves controlled submucosal tongue-base ablation.[35] A coblator wand (Coblator II, Arthrocare Corp, Sunnydale, CA) is passed into a midline stab incision, 1 cm anterior to circumvallate papillae. Tissue within 1 cm of the midline on either side is ablated, and the incision is then left open for drainage. Pretreatment identification of the lingual artery course by Doppler ultrasonography is required. SMILE is a better option than RFA for patients with severe apnea (AHI > 30) with airway obstruction by large tongue base.

Tongue Base Suspension

The aim of this technique is to stabilize the tongue base and prevent it from collapsing during sleep. This is accomplished by a suture that is looped around the posterior base of the tongue and tied after being passed through the hole on the mandible. The first step is to make a 2-cm submental incision and drill a hole through the inferior part of the mandible. Then, the suture is passed through the hole and carried to the tongue base with the help of a simple suture carrier. The suture comes out at the posterior base of the tongue, is passed to the next side of the tongue submucosally by the help of a free needle, and is carried back to the mandible by the help of a second guide suture. Finally, the suture is tied around the mandible. This minimally invasive technique is highly successful at 82% when combined with UPPP in patients with severe OSA with multilevel airway collapse.[36]

Genioglossal Suspension

Genioglossal suspension involves looping a suture through the tongue base and securing it on a titanium screw that is anchored onto the lingual surface of the mandible. The procedure effectively advances and stabilizes the tongue base, reducing postlingual collapsibility. It is best suited for nonobese patients with normal sized tongues and is generally used as part of a multilevel approach.[37]

Genioglossal Advancement

Genioglossal advancement is a procedure that repositions the tongue anteriorly by creating parasagittal mandibular osteotomies and advancing the genial tubercle forward on the mandible. It is generally used as part of a multilevel approach to enlarge the retrolingual airway.

Hyoid Myotomy and Suspension

Hyoid myotomy and suspension effectively immobilizes the tongue base by releasing infrahyoid musculature, repositioning the hyoid anteriorly, and suspending it to the thyroid cartilage, lingual surface of the mandible, or a bone-anchored suture-suspension system. It may be used alone but is frequently combined with genioglossal advancement or suspension. Procedure-related complications are uncommon, but tongue edema and neck seromas, despite drain placement, have been reported.[38]

Maxillomandibular Advancement

Maxillomandibular advancement (MMA) is a multilevel procedure that enlarges the retrolingual and retropalatal airway by establishing LeFort I and bilateral sagittal split ramus osteotomies and advancing the maxilla, mandible, and hyoid bone along with their attached anterior pharyngeal tissues (i.e., soft palate, tongue base, and suprahyoid musculature). Osteotomies are then stabilized with plates, screws, or bone grafts.

MMA is indicated for patients with severe OSA who cannot tolerate or are unwilling to adhere to CPAP therapy and when OAs, which are more often appropriate in mild to moderate OSA, have been considered ineffective or undesirable.[39] MMA is considerably successful at reducing the AHI to less than 10, especially among younger (age < 40 years) nonobese patients; however, it is associated with a substantially longer recovery time compared with other surgical procedures used to treat OSA.

Potential complications include bony nonunion, malocclusion, nerve damage (facial paresthesias), tooth injury, and facial deformity.[29,39] MMA is a technically challenging and protracted procedure that is often employed as a final surgical approach in a stepwise or phased multiple-level surgery, but it may be considered as an initial surgical approach in certain individuals who have been deemed appropriate candidates by a multidisciplinary team.[39]

Multilevel Surgery

Because airway collapse can occur at multiple sites, a multilevel surgical approach in the treatment of OSA is often recommended.[26] MMA is the most successful single multilevel surgery, but it may lack availability, patient acceptance, and insurance coverage. Alternatively, multiple operations can be performed (either concurrently or staged sequentially) to address various airway sites. Multilevel surgery includes a range of procedures that both enlarge the lumen and reduce the collapsibility of the upper airway. Combinations commonly include UPPP with a surgical procedure that involves the tongue and occasionally the hyoid. Currently, there is no readily defined standard by which to decide which combinations of procedures work best for a given patient. Surgical decision making is influenced by physiologic variables (e.g., BMI), anatomic factors (e.g., craniofacial structure and tongue and tonsil size), OSA severity, findings on upper airway fiber-optic endoscopy, and patient preference.[38]

Tracheostomy

Although tracheostomy is nearly uniformly successful in completely bypassing regions of upper airway obstruction, it involves considerable economic and quality-of-life consequences and carries a significant long-term risk of permanent tracheal damage (tracheomalacia/stenosis). Therefore, it is reserved for patients who have failed or refused other options or when other options do not exist and the operation is necessary urgently.[39]

Conclusions

OSA is a common sleep disorder that often requires surgical treatment when noninvasive therapies fail. Surgical success is based on patient and procedure selection. Accurate identification of the site of airway collapse in patients with OSA improves surgical outcomes by allowing for precise procedure selection. Future studies are needed to help better define patient factors that may be predictive of successful outcomes and to evaluate the most effective method of preoperative airway evaluation.

References

1. Sleep-related breathing disorders in adults: recommendations for syndrome definition and measurement techniques in clinical research. The Report of an American Academy of Sleep Medicine Task Force. Sleep 1999;22(5):667–689
2. Young T, Palta M, Dempsey J, Skatrud J, Weber S, Badr S. The occurrence of sleep-disordered breathing among middle-aged adults. N Engl J Med 1993;328(17):1230–1235
3. Punjabi NM. The epidemiology of adult obstructive sleep apnea. Proc Am Thorac Soc 2008;5(2):136–143
4. Drager LF, Genta PR, Pedrosa RP, et al. Characteristics and predictors of obstructive sleep apnea in patients with systemic hypertension. Am J Cardiol 2010;105(8):1135–1139

5. Russell T, Duntley S. Sleep disordered breathing in the elderly. Am J Med 2011;124(12):1123–1126

6. Chan W, Coutts SB, Hanly P. Sleep apnea in patients with transient ischemic attack and minor stroke: opportunity for risk reduction of recurrent stroke? Stroke 2010;41(12):2973–2975

7. Vasu TS, Grewal R, Doghramji K. Obstructive sleep apnea syndrome and perioperative complications: a systematic review of the literature. J Clin Sleep Med 2012;8(2):199–207

8. Tregear S, Reston J, Schoelles K, Phillips B. Obstructive sleep apnea and risk of motor vehicle crash: systematic review and meta-analysis. J Clin Sleep Med 2009;5(6):573–581

9. Marin JM, Carrizo SJ, Vicente E, Agusti AG. Long-term cardiovascular outcomes in men with obstructive sleep apnoea-hypopnoea with or without treatment with continuous positive airway pressure: an observational study. Lancet 2005;365(9464):1046–1053

10. Campos-Rodriguez F, Martinez-Garcia MA, de la Cruz-Moron I, Almeida-Gonzalez C, Catalan-Serra P, Montserrat JM. Cardiovascular mortality in women with obstructive sleep apnea with or without continuous positive airway pressure treatment: a cohort study. Ann Intern Med 2012;156(2):115–122

11. Avlonitou E, Kapsimalis F, Varouchakis G, Vardavas CI, Behrakis P. Adherence to CPAP therapy improves quality of life and reduces symptoms among obstructive sleep apnea syndrome patients. Sleep Breath 2012;16(2):563–569

12. Tregear S, Reston J, Schoelles K, Phillips B. Continuous positive airway pressure reduces risk of motor vehicle crash among drivers with obstructive sleep apnea: systematic review and meta-analysis. Sleep 2010;33(10):1373–1380

13. Rennotte MT, Baele P, Aubert G, Rodenstein DO. Nasal continuous positive airway pressure in the perioperative management of patients with obstructive sleep apnea submitted to surgery. Chest 1995;107(2):367–374

14. Fujita S, Conway W, Zorick F, Roth T. Surgical correction of anatomic abnormalities in obstructive sleep apnea syndrome: uvulopalatopharyngoplasty. Otolaryngol Head Neck Surg 1981;89(6):923–934

15. Friedman M, Ibrahim H, Joseph NJ. Staging of obstructive sleep apnea/hypopnea syndrome: a guide to appropriate treatment. Laryngoscope 2004;114(3):454–459

16. Mallampati SR, Gatt SP, Gugino LD, et al. A clinical sign to predict difficult tracheal intubation: a prospective study. Can Anaesth Soc J 1985;32(4):429–434

17. Epstein LJ, Kristo D, Strollo PJ Jr, et al; Adult Obstructive Sleep Apnea Task Force of the American Academy of Sleep Medicine. Clinical guideline for the evaluation, management and long-term care of obstructive sleep apnea in adults. J Clin Sleep Med 2009;5(3):263–276

18. Ghegan MD, Angelos PC, Stonebraker AC, Gillespie MB. Laboratory versus portable sleep studies: a meta-analysis. Laryngoscope 2006;116(6):859–864

19. Giles TL, Lasserson TJ, Smith BJ, White J, Wright J, Cates CJ. Continuous positive airways pressure for obstructive sleep apnoea in adults. Cochrane Database Syst Rev 2006;(1):CD001106

20. Lim J, Lasserson TJ, Fleetham J, Wright J. Oral appliances for obstructive sleep apnea. Cochrane Database Syst Rev 2006;25:CD004435

21. Chan AS, Lee RW, Cistulli PA. Dental appliance treatment for obstructive sleep apnea. Chest 2007;132(2):693–699

22. Clark GT, Sohn JW, Hong CN. Treating obstructive sleep apnea and snoring: assessment of an anterior mandibular positioning device. J Am Dent Assoc 2000;131(6):765–771

23. Richard W, Venker J, den Herder C, et al. Acceptance and long-term compliance of nCPAP in obstructive sleep apnea. Eur Arch Otorhinolaryngol 2007;264(9):1081–1086

24. Kezirian EJ. Drug-induced sleep endoscopy. Operative Techniques in Otolaryngology 2006;17:230–232

25. Gillespie MB, Smith JE, Clarke J, Nguyen SA. Effectiveness of Pillar palatal implants for snoring management. Otolaryngol Head Neck Surg 2009;140(3):363–368

26. Caples SM, Rowley JA, Prinsell JR, et al. Surgical modifications of the upper airway for obstructive sleep apnea in adults: a systematic review and meta-analysis. Sleep 2010;33(10):1396–1407

27. Sher AE. Upper airway surgery for obstructive sleep apnea. Sleep Med Rev 2002;6(3):195–212

28. Kezirian EJ, Goldberg AN. Hypopharyngeal surgery in obstructive sleep apnea: an evidence-based medicine review. Arch Otolaryngol Head Neck Surg 2006;132(2):206–213

29. Franklin KA, Anttila H, Axelsson S, et al. Effects and side-effects of surgery for snoring and obstructive sleep apnea—a systematic review. Sleep 2009;32(1):27–36

30. Powell N, Riley R, Guilleminault C, Troell R. A reversible uvulopalatal flap for snoring and sleep apnea syndrome. Sleep 1996;19(7):593–599

31. Woodson BT, Robinson S, Lim HJ. Transpalatal advancement pharyngoplasty outcomes compared with uvulopalatopharyngoplasty. Otolaryngol Head Neck Surg 2005;133(2):211–217

32. Pang KP, Tan R, Puraviappan P, Terris DJ. Anterior palatoplasty for the treatment of OSA: three-year results. Otolaryngol Head Neck Surg 2009;141(2):253–256

33. Woodson BT, Karakoc O. Expansion sphincter pharyngoplasty for obstructive sleep apnea. In: Yaremchuk Kathleen L, Wardrop PA, eds. Sleep Medicine. San Diego: Plural Publishing Inc, 2011:301–311

34. Farrar J, Ryan J, Oliver E, Gillespie MB. Radiofrequency ablation for the treatment of obstructive sleep apnea: a meta-analysis. Laryngoscope 2008;118(10):1878–1883

35. Friedman M, Soans R, Gurpinar B, Lin HC, Joseph N. Evaluation of submucosal minimally invasive lingual excision technique for treatment of obstructive sleep apnea/hypopnea syndrome. Otolaryngol Head Neck Surg 2008;139(3):378–384, discussion 385

36. Omur M, Ozturan D, Elez F, Unver C, Derman S. Tongue base suspension combined with UPPP in severe OSA patients. Otolaryngol Head Neck Surg 2005;133(2):218–223

37. Fernández-Julián E, Muñoz N, Achiques MT, García-Pérez MA, Orts M, Marco J. Randomized study comparing two tongue base surgeries for moderate to severe obstructive sleep apnea syndrome. Otolaryngol Head Neck Surg 2009;140(6):917–923

38. Gillespie MB, Ayers CM, Nguyen SA, Abidin MR. Outcomes of hyoid myotomy and suspension using a mandibular screw suspension system. Otolaryngol Head Neck Surg 2011;144(2):225–229

39. Aurora RN, Casey KR, Kristo D, et al; American Academy of Sleep Medicine. Practice parameters for the surgical modifications of the upper airway for obstructive sleep apnea in adults. Sleep 2010;33(10):1408–1413

Index